Current Topics in General Thoracic Surgery
An International Series

VOLUME 2: PERIOPERATIVE CARE

Current Topics in General Thoracic Surgery
An International Series

Current Topics in General Thoracic Surgery
An International Series

VOLUME 2

PERIOPERATIVE CARE

Edited by

Richard M. Peters
Professor of Surgery Emeritus
University of California San Diego;
Oceania Healthcare Systems
325 Lytton Avenue, Suite 400
Palo Alto, CA 94301, USA

Jose Toledo
Chief Thoracic Surgeon
Thoracic Surgery
Doce de Octubre Hospital
Ctra. Andalucia Km 5.400
28041 Madrid
SPAIN

1992

ELSEVIER
AMSTERDAM • LONDON • NEW YORK • TOKYO

ELSEVIER SCIENCE PUBLISHERS B.V.
Sara Burgerhartstraat 25
P.O. Box 211, 1000 AE Amsterdam, The Netherlands

Library of Congress Cataloging-in-Publication Data

Perioperative care / edited by Richard M. Peters, Jose Toledo
p. cm. -- (Current topics in general thoracic surgery; v.2)
Includes bibliographical references and index.
ISBN 0-444-89660-0 (alk. paper)
1. Chest-Surgery. 2. Therapeutics, Surgical. 3. Perioperative care.
4. Postoperative care. I. Peters, Richard M., 1922- . II. Toledo, Jose. III. Series.
[DNLM: 1. Intraoperative Care. 2. Postoperative Care.
3. Preoperative Care. 4. Thoracic Surgery. WF 980 P445]
RD536.P47 1992
617.5'4059--dc20
DNLM/DLC
for Library of Congress 92-49794
CIP

ISBN: 0 444 89660 0

This book is printed on acid-free paper.

Printed in The Netherlands

Foreword to the Series

Current Topics in General Thoracic Surgery: An International Series is the successor to *International Trends in General Thoracic Surgery*; the latter is six years and eight volumes old. Volume 1 represented the passing of the series into new hands, new series editors, and a new publisher, Elsevier Science Publishing Company, Inc. (from Volume 2 on: Elsevier Science Publishers B.V.).

The world has been made progressively smaller by our technological advances in travel. The jumbo jet assures that any physician may have a patient with disease acquired in any part of the world and patients of any race, nationality, and language. Compendiums of medical knowledge have an international readership and, we believe, should include the views of the international medical community. The electronic communications revolution is giving us new exciting tools for dissemination of knowledge and communication between individuals. These improved communications methods may speed discourse between editors and authors but the task of assembling medical knowledge from an international group of medical experts (even with the FAX) still requires arduous work by devoted and underpaid editors and authors. This series exists because dedicated editors and authors believe this task is part of their obligation as medical experts.

In the foreword to the first volume of the *International Trends in General Thoracic Surgery* series, Drs. Norman Delarue and Henry Eschapasse indicated that "A void exists in the sphere of information transfer within the specialty of general thoracic surgery." This void persists and there remains "an obvious need to fill the resultant vacuum." The developers of the *International Trends in General Thoracic Surgery* series wanted to reach a wide international audience. Recognizing that most individuals with English as a native language are unilingual, they chose English as the language for the series. "In order to foster international dialogue" they established the format that "the contributions from one medical culture" have been, and will continue to be, discussed "by representatives ... from another part of the world."

The first volume published within the *Current Topics in General Thoracic Surgery: An International Series* series was conceived by the *International Trends in General Thoracic Surgery* Series Editors and guided to publication by their careful and diplomatic supervision. They stimulated the volume editors to gather an outstanding group of contributors and gave invaluable aid to the new Series Editors and the publisher in bringing that volume to publication.

Co-editors from North America and Europe are responsible for the contents of this volume. We hope in the future to include more contributors from Russia, Eastern Europe, the Southern Hemisphere, and Asia to catalyze a broader authorship and leadership.

The *Current Topics in General Thoracic Surgery: An International Series* Series Editors know we have a challenge to meet the standards set by Drs. Norman Delarue and Henry Eschapasse. With their continued counsel and the excellent help of the staff at Elsevier we hope to be able to continue to provide a high quality series.

Richard M. Peters, MD

Preface

This volume is number 9 in the series which started as *International Trends in General Thoracic Surgery.* It represents the last of the books that were initiated under the auspices of the original Series Editors Norman Delarue and Henry Eschapasse. They shepherded this international series with the hope that "by emphasizing ... international input ... important new trends in thoracic surgery will be drawn to the attention of the broadest possible audience at the earliest possible moment." This volume, *Perioperative Care,* is the second volume in the new series designated *Current Topics in General Thoracic Surgery: an International Series.*

Books about the non-surgical care of surgical patients are usually entitled pre- and postoperative care. Pre is defined in Webster's Dictionary as "before, in front of, prior to". Post is defined as "after, subsequent to". The patient is, and the surgeon certainly should be, as interested in the non-surgical care during surgery as the care before and after surgery. The word peri standing alone is defined as "1. one of a large group of beautiful fairy-like beings of Persian mythology 2. any lovely, graceful creature". Peri as a prefix is less exciting; it means "about, around, enclosing". This book then tries to enclose the non-surgical care of the patient being prepared for general thoracic surgery, undergoing a thoracotomy for a general thoracic condition, and being cared for during recovery from general thoracic surgery. The continuity of this care will improve the chance that the process would emulate the potential of providing for a "lovely and graceful" outcome. We hope that in the choice of subjects and their presentation we have given the reader a chance to understand the continuity necessary to prevent and/or anticipate complications of general thoracic surgery. Comments are provided for more than half of the chapters to broaden the perspectives offered.

A monograph of this length cannot be exhaustive and this one is not. The subject matter was chosen by the editors to cover areas where the presented information could have significant effect on patient welfare. Evaluation of heart and lung function, control of infection, postoperative pain and prevention of pulmonary complications are examples of the subject matter. Each chapter can be read as an independent monograph, or the book can serve as an overall review of significant areas of knowledge about perioperative care.

This volume has had a difficult perioperative course. It has been victim to the craze of acquisition and sale of publishing houses. The contributing authors have been patient and helpful as the Series Editors and Editorial Board dealt with this manifestation of the instabilities of the book publishing industry caused by the brokers who made decisions on the basis of immediate financial return. During this book's pre-planning and preparation it had to have its development put on hold while the series went through three and a half publishers. We now have moved from a USA publisher through a New York office of an international publisher to our present publishers, the Amsterdam Office of Elsevier Science Publishers BV. When the red tape of getting rights transferred and a contract signed was accomplished the publishers made extra efforts to put the book on a fast track. We hope that we will have the next volume in this series within the year and then at 6 to 9 month intervals thereafter.

This book would not have gotten to the publishers without Susan Seigel's care in accomplishing all of the difficult tasks of keeping track of the progress of the book, helping with the editors' efforts to make the book coherent, and acting as the primary person to read the proofs. Thanks is also due to one of the Series Editors, Earle W. Wilkins Jr., for helping with extensive editing of some chapters and providing comments within very short time frames.

In order to gain back some of the time lost and to speed up the publication of this book all the proofs have been read only by the series editor (RMP). Any mistakes introduced in the publishing process are not the errors of the authors but are the responsibility of the copy editors and the series editor.

Richard M. Peters, Palo Alto, California, USA
Jose Toledo, Madrid, Spain

CONTENTS

CONTRIBUTORS

Dr. E. Anyanwu
Thoraxklinik der LVA Baden, Heidelberg-Rohrbach, Amalienstr. 5, Haupteingang Schelklystrasse, 6900 Heidelberg 1, Germany

Robert H. Bartlett, MD
University of Michigan Medical Center, TC-/920/0331, Ann Arbor, Michigan 48109, USA

Arthur E. Baue, MD
Professor of Surgery, Saint Louis University School of Medicine, Department of Surgery, 3635 Vista, P.O. Box 15250, St. Louis, Missouri 63110-0250, USA

John R. Benfield, MD
Professor and Chief, Division of Cardiothoracic Surgery, Vice-Chairman, Department of Surgery, University of California Davis Medical Center, School of Medicine, Sacramento, California 95817, USA

James A. Bennett, MD
Division of Cardiothoracic Surgery, Albany Medical College, Albany, New York 12208, USA

Jonathan L. Benumof, MD
Professor of Anesthesiology, Department of Anesthesia, T-001, UCSD Medical Center, 225 Dickinson Street, San Diego, California 92103, USA

Dr. José Mª. Borro
Thoracic Surgery Service, La Fe University Hospital, 46009 Valencia, Spain

Dr. C. Chopin
Thoracic Unit, Hôpital Albert Calmetto, F 59037 Lille Cedex, France

Jack L. Clausen, MD
Assistant Clinical Professor, Department of Medicine, HH-772-F, UCSD Medical Center, 225 Dickinson St., San Diego, CA 92103, USA

F. Hammond Cole Jr., MD
University Physicians Foundation, 956 Court Ave., #G226, Memphis, Tennessee 38163, USA

Dr. Ph. Dartevelle
Thoracic and Vascular Department, Marie Lannelongue Hospital, 133 Avenue de la Resistance, Le Plessis Robinson, France

Claude Deschamps, MD
Mayo Clinic, 200 First Street SW, Rochester, Minnesota 55905, USA

P. Drings, MD
Krankenhaus Rohrbach, Klinik für Thoraxerkrankungen, Heidelberg 6900, Germany

Dr. S.R. Dunn
Consultant Anaesthetist, Humberside Cardiothoracic Surgical Centre, Castle Hill Hospital, Cottingham, North Humberside, HU16 5JQ, UK

Martín Escribano P., MD
c/o Jose Toledo, MD Thoracic Surgery, Doce de Octubre Hospital, Ctra Andalucia Km 5.400, 28041 Madrid, Spain

Dr. Mª.J. Gallo
Consultant of Anesthesiology, Anesthesiology Service, Hospital Universitario, Valladolid, Spain

Robert J. Ginsberg, MD
Chief, Thoracic Surgery, Memorial Sloan-Kettering Cancer, 1275 York Ave., Suite C-881, New York, New York 10021, USA

Melvyn Goldberg, MD
Thoracic Surgery, Memorial Sloan-Kettering Cancer, 1275 York Ave., Suite C-881, New York, New York 10021, USA

Renato Guerricchio, MD
Cardiothoracic Surgery, Universita Degli Studi Di Roma "La Sapienza", 1 Scuola Di Spezializzazione, Policlinico Umberto 1, Rome, Italy

Hani A. Hennein, MD
Division of Cardiothoracic Surgery, University of California, San Francisco School of Medicine, San Francisco, California 94143-0304, USA

Dr. Ph. Icard
Thoracic and Vascular Department, Marie Lannelongue Hospital, 133 Avenue de la Resistance, Le Plessis Robinson, France

Dr. Ph. Levasseur
Head, Thoracic and Vascular Department, Marie Lannelongue Hospital, 133 Avenue de la Resistance, Le Plessis Robinson, France

Daniel P. Link, MD
Division of Cardiothoracic Surgery, Department of Surgery, University of California Davis Medical Center, School of Medicine, Sacramento, California 95817, USA

A. López-Encuentra, MD
Associated Professor, Ocana 120, 30 B, 28047 Madrid, Spain

J. Allen McCutchan, MD
Associate Professor in Residence, Department of Medicine H-208, UCSD Medical Center, 225 Dickinson St., San Diego, California 92103, USA

Martin F. McKneally, MD
Division of Cardiothoracic Surgery, Albany Medical College, Albany, New York 12208, USA

Mario J. Milano, MD
Instituto Nacional de la Salud, Ctra Andalucia Km 5.400, 28041 Madrid, Spain

Joseph I. Miller, MD
Emory University Clinic, 25 Prescott St., Suite 2424, Atlanta, Georgia 30308, USA

K. Moghissi, MD
Consultant Cardiothoracic Surgeon to Humberside Cardiothoracic Surgical Centre, Castle Hill Hospital, Cottingham, Hull, North Humberside HU16 5JG, UK

Gordon F. Murray, MD
Professor and Chairman, Department of Surgery, West Virginia University, Health Sciences Center, Morgantown, West Virginia 26506, USA

Peter C. Pairolero, MD
Professor of Surgery, Mayo Clinic, 200 First Street SW, Rochester, Minnesota 55905, USA

Dr. Francisco París
Thoracic Surgery Service, La Fe University Hospital, 46009 Valencia, Spain

James W. Pate, MD
University Distinguished Professor and Chairman, Cardiothoracic Surgery, University of Tennessee College of Medicine, 956 Court Avenue, Memphis, Tennessee 38163, USA

Richard M. Peters, MD
Professor of Surgery Emeritus, University of California, San Diego; Oceania, 325 Lytton Ave., Suite 400, Palo Alto, California 94301, USA

Dr. G. Ramos
Professor of Thoracic Surgery and Chairman, Department of Surgery, Hospital Universitario, Valladolid, Spain

Dr. J.F. Regnard
Thoracic and Vascular Department, Marie Lannelongue Hospital, 133 Avenue de la Resistance, Le Plessis Robinson, France

Erino A. Rendina, MD
Cardiothoracic Surgery, Universita Degli Studi Di Roma "La Sapienza", 1 Scuola Di Spezializzazione, Policlinico Umberto 1, Rome, Italy

Dr. M. Ribet
Chief Thoracic Unit, Hôpital Albert Calmetto, F 59037 Lille Cedex, France

Costante Ricci, MD
Professor and Chief, Cardiothoracic Surgery, Universita Degli Studi Di Roma "La Sapienza", 1 Scuola Di Spezializzazione, Policlinico Umberto 1, Rome, Italy

V. Schulz, MD
Department of Pneumology, Clinic for Thoracic Diseases, Heidelberg-Fohrbach, Germany

Julie A. Swain, MD
Professor and Chief, Division of Cardiothoracic Surgery, University of Nevada School of Medicine, 2040 West Charleston Boulevard, Suite 601, Las Vegas, Nevada 89102, USA

Dr. Vicente Tarrazona
Thoracic Surgery Service, La Fe University Hospital, 46009 Valencia, Spain

Jose Toledo, MD
Thoracic Surgery, Doce de Octubre Hospital, Ctra. Andalucia Km 5.400, 28041 Madrid, Spain

Victor F. Trastek, MD
Mayo Clinic, 200 First Street SW, Rochester, Minnesota 55905, USA

G. Varela, MD
Thoracic Surgery, Doce de Octubre Hospital, Ctra. Andalucia Km 5.400, 28041 Madrid, Spain

Federico Venuta, MD
Cardiothoracic Surgery, Universita Degli Studi Di Roma "La Sapienza", 1 Scuola Di Spezializzazione, Policlinico Umberto 1, Rome, Italy

Professor I. Vogt-Moykopf, MD
Arztlicher Direktor, Thoraxklinik der LVA Baden, Heidelberg-Rohrbach, Amalienstr. 5, Haupteingang Schelklystrasse, 6900 Heidelberg 1, Germany

Earle W. Wilkins Jr, MD
Clinical Professor of Surgery Emeritus, 240 South St., Box 593, Williamstown, Massachusetts 01267, USA

Martin J. Wood, FRCP
Consultant Physician, Department of Communicable and Tropical Disease, East Birmingham Hospital, Bordesley Green East, Birmingham B9 5ST, UK

Part I

Preoperative evaluation of the surgical risk

Current Topics in General Thoracic Surgery: An International Series, Vol. 2
Perioperative Care, edited by R.M. Peters and J. Toledo

Chapter 1

Assessment of pulmonary function

Jack Clausen

GLOSSARY

ARDS	acute respiratory distress syndrome
BC	bronchogenic carcinoma
CAO	chronic airway obstruction
COHB	carboxyhemoglobin
CT scan	computed tomography scan
DLCO	lung diffusion test for carbon monoxide
FEF_{25-75}	average forced expiratory flow between 25 and 75% of vital capacity
FEV_1	forced expiratory volume in the first second
FEV_1/FVC	ratio of forced expiratory volume in the first second to forced vital capacity
FRC	functional residual capacity
FVC	forced vital capacity
MBC	maximum breathing capacity
MEFR	maximal expiratory flow rate
MEP	maximum expiratory pressure
MIP	maximum inspiratory pressure
MV	minute volume
NMR	nuclear magnetic resonance imaging
QPLS	quantitative perfusion lung scanning
P_aCO_2	arterial partial pressure of carbon dioxide
p_aH	arterial pH
P_aO_2	arterial partial pressure of oxygen
PAP	pulmonary artery pressure
PFTs	pulmonary function tests
PPF	predicted postoperative FEV_1
PVR	pulmonary vascular resistance
RV	right ventricular
TLC	total lung capacity
VC	vital capacity
$V_{E, max}$	maximum ventilatory volume
$\dot{V}_{O_2, max}$	ratio of $V_{E, max}$ to MBC, or maximum oxygen consumption

1. INTRODUCTION

The lungs play a key role in intra-operative complications and mortality. In a patient with normal lungs, alterations of lung function during anesthesia may result in life-threatening operative complications because of interruption of oxygenation or alterations of acid–base balance. In patients with pre-existing, acute, or chronic lung dysfunction, worsening of oxygenation acid–base function may occur during anesthesia.

The lungs also play a critical role in the postoperative period, not only because of the challenges of restoration of effective lung function as the anesthetic wears off, but also because of the propensity for lungs to act as an incubator of serious infections postoperatively. The likelihood of pulmonary complications is magnified in the intra- and postoperative course in patients undergoing thoracotomy, which violates the integrity of the chest wall, pleural space, and respiratory muscles.

Not unexpectedly, because of the important role of the lungs in determining the outcome of many surgical procedures, substantial attention has been directed to the preoperative recognition of lung dysfunction. The purposes of such preoperative evaluations vary. Some are determinations of whether the expected beneficial outcome from surgery outweighs the predicted risks of surgery; some seek to identify patients at high risk for complications which may be avoided if appropriate preventive measures are taken. In patients for whom resection of pulmonary tissue is planned, preoperative evaluations may be used to predict the extent of resection which can be done without postoperative ventilator dependency or long-term limitations in normal physical activities.

This chapter will review the pathophysiologic basis of postoperative pulmonary complications, currently available methods for assessing pulmonary function preoperatively, and general recommendations for preoperative assessment of pulmonary function for the major types of thoracic surgery.

2. PATHOPHYSIOLOGIC BASIS FOR PULMONARY COMPLICATIONS OF THORACIC SURGERY

The physiologic basis of lung dysfunction after surgery will not be reviewed in depth here. Readers desiring more information should read the excellent review by Tisi [1].

The pathophysiologic basis of perioperative pulmonary complications involves interactions of a number of factors. Decreases in the functional residual capacity (FRC) can occur after induction of general anesthesia [2,3], which is in part responsible for atelectasis. These decreases in lung volumes during tidal breathing may cause widening of the alveolar-arterial oxygen gradient from compression and closure of smaller airways and changes in lung compliance and resistance and the resulting mismatching of ventilation and perfusion [3].

Intraoperative alterations may persist into the postoperative period because of a number of interacting factors. Atelectasis may develop as a result of limitations in maximal inspiration and coughing from pain; altered respiratory muscle function [4]; restriction of mobility; accumulations of secretions within airways; alterations of intrapulmonary fluid; and, possibly, alterations in surfactant function.

Disruptions of respiratory muscle function during anesthesia, due to postoperative incisional pain, pain control medications, and restrictive wound dressings, all play a role in the interruption of the normal cycles of sighs which prevent decreases in compliance and localized areas of airspace collapse.

When lung structure is normal, this marvelously effective combination of airways and gas exchanging airspaces and capillaries results in the necessary exchange of oxygen and carbon dioxide with minimal work of breathing. These functions, however, are very susceptible to significant derangements when the airspaces or adjoining interstitial structures accumulate fluids, which can occur because of increases in capillary hydrostatic pressures (as may occur with congestive heart failure) or secondary to lung injury. Postoperative acute respiratory distress syndrome (ARDS) capillary injury may also play an underestimated role in more localized dysfunction usually attributed to pneumonia or atelectasis. The specific mechanisms of diffuse or localized ARDS are currently not well understood.

Complex and poorly understood factors may decrease the effectiveness of the normal mechanisms which protect the lung from infections, or limit the dissemination of infections via the large capillary/air space surface through which lungs interact with the environment.

3. RATIONALE FOR PREOPERATIVE ASSESSMENTS OF PULMONARY FUNCTION

Recognition of the high incidence of perioperative pulmonary complications has led to major efforts to identify optimal methods of recognizing patients who should not undergo surgery or who would benefit from special procedures to reduce the risks of pulmonary complications. The increasingly complex (and often expensive) options for the diagnostic and functional evaluation of patients are in conflict with increasing pressure to limit preoperative evaluations to those components demonstrated to be 'cost-effective' or of demonstrated clinical usefulness. Discerning, however, what aspects of preoperative evaluations are clinically effective (or 'cost-effective') is not easy.

The many published studies which sought to define optimal preoperative assessment of pulmonary function have reached conflicting conclusions. The numerous factors contributing to these differences of opinion include: the age and general health of patient populations; the stage of disease; the availability of past medical histories and results of physical examinations; the quality of the preoperative tests; screening of patients by their primary care physicians prior to referrals for surgery; the type of surgery performed; the number of patients with significant complications or mortality; and the quality of the peri- and postoperative care. Most published studies have been retrospective rather than prospective. Very few have randomized patients to different types of preoperative assessment.

In some hospitals, the current methods for postoperative care of all patients include procedures which 10–15 years ago were reserved only for patients preoperatively recognized to have significant pulmonary disease. These methods include preoperative training in deep inspirations and periodic coughs; postoperative monitoring and/or assistance with these prophylactic exercises; early ambulation; better pain control so periodic deep inspirations and coughs are not inhibited.

TABLE 1.1
Baseline and preoperative PFT data from a patient with a history of increased shortness of breath shortly prior to preoperative evaluation for resection of lung carcinoma

Date	VC (l)	FEV_1 (l)	FEV_1/FVC	FRC (l)	TLC (l)
18/06/82 (clinic baseline)	2.7	1.8	66%	3.3 (107%)	5.6 (111%)
27/12/82 (preop)	1.2	0.6	50%	6.4 (205%)	7.4 (149%)
29/12/82 (p 2 days treatment)	2.1	1.5	71%	–	–

Differences in perioperative care can have a major impact on whether or not of preoperative assessment of pulmonary function is effective.

Differences of opinion regarding the preoperative evaluation of patients may also arise because of basic differences in hospital practices, resources, and patient populations. The preoperative evaluation which is optimal for patients undergoing coronary bypass surgery in a sophisticated urban hospital serving an upper-class patient population may be much different from that which is optimal for a hospital with less resources for postoperative management which delivers care to an indigent immigrant population with a high prevalence of active and inactive tuberculosis.

The diversity of the practice of medicine makes impossible a goal of developing specific recommendations which are applicable to all situations. The following sections will review available options for preoperative assessment of pulmonary function in the patient undergoing thoracic surgery and will conclude with some general recommendations.

4. METHODS OF ASSESSMENT

Patients histories can play an important role in the preoperative evaluation of patients and determining the need for special preoperative tests of function. The time course of symptoms may indicate whether the function observed with testing describes chronic function or transiently poor function which may improve with time or appropriate therapy. Table 1.1 shows data from a patient with pulmonary function tests prior to the preoperative evaluation. The preoperative first-second forced expiratory volume (FEV_1) of 0.6 l compared to baseline value of 1.8 l corroborated the history which suggested subacute deterioration of function over the last two weeks. Based on this history and significantly better function observed on baseline studies, surgery was postponed until aggressive bronchodilator therapy had returned the patient's function to near baseline. Note also the large increase in functional reserve capacity (FRC) and total lung capacity (TLC), physiologic changes which might have further compromised the patient's postoperative course if function had not been improved prior to surgery.

The most important functional symptom is usually shortness of breath at rest or during exercise. Because perceptions of increasing dyspnea with exercise commonly accompany the normal aging process, it is often necessary to ask patients to compare their exercise tolerance with companions of their same age without disease, or to ask them about the time course of changes in their exercise tolerance. Not infrequently, direct observation of a patient during exercise is needed in order to interpret patients' perceptions of abnormal dyspnea on exertion.

Chronic cough is most frequently associated with chronic bronchitis, but can occur as the sole indicator of otherwise unsuspected asthma. The causes of chest pain are multifactorial but primarily include disease of the heart and pericardium, pleural space, thoracic cage, and esophagus. Although pulmonary emboli may cause pleuritic pain, they may also cause vague chest discomfort which may be the only indication of possible embolic disease. A history of thrombophlebitis may also be important clues that limitations in cardiorespiratory function are secondary to pulmonary emboli.

Currently used medications, and a past history of pulmonary disease, thoracic surgery or trauma are all of obvious importance, especially when interpreting preoperative tests of function.

Cigarette smoking increases the risk of postoperative complications. Preoperative cessation of smoking may: improve the oxygen-carrying capacity of the blood by decreasing carboxyhemoglobin[5]; improve airflows; reduce airway reactivity to irritants; decrease airway secretions; restore depressed ciliary function, enhancing clearance of secretions.

A number of studies show small improvements in measured pulmonary function in subjects retested months after cessation of cigarette smoking, but few studies have observed physiological improvements soon after cessation. It has been shown that ciliary function can improve within days of smoking cessation. Levels of carboxyhemoglobin, which can be 10% or higher in heavy smokers, also decrease rapidly after stopping smoking.

Though the time course of restoration of physiologic functions after cessation of cigarette smoking is of interest, more relevant is the relationship between decreases of postoperative complications and the interval between smoking cessation and surgery. Warner and colleagues[6] observed that the pulmonary complication rate was lowered only if patients stopped smoking at least 8 weeks prior to surgery. Although thought-provoking, the study is not definitive because of its retrospective noncontrolled design which relied on self-reporting of smoking cessation. Until better studies become available, it seems justified to encourage patients to stop cigarette smoking even if planned surgery is only one or two days in the future.

4.1. Physical examination

In addition to anatomic signs which indicate abnormal lung function such as asymmetry of the chest, percussive signs of fluid, masses or consolidation, a number of dynamic physical signs may provide clues of deranged pulmonary function.

A localized wheeze may be the only clue of an endobronchial tumor; signs of lobar collapse may be present in cases of complete obstruction. Diffuse wheezes on inspiration may be the best sign of suboptimal bronchodilator therapy; expiratory wheezes are less significant and frequently persist in patients with chronic obstructive lung disease even with optimal bronchodilator therapy. A rub may suggest the presence of pleural inflammation associated with metastatic disease, pneumonia, or pulmonary emboli and infarction; diffuse rales may be the only indication of airway dysfunction associated with congestive heart failure. Percussion can identify failure of the diaphragms to move appropriately with respiration, indicating diaphragmatic paralysis.

An increase in minute ventilation at rest is a common but nonspecific indication of lung dysfunction, but even the best of observers have difficulty in visually detecting an abnormal increase in tidal volume. An elevated respiratory rate counted when the patient is at rest and relaxed is a more readily detected sign of underlying lung dysfunction (e.g., hypoxemia, increased physiologic dead space). Extension of tumor to the mediastinum may be indicated by prominence of the superficial veins of the thorax, a sign of impaired venous function, or hoarseness due to metastatic tumor disrupting the recurrent laryngeal nerve.

An optimal physical examination can often detect patients with severe functional abnormalities, obviating the need for more expensive laboratory tests. However, even the most skilled of observers can miss significant dysfunction on physical examination.

4.2. Radiographic evaluation of pulmonary function

Standard chest radiographs [7], CT scans and NMR [8,9] for the preoperative assessment of anatomic abnormalities in patients undergoing thoracic surgery often help interpretation of lung function studies. The presence of atelectasis, pleural disease, bullae, and their lateralization to potential surgical disease are of critical importance. Additional indices, such as the diameter of the descending branch of the right pulmonary artery or the ratio of the hilar width to transverse diameter of the thorax, may identify patients with pulmonary hypertension [10], but are of limited value for quantitating the pulmonary artery pressure (PAP) accurately. Standard P–A and lateral chest radiographics can provide good estimates of the total lung capacity [11], but such assessments are seldom of value for the preoperative assessment of patients. Radiographic lung volumes may be useful for the rare case in which a patient's total lung capacity is inexplicably low and analysis of previous chest radiographs may indicate whether or not this abnormal function represents a change or a chronic condition.

The observation of an elevated diaphragm on a chest radiograph is an important clue of primary diaphragmatic dysfunction, but even more involved assessments such as sniff tests under fluoroscopy have a significant false negative rate [12].

In patients with bronchiectasis being considered for resectional surgery, pulmonary functional tests can assess overall ventilatory reserve. Bronchograms are useful for accurately documenting the extent of disease. Newer CT scanning technology may negate the need for bronchograms in the future. To date there is still controversy about the sensitivity of CT for identifying tubular bronchiectasis [13], but reduced slice thickness and intervals increase the sensitivity of CT scans [14]. In our institution it is the current impression that newer generation high resolution CT techniques are as good as bronchograms. The role of CT for detection and functional evaluation of patients with obstructive lung disease in general is limited [15].

4.3. Physiologic tests of pulmonary function

Spirometry has been used clinically for over 100 years and remains one of the most useful tests of lung function. In the 1840s the British surgeon, John Hutchinson, was one of the first to call attention to the clinical value of measurements of vital capacity for the detection of lung disease. In the 1950s, Gaensler made a major contribution by demonstrating the usefulness of measurements of expiratory flow rates to detect obstructive lung disease.

Spirometry can measure the vital capacity and subdivisions (e.g., expiratory reserve volume, inspiratory reserve capacity); minute ventilation from measurements of tidal volume and respiratory rate; maximal expiratory flow rates including the volume expired in the first second of expiration (FEV_1), the FEV_1/FVC (forced vital capacity) ratio, the forced expiratory flow FEF_{25-75} (a measure of the average flow between 25 and 75% of the VC); numerous instantaneous flows at specific lung volumes (e.g., $FEF_{75\%}$ – the forced expiratory flow when 75% of the FVC has been exhaled); maximal inspiratory flow rates; and the maximal breathing capacity (MBC or MMV) – the total volume which is inspired and expired during maximal efforts of hyperventilation over 15 seconds (expressed in terms of 60 seconds of hyperventilation).

From this confusing number of options, FVC, FEV_1, and FEV_1/FVC ratio are most useful in preoperative assessments. Few studies [16] have found volume-specific forced expiratory flow rates (e.g., the FEF_{25-75} or the $FEF_{50\%}$) to be of more use than the FEV_1 for identification of patients with increased risk for surgery.

Measurements of maximal inspiratory flow rates are valuable for the detection of localized upper airway obstruction, for example in vocal cord paralysis where expiratory flows may be normal. The relative rarity of upper airway dysfunction and the likelihood of history or physical exam calling attention to this possibility appear to obviate the need for routine preoperative measurement of inspiratory flows.

In 1955, Gaensler and co-workers [17] reported on the value of preoperative spirometry for predicting postoperative pulmonary complications: in 460 patients with advanced pulmonary tuberculosis who underwent surgical resection or collapse therapy, all 8 patients who died of postoperative respiratory failure had preoperative maximal breathing capacities less than 45 l/min and VC less than 2.0 l.

In 1962, Stein and colleagues [18] reported that in 30 randomly selected preoperative patients who had normal maximal expiratory flow rates (MEFR), only one had postoperative complications. In contrast, 20 of 29 patients with decreased MEFR had complications. Of the pulmonary function tests utilized, the MEFR was the most useful spirometric measurement for identifying patients at risk. In 1970 Stein and Cassaro [19] did another study in which 48 patients identified as high-risk by pulmonary function testing were randomly divided into those receiving intensive pre- and postoperative pulmonary therapy and those who did not receive it unless it was specifically requested postoperatively. In the prophylactic treatment group there was a 22% pulmonary complication rate and no deaths, in contrast with a 60% pulmonary complication rate and 17% mortality rate in the controls. The average length of hospital stay was 12 days in the treatment group and 24 days in the survivors of the control group. This study remains as one of the most conclusive in support of the value of preoperative screening for lung disease followed by appropriate prophylactic measures in those identified as high-risk patients.

More recently, Cain et al. [20] presented conflicting conclusions in their study of 106 patients who underwent cardiovascular surgery. They could not define specific quantitative limits of pulmonary function that were predictive of postoperative problems, although low FVC, FEV_1 and MEFR correlated with postoperative complications. It is not clear whether these negative results were because of screening of patients by physicians referring patients for surgery, a high level of postoperative pulmonary care of all patients, or because spirometry is indeed of limited screening value in this particular patient population.

Olsen et al. [21] addressed the concept that spirometry is useful for predicting limits of lung resection; they recommended that the predicted postoperative FEV_1 should be no less than 800 ml. In a more recent review, Gass and Olsen [22] raised concerns that such fixed threshold values may be inappropriate for patients with smaller than average predicted lung volumes and FEV_1 as would be seen, for example, in short, elderly females. They suggested consideration of threshold criteria based on percent of predicted. Studies which validate such threshold criteria will hopefully be forthcoming.

A number of investigators [16,17,23] have found the maximum breathing capacity (MBC) to be a useful predictor of postoperative complications. The test is, however, relatively nonspecific; it can be low from respiratory muscle weakness, lack of effort, or obstructive airway disease.

4.4. Maximal respiratory pressures

Measurements of vital capacity and MBC are commonly used for the assessment of respiratory muscle function. However, measurements of maximal inspiratory and maximal expiratory pressures (MIP and MEP) allow more direct assessment of respiratory muscles, especially in patients with both muscle weakness and intrinsic lung disease. Measurements of MIP and MEP are simple to make and have played an important role in the assessment of patients on ventilators being considered for weaning, but have not been widely used for routine preoperative evaluations. In a study which did include these parameters, Peters et al.[24] noted that a combination of two tests, the FEF_{75-85} and maximal expiratory pressure (MEP), was able to predict success or failure in weaning within 24 hours postoperatively in over 90% of cases. This combination had a higher predictive value than any of the individual spirometer or maximal respiratory pressure parameters including MBC. Klidjian[25] suggests that muscle weakness in general may be a significant risk factor and that the predictive powers of MIP and MEP measurements may be related more to generalized physical fitness or nutritional status than specific limitations with ventilation.

4.5. Blood gases

Several studies have noted higher postoperative mortality and morbidity in patients with elevations of arterial P_aCO_2[1,18,20,26]. For example, in Cain's study[20] of patients undergoing cardiovascular surgery, four patients with P_aCO_2 greater than 45 had complications and two died. Interestingly, the arterial P_aCO_2 did not significantly correlate with postoperative complications despite the predictive power of elevated P_aCO_2 in individual patients. Although any elevation of P_aCO_2 above normal (e.g., 45 mmHg) places a patient in a much higher risk group, it has also been repeatedly demonstrated that selected patients with elevated P_aCO_2 can survive general anesthesia and thoracic surgery.

One might expect that elevations of P_aCO_2 during exercise would indicate limited pulmonary reserve and hence be a useful predictor of postoperative morbidity and mortality, but few published reports have assessed the usefulness of this test. In a study of exercise in 50 consecutive patients undergoing lung resection, Bechard and Wetstein[27] implied that elevation of P_aCO_2 during exercise was not predictive of complications of mortality, but they did not present specific data or statistics regarding this conclusion. Despite the paucity of literature to support or disprove measurements of P_aCO_2 during exercise as useful predictors of postoperative problems, elevations of P_aCO_2 during exercise should be considered as warning signs indicating a need for more extensive consideration of surgical risks or limits of resectability.

An elevation of P_aCO_2 (e.g., $P_aCO_2 > 45$ mmHg) during resting conditions is one of the most respected indicators that a patient is at risk and deserves careful consideration before proceeding with general anesthesia or thoracic surgery. Nevertheless, we cannot assign a specific threshold value for P_aCO_2 which by itself indicates prohibitive risk. This is because surgical risk is most commonly defined by multiple factors, some of which may be interactive, and because of the paucity of studies in which significant numbers of high-risk patients with elevations of P_aCO_2 have undergone thoracic surgery. Thus, those who seek a magic number for P_aCO_2 which will clearly separate those who will and will not survive surgery or have major complications, will be disappointed. Clearly, however, even a slight elevation of

P_aCO_2 (e.g., $P_aCO_2 = 48$ mmHg) can indicate respiratory failure and a markedly increased surgical risk.

In contrast with P_aCO_2, P_aO_2 is a relatively insensitive and nonspecific predictor of postoperative complications unless the P_aO_2 is profoundly low (e.g., < 45) and does not rise appreciably with oxygen supplementation. The limited predictive value of moderately decreased P_aO_2 is probably because the P_aO_2 on room air can be significantly reduced by shunting which may be occurring in only a small portion of the lung.

Significant derangements of p_aH (e.g., < 7.25 or > 7.55) are infrequently mentioned as a specific preoperative risk factor, but they indicate a need for careful consideration of underlying acid–base problems prior to proceeding with surgery.

Preoperative patients are seldom screened for elevations of carboxyhemoglobin. Goldzimer et al.[5] pointed out that although the risks of elevated intraoperative COHb levels are not established, operative levels of COHb can be significant in those who continue to smoke cigarettes until immediately prior to surgery.

4.6. Lung volumes

Restrictive lung disease is usually defined physiologically by decreased values for total lung capacity (TLC). The number of specific diseases causing restriction of lung volumes is large, but the basic mechanisms for restrictive changes can be divided into five general categories (which fit the mnemonic PAINT): pleural (effusion, fibrosis); alveolar filling processes (pneumonia, tumor); interstitial (idiopathic fibrosis, early congestive heart failure); neuromuscular (diaphragmatic paralysis, myasthenia gravis); thoracic cage (kyphoscoliosis, obesity).

If a patient has restrictive lung disease, the vital capacity is usually reduced along with the reduced TLC. Spirometric findings of a reduced VC and normal or supranormal maximal expiratory flow rates strongly suggest the presence of a restrictive disorder and often obviate the need to directly measure TLC. Note, however, that with reduced lung volumes, the instantaneous maximal expiratory flow rates (FEF_{25-75}; $FEF_{50\%}$) may be reduced solely because of the small lung volumes and corresponding reductions in airway caliber, thereby misleadingly suggesting the diagnosis of obstructive airway disease. Although in these circumstances, a normal FEV_1/FVC ratio strongly suggests restriction as a cause of the reduced VC, it is only with measurements of TLC that the presence of a restrictive disorder can be established. Similarly, when the FEV_1/FVC ratio is below predicted and there are marked reductions of the VC, direct measurements of TLC may be necessary to recognize restrictive lung disease superimposed on obstructive airway disease. Table 1.1 illustrates a case with subacute deterioration of function in whom plethysmographic measurements of TLC demonstrated that the observed decrease in VC was secondary to hyperinflation without any evidence for superimposed restrictive problems.

TLC can be measured by three different techniques: gas dilution or wash-out; body plethysmography; and radiographic estimates from standard P–A and lateral chest radiographs. All three methods give comparable results in groups of normal subjects [11]. In patients with obstruction, gas dilution or wash-out techniques often underestimate TLC, thereby incorrectly suggesting a restrictive disorder. Utilization of gas dilution techniques for measuring TLC in studies of preoperative assessment of pulmonary function [21,28,29] limits the conclusions which can be drawn regarding the usefulness of TLC measurements for predicting postoperative problems.

Measurements of TLC may be clinically useful preoperatively in patients with chronic obstructive pulmonary disease whose low plethysmographic TLC may be the first clue of superimposed neuromuscular disease involving respiratory muscles. Evidence does not support the use of measurements of TLC in routine preoperative screening.

4.7. DLCO (lung diffusion test for carbon monoxide)

The DLCO may be a useful, albeit non-specific, clue indicating the presence of lung dysfunction. It is commonly reduced in patients with diffuse interstitial fibrosis, emphysema, or pulmonary emboli; it can be elevated in patients with alveolar hemorrhage, polycythemia, and in some asthmatics. In a patient with unexplained dyspnea on exertion, low values for DLCO are good evidence of lung dysfunction that warrants further evaluation. Values within normal limits do not, however, exclude significant disease. There is no evidence to support the use of DLCO in routine preoperative screening [28].

5. EXERCISE TESTING

As a preoperative test of function, exercise testing offers the potential for evaluating cardiac as well as pulmonary function. It also offers the opportunity to test the amount of cardiopulmonary reserve.

For preoperative evaluations, exercise tests can be divided into three broad categories as modified from those categories described by Olsen [30]: (1) those that utilize completion of target levels of exercise as a predictor of mortality and/or morbidity [29]; (2) those that use measurements of respiratory function during maximal exercise (e.g., $\dot{V}_{O_2,\,max}$; ratio of maximum ventilatory volume, $V_{E,\,max}$, to MBC) as a predictor of mortality and morbidity [17,31]; and (3) those that monitor the development of pulmonary hypertension during exercise as a predictor [21].

Reichel [29] recommended the use of a standardized treadmill test with increasing speeds and grades to predict operative risk for pneumonectomy. In his series there were no mortalities or significant pulmonary complications in the 11 patients who completed this exercise protocol. In contrast, there were 3 mortalities and 5 additional patients with pulmonary complications in the 13 patients who could not complete the exercise protocol. Similar results were reported by Berggren et al. [32]: abilities to reach defined levels of incremental exercise testing with a bicycle ergometer were predictive of 6-week mortality in 82 patients aged 70 and over. Spirometry alone was also lower in the group with complications, but this study did not report whether exercise testing added to the predictive powers of spirometry alone.

In contrast, Bagg[33] observed that measuring the distance walked in 12 minutes and the severity of preoperative dyspnea in 22 patients was not useful for identifying the 7 patients who had postoperative pulmonary complications. It is possible that these negative results were because of patient selection criteria (consecutive cases of carcinoma of the bronchus "thought to be suitable for resection"), the small number of patients with major ventilatory complications, or other factors.

In the report from the clinical physiology laboratory which was an integral part of their thoracic surgery service, Gaensler and colleagues[17] noted that although the minute ventilation during walking at 180 feet per minute did not correlate with surgical mortality, the ratio of this minute ventilation to the patient's MBC (the 'walking dyspnea index') did correlate. All 8 patients who died of respiratory failure postoperatively (within 30 days of surgery) had a walking dyspnea index greater than 35%.

The usefulness of determinations of oxygen consumption during maximal exercise was studied by Eugene et al.[31], who noted that a threshold criterion for maximal oxygen consumption ($\dot{V}_{O_2,\max}$) of 1.0 l/min was useful for predicting operative outcome. In the 15 patients with $\dot{V}_{O_2,\max}$ greater than 1.0 l/min, there were no mortalities after lung resection. Of the 4 patients with $\dot{V}_{O_2,\max}$ less than 1.0 l/min, 3 died postoperatively ($p < 0.005$).

In contrast, in a prospective study of 59 candidates for lung resection, Colman et al.[34] concluded that exercise testing and measurements of $\dot{V}_{O_2,\max}$ did not enhance decision making about suitability for lung resection, nor were they predictive of postoperative complications. The fact that the $\dot{V}_{O_2,\max}$ from this study were not adjusted for patients' weights may be a possible explanation for the negative results.

Smith et al.[35] studied the power of preoperative measurements of both $\dot{V}_{O_2,\max}$ and $\dot{V}_{O_2,\max}$/wt for predicting postoperative complications attributable to limitations in cardiopulmonary reserve in 22 patients. $\dot{V}_{O_2,\max}$ was significantly lower in those who had complications (mean = 1.00 l/min) when compared with those without complications (mean = 1.59 l/min). The association was even more significant when $\dot{V}_{O_2,\max}$ was adjusted for the patient's weight. All 6 patients with $\dot{V}_{O_2,\max} < 15$ ml/kg/min had postoperative cardiopulmonary complications, whereas 9/10 with $\dot{V}_{O_2,\max} > 20$ ml/kg/min had an uncomplicated course. Of the two mortalities in this series, one patient with $\dot{V}_{O_2,\max} > 20$ ml/kg/min died of pneumonia; the other had preop $\dot{V}_{O_2,\max} < 15$ ml/kg/min and died of respiratory insufficiency.

5.1. Unilateral balloon occlusion of the pulmonary artery during exercise

This approach may be useful for further evaluation of patients who otherwise would not qualify for surgery on the basis of spirometry and quantitative perfusion scans. According to the results of the study by Olsen et al.[21], the primary functional criterion which suggests inoperability is a main pulmonary artery pressure of greater than 35 mmHg after balloon occlusion of the lobe or lung during supine exercise using a bicycle ergometer. Another criterion suggesting inoperability was if the arterial oxygen tension fell to 45 mmHg or less under the same testing. The technical demands of this procedure appreciably limit its use[22].

5.2. Measurements of pulmonary vascular resistance during exercise

Because of the expected elevations of pulmonary vascular resistance (PVR) after resection of lung tissue, and limitations in the ability of the right ventricle to respond to elevated pressures (especially acutely postoperatively), measurements of PVR at rest and during exercise have been hypothesized to be useful predictors of postoperative problems after lung resection. In the retrospective analysis reported by Fee et al.[36], it was noted that in their 5 patients who died of respiratory failure after undergoing lobectomy or pneumonectomy, all had PVR > 190 dynes/sec/cm^{-5} during exercise in the upright position. The importance of measuring PVR during exercise was underlined by the observation that in 9 patients with PVR greater than 190 dynes/sec/cm^{-5} at rest with decreases to less than 190 dynes/sec/cm^{-5} during exercise, all survived resection.

Although measurements of PVR at rest and exercise by Swan–Ganz catheterization are easier and safer than intravascular balloon occlusion studies, the invasiveness of the test may have contributed to the paucity of subsequent papers on this test for assessing patients with marginal function as determined by conventional pulmonary function tests. Acceptance of PVR measurements at rest and exercise as clinically useful predictors of operability should await confirmation of the results of Fee et al.[36] with prospective studies[22]. If less invasive assessments of right ventricular function and pulmonary vascular pressures by radionucleotide or Doppler methods improve, perhaps these approaches will increase the clinical usefulness of assessments of pulmonary vascular function for preresection evaluations of functionally marginal patients.

5.3. Conclusions regarding exercise testing

As is the case with many other potential predictors of postoperative morbidity and mortality, reports in the literature differ regarding the predictive power of specific tests of exercise performance. It is unlikely that any one criterion from exercise testing will allow accurate prediction of morbidity and/or mortality. Such parameters are probably of more predictive value when integrated with other factors which may affect mortality such as age, pulmonary function, underlying illnesses, obesity. Exercise testing is most appropriate for the further evaluation of patients with pulmonary function testing results which are marginal or suggest inoperability. Currently, patients should not be declared ineligible for thoracotomy on the basis of exercise testing alone[35]. There is some evidence from Bechard and Wetstein's study[27], however, that a $\dot{V}_{O_2,max} < 10$ ml/kg/min may indicate prohibitive risks even if spirometry is within acceptable limits. On the basis of his comprehensive review of published studies, Olsen[30] concluded that those studies which exercised subjects to the highest work rate have demonstrated the strongest predictors of postoperative results but that the specific levels which define inoperability remain to be defined. The exact role of exercise testing, and especially assessments of pulmonary vascular pressures and right ventricular performance during exercise for defining resectability, will hopefully be more clearly defined by prospective studies in the future.

6. REGIONAL ASSESSMENT OF FUNCTION

Although physiologic testing is of value for defining whether or not a patient has sufficient functional reserve to sustain resectional surgery of the lung, conventional tests are limited in the ability to assess regional differences in function. In patients with functional limitations of sufficient magnitude to preclude resection, it is often important to predict the functional contribution of the portion of lung to be resected. Estimates of functional limitation from conventional radiographs may underestimate regional function, especially in cases where the proximity of tumor to airways or pulmonary vasculature may limit regional function.

There are a number of methods for estimating regional function of the lungs: selective bronchospirometry, quantitative ventilation and perfusion lung scans, the lateral position test, balloon occlusion of the pulmonary arteries, and pulmonary angiography.

6.1. Selective bronchoscopy

Selective bronchospirometry using a Carlens double lumen endotracheal tube requires considerable technical expertise. In addition, the patient's discomfort or need for general anesthesia associated with this procedure has markedly contributed to the decline in its use. It can be used to assess regional lung function from measurements of VC and oxygen consumption of each lung[37].

6.2. Ventilation and perfusion lung scans

For regional assessment of function, radionucleotide scans of ventilation and perfusion offer the significant advantages of limited invasiveness, show good correlation of regional function as assessed by regional oxygen uptake measurements using bronchospirometry[38], and are useful for predicting operability in patients who might otherwise be considered inoperable by history, physical examination, and pulmonary function tests (PFTs) alone [21]. As demonstrated by Wernly et al. [39], predictions of postoperative pulmonary function based on simple quantitative perfusion scans are as useful as those based on matched ventilation and perfusion scans (or ventilation scans alone), probably because of compensating mechanisms which reduce ventilation in regions with gross reductions of perfusion. In their series of patients undergoing lung resection for carcinoma, the FEV_1 after lobectomy could be predicted with a mean error of less than 10% with the combined use of spirometry and quantitative perfusion scans. Of 45 patients whose postoperative FEV_1 was predicted to be greater than 1.0 l according to the combined spirometry and perfusion scan studies, 22 patients had a preoperative FEV_1 less than 2.0 l and might not have been considered candidates for pneumonectomy if the function of each lung was assumed to be equal. There were no cases of respiratory insufficiency or postoperative mortality attributable to surgery in the patients selected by these combined procedures despite the fact that 7 patients had preoperative FEV_1 less than 1.0 l. Wernley's article [39] presents an informative comparison of different approaches for quantitating regional function which included visual estimates of lobar function as well as computer calculations based on regional differences in gamma camera output. Combined with appropriate pulmonary function tests, perfusion scans have also been shown of value for predicting postresectional values of MBC, DLCO, and exercise capacity.

6.3. Lateral position test

The lateral position test was described by Bergan [40] as an alternative to quantitative lung scans for assessing regional differences in lung function. Recording changes in FRC during changes from supine to right and left lateral positions is felt to reflect the relative distribution of minute ventilation and oxygen uptake of the right and left lungs [41]. In addition to being limited to assessing right versus left differences in function, and to having a somewhat poorer correlation with bronchospirometry than perfusion scan estimates of postoperative function [38], the intrasubject variability of test results may also limit its clinical usefulness [42].

6.4. Unilateral balloon occlusion of the pulmonary artery

As discussed in Section 5 on exercise testing, the technical demands and invasive nature of this testing have limited its clinical use. This approach may be of some use for predicting post-resection problems by directly assessing the impact of changes in regional blood flow.

7. GENERAL RECOMMENDATIONS IN TERMS OF SPECIFIC PROCEDURES

7.1. Screening tests of pulmonary function: When? What tests?

As noted in Tisi's comprehensive review of preoperative evaluation, many authors have recommended limited screening tests of pulmonary function (e.g., spirometry and an arterial blood gas) for all patients undergoing thoracic surgery [1]. Others base the indications for preoperative screen studies on specific risk factors, symptoms, or signs suggestive of pulmonary disease (e.g., spirometry preoperative for: productive cough; age over 60; 20 pack/yr or greater smoking history; history or physical findings of cardiopulmonary disease; or obesity [43]. From their retrospective study of 106 patients who underwent major cardiovascular surgery, Cain and colleagues [20] raised questions about the usefulness of routine screening spirometry. They noted significant correlations of spirometry with postoperative complications, but could not identify specific spirometric criteria which served as effective predictors of postoperative complications. They suggested that careful clinical assessment may be as good as preoperative pulmonary function tests for managing patients undergoing cardiovascular surgery.

One can argue that routine screening pulmonary function tests may not be warranted for all thoracic surgery patients in a contemporary setting of careful clinical assessments and rigorous postoperative pulmonary care. Because of the earlier evidence of efficacy in one of the rare randomized prospective studies [19], and since spirometry is noninvasive and usually reasonable in cost ($<$ \$40 in our institution), I recommend spirometry as a screening test for most thoracic surgery patients, specifically those with: $>$ 20 pack/yr cigarette smoking history; any symptoms or history suggesting pulmonary disease or dysfunction; patients over the age of 60. (Obesity itself is an important risk factor, but in the absence of cigarette smoking history or signs or symptoms of pulmonary dysfunction, screening spirometry and ABGs are not routinely necessary in obese patients prior to thoracotomy, in part because of the evidence presented by Crapo et al. [44] regarding the lack of predictive value of these tests in these patients undergoing abdominal surgery.)

Whether or not an arterial blood gas determination should routinely accompany screening spirometry or should be done only in those with abnormal spirometry cannot be answered from studies in the literature. Significant elevations of P_aCO_2 are uncommon in patients with normal spirometry results; significant hypoxemia, however, can clearly occur in patients whose spirometric parameters are within normal limits. Milledge and Nunn [26] concluded that FEV_1 of less than 1.0 l identifies those patients who need follow-up blood gases. However, because this conclusion was based on a study of only 12 patients their conclusion should be considered interesting and provocative but not conclusive until confirmed by studies of larger numbers of patients. Therefore, I recommend that an arterial blood gas determination accompany simple spirometry as the standard preoperative function screening test for thoracic surgery patients with the risk factors defined above for spirometry.

There is some evidence that measurements of maximal respiratory pressures are useful preoperative screening tests for predicting success in weaning from ventilators postoperatively [24]. As may be the case with spirometric measurements of maximal breathing capacity (MBC or MVV), measurements of maximal respiratory pressures may be useful predictors of postoperative complications more because they relate to patients' cooperation, vigor, physical fitness and nutritional status rather than because they detect diseases causing respiratory muscle dysfunction. Nevertheless, currently there is insufficient evidence to recommend measurements of maximal respiratory pressures for preoperative screening of all patients. Similarly, although appropriate as part of prospective studies defining limits of operability, in the ordinary clinical setting there is no evidence to support routine screening measurements using more complex tests such as lung volumes by plethysmography or the diffusion capacity. If there is suspicion of lung dysfunction from the history or other clinical findings (e.g., unexplained dyspnea), more extensive functional testing may be indicated.

7.2. Are there functional indices which indicate prohibitive risks of surgery?

The search for single values of pulmonary function which will cleanly separate patients into those who are and are not able to tolerate thoracotomy is unlikely to be productive. In part this is because determinants of postoperative complications and survival are multifactorial. A clinician's usual approach to determining operability is clearly multifactorial, and in addition to 'hard' data such as spirometry and blood gases, includes unconscious if not conscious consideration of 'soft' data such as general physical condition, physical rather than chronological age, associated diseases, normal activity level, and anticipated complexity and duration of surgery.

Attempts to assess the clinical utility of preoperative function tests may be enhanced by incorporating such multifactorial approaches in the statistical analyses. For example, in a study which attempted to predict the need for postoperative mechanical ventilation in patients with myasthenia gravis, a history of respiratory disease and the magnitudes of the vital capacities were two of the four factors which did effectively predict respiratory outcome when used as part of multivariate discriminant analysis [45].

Although one can predict that the postoperative mortality rate for thoracotomy is increased in a group of patients with P_aCO_2 of 48 mmHg, if one considers other factors (e.g., presence of right ventricular (RV) failure, severe hypoxemia, reductions of VC, low $\dot{V}_{O_2,\max}$ during exercise), the predicted mortality rate for *individual* patients with and without these added risk factors may vary from 10 to 90%.

The search for a specific functional criterion which defines inoperability is also unlikely to be rewarding because of the inherent diversity of operative risks and

TABLE 1.2
Screening PFT values which indicate elevated risks for thoracotomy

(1)	$P_aCO_2 > 45$ mmHg
(2)	$P_aO_2 < 55$ mmHg
(3)	pH < 7.25, pH > 7.55
(4)	VC(FVC) < 2.0 l or $< 60\%$ of predicted
(5)	$FEV_1 < 2.0$ l or $< 60\%$ of predicted

surgical outcomes within groups of patients who have similar levels of dysfunction in those tests available to us.

Utilization of multiple interactive criteria of operability may increase our ability to establish 'objective' criteria of operative risks. However, we will probably always need to rely on some degree of clinical intuition and will never achieve both 100% sensitivity and specificity in our predictions from specific criteria.

Thus, instead of seeking absolute criteria of prohibitive risk for thoracotomy from screening tests, I prefer to seek screening criteria which define higher-risk patients who need careful consideration and perhaps further tests prior to final decisions regarding surgery. Table 1.2 lists my selection of these screening criteria. Some criteria, such as elevation of P_aCO_2, are clearly more predictive of problems than others. If these screening tests are all to the normal side of these threshold values, more extensive functional evaluation may still be indicated, as for instance in a patient who has inexplicably severe dyspnea on exertion or who has evidence of severe bullous lung disease on chest radiographs.

7.3. What follow-up tests? When to use them?

In patients being considered for thoracotomy, if one or more of the screening tests are abnormal, or if the clinical evaluation suggests otherwise undefined lung dysfunction, the optimal follow-up evaluation will vary according to the type of surgery considered and other factors which define surgical risk such as age, physical and nutritional condition, presence of associated disease.

In an elderly female with a vital capacity just below 2.0 l, a P_aO_2 of 70 mmHg and a P_aCO_2 of 37 mmHg, a simple confirmation that the patient has a long history of stable interstitial fibrosis of the lung and a history of near normal exercise tolerance for her age may suffice before proceeding with coronary bypass surgery. Conversely, if on review of the same screening results, the patient has a long history of interstitial fibrosis but had worsening of dyspnea on exertion in the last month, prior to assessing her risks of semi-elective cardiac surgery, the follow-up assessment should include one or more of the following tests: comparison of spirometry and possibly lung volumes and DLCO with previous measurements made prior to the worsening of dyspnea; response to bronchodilator therapy if there is evidence of obstructive airway dysfunction; measurements of maximal respiratory pressures; V/Q scan to rule out pulmonary emboli; assessment of maximal exercise levels; measurement of blood gases and/or oxygen consumption during maximal exercise; and possible measurement of pulmonary artery pressures at rest and with exercise.

Results from spirometry and blood gases that fall within normal limits do not rule out the need for further follow-up functional evaluation. In a patient with normal spirometry and blood gases but otherwise unexplained dyspnea on exertion, follow-up evaluation of function is necessary before clearing the patient for anything other than emergency surgery.

Which specific follow-up tests are most useful depends in part upon the specific clinical picture, and in part upon the resources of expertise and equipment available. Additional prospective studies are needed for more objective identification of optimal follow-up tests for defining surgical risk in patients with abnormalities on screening tests. Likewise, the specific levels of dysfunction which separate reasonable from high or prohibitive surgical risks are not firmly established and await further evaluation by prospective studies.

8. PREDICTING LIMITS OF LUNG RESECTION

If the results of spirometry and an arterial blood gas are near normal, these tests will usually suffice for clearing a patient for pneumonectomy unless there are signs or symptoms of significant lung dysfunction. If these screening tests indicate compromised function, then assessments of regional function become important. The criteria defining higher-risk patients cited in Table 1.2 can also be used for identifying subjects needing regional assessments of function.

In some cases (e.g., total collapse of the lobe to be resected), the chest radiographs may provide the necessary information. Usually more specific tests of regional function are needed, especially in patients with intrathoracic tumors which may interfere with pulmonary ventilation or blood flow without such dysfunction being suspected from chest radiographs. In most centers, because of the invasiveness and technical demands of selective bronchospirometry and balloon occlusion of pulmonary arteries, radionucleotide assessment of the distribution of pulmonary perfusion is the best option for regional assessment of function.

In addition to demonstrating that perfusion scans alone were as effective for predicting postoperative function as ventilation or combined ventilation and perfusion scans in patients undergoing pneumonectomy, Wernly et al.[39] also demonstrated that the loss of function from lobectomy could be predicted by simply multiplying the preoperative FEV_1 by the fraction of the number of functional segments in the lobe to be resected divided by the total number of segments in both lungs. This approach in lobectomy patients was as accurate for predicting morbidity as more complex formulae which incorporated the distribution of perfusion from radionucleotide scans. However, the small number (14) of patients in that study prevents us from concluding whether or not perfusion scans may be useful for more accurately predicting postoperative function and complications in specific patients undergoing lobectomy.

In cases where only a limited resection is planned, it is still usually advisable to make a decision preoperatively whether a patient could undergo more extensive resection in the event that during surgery the limits of resection need to be expanded.

The following minimum spirometric criteria have been recommended for identifying patients appropriate for consideration for lung resection[46]: for pneumonectomy, a preoperative $FEV_1 > 2.0$ l or a predicted postoperative $FEV_1 > 0.8$ l; for lobectomy, a preoperative $FEV_1 > 1.0$ l; for wedge or segmental resection, preoperative $FEV_1 > 0.6$ l. Such limits should not, however, be considered as absolute criteria since additional clinical data in individual patients may predict a tolerable or intolerable risk of resection.

Using exercise testing as a guide, Bechard[27] concluded that a $\dot{V}_{O_2,max}$ of less than 10 ml/kg/min was associated with significant elevations of morbidity and mortality. In contrast, there were no complications in the 17 patients undergoing lung resection who were able to attain $\dot{V}_{O_2,max}$ greater than 20 ml/kg/min. Using measurements of pulmonary vascular resistance during exercise, Fee et al.[36] suggested that a PVR greater than 190 dynes/sec/cm^{-5} during exercise was an indicator of unacceptable morbidity and mortality rate after surgery.

Olsen's comprehensive review[30] recommends exercise testing for predicting resectability, but more data from prospective studies are needed before these tests and specific criteria of resectability can be recommended for general use.

For surgical patients who also undergo radiation therapy to the lungs or chemotherapy with drugs with known pulmonary toxicity, appropriate prior evaluation of function should be done. In patients with limited function, such evaluations may reduce complications by limiting the amount of radiation. The availability of baseline values may also increase the sensitivity for detecting pulmonary drug toxicity should the patient develop suggestive signs or symptoms.

9. BULLECTOMY

Although in the future we may see less invasive treatment approaches such as the tube deflation and glue approach[47], surgery to deflate or resect bullae and reinflate functional lung currently offers an important option for patients with respiratory insufficiency secondary to enlarging bullae.

One suggested criterion for selecting surgical patients is that bullous lesions be greater in size than 30% of a hemithorax[48,49]. Although CT scans, bronchograms and pulmonary angiograms[50–52] may be useful for identifying compressed lung tissue, their usefulness for identifying lung tissue which upon reinflation will contribute significant gas-exchange function is problematic.

Currently we are most likely to identify good bullectomy candidates when patients complain of subacute (i.e., 1–12 months) worsening of dyspnea and functional tests done relatively recently before the deterioration are available. A previous CT scan may provide additional evidence that a new compressed region of the lung recently contained functional tissue. Without such baseline data, the reliable prediction of outcome from bullectomy in a patient with seemingly prohibitive function (e.g., $P_aCO_2 = 55\,mmHg$, $FEV_1 = 0.6\,l$) is very difficult. Periodic CT scans and assessments of function in patients with progressive bullous disease should make possible better conclusions in the future regarding the utility of such data for optimal selection of patients likely to benefit from surgery.

10. CARDIAC AND LUNG TRANSPLANTS

A thorough discussion of pulmonary criteria for minimizing risks of cardiac and lung transplantation is beyond the scope of this chapter. The relatively narrow spectrum of lung disease in patients who have undergone cardiac transplantation limits conclusions about minimal acceptable pulmonary function criteria. Because of reports of transplanted normal right ventricles not adapting acutely to high pulmonary resistances postoperatively, the importance of pulmonary vascular resistance is widely recognized. For example, elevations of PVR above 480 to 640 $dynes/sec/cm^{-5}$ are considered by some as absolute contraindications for cardiac transplantation [53].

For lung transplants, pulmonary assessment of prospective donors is usually very limited. Criteria often include: a preference for donors under age 50; negative histories of drug abuse or heavy cigarette smoking; essentially normal radiographs of the lungs. Direct functional testing may be limited to demonstrating acceptable gas exchange (e.g., $P_aO_2 > 300\,mmHg$ on 100% O_2 with a PEEP of 5) [53].

The impact of chronic elevations of pulmonary artery pressures on right ventricular (RV) function of the recipient's heart is important in candidates for lung transplantation, but the limits for recovery of RV function after reduction of pulmonary artery pressures by lung transplantations are not known. Criteria reported by the Toronto group for lung transplantation require a RV ejection fraction of 20% or greater as measured by first-pass nuclear angiography. Noninvasive Doppler techniques were used for estimates of mean P–A pressures preoperatively, replacing direct measurements formerly made using pulmonary artery catheters [54].

Although some have experimented with radiographic measurements of lung volumes for optimal matching of the donor lung to the recipient, the Toronto group has reported primary reliance on vertical and transverse dimensions from chest radiographs in combination with some consideration of heights, weights, and chest circumference [55]. More recently, the same group indicated a surprisingly rapid return of thoracic configurations towards normal after lung transplantation in patients who formerly had marked hyperinflation secondary to COPD [55]. Accordingly, donor lungs are sought of a size estimated to be appropriate for the height and ideal weight of the recipient.

11. SUMMARY

The lungs are a major source of postoperative complications after thoracic surgery. Functional evaluation of patients preoperatively is useful for identifying those patients who need careful consideration before proceeding with surgery. The cost-effectiveness of screening tests varies with patient populations, types of surgery, and the type of postoperative care offered routinely. Simple screening tests such as spirometry and an arterial blood gas are useful for identifying patients at higher risk for surgery, for whom more extensive follow-up tests may be indicated. Specific follow-up tests which are optimal, and the exact levels of function which predict prohibitive surgical risk, are currently not well defined. Radionucleotide perfusion scans are sufficiently noninvasive to have replaced bronchospirometry and intravascular balloon occlusion techniques for assessing regional distribution of lung function in patients being considered for lung resection. Exercise studies hold special promise for better defining operability in high-risk patients. Hopefully, prospective studies in the future will help answer some of the questions that remain for the preoperative assessment of the challenging patients with borderline function.

REFERENCES

1 Tisi GM. Preoperative evaluation of pulmonary function. State of the art. Am Rev Respir Dis 1979; 119: 292–310.
2 Don HF, Wahba WM, Craig DB. Airway closure, gas trapping and the functional residual capacity during anesthesia. Anesthesiology 1972; 36: 533–539.
3 Dueck R, Prutow RJ, Davies JH, Clausen J, Davidson TM. The lung volume at which shunting occurs with inhaled anesthesia. Anesthesiology 1988; 69: 854–861.
4 Ford GT, Whitelaw WA, Rosenal TW, Cruse PJ, Guenter CA. Diaphragm function after upper abdominal surgery in humans. Am Rev Respir Dis 1983; 127: 431–436.
5 Goldzimer EL, Parton ME, Kane EW. Elevated intraoperative carboxyhemoglobin levels. Anesth Analg 1984; 63: 698.
6 Warner MA, Civertie MB, Tinker JH. Preoperative cessation of smoking and pulmonary complications in coronary artery bypass patients. Anesthesiology 1984; 60: 380–383.
7 Charpak Y, Blery C, Chastang C, Szatan M, Fourgeaux B. Prospective assessment of a protocol for selective ordering of preoperative chest X-rays. Can J Anaesth 1988; 35: 259–264.
8 Patterson GA, Ginsberg RJ, Poon PY, et al. A prospective evaluation of magnetic resonance imaging, computed tomography, and mediastinoscopy in the preoperative assessment of mediastinal node status in bronchogenic carcinoma. J Thorac Cardiovasc Surg 1987; 94: 678–684.
9 Gamsu G, Sostman D. Magnetic resonance imagine of the thorax; state of the art. Am Rev Respir Dis 1989; 139: 254–274.
10 Chetty KG, Brown SE, Light RW. Quantification of pulmonary hypertension in chronic obstructive pulmonary disease from routine chest radiographs. Am Rev Respir Dis 1982; 126: 338–341.
11 Clausen JL, Zarins LP. Estimation of lung volumes from chest radiographs. In: Clausen J (ed.). Pulmonary Function Testing, Guidelines and Controversies. New York, Academic Press 1982.
12 Newsom Davis J, Goldman M, Loh L, Casson M. Diaphragm function and alveolar hypoventilation. Q J Med 1976; 177: 87–100.

13 Cooke JC, Currie DC, Mortgan AD, Kerr IH, et al. Role of computed tomography in diagnosis in bronchiectasis. Thorax 1987; 42: 272–277.
14 Joharjy IA, Bashi SA, Adbullah AK. Value of medium-thickness CT in the diagnosis of bronchiectasis. AJR 1987; 149: 1133–1137.
15 Sider L, Dennis L, Smith LJ, Dunn MM. CT of the lung parenchyma and the pulmonary function test. Chest 1987; 92: 406–610.
16 Gracey DR. Divertie MB, Didier EP. Preoperative pulmonary preparation of patients with chronic obstructive pulmonary disease, a prospective study. Chest 1979; 76: 123–129.
17 Gaensler EA, Cugell DW, Lindgren I, et al. The role of pulmonary insufficiency in mortality and invalidism following surgery for pulmonary tuberculosis. J Thorac Cardiovasc Surg 1955; 29: 163–187.
18 Stein M, Koota GM, Simon M, Frank HA. Pulmonary evaluation of surgical patients. JAMA 1962; 181: 765–770.
19 Stein M, Cassara EL. Preoperative pulmonary evaluation and therapy for surgery patients. JAMA 1970; 211: 787–790.
20 Cain HD, Stevens PM, Adaniya R. Preoperative pulmonary function and complications after cardiovascular surgery. Chest 1979; 76: 130–135.
21 Olsen GN, Block AJ, Swenson EW, Castle JR, Wynne JW. Pulmonary function evaluation of the lung resection candidate: a prospective study. Am Rev Respir Dis 1975; 111: 379–387.
22 Gass GD, Olsen GN. Preoperative pulmonary function testing to predict postoperative morbidity and mortality. Chest 1986; 89: 127–135.
23 Miller WF, Wu N, Johnson Jr RL. Convenient method of evaluating pulmonary ventilatory function with a single breath test. Anesthesiology 1956; 17: 480–493.
24 Peters RM, Brimm JE, Utley JR. Predicting the need for prolonged ventilatory support in adult cardiac patients. J Thorac Cardiovasc Surg 1979; 77: 175–182.
25 Klidjian AM, Foster KJ, Dammerling RM, Cooper A, Karran SJ. Relation of anthropometric and dynamometric variables to serious postoperative complications. Br Med J 1980; 281: 899–901.
26 Milledge JS, Nunn JF. Criteria of fitness for anaesthesia in patients with chronic obstructive lung disease. Br Med J 1975; 3: 670–673.
27 Bechard D, Wetstein L. Assessment of exercise oxygen consumption as preoperative criterion for lung resection. Ann Thorac Surg 1987; 44: 344–349.
28 Lockwood P, Lloyd MH, Williams GV. The value of a wide range of tests in the assessment of lung function in carcinoma of the bronchus. Br J Dis Chest 1980; 74: 253–258.
29 Reichel J. Assessment of operative risk of pneumonectomy. Chest 1972; 62: 570–576.
30 Olsen GN. The evolving role of exercise testing prior to lung resection. Chest 1989; 95: 218–225.
31 Eugene J, Brown SE, Light RW, Milne NE, Stemmer EA. Maximum oxygen consumption: a physiologic guide to pulmonary resection. Surg Forum 1982; 33: 260–262.
32 Berggren H, Ekroth R, Malmberg R, Naucler J, William-Olsson G. Hospital mortality and long-term survival in relation to preoperative function in elderly patients with bronchogenic carcinoma. Ann Thorac Surg 1984; 38: 633–636.
33 Bagg LR. The 12 minute walking distance: its use in the preoperative assessment of patients with bronchial carcinoma before lung resection. Respir 1984; 46: 342–345.
34 Colman NC, Schraufnagel DE, Rivington RN, Pardy RL. Exercise testing in evaluation of patients for lung resection. Am Rev Respir Dis 1982; 125: 604–606.
35 Smith TP, Kinasewitz GT, Tucker WY, Spillers WP, George RB. Exercise capacity as a predictor of post-thoracotomy morbidity. Am Rev Respir Dis 1984; 129: 730–734.
36 Fee HJ, Holmes EC, Gewirtz HS, Ramming KP, Alexander JM. Role of pulmonary vascular resistance measurements in preoperative evaluation of candidates for pulmonary resection. J Thorac Cardiovasc Surg 1978; 75: 519–525.
37 Snider GL, Shaw AR. A critical evaluation of bronchospirometric measurement in predicting loss of ventilatory function due to thoracic surgery. J Lab Clin Med 1964; 64: 321–329.

38 DeMeester TR, Van Heertum RL, Karas JR, Watson RL, Hansen JE. Preoperative evaluation with differential pulmonary function. Ann Thorac Surg 1974; 18: 61–70.
39 Wernly JA, DeMeester TR, Keahner PT, Myerrowitz PD, et al. Clinical value of quantitative ventilation–perfusion lung scans in the surgical management of bronchogenic carcinoma. J Thorac Cardiovasc Surg 1980; 80: 535–543.
40 Bergan F. A simple method for determination of the relative function of the right and left lung. Acta Chir Scand Suppl 1960; 253: 58–63.
41 Hazlett JDR, Watson RL. Lateral position test: a simple, inexpensive, yet accurate method of studying the separate functions of the lungs. Chest 1971; 59: 276–279.
42 Schoonover GA, Olsen GN, McLain III WC, Habibian MR, et al. Lateral position test and quantitative lung scan in the preoperative evaluation for lung resection. Chest 1984; 86: 854–859.
43 Jackson CV. Preoperative pulmonary evaluation. Arch Intern Med 1988; 148: 2120–2127.
44 Crapo RO, Kelly TM, Elliott CG, Jones SB. Spirometry as a preoperative screening test in morbidly obese patients. Surgery 1986; 99: 765–767.
45 Leventhal SR, Orkin FK, Hirsh RA. Prediction of the need for postoperative mechanical ventilation in myasthenia gravis. Anesthesiology 1980; 53: 26–30.
46 Miller JI, Grossman GD, Hatcher CR. Pulmonary function test criteria for operability and pulmonary resection. Surg Gynecol Obstet 1981; 153: 893–895.
47 Uyama T, Moden Y, Harada K, Kimura S, Toshikatsu T. Drainage of giant bulla with balloon catheter using chemical irritant and fibrin glue. Chest 1988; 94: 1289–1290.
48 Pearson MG, Oglivie C. Surgical treatment of emphysematous bullae: late outcome. Thorax 1983; 38: 134–137.
49 FitzGerald MX, Keelan PJ, Cugell DW, Gaensler EA. Long-term results of surgery for bullous emphysema. J Thorac Cardiovasc Surg 1974; 68: 566–587.
50 FitzGerald MX, Keelan PJ, Gaensler EA. Surgery for bullous emphysema. Respir 1973; 30: 187–200.
51 Ptogieter PD, Benatar SR, Hewitson RP, Ferguson AD. Surgical treatment of bullous lung disease. Thorax 1981; 36: 885–890.
52 Jensen KM, Miscall L, Steinberg I. Angiocardiography in bullous emphysema: its role in selection of the case suitable for surgery. Am J Roent Rad Ther Nucl Med 1961; 85: 229–245.
53 Andreone PA, Olivari MT, Ring WS. Clinical considerations of cardiac transplantation in organ transplantation: preoperative and postoperative evaluation. Radiol Clin North Am 1987; 25: 357–366.
54 Toronto Lung Transplant Group. Experience with single-lung transplantation for pulmonary fibrosis. JAMA 1988; 259: 2258–2262.
55 Cooper JD, Patterson GA, Grossman R, Maurer J, Toronto Lung Transplant Group. Double-lung transplant for advanced chronic obstructive lung disease. Am Rev Respir Dis 1989; 139: 303–307.

Current Topics in General Thoracic Surgery: An International Series, Vol. 2
Perioperative Care, edited by R.M. Peters and J. Toledo

Prediction of pulmonary function after lung resection

Discussion of "Assessment of pulmonary function" by Jack Clausen

A. López-Encuentra

1. INTRODUCTION

Clausen's work is an excellent up to date review of the preoperative evaluation of pulmonary function. As he says, we know more about the physiology and the ways of preventing clinical problems but we remain where we were 11 years ago, when Tisi showed the nonexistence of 'magic values' to establish the patient's operability or inoperability [1]. We fully agree on the fact that from the point of view of clinical practice it is not usually easy to decide which techniques are clinically useful or cost-effective.

Among the problems concerning preoperative pulmonary function, there is a clinical situation of great importance regarding decision making: Analysis of operability on patients with bronchogenic carcinoma (BC) and ventilatory insufficiency. This ventilatory insufficiency is secondary to a large extent to the coexistence of chronic airways obstruction (CAO). This is a frequent situation since 73.5% of all lung resections in our hospital are due to BC and 86% of these show associated CAO. Besides, the average age of patients with BC is 60 years, and most of them are or have been smokers.

For lung resection to be oncologically useful, it is necessary to remove functional lung tissue, and this is a usual practice. That implies that surgical complications increase in this group of patients, who are already at risk from other different causes.

One of the methods employed for discriminate evaluation of surgical risk in these resected patients consists of prediction of postoperative function. For several decades, individualized prediction of postoperative pulmonary function in patients with preoperative intermediate values was considered to be useful, and this has been widely followed.

It has been assumed that the different degrees of predicted postoperative lung function could be related to the risk of immediate complications, the limitations of ventilatory insufficiency or the prediction of the decrease in life expectancy related to the new ventilatory situation. The clinical usefulness of this information could result in an intensification of the preoperative use of resources in high-risk cases, or in the quantified evaluation of the risk/benefit balance in surgical decisions concerning individual patients.

In this discussion, we state our opinion about the possibilities and limitations of some methods of prediction of postoperative pulmonary function when pulmonary resection is indicated as treatment for BC.

2. METHODS OF PREDICTION OF POSTOPERATIVE PULMONARY FUNCTION

As Clausen reports, there are numerous methods for the regional evaluation of the pulmonary function, which can help to predict the postoperative function. Quantitative perfusion lung scanning (QPLS) [2] is the most used. In spite of all reservations, this method has been defended by many authors as the most useful procedure since it combines comfort, accessibility, acceptable clinical precision and reproducibility [3–8]. QPLS has been used in the United States [2,3,6], Europe [7,9,10–12], Japan [13,14] and Australia [15], and we have witnessed a continuous communication of results over several decades up to the present time. The evaluating parameter is forced expiratory volume at 1 second (FEV_1), and basically this has been used to predict the function after pneumonectomy due to BC. If we compare the data of QPLS with those obtained by ventilation scanning, the correlation coefficient is between 0.80 and 0.96 in six different series [7,16–20], and 0.95 when comparing it with bronchospirometry [6].

Technical resources are too frequently limited and access of all patients to all investigative methods is not always guaranteed; that is why the use of simpler techniques should be encouraged, as long as they are scientifically precise and reliable.

In the last few years several simpler methods have been described. These attempt to predict the postoperative function by subtracting from the preoperative FEV_1 the information about the number of functional segments to be resected taking into account radiological or endoscopic observation of the bronchi obstructed by tumor [19,21–22]. Although these methods have been used for every type of resection, it is possible that their main utility is for lobectomies.

QPLS is the most used complex method to predict the postoperative pulmonary function. The simplest method is to combine spirometric, radiologic and/or bronchoscopic data to make a clinical estimate of predicted post lung resection function.

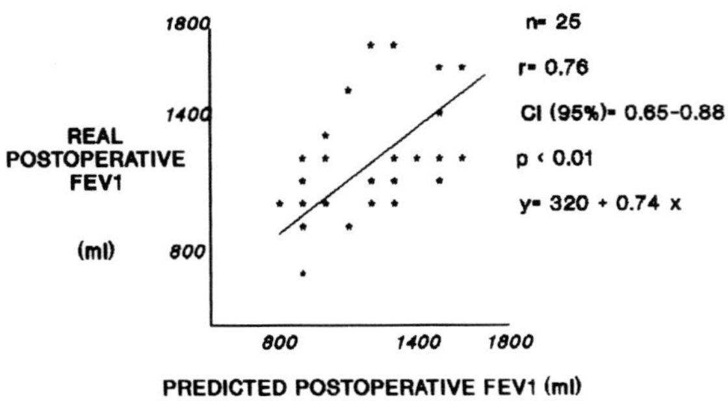

FIGURE D1.1. Correlation between the real postoperative FEV_1 and the predicted postoperative FEV_1: *n*, number of cases; *r*, correlation coefficient; CI, confidence interval; *p*, probability.

3. QUANTITATIVE PERFUSION LUNG SCANNING (QPLS)

In our experience, QPLS has been useful in the prediction of function after pneumonectomies[23]. A study was carried out on 40 patients who underwent pneumonectomy for BC, all cases having a preoperative FEV_1 between 1000 and 2000 ml. They were considered operable and resectable according to our own prospective protocol of BC study[24,25]. The mean age was 62 years (SD=5.7). The mean preoperative FEV_1 was 1645 ml (SD=228) and 59%(±2.3) in relation to the theoretical FEV_1[26].

The methodology used is that described by Olsen[2,16,18,27]. The postoperative spirometry was carried out from the third month after surgery, since this period of time was considered enough to get a stable function[28,29]. A patient was considered operable when the predicted postoperative FEV_1 (PPF), calculated by this method, was above 800 ml, according to well-known criteria[27–30]. It is assumed that FEV_1 values below 800 ml lead to a significant increase in annual mortality due to respiratory failure[31].

The operative mortality rate of this group was 7.5%. The ages of the three deceased patients ranged between 55 and 65 years, with actual preoperative FEV_1 between 1340 and 1800 ml (42% to 70% of the theoretical). The percentage of perfusion of the lung to be resected was very variable in relation to the whole (8.8%, 25.7%, 48.7%). The PPFs were between 965 and 1220 ml.

Valid postoperative data were available in 25 patients; a correlation between the PPF and actual postoperative FEV_1 was studied. The results are shown in Fig. D1.1.

TABLE D1.1
Correlation between predicted postoperative FEV_1 and real postoperative FEV_1 [a]

Reference	No. of cases[b]	Year	Correlation coefficient
2	13	1974	0.72
19	23	1980	0.81
28	NA	1980	0.83
11	13	1982	0.85
9	NA	1986	0.70
3	28	1987	0.86
32	9	1987	0.80
33	11	1988	0.66
13	26	1988	0.81
15	18	1989	0.51
12	8	1989	0.69
23	25	1989	0.75

[a] Calculation for pneumonectomies by perfusion lung scanning. All correlations are calculated on the absolute values of FEV_1 except those for reference 3.
[b] NA, not available.

The study shows that there is a 4% probability of having a postoperative FEV_1 lower than 800 ml. The mean of the differences between proven postoperative FEV_1 and the PPF is 152 ml, with intervals between 4 and 340 ml. In 45% of the cases the PPF was lower than the actual postoperative FEV_1 and in 52% it was higher. Both values were identical in one of the cases.

The experience gathered in the literature published since 1974 is summarized in Table D1.1. The series in which PPF after pneumonectomy was calculated by means of QPLS were selected. The indication for resection was always BC in all reports but two, in which BC cases were 84% [9] and 93% [32] of totality. For Leblanc's group [33] and our own [23], the cases chosen for the study had a preoperative FEV_1 between 1000 and 2000 ml. In the remaining series the preoperative function was variable, including cases with a preoperative FEV_1 over 2000 ml. In 10 out of the 11 studies the correlation coefficient was between 0.66 and 0.86, and therefore within the confidence intervals at 95% of our own study.

Several reports show the presence of error margins of 10% between the PPF and the real postoperative FEV_1 [13,19]. Speaking in terms of absolute values, differences greater than a standard deviation were described in 23% of the patients studied [9]. Also, differences greater than 150 ml were found in 45% of the patients using ventilation and perfusion scanning [34]. Most of the time the real postoperative FEV_1 was higher than the calculated one [2,3,20,34], although in others, including our experience, the probabilities of underestimation and overestimation were similar [9].

Experience in perfusion scanning as a method of calculating PPF in cases of lobectomy is much smaller. The degree of correlation between PPF and actual postoperative FEV_1 is reported to be very high in several of the papers published. Correlation coefficients such as 0.97 [28], 0.95 [19], 0.89 [15] and 0.88 [20] have been reported.

On analyzing a series of resected patients according to the criteria mentioned above, it was found that 21 of the 28 surgical survivors lived a year or more; 15 of these were without respiratory insufficiency [18]. After four years, the same group evaluated the experience with 38 pneumonectomy cases [35]. In the first year, 15 of the 38 patients died, but only one had succumbed to respiratory failure. Throughout the years, they found out the cause of death in 29 of the 31 patients that had died: 20 died due to BC and 5 because of respiratory failure. In short, it could be considered that 17% of this group of patients with known cause of death died as a result of respiratory failure. In another series, in which a number of patients were evaluated by means of ventilation and perfusion scanning, no dyspnea was found after pneumonectomy [34].

3.1. Limitations of the PPF calculation by QPLS

PPF calculation by QPLS is easily used in the clinical practice. The correlation coefficients with real postoperative values are acceptable, but not excellent; that is why it is necessary to look for factors that can affect the calculation.

One of the possible explanations for the observed differences is the absence of an absolute connection between the two main parameters used in the calculation: ventilation (FEV_1) and perfusion parameters. It has been found that 28% of the cases with BC show a poor relation between ventilation and perfusion, with ventilatory defects greater than those of perfusion in 18% of the cases and the opposite in the remaining 10% [36].

For the preoperative FEV_1 there is an individual variability in its determination [9], as well as the possibility of FEV_1 not being the most appropriate ventilatory parameter since it can be altered by the presence of proximal bronchial obstruction with a 'valve effect'. In cases of unilateral diaphragm paralysis, as FEV_1 is established in a sitting-up position and the regional perfusion parameters in decubitus, these different positions might be the cause of a discordance in values [9].

Pulmonary perfusion data obtained by gammagraphy can be regionally altered by the associated presence of bullas or pulmonary thromboembolism without any parallel alteration in the ventilation. Likewise a tumor which can affect the hilar vascular vessels can produce a similar effect. In case of pleural effusion, its interposition between the lung and the counter can cause false data in the determination of ipsilateral perfusion.

Finally, this calculation system presumes unilateral homogeneity in the distribution of perfusion. This may not be so in case of alteration of the thoracic cage (thoracoplasty or kyphoscoliosis), in cases of cardiomegaly [37] or when there are large pulmonary consolidations due to BC; in this the extent of anterior perfusion may be greater than the posterior one, or vice versa.

Although a few papers report calculations obtained by means of perfusions of both anterior and posterior projections [7,9,17], the majority of calculations uses only the posterior projection. In theory, when pulmonary consolidation is entirely or predominantly posterior, the posterior projection may undervalue the lung contribution to total pulmonary function; just the opposite is true for anterior projection [38]. This was studied on 70 patients, performing two scanning determinations in each case (an anterior and a posterior one). The data were compared to the analysis of the lateral chest roentgenograms. The gammagraphical and radiological results were read in a blind way, and we studied the interobserver concordance in the description of localization and size of the radiological image between two observers by Kappa's index calculation [39]. This index was 0.74 for image visibility, 0.80 for asymmetric description (anterior or posterior), and 0.96 for the degree of radiological extent in the anterior and posterior half. The study was carried out on 42 cases with radiological consolidation which was visible and asymmetric (anterior or posterior) with interobserver concordance in all the parameters which have been used.

The probability that perfusion in the posterior projection was greater than that obtained in the anterior projection in relation with the localization and the size of the radiological consolidation was studied. That probability is greater if the consolidation is anterior ($p = 0.10$ in comparison with the consolidation of posterior localization). The probability increases when the consolidation is higher than 25% of the posterior or anterior half of the thorax in the lateral radiological image, a significant difference ($p < 0.02$; $n = 21$). In 5 cases (12%), one projection estimated PPF above 800 ml and another projection below. An identical percentage resulted for the analysis of FEV_1 relative to the theoretical value. Further research is necessary in order to establish which projection, or combination of both, is more predictive of the real postoperative FEV_1.

The introduction of this factor should be qualitative since there is not a direct connection between the size of the radiological consolidation and the gammagraphic defects. The defects in ventilatory scanning were considered greater than expected by radiology in 48% of the cases [36]. Likewise, 23% had perfusion defects greater than radiologically expected; this occurred more frequently in cases affected by hilar or mediastinal tumors (84%) [40].

3.2. Limitations of the operability criterion for pneumonectomy

For years it has been reported that the absolute value of the PPF could be adjusted towards reality by correcting for the age, the height and the sex of each patient [3,10,41,42].

An additional problem is that of reference values for older patients. Comparing CECA values for people over 70 years of age [26] with those most recently published for this age group [43], CECA values could be overrated up to 25–30%.

Our experience has been analyzed (Fig. 2) in order to weigh possible implications of the change of operability criteria. We studied 89 patients with a preoperative

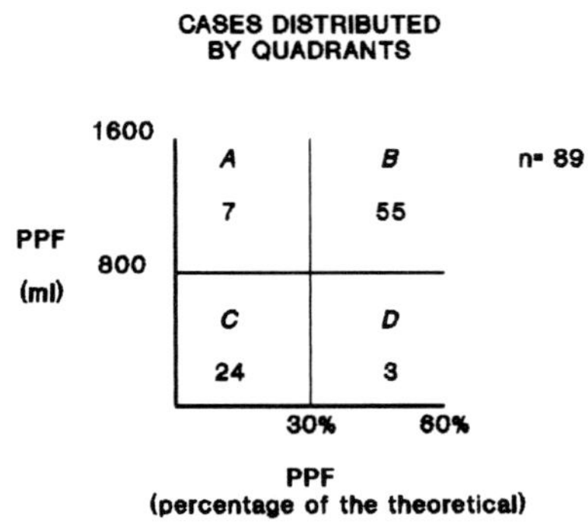

FIGURE D1.2. Operability by calculation of the predicted postoperative FEV_1 (PPF) in absolute value or percentage of the theoretical. Comparison of operability criteria: PPF over 800 ml or over 30% of the theoretical.

FEV_1 below 2000 ml. As can be seen in the figure, there are 10 cases (11%) in an undefined area. The 3 cases in quadrant D were considered inoperable from 1978 to 1982. This circumstance has not been a criterion of inoperability in our group since 1984 [10]. We performed a thoracotomy with no operative mortality on 6 out of the 7 cases in quarter A. The other patient refused surgery. In our opinion, these data suggest that the operability criterion, which is based on the PPF as a percentage of the theoretical one, must be considered when the PPF, in absolute values, is under 800 ml.

4. USE OF METHODS BASED ON SPIROMETRY, THORACIC RADIOLOGY AND BRONCHOSCOPY TO CALCULATE THE POSTOPERATIVE PULMONARY FUNCTION

Several methods to calculate the PPF have been described in the last decade, taking as a basis the data of simple spirometry, thoracic radiology, bronchography and bronchoscopy [19,21,22].

In one of our studies, we analyzed 152 pulmonary resections of any extent, due to BC; they were carried out between 1986 and 1989 at our hospital. The PPFs were calculated according to the formulas described by Wernly et al. [19], Nakahara et al. [21] and Egeblad et al. [22], and they were compared with the real postoperative FEV_1 collected between 3–12 months after surgery. The calculations were done with the preoperative FEV_1 and the collected data on the estimation of the segmental and subsegmental obstruction detected in bronchoscopy.

The correlation between the PPF and the real postoperative FEV_1 of this group had a coefficient of 0.80 (CI 95%: 0.74–0.85) according to Wernly's formula [19] and 0.81 (CI 95%: 0.75–0.86) for Nakahara's [21] and Egeblad's [22].

The coefficient of determination oscillated between 0.64 and 0.66 for the three calculations. The coefficient of correlation that Wernly [19] found in lobectomy was 0.96 (14 cases). Nakahara [21] reported different degrees of correlation depending on the type of resection accomplished. In the whole group of 52 patients, the correlation coefficient was 0.82. When only the pneumonectomy cases ($n = 13$) were considered, the correlation was 0.72. In right upper lobectomy and left upper lobectomy, the coefficients were 0.88 and 0.90 respectively. In 1986, Egeblad [22] reported a correlation of 0.84 in a group of 30 patients. Finally, Pereira-Vega et al. [44], using Egeblad's formula, reported a correlation of 0.97 in 20 patients; 15 of these cases were lobectomies; 25% of the patients had no BC.

Considering all these studies, we can deduce that the use of these simple calculation methods yields correlations with real postoperative values which are similar to more sophisticated methods. Besides, the techniques needed are easily accessible (simple spirometry) or otherwise necessary to diagnose disease (bronchoscopy). The coefficient of determination of these calculations, according to these formulae, shows that only 64%–66% of the PPF forecast is controlled with the suggested formula, so other factors must be introduced. Nakahara's study [45] shows that there is a connection between the PPF calculated by his method and the probability of complications. This clinical utility must be verified in the light of new experiences.

5. CONCLUSIONS

In the group with BC and ventilatory insufficiency, frequently aggravated by the coexistence of CAO, the prediction of postoperative pulmonary function may have different clinical uses. One of these is its value as a criterion in the evaluation of surgical risk as regards probability of mortality or postoperative morbidity. Likewise, it could be useful in establishing the prognosis in the long term by contemplating both the probability of survival depending on the tumor [46] and that related to diminished lung function after resection in cases of CAO [47,48]. It could also be useful for the prediction of pulmonary function after thoracic radiotherapy [49].

The methods that have been used for this prediction are numerous but the most frequently used consists of the regional calculation of the function by means of quantitative perfusion lung scanning (QPLS). In our study, if the PPF calculation by this method is over 800 ml, the operative mortality rate is 7.1% for pneumonectomy, and the correlation to the real postoperative values is acceptable. We need to know the limitations of the method when using it with specific patients. In this respect, it should be used carefully when there is a pulmonary consolidation in the anterior or posterior half of the hemithorax.

Some other, simpler methods use only the information from the preoperative FEV_1 and the degree of bronchial obstruction detected in bronchoscopy. They can reach levels of efficacy similar to those in isotopic studies. New variables must be introduced to improve the predictions of these methods.

Finally, certain precautions must be taken when using these parameters as operability criteria. The value of the prediction of pulmonary function and predictions related to the incidence of immediate and late complications in relation to the PPF must be validated in further studies. Likewise, the data of calculated postoperative pulmonary function must be considered with other clinical criteria, age, weight, associated disease, other lung-function and hemodynamics tests. All this should be combined within a multifactorial analysis of risk evaluation.

With all the precautions already indicated, recommendations have been made recently for reaching a decision in the preoperative evaluation in patients who need to undergo thoracic surgery[50]. After a critical review of the literature, a systematic sequence of preoperative studies is advocated. Perfusion scanning for the calculation of postoperative pulmonary function comes after performing simple tests of lung function. In some situations, this calculation must be complemented by other study procedures (exercise test, hemodynamic studies).

The absence of ‘magic values’ persists but nevertheless there is a progressive improvement in the measurement of uncertainty with a more precise knowledge of the quantified probabilities of risk. Admitting the limitations and the need for further research, this information is basic for correct decision making, for patients as well as for physicians.

REFERENCES

1 Tisi GM. Preoperative evaluation of pulmonary function. Validity, indications, and benefits. Am Rev Respir Dis 1979; 119: 293.

2 Olsen GN, Block AJ, Tobias JA. Prediction of postpneumonectomy pulmonary function using quantitative macroagregate lung scanning. Chest 1974; 66: 13.

3 Gass GD, Olsen GN. Preoperative pulmonary function testing to predict postoperative morbidity and mortality. Chest 1986; 89: 127.

4 Brown LK. Surgical considerations: Effects of surgery on lung function; preoperative evaluation. In: Miller A (ed.). Pulmonary function tests in clinical and occupational lung disease. Orlando, FL, Grune-Stratton 1986: pp 341–352.

5 López-Encuentra A, Varela-Simo G. Predicción del VEMS postoperatorio. Cirugía Española 1989; 46: 46.

6 DeMeester TR, Van Heertum RL, Karas JR, Watson RL, Hansen JE. Preoperative evaluation with differential pulmonary function. Ann Thorac Surg 1974; 18: 61.

7 Corris PA, Ellis DA, Hawkins T, Gibson GJ. Use of radionuclide scanning in the preoperative estimation of pulmonary function after pneumonectomy. Thorax 1987; 42: 285.

8 Usseti P, Agusti AGN, Roca J, et al. Toracotomia: Morbilidad cardiorespiratoria precoz. Analisis multivariante de los factores de riesgo. Arch Bronconeumol 1988; 24: 54.

9 Le Roy Ladurie M, Ranson-Bitker B. Uncertainties in the expected value for forced expiratory volume in one second after surgery. Chest 1986; 90: 222.

10 López-Encuentra A, Varela G, Martin-Escribano P, et al. Operabilidad en el carcinoma broncogénico. Valoración por estudio gammagrafico pulmonar de perfusion, cuantitativo y diferencial. Arch Bronconeumol 1984; 20: 181.
11 Ellis DA, Hawkins T, Gibson GJ, Nariman S. Prediction of lung function after pneumonectomy for bronchial carcinoma. Thorax 1982; 37: 786.
12 Usseti P, Agusti AGN, Roca J, Rodriguez-Roisin R, Sanchez-Lloret J, Agusti-Vidal A. Resección pulmonar: Predicción de la perdida de función. Arch Bronconeumol 1989; 25: 9.
13 Novoyama A, Saito Y, Umamoto M, Ohmoto K, Kagama T. Prediction of postpneumonectomy pulmonary function using perfusion lung scanning. Lung Cancer 1989; 4: A89.
14 Hara F, Kanetou S, Watanabe T, et al. Prediction of postoperative pulmonary function in lung cancer patient using corrected lateral lung scan image. Lung Cancer 1986; 2: 66.
15 Markos J, Mullan BP, Hillman DR, et al. Preoperative assessment as a predictor of mortality and morbidity after lung resection. Am Rev Respir Dis 1989; 139: 902.
16 Schoonover GA, Olsen GN, McLain WC, Habibian MR, Edwards DG, Spurrier P. Lateral position test and quantitative lung scan in the preoperative evaluation for lung resection. Chest 1984; 86: 854.
17 Lipscomb DJ, Pride NB. Ventilation and perfusion scans in the preoperative assessment of bronchial carcinoma. Thorax 1977; 32: 720.
18 Boysen PG, Block AJ, Olsen GN, Moulder PV, Harris JO, Rawitscher RE. Prospective evaluation for pneumonectomy using the ^{99m}technetium quantitative perfusion lung scan. Chest 1977; 72: 422.
19 Wernly JA, DeMeester TR, Kirchner PT, Myerowitz PD, Oxford DE, Golomb HM. Clinical value of quantitative ventilation–perfusion lung scans in the surgical management of bronchogenic carcinoma. J Thorac Cardiovasc Surg 1980; 80: 535.
20 Bria WF, Kanarek DJ, Kazemi H. Prediction of postoperative pulmonary function following thoracic operations. Value of ventilation–perfusion scanning. J Thorac Cardiovasc Surg 1983; 86: 186.
21 Nakahara K, Mouden Y, Ohno K, Miyoshi S, Maeda H, Kawashima Y. A method for predicting postoperative lung function and its relation to postoperative complications in patients with lung cancer. Ann Thorac Surg 39: 260: 1985.
22 Egeblad K, Ausholt A, Funder V, Nielsen PH. A simple method for predicting pulmonary function after lung resection. Scand J Thorac Cardiovasc Surg 1986; 20: 103.
23 Diaz-Atauri J, López-Encuentra A, Gutierrez ME, Sanz-Sanchez ML, Cabanillas-Martin JJ, Martin-Escribano P. Predicción del VEMS postoperatorio para neumonectomia por carcinoma broncogénico. Arch Bronconeumol 1989; 25: 13.
24 López-Encuentra A, Martinez-Gonzalez J, Cortes-Funes H. Protocolo para el estudio y el tratamiento del carcinoma broncogénico (I). Med Clin (Barcelona) 1979; 72: 321.
25 López-Encuentra A. Carcinoma broncogénico. In: Martin-Escribano P, López-Encuentra A (eds.). Diagramas Neumologia. Madrid, IDEPSA 1989.
26 Denolin H, Sadoul P, Orie NGM. Établissement des Normes Physiologiques. L'Exploration Fonctionnelle Pulmonaire. Paris, Medicale Flammarion 1964.
27 Olsen GN, Block AJ, Swenson EW, Castle JR, Wynne JW. Pulmonary function evaluation of the lung resection candidate: A prospective study. Am Rev Respir Dis 1975; 111: 379.
28 Ali MK, Mountain CF, Ewer MS, Johnston D, Haynie TP. Predicting loss of pulmonary function after pulmonary resection for bronchogenic carcinoma. Chest 1980; 77: 337.
29 Legge JS, Palmer KNV. Effect of lung resection for bronchial carcinoma on pulmonary function in patients with and without chronic obstructive bronchitis. Thorax 1975; 30: 563.
30 Peters RM. Special problems in preoperative and postoperative management. In: Delarue NC, Eschapasse H (eds.). International Trends in General Thoracic Surgery, Vol 1, Lung Cancer. Philadelphia, PA, WB Saunders 1985.
31 Burrows B, Strauss RN, Niden AH. Chronic Obstructive Lung Disease III. Interrelationships of pulmonary function data. Am Rev Respir Dis 1965; 91: 861.
32 Julius AJ, DeJong D, Van Detekom H, Heidendal GAK, Otter G, Kester ADM. The value of ^{99m}Tc macroaggregated albumin lung perfusion scanning in the prediction of postpneumonectomy function and pulmonary artery pressure. Scan J Thorac Cardiovasc Surg 1987; 21: 81.

33 Leblanc P, Pelletier C, Rosseau M. Is the prediction of postpneumonectomy FEV_1 by lung perfusion scan really accurate?. Am Rev Respir Dis 1988; 137: 214.

34 Williams AJ, Cayton RM, Harding LK, Mostafa AB, Matthews HR. Quantitative lung scintigrams and lung function in the selection of patients for pneumonectomy. Br J Dis Chest 1984; 78: 105.

35 Boysen PG, Harris JO, Block AJ, Olsen GN. Prospective evaluation for pneumonectomy using perfusion scanning. Follow-up beyond one year. Chest 1981; 80: 163.

36 Libert P, Ravez P, Chattou O, Richez M, Delwarte J, Godart G, Robience YJ. Radioaerosol scans in lung cancer. Lung Cancer 1986; 2: 72.

37 Wiener ChM, McKenna WJ, Myers MJ, Lavender JP, Hughes JMB. Left lower lobe ventilation is reduced in patients with cardiomegaly in the supine but not the prone position. Am Rev Respir Dis 1990; 141: 150.

38 Cassen B. Principles of measurement of radioactivity. In: Blahd WH (ed.). Nuclear Medicine. New York, McGraw-Hill 1965.

39 Department of Clinical Epidemiology and Biostatistics, McMaster University. Clinical Disagreement: How often it occurs and why. Can Med Ass 1980; 123: 499.

40 Macunber HH, Calvin JW. Perfusion lung scan patterns in 100 patients with bronchogenic carcinoma. J Thorac Cardiovasc Surg 1976; 72: 299.

41 Johnson B. Discussion of special problems in preoperative and postoperative management. In: Delarue NC, Eschapasse H (eds.). International Trends in General Thoracic Surgery, Vol 1, Lung Cancer. Philadelphia, PA, WB Saunders 1985.

42 Mountain CF. Biologic, physiologic and technical determinants in surgical therapy for lung cancer. In: Strauss MJ (ed.). Lung Cancer. Clinical Diagnosis and Treatment. New York, Grune-Stratton 1983.

43 Burr ML, Phillips KM, Hurst DN. Lung function in the elderly. Thorax 1985; 40: 54.

44 Pereira-Vega A, Capote-Gil F, Castillo-Gomez J, Ureta-Toslada MP, Rodriguez-Panadero F, Torres-Cansino M. Estimación de la función pulmonar tras la exeresis. Análisis de un método sencillo. Arch Bronconeumol 1990; 26: 195.

45 Nakahara K, Ohno K, Hashimoto J, et al. Prediction of postoperative respiratory failure in patients undergoing lung resection for lung cancer. Ann Thorac Surg 1988; 46: 549.

46 Mountain CF. New international staging system for lung cancer. Chest Suppl 1986; 89: 225S.

47 Traver GA, Cline MG, Burrows B. Predictors of mortality in Chronic Obstructive Pulmonary Diseases. A 15 years follow-up study. Am Rev Respir Dis 1979; 119: 895.

48 López-Encuentra A. Clasificación anatomica del tumor y clasificación clinica del paciente. Decisiones individualizadas en situación clínical desfavorable. In: López-Encuentra A (ed.). Abordaje Multidisciplinario del tratamiento del Cancer Primitivo de Pulmon. Proc I Congr Luso-Español de Neumologia. Lisboa, Sociedad Portuguesa de Patologia Respiratoria 1989.

49 Choi NC. Prospective prediction of postradiotherapy pulmonary function data: promise and pitfalls. Int J Radiot Oncol Biol Phys 1988; 15: 245.

50 American College of Physicians. Preoperative pulmonary function testing. Ann Intern Med 1990; 112: 793.

Current Topics in General Thoracic Surgery: An International Series, Vol. 2
Perioperative Care, edited by R.M. Peters and J. Toledo

Chapter 2

Preoperative cardiac assessment

Hani A. Hennein and Julie A. Swain

GLOSSARY

ACT	activated clotting time	MAT	multifocal atrial tachycardia
AHA	American Heart Association	MR	mitral regurgitation
APTT	activated partial thromboplastin time	MVP	mitral valve prolapse
		NYHA	New York Heart Association
AR	aortic regurgitation	PAT	paroxysmal atrial tachycardia
CAD	coronary artery disease	PT	prothrombin time
CHF	congestive heart failure	PVC	premature ventricular complex
CXR	chest X-ray	PVD	peripheral vascular disease
DC	direct current (cardioversion)	W s	watt seconds (energy level)
ETT	exercise tolerance test		

1. INTRODUCTION

An increasing number of elderly patients are undergoing general thoracic operations. This is due to both a higher percentage of older patients in the population, and a greater number of operations being performed. The prime risk to operation in the elderly population is generally considered to be cardiac in origin [1]. There is not only an increased prevalence of most cardiovascular diseases in the elderly, but aging also causes a progressive decline in the maximum heart rate, oxygen consumption, stroke work, and cardiac output [2,3]. Recent improvements made in anaesthetic techniques and intensive care facilities, however, have allowed many high-risk patients to undergo safe non-cardiac operations [4]. This improvement has been in part ascribed to the use of perioperative hemodynamic monitoring with pulmonary and systemic arterial catheters, and interventions made based on these continual measurements [5].

Preoperative cardiac risk factors associated with subsequent cardiovascular events after non-cardiac surgery include presence of signs of heart failure, the occurrence of a myocardial infarction within six months of operation, the presence

TABLE 2.1
Goldman and Caldera cardiac risk index

Criteria[a]	Points
(1) History	
(a) Age > 70 yr	5
(b) MI in previous 6 mo	10
(2) Physical examination	
(a) S_3 gallop or JVD	11
(b) important VAS	3
(3) Electrocardiogram	
(a) Rhythm other than sinus or PAC's on last preoperative ECG	7
(b) > 5 PVC's/min documented at any time before operation	7
(4) General status	
$P_aO_2 < 60$ or $P_aCO_2 > 50$ mmHg, K < 3.0 or $HCO_3 < 20$ meq/l, BUN > 50 or Cr > 3.0 mg/dl, abnormal SGOT, signs of chronic liver disease or patient bed-ridden from noncardiac causes	3
(5) Operation	
(a) Intraperitoneal, intrathoracic or aortic operation	3
(b) Emergency operation	4

[a] Notation: MI, myocardial infarction; JVD, jugular venous distention; VAS, valvular aortic stenosis; PAC's, premature atrial contractions; pO_2, partial pressure of oxygen; pCO_2, partial pressure of carbon dioxide; K, potassium; BUN, blood urea nitrogen; Cr, creatinine; SGOT, serum glutamic oxalacetic transaminase.

TABLE 2.2
Goldman and Caldera cardiac risk index

Class	Points	Risk (%)		
		None or minor	Major[a]	Deaths
I	< 5	99	< 1	< 1
II	6–12	93	5	2
III	13–25	86	11	2
IV	> 26	22	22	56

[a] Documented intraoperative or perioperative myocardial infarction, pulmonary edema, or ventricular tachycardia without progression to cardiac death.

of a rhythm other than sinus, the presence of aortic stenosis, the patient's age, the type of planned surgery (including whether it is an emergency or elective procedure), and the patient's general medical condition[6]. Each factor can be assigned points based on its statistical relevance to postoperative events (Table 2.1), and the number of points can give an estimate of the risk of cardiovascular events following major non-cardiac operations (Table 2.2). It is important to note that some of these risk factors, such as signs of heart failure and the interval of time following a myocardial infarction, can be reversed in

TABLE 2.3
Factors not independently associated with increased cardiac risk

Hyperlipidemia	Peripheral vascular disorders
Smoking	Old MI by history
Diabetes	ST segment or T wave changes
Hypertension	Cardiomegaly
Stable angina	Mitral valve disease
Bundle branch blocks	CHF without S_3 or JVD

the preoperative period. Additionally noteworthy are factors not found to be independently significant predictors of postoperative cardiac events, such as the presence of risk factors associated with coronary artery disease, old myocardial infarctions, and heart failure without an S_3 gallop or jugular venous distention (Table 2.3). Preoperative exercise testing or cardiac catheterization to assess risk are not routinely indicated, but perioperative hemodynamic monitoring to improve management is recommended in patients at high risk. Postoperative hypertension, arrhythmias, and heart failure commonly occur in the first 2 days after surgery, but the risk of myocardial infarction persists for at least 5 or 6 days after surgery [7].

In addition to coronary artery disease and heart failure, this chapter summarizes the preoperative assessment and management of patients with other forms of cardiac disease, such as valvular heart disease, conduction disturbances, and arrhythmias. Guidelines regarding the perioperative management of cardiac medications, prophylactic antibiotics, and pacemakers are also discussed.

2. CORONARY ARTERY DISEASE

2.1. Asymptomatic patients

The perioperative myocardial infarction rate is variously reported to be between 0.08 to 2.4% in patients with no known coronary artery disease (CAD) [8,9,10,11]. A careful history is probably the only method that is useful in assessing the presence of important CAD in asymptomatic patients. Symptoms of exertional ischemia should be carefully sought. Chest, jaw or arm pain, tightness, pressure or discomfort brought on by either physical or emotional stress are suspect for underlying coronary artery disease. Similar sensations brought on by either large meals or cold weather may also signify underlying disease.

Peripheral vascular disease (PVD) is highly associated with CAD [12,13]. For example, 75 to 90% of patients with abdominal aortic aneurysm have CAD on angiography, while 50% of these patients have severe CAD. Very often patients with vascular disease do not manifest symptoms of CAD, due to limitations in exercise capacity brought on by their vascular disease. In such patients, dipyridamole–thallium imaging is a potentially useful method in assessing operative risk [14,15], by demonstrating anatomical perfusion abnormalities. The principal limitation of this method is that it does not delineate the physiologic severity of the lesion, however it remains a useful method to evaluate patients in whom other noninvasive tests are not helpful [16]. The operative mortality rate in patients with PVD is high (6–8%) [17], and is primarily due to CAD. This compares to an expected rate of about 1% in the general thoracic population.

Cardiac risk factors alone, such as hyperlipidemia, smoking, diabetes, and hypertension, generally do not increase the incidence of perioperative cardiac events [6] (see Table 2.3). Preoperative exercise tolerance testing (ETT) may be helpful in judging operative risk [18], although it is fraught with a high rate of false positive and false negative results in otherwise asymptomatic patients [19]. Interpretation of exercise testing in patients with PVD may likewise be difficult, in that such patients may be unable to exert themselves. In general, asymptomatic patients who have no apparent coronary artery or peripheral vascular disease after a careful history, have a low incidence of perioperative infarction and mortality. Exercise testing may occasionally be useful, but further diagnostic procedures are generally not indicated.

2.2. Stable angina

Patients with chronic stable angina who have had no previous myocardial infarction likewise have a low risk for perioperative myocardial infarction and cardiac death [6,20,21]. In this group of patients an exercise stress test may be helpful in assessing the patient's exercise tolerance and the probability of developing preoperative ischemia [22,23]. Cardiac catheterization and other cardiac diagnostic tests are generally not indicated. Patients whose symptoms are controlled with beta blockers or calcium channel blockers should have these medications continued up to and including the day of operation. Discontinuing such medications prior to operation may result in rebound tachycardia, myocardial ischemia, and infarction [24].

2.3. Unstable angina

Unstable angina poses an unpredictable preoperative risk due to the paucity of data on its influence on postoperative cardiac events. This is primarily due to a general reluctance to operate on patients with unstable angina. The risk is probably very high, and may signify the highest risk group in patients with CAD. Patients in this group should have cardiac catheterization and, if indicated, myocardial revascularization prior to elective non-cardiac surgery. Patients who cannot undergo myocardial revascularization prior to non-cardiac surgery may be temporarily supported by either intra-aortic balloon counterpulsation or percutaneous cardiopulmonary bypass [25] either prophylactically or if hemodynamic instability ensues. Mechanical techniques for circulatory support have been successfully used as prophylactic measures during invasive cardiac procedures, such

TABLE 2.4
Mayo Clinic studies of reinfarction rates and mortality in patients with a prior MI

Study	Patients	Previous MI	Reinfarction rate				Reinfarction mortality
			0–3 mo	3–6 mo	> 6 mo	no prior MI	
1971 [9]	32877	422	37%	16%	4–5%	0.13%	–
1978 [21]	73321	587	27%	11%	4–5%	–	69%

as coronary angioplasty and aortic valvuloplasty [26], but no reports of their use during non-cardiac procedures have as yet appeared.

2.4. Previous myocardial infarction

As many as 10% of the population over 40 years of age have had a myocardial infarction [6,10]. The relationship between previous myocardial infarction and perioperative reinfarction has been well studied (Table 2.4) [9,23]. Patients with a history of a previous myocardial infarction have an overall rate of reinfarction of 6% when undergoing non-cardiac surgery, while patients with no history of previous infarction had a perioperative myocardial infarction rate of approximately 1%. Infarctions occurring within three months of operation carry a reinfarction rate of 27 to 37%, a rate considered virtually prohibitive for elective operations. From three to six months after myocardial infarction the risk of reinfarction decreases to 11 to 16%, and beyond six months the reinfarction rate declines further to a chronic basal rate of 4 to 5%.

Additional risk factors that may be important in predicting perioperative reinfarction include: (1) the site of operation, (2) the duration of anesthesia, (3) associated congestive heart failure (CHF), (4) intraoperative hypotension or hypertension and (5) tachycardia [5]. Neither the site nor the type of a previous infarction are significant predictors of perioperative reinfarction. Patients with previous subendocardial infarcts have the same propensity for reinfarction as those with transmural infarcts. Furthermore, infarctions in an anterior, anteroinferior, or inferior location are associated with the same risk of reinfarction. The site of operation, conversely, is a primary determinant of risk, with patients undergoing operations on the great vessels having the greatest risk, followed by other intrathoracic and upper abdominal operations. The duration of anesthesia is an added risk factor, but is dependent on the site of operation, with greater anesthetic times being required for higher-risk operative sites. The type of anesthetic (spinal or general) being used, however, does not appear to be an additional risk factor.

Perioperative reinfarctions carry a very high mortality rate, variously reported between 55 to 70% [7,27,28], as compared to less than a 30% mortality for myocardial infarctions that occur without attendant operation or anesthesia. Reinfarctions occur most frequently during the third postoperative day, and because they may be masked by narcotic management of postoperative pain, 21 to more than 60% may be silent [8,9,21]. Common presenting signs are cardiovascular collapse, hypotension, arrhythmias, congestive failure, and sudden death [5,9,11,21]. The relatively high risk of reinfarction and mortality in patients with a history of previous myocardial infarction can be significantly reduced with myocardial revascularization [12,29]. This has been demonstrated following aortocoronary bypass, but should be expected to yield similar results following percutaneous coronary angioplasty (PTCA) if subsequent complete revascularization (defined as no remaining lesion greater than 70%), has been accomplished.

In summary, asymptomatic patients and patients with only risk factors for coronary artery disease do not appear to be at significant risk for perioperative myocardial infarction. Further invasive or noninvasive evaluation for CAD is generally not indicated. Patients with chronic stable angina also appear to not be at significant risk, but the risk may be better defined with exercise tolerance testing. Although there is a paucity of data on the risk of new or unstable angina, such patients are probably at high risk for sustaining a myocardial infarction, and should undergo appropriate non-invasive and invasive testing prior to elective intrathoracic operation. Finally, elective surgery should be postponed for three months following myocardial infarction, since the rate of reinfarction and mortality are high.

Patients at high risk of myocardial ischemia during major operative procedures are those with new or unstable angina or those who have had a myocardial infarction within three months of operation. All such patients should be monitored by telemetry in the perioperative period, along with being monitored by systemic and pulmonary artery catheters in the operative and immediate postoperative period. This will allow for the early detection and treatment of hypotension, hypertension, intravascular fluid imbalance, ischemic electrocardiographic changes, and arrhythmias.

3. CONGESTIVE HEART FAILURE

A primary determinant of postoperative cardiac complications and death is the presence of uncompensated heart failure in the preoperative period [7]. It is important to identify both the underlying cause of heart disease as well as precipitating causes of left ventricular dysfunction. Congestive heart failure may be caused by any of the cardiac lesions or conditions discussed in this chapter, while precipitating causes may include anemia, thyrotoxicosis, sepsis, emotional or physical stress, pulmonary embolus, and renal, hepatic, or multiorgan failure. Signs and symptoms of overt CHF include dyspnea, orthopnea, paroxysmal nocturnal dyspnea, tachycardia, jugular venous distension, ventricular (S_3) gallop, pulsus alternans, basilar pulmonary rales, and peripheral edema. Subtle signs of diminished cardiac reserve and possible cardiac decompensation following major surgery include unexplained fatigue, a nocturnal cough, irritability, or insomnia. In addition, signs of increased sympathetic tone may be present, including persistent sinus tachycardia, restlessness, and increased perspiration. The chest roentgenogram typically shows cardiomegaly and signs of pulmonary venous congestion.

3.1. Preoperative considerations

The risk of heart failure is decreased if the failure is compensated prior to operation [10,30]. The usual measures to achieve this goal include rest, salt and water restriction, and the use of digoxin, diuretics, along with afterload (hydralazine or captopril) and/or preload (nitroglycerine) reduction. Emotional and physical rest continue to be the cornerstone of treatment of patients with CHF. Adequate preoperative teaching, informed consent, and counseling are important for both the patient and family. Judicious use of sedatives and tranquilizers may occasionally be warranted. The prophylactic use of digoxin in CHF is especially important for the patient with a history of symptomatic supraventricular tachycardia, but is recommended for other high-risk patients, such as those with aortic stenosis who do not tolerate supraventricular tachyarrhythmias well. Non-urgent operations should be postponed if further diagnostic and therapeutic modalities are required to alleviate symptoms of CHF.

3.2. Operative and postoperative considerations

Perioperative monitoring of the systemic pressure, pulmonary arterial pressure and oxygen saturation, and telemetry are recommended for patients with a history of prior CHF or who are at risk of developing cardiac decompensation with major operation and anesthesia [5]. These measures will allow for both more accurate fluid and drug administration, in addition to serving as early indicators of impending cardiac failure.

Treatment of congestive failure in the postoperative period follows the same guidelines as in the preoperative period, except that treatment must usually be initiated rapidly and definitively. Diuretic and nitroglycerine preparations may be administered intravenously, and morphine may be used to treat pulmonary edema. Inotropic agents such as dolbutamine, dopamine and amrinone may be beneficial in increasing cardiac output and decreasing cardiac size. Aggressive treatment of arrhythmias is also indicated (see Section 6). Intra-aortic balloon counterpulsation or percutaneous cardiopulmonary bypass are adjunctive mechanical measures in temporarily supporting cardiac performance in severe cases of cardiac failure [25,26].

4. AORTIC VALVE DISEASE

4.1. Aortic stenosis

The presence of aortic stenosis significantly increases the mortality of non-cardiac surgery. An overall 13–20% mortality has been found in patients with aortic stenosis undergoing non-cardiac operations, as compared to a 1.9% mortality in patients with other valve lesions [10,30].

Isolated valvular aortic stenosis is most often caused by a bicuspid aortic valve in patients under 65 years, and by fibrosis and calcification of a trileaflet valve in patients over 65 years. Classic symptoms of significant aortic stenosis are exertional angina, syncope, and congestive heart failure. Many patients, however, remain asymptomatic with advanced disease. Physical findings include a narrow pulse pressure with a slow upstroke of the carotid pulse. The apical impulse is usually non-displaced, and auscultation usually reveals a crescendo–decrescendo systolic murmur over the aortic area that is transmitted to both carotid arteries. The ECG typically shows left ventricular hypertrophy, while the chest X-ray (CXR) may show mild enlargement of the cardiac silhouette along with poststenotic dilatation of the ascending aorta. Exercise tolerance testing in patients suspected of having aortic stenosis may occasionally result in syncope, injury, or sudden death, and should be avoided. Two-dimensional echocardiography is diagnostic in most cases, and will yield important structural information, while Doppler ultrasonography may be used as a relatively accurate guide to the valve gradient. Patients with mild to moderate symptoms and ECG evidence of left ventricular hypertrophy should be cleared for operation by echocardiography and thallium angiography. Patients with low aortic valve gradients by Doppler ultrasonography, and no reperfusion defects by thallium angiography have relatively low cardiac risk factor. Cardiac catheterization, however, remains the standard method of assessing the significance of the aortic stenosis, and should be performed in all symptomatic patients.

Indications for aortic valve replacement include symptomatic patients with a valve gradient of 50 mmHg or greater, or a calculated valve area less than 0.75 cm^2, and should be performed prior to elective thoracic surgery. Prosthetic valve replacement is the treatment of choice in almost all cases. Patients with coronary artery disease and aortic stenosis should undergo concomitant coronary artery bypass grafting.

4.1.1. Preoperative considerations

All patients with known aortic stenosis, and those who have undergone either aortic valve repair or replacement should receive antibiotic prophylaxis as high-risk patients (See Section 7).

Preoperative monitoring is an essential part of the preoperative care. Patients with aortic stenosis require a properly timed atrial contraction for left ventricular filling. Advanced left ventricular hypertrophy causes diastolic dysfunction manifested by a non-compliant left ventricular wall, and a normal to slightly reduced left ventricular end diastolic volume. In this setting, left atrial contraction may contribute as much as 30% of the left ventricular volume, as compared to about 15% in the normal population. Supraventricular tachyarrhythmias may therefore cause severe hemodynamic deterioration [31], and is best treated with either DC cardioversion or verapamil (see Section 6).

It is important to avoid medications that may cause a decreased preload, such as venodilators, sedatives and diuretics. Such medications could effect a large decrease in left ventricular diastolic filling, with a subsequent decrease in left ventricular pressure, stroke volume, and cardiac output. Nitrates may also decrease aortic diastolic pressure, subsequently reducing coronary perfusion. They should ordinarily not be used in the preoperative period. Preoperative anesthetic premedications not only decrease preload, but are also associated with hypoxemia, which may further decrease myocardial oxygen delivery.

4.1.2. Operative and postoperative considerations

Most patients with aortic stenosis should have a pulmonary artery catheter placed prior to major non-cardiac surgery. Similar guidelines as stated above for the use of preload reducing agents also apply in the postoperative period. Nitrates, diuretics, and beta blockers should be avoided or used with great caution as they may precipitate myocardial ischemia and cardiac failure. Factors that may predispose to tachyarrhythmias should be corrected, and hemodynamically significant arrhythmias should be treated definitively (see Section 6). Antibiotic prophylaxis should be continued for 24–48 hours postoperatively.

4.2. Aortic regurgitation

Aortic regurgitation (AR) may be due to either valvular dysfunction, as in rheumatic valve disease or endocarditis, or by processes that dilate the aortic root, such as occurs with Marfan's syndrome or syphilis. Patients typically remain asymptomatic until late in the course of the disease, and emergence of symptoms may signify advanced ventricular dysfunction. Symptoms include dyspnea on exertion, orthopnea, and paroxysmal nocturnal dyspnea, while angina, and to a greater degree, heart failure, signify severe left ventricular dysfunction, and a subsequent high cardiac risk.

The physical examination in aortic regurgitation usually reveals an exaggerated arterial pulse, with both a rapid upstroke and quick descent. The diastolic pressure is usually below 60 mmHg, while the systolic pressure is typically high (over 160 mmHg). The sine qua non of aortic regurgitation is an early decrescendo diastolic (blowing) murmur, which is heard best at the left sternal border. The murmur is intensified by having the patient lean forward and hold respiration at the end of a complete expiration, or by isometric exercises. The ECG shows left ventricular hypertrophy in most cases. The chest X-ray typically shows cardiomegaly due to left ventricular dilatation, but may also reveal a dilated ascending aorta, a calcified aortic valve, or pulmonary venous distention. Echocardiography is most useful in the long-term follow-up and timing of operative intervention in patients with AR, while cardiac catheterization is usually reserved for patients who are operative candidates.

Many patients with significant aortic regurgitation require peripheral vasodilator therapy for systolic hypertension. Medical therapy is otherwise expectant. Although somewhat controversial, indications for corrective operation prior to major elective non-cardiac operations include all symptomatic patients, and those asymptomatic patients with echocardiographic evidence of (1) an end-systolic dimension of 55 mm or greater [32], or (2) a fractional shortening of 30% or lower [33].

4.2.1. Preoperative considerations

Patients with aortic regurgitation require appropriate antibiotic prophylaxis, which should follow the AHA guidelines for high-risk patients (see Section 7). Bradycardia is generally poorly tolerated, and should be avoided. In addition, such patients are generally quite sensitive to vasodilator therapy, which may lead to large decreases in diastolic coronary perfusion pressure. Patients with significant aortic regurgitation should be continually monitored with telemetry, and special reference made to ECG lead V_5[34] for signs of subendocardial ischemia.

4.2.2. Operative and postoperative considerations

Most patients with significant aortic regurgitation should be managed in the perioperative period with telemetry and continual monitoring of systemic and pulmonary arterial pressures. Similar considerations as given above regarding the use of vasodilator therapy, and avoiding both bradycardia and diastolic hypotension should be given. Occasionally, the stress of the postoperative period may result in large increases in systemic and pulmonary resistance, leading to decreased forward flow and high pulmonary wedge pressures. Such episodes are best treated with a continuous infusion of sodium nitroprusside, usually at a low concentration. Maintaining an adequate end-diastolic pulmonary pressure while avoiding low systemic diastolic pressures are important consideration in avoiding hemodynamic instability.

5. MITRAL VALVE DISEASE

5.1. Mitral stenosis

Mitral stenosis is virtually always due to rheumatic heart disease, classic symptoms of which include exertional dyspnea, fatigue, and nocturnal dyspnea. Hemoptysis, palpitations, and a history of stroke due to embolization of left atrial clot are not uncommon. The physical exam in pure mitral stenosis is typified an irregularly irregular pulse, jugular venous distension, a normal carotid pulse, mild to moderate pulmonary edema, and peripheral edema or ascites in advanced disease. The characteristic auscultatory findings are those of an opening snap in early diastole, followed by a diastolic low-pitched rumble. The ECG characteristically shows left atrial enlargement or atrial fibrillation and a normal left axis. The chest roentgenogram usually shows cardiomegaly due to left atrial enlargement, elevation of the left main stem bronchus, and evidence of pulmonary venous hypertension.

The echocardiogram is diagnostic, and may also be used as a screening device. Typical findings include thickened mitral valve leaflets, shortened chordae tendinea, and commissural fusion. A mitral valve area can often be approximated using the two-dimensional study, and a valve gradient can be estimated using continuous wave Doppler. A valve area less than $1.2\,cm^2$ or a mean valve gradient greater than 10 mmHg may warrant further investigation and postponement of elective operations. Cardiac catheterization is usually reserved for patients whose symptoms are difficult to control while on medical management, or who are being considered for percutaneous or operative mitral valve procedures. In severe disease, catheterization typically shows elevated pulmonary arterial pressures, a gradient across the mitral valve, a depressed cardiac output, and normal to slightly decreased left-sided pressures.

Indications for either percutaneous or operative correction of mitral stenosis prior to non-cardiac operations include New York Heart Association (NYHA) functional class III or IV symptoms, failure of medical management to control symptoms, the presence of a significant rise in the pulmonary vascular resistance, or recurrent episodes of arterial emboli [35].

5.1.1. Preoperative considerations

Antibiotic prophylaxis should follow the AHA guidelines (see Section 7). Patients with mitral stenosis are at risk for a depressed cardiac output, which is best treated by controlling atrial fibrillation or tachycardia, optimizing the fluid status, and discontinuing all nonessential medications. If optimization of medical therapy fails to improve the patient's symptoms, consideration must be given to preoperative balloon valvuloplasty or operative mitral valve repair or replacement.

Pulmonary hypertension (PHTN) is often hard to assess accurately without right heart catheterization, and may be aggravated by lobectomy or pneumonectomy. Historically, patients with symptoms predominantly of fatigue, as opposed to dyspnea or orthopnea, are more likely to manifest PHTN. Physical signs of right ventricular failure and PHTN include a right ventricular heave, ascites, refractory edema, and a pulmonary artery flow murmur. Chest roentgenography may disclose obliteration of the anterior mediastinal window on lateral projection, pulmonary artery distension, or chronic interstitial changes. Pulmonary arterial pressures may rise after lobectomy or more extensive procedures if PHTN is present, and may precipitate severe right ventricular failure and cardiogenic shock.

5.1.2. Operative and postoperative considerations

Anesthetic agents are particularly deleterious in patients with mitral stenosis, both by acting as primary myocardial depressants, and by reducing preload. The tendency to administer intravenous fluids to offset this situation must be balanced with the propensity of aggravating or developing severe PHTN and right ventricular failure with fluid overloading. This is especially important if pulmonary resections greater than a single lobectomy are performed, which may further aggravate PHTN. Patients with symptomatic mitral stenosis are best managed intraoperatively by continuous systemic and pulmonary arterial monitoring, frequent measurement of cardiac output, and definitive treatment of hemodynamically significant arrhythmias.

Acute pulmonary edema is not uncommon in the postoperative period in patients with unrecognized mitral stenosis, and most commonly occurs within 30 minutes after the anesthetic is discontinued [36]. Aggressive treatment, including the use of intravenous furosemide, continuous infusion of inotropic agents such as dopamine, and definitive treatment of hemodynamically significant arrhythmias, should decrease the mortality of this complication. Agents which decrease pulmonary hypertension, such as isoproterenol, may need to be administered if PHTN is present. Emergent percutaneous valvuloplasty or mitral valve replacement may be required, albeit rarely, in patients who do not respond to medical management. These procedures would, however, be expected to carry a high operative morbidity and mortality.

Digoxin should be restarted if it had been given preoperatively. Heparin anticoagulation should be restarted approximately 12 hours following operation, after assurance that adequate hemostasis has been accomplished. Adequate anticoagulation can usually be attained with a continuous infusion of heparin as discussed below.

5.2. Mitral regurgitation

Mitral regurgitation (MR) causes a volume overload to the left ventricle, and may be caused by a variety of lesions such as rheumatic heart disease, coronary artery disease, or myxomatous degeneration of the mitral valve leaflets and supporting structures. Chronic mitral regurgitation, even when severe, is often asymptomatic for many years. Once symptoms do appear, there is usually a gradual progression of their severity, and the onset of rapid symptomatic deterioration usually connotes the onset of atrial fibrillation, ruptured chordae tendineae, or infective endocarditis.

The physical exam may reveal mild to moderate jugular venous distension with pulmonary edema depending on the progression of the underlying disease. The cardiac exam reveals an apical, high-pitched, holosystolic murmur that may radiate to the axilla. In severe mitral regurgitation there may be a third heart sound with or without a diastolic rumble. The ECG usually reveals left atrial and left ventricular enlargement, and may show atrial fibrillation. The chest roentgenogram typically shows cardiomegaly (primarily due to left atrial enlargement), but may also reveal pulmonary venous distension. Two-dimensional echocardiography may reveal important clues as to the etiology of the disease, but is most useful in following left ventricular size [37]. While Doppler ultrasonography and color flow mapping can assess the degree of regurgitation, cardiac catheterization remains the procedure of choice in defining the severity of the regurgitation.

Patients with well compensated mitral regurgitation have a small increased risk with non-cardiac surgery [38]. Operative mitral annuloplasty or valve replacement prior to elective non-cardiac operation is indicated for patients with NYHA functional class III or IV symptoms, and for patients with NYHA functional class I or II symptoms who develop left ventricular dysfunction or dilatation [39].

5.2.1. Preoperative considerations

Patients with mitral regurgitation require appropriate antibiotic prophylaxis as outlined below. In addition, chronic and acute anticoagulation is indicated in patients with rheumatic mitral regurgitation who have concomitant atrial fibrillation, left ventricular dysfunction, or documented left atrial thrombi (see Section 6).

Hemodynamically, patients with mitral regurgitation have decreased forward flow accompanied by a compensatory increase in systemic vascular resistance. The proportion of flow that is directed to the systemic circulation is partially dependent on the systemic vascular resistance. Hence, afterload reducing agents, such as sodium nitroprusside, oral prasozin, hydralazine, or captopril, are often associated with marked hemodynamic improvement [40,41].

Patients with mitral regurgitation depend less on a properly timed atrial contraction for adequate left ventricular filling as compared to patients with mitral stenosis. Controlling the ventricular rate of atrial fibrillation, however, would be expected to improve left ventricular diastolic filling and forward flow (see Section 6).

5.2.2. Operative and postoperative consideration

Most patients with significant mitral regurgitation undergoing major non-cardiac operations should be managed perioperatively with telemetry and continuous systemic and pulmonary arterial pressure monitoring. This will allow for the early detection and treatment of arrhythmias and conduction disturbances, pulmonary hypertension, decreased cardiac output, and increased systemic vascular resistance.

In addition to the beneficial effects of peripheral vasodilatation as discussed above, positive inotropic agents (such as dopamine) are useful in reducing cardiac size, and may decrease the amount of regurgitation due to cardiac enlargement. In severe cases of left ventricular dysfunction, vasodilator therapy, inotropic support, and intra-aortic balloon counterpulsation may be required to support cardiac output.

5.3. Mitral valve prolapse

Mitral valve prolapse (MVP) is a common cause of mitral regurgitation, which especially affects young women. The lesion is most often asymptomatic, and on auscultation is characterized by a mid-systolic click followed by a late systolic murmur. Echocardiography is diagnostic, often revealing posterior bowing of one or both mitral valve leaflets.

Mitral valve prolapse is of little hemodynamic significance, unless the left ventricular ejection fraction falls below 30% [42]. Perioperative considerations are

TABLE 2.5
Recommendation of the American Heart Association–American Dental Association for antibiotic prophylaxis during surgical procedures

	Low risk	High risk[a]
No PCN allergy[b]	PCN V 2.0 g PO one hour prior to procedure, then 1.0 g six hours after initial dose	AMP 1.0–2.0 g + GENT 1.5 mg/kg IM or IV 30 minutes prior to procedure, then PCN V 1.0 g PO six hours after initial dose.
PCN allergy[b, c]	PCN Erythromycin 1.0 g PO one hour prior to procedure, then 500 mg six hours after initial dose	Vancomycin 1.0 g IV over 60 minutes, starting 60 minutes prior to procedure. No repeat dose necessary

[a] Especially those with prosthetic heart valves.
[b] Notation: PCN V, penicillin V; AMP, ampicillin; GENT, gentamicin; PO, orally; IM, intramuscular; IV, intravenous; g, gram; mg, milligram.
[c] May also be selected for those receiving oral PCN as continuous rheumatic fever prophylaxis.

principally those of antibiotic prophylaxis, which should follow the AHA guidelines for high-risk patients (Table 2.5). There is an increased frequency of supraventricular arrhythmias in patients with MVP, and patients with a history of such arrhythmias are best monitored by telemetry in the perioperative period. Any hemodynamically significant arrhythmias should be treated definitively as discussed in Section 6, below.

6. ARRHYTHMIAS AND CONDUCTION DEFECTS

Disturbances of cardiac rate and rhythm can potentially precipitate or aggravate heart failure and interfere with cardiac performance. Ventricular arrhythmias may be entirely benign, although they often signify decreased cardiac performance. Supraventricular tachyarrhythmias decrease diastolic filling of the left ventricle and may lead to a severely reduced cardiac output. Bradyarrhythmias may also decrease cardiac output in the failing or nonconditioned heart, and may precipitate presyncope or syncope.

6.1. Sinus tachycardia

Sinus tachycardia is the most common arrhythmia, and is usually defined as a sinus node generated rate greater than 100 beats per minute. The most frequent causes in the perioperative period are due to increased sympathetic or decrease parasympathetic tone and include pain, hypoxemia, hypovolemia, inotropic medications, infection, cardiac failure, anemia, myocardial ischemia, and shivering. Sinus tachycardia is best treated by correcting the underlying cause, and not by the addition of a beta-blocking drug or a cardiac glycoside.

6.2. Atrial tachycardia

Atrial tachycardia is defined as greater than 6 consecutive premature atrial complexes, and may be related to the patient's overall medical condition [43]. When occurring in paroxysms, it is referred to as paroxysmal atrial tachycardia (PAT), the rate of which is usually 150 to 220 beats per minute. The QRS complex is usually normal, although the P wave may be buried in the T-wave configuration. Atrial tachycardia may be due to cardiac causes, such as rheumatic heart disease, Wolff–Parkinson–White (WPW) syndrome, and myocardial infarction, or to non-cardiac causes such as excessive caffeine or nicotine intake, ischemia, or anxiety. PAT with AV block is frequently a complication of digoxin toxicity. Multifocal atrial tachycardia (MAT), in which there is a variation in both the P-wave contour and the rate of atrial depolarization, is often seen in patients with severe chronic obstructive pulmonary disease.

Long-term treatment for PAT or MAT is usually aimed at correcting the underlying cause, but many patients may require digoxin, beta-blocking agents, or calcium-channel blockers to decrease or eliminate further paroxysms. PAT with AV block requires withdrawing digoxin and potassium-wasting diuretics, continuous ECG monitoring, and careful administration of potassium and/or beta blockers as indicated.

6.3. Atrial flutter and fibrillation

6.3.1. Atrial flutter

Atrial flutter is caused by an ectopic atrial pacemaker that depolarizes at a rate faster than 220 beats per minute, and usually at a rate of approximately 300 beats per minute. Since the AV node cannot conduct impulses to the ventricles with such rapidity, every second to every fifth impulse produces ventricular depolarization, yielding a 2:1 to 5:1 block. Atrial flutter is characterized by an undulating or saw-toothed baseline with a regular ventricular response. Atrial flutter is usually an unstable rhythm, and is best treated with aggressive pharmacological therapy or DC cardioversion using low energy levels (25–50 W s).

6.3.2. Atrial fibrillation

Atrial fibrillation occurs when atrial depolarization exceeds 400 beats per minute, creating an irregular, chaotic baseline, and when untreated often leads to a variable and rapid ventricular response (140 to 180 beats per minute). Among the many organic causes of atrial fibrillation are significant mitral valve disease (regurgitation or stenosis), coronary artery disease, pericarditis, and atrial septal defect. Non-organic causes are related to thyrotoxicosis, severe stress, fatigue, and excessive cigarette, caffeine, and alcohol consumption.

The hemodynamic significance of atrial fibrillation depends on the rapidity of the ventricular response, the underlying cardiac abnormality, and the significance of atrial systole on left ventricular function. Surgical mortality is increased to 13 to 18% in patients with acute atrial fibrillation [10,44], especially if the ventricular response is rapid or poorly controlled. In contrast, patients with chronic atrial fibrillation and a controlled ventricular response do not appear to suffer from increased operative morbidity or mortality [45].

Treatment of hemodynamically unstable atrial fibrillation consists of DC cardioversion to normal sinus rhythm. The most efficacious starting dose appears to be 200 W s [46]. Relative contraindications to DC cardioversion include digoxin toxicity (which may lead to refractory ventricular tachycardia and fibrillation), underlying heart block, and a left atrial size greater than 50 mm by echocardiography. Digoxin serum levels should be monitored, and the digoxin discontinued 24 hours prior to cardioversion. A class I antiarrhythmic agent, such as quinidine or procainamide, should be present in therapeutic plasma concentrations at the time of cardioversion. As a further precautionary guide against traumatic hemorrhage at the time of cardioversion, coumadin should be withdrawn 2 to 3 days prior to cardioversion, and replaced with a continuous heparin infusion. Heparin can be stopped 4 to 6 hours prior to cardioversion, and restarted immediately following cardioversion.

Digoxin is the treatment of choice for controlling the ventricular response to atrial fibrillation, provided that urgent DC cardioversion is not indicated. The goal of digitalization is a ventricular response of 90 to 100 beats per minute. Occasionally a beta-blocking agent or verapamil may be required for additional rate control, but the negative inotropic and hypotensive side effects of these medications preclude their routine or injudicious use. Atrial fibrillation with a ventricular response below 90 beats per minute may require no therapy. Digoxin toxic rhythms, such as PAT with block, junctional escape beats, sick sinus (brady–tachy) syndrome, and ventricular rates below 70 beats per minute, should be treated with careful withdrawal of the medication.

6.4. Premature ventricular complex

Premature ventricular complexes (PVC) arise from an ectopic ventricular focus that interrupts normal sinus rhythm, and are characteristically followed by a compensatory pause. The QRS morphology of a PVC is typically wide, since depolarization and repolarization occur along abnormal pathways. Bigeminy occurs if every other ventricular complex is premature, and trigeminy occurs if every third complex is premature. Multifocal PVCs originate from multiple ventricular sites and are variant in morphology, as opposed to unifocal PVCs which are of identical morphology.

Patients with greater than 10 PVCs per minute, PVCs that occur on or close to the apex of the T wave (R-on-T phenomenon), multifocal PVCs, and those occurring in pairs or triplets, have increased risk for perioperative cardiac complications [30]. These so-called malignant PVCs carry a 14% rate of operative mortality, especially when associated with coronary artery disease [47]. Arrhythmias are associated with the same postoperative complications typically seen with ischemic and congestive heart disease, and therefore serve as sensitive markers of more serious underlying coronary artery disease and ventricular dysfunction [48,49]. Unifocal PVCs do occur in otherwise healthy patients with no evidence of heart disease [50], and in this setting would not be expected to carry an additional risk to operation.

When malignant PVCs are associated with coronary artery disease, aggressive management is indicated [48]. Lidocaine is the preferred method of initial management. Central nervous system side effects, such as lightheadedness, lethargy, paresthesia, and seizures may occur, and are more common in the elderly, those with liver dysfunction, reduced cardiac output, or when given with a general anesthetic. Procainamide is a suitable alternative in patients who suffer from the CNS side effects of lidocaine. Hypotension, a not uncommon side effect of procainamide, may require adjustment of the dose.

Patients with refractory arrhythmias due to either severe myocardial dysfunction or myocardial infarctions have a high rate of operative morbidity and mortality [10]. Preoperatively, such patients should be considered for electrophysiologic (EP) studies. Treatment strategies include optimization of medical management, cryo- or operative ablation of suspected subendocardial tissue [51], and/or implantation of an automatic internal cardiac defibrillator [52,53].

6.5. Conduction disturbances

Prophylactic pacemakers are recommended for all preoperative patients with second- and third-degree heart block, regardless of whether the block is in the AV node or the trifascicular conduction system [54]. Patients with symptoms of presyncope or syncope and who are at risk of developing trifascicular block should also have a transvenous pacemaker implanted prior to operation. Asymptomatic patients, however, do not require a pacemaker, but should be under close observation with adequate monitoring in the perioperative period.

6.6. Management of patients with pacemakers

Many patients with permanently implanted pacemakers undergo major thoracic operations. Important information to be known prior to the operation include the type and severity of the underlying rhythm or conduction defect, and the manufacturer, type, age, location, and the pacing mode of the pacemaker. Evaluation of pacing threshold energy requirements and evaluation of the sensing circuit should be obtained prior to operation. If these studies indicate that the pulse generator is nearing end-of-life, inappropriately sensing, or if the resistance in the pacing leads is excessively high, the pulse generator and/or the pacing leads should be changed prior to operation.

There is a small but potentially serious risk of pacemaker shutdown at the time of operation secondary to electrocauterization [55]. This risk can probably be reduced by ensuring that the electrocautery unit is properly grounded, and by avoiding electrocauterization in the immediate vicinity of the pulse generator. It is essential to have a magnet in the operating room immediately available to convert a demand pacemaker to a fixed-rate mode. A programmable pacer is most advantageous in this regard, as it will allow for the programming of an increased ventricular response when necessary. Patients who are pacemaker dependent or who have an underlying hemodynamically unstable arrhythmia or conduction defect should be given serious consideration for the preoperative placement of temporary pacing wires or a pulmonary artery catheter equipped with a pacing port and connected to an external pacemaker.

7. ANTIBIOTIC PROPHYLAXIS

Judicious use of prophylactic antibiotics is imperative for the prevention of valvular or prosthetic endocarditis in patients at risk. Occasional failures do occur, even when the infecting organism is susceptible to the antibiotics used [56], however adherence to chemoprophylactic guidelines should yield excellent overall results [57]. The American Heart Association (AHA) presented their initial recommendation for chemoprophylaxis in 1977 [58], and made revisions in 1985 [59] (see Table 2.5). Compliance to the initial AHA guidelines had been noted to be low [60], especially in conditions such as mitral valve prolapse where the risks are not certain. The revised AHA recommendations should improve the compliance rate, and should be followed closely by medical practitioners [61]. For the present time, chemoprophylactic methods that differ from those of the AHA offer no clear advantages, and may in fact have some adverse effects on patients receiving cardiac agents or anticoagulants [62].

In a survey of London medical practitioners [63], chemo-prophylactic regimens and dosing schedules being used were found to differ markedly from published guidelines. In the United Kingdom and Europe simple oral chemoprophylaxis has also been recommended by both the BSAC Endocarditis Working Party and the European Society of Cardiology [64]. These recommendations consist of a single 3-gram oral dose of amoxycillin one hour before the procedure, or two doses of erythromycin for persons allergic to penicillin. Antibiotic prophylaxis in European countries should in general follow the recommendations of the BSAC Endocarditis Working Party or the European Society of Cardiology for similar reasons as stated above.

8. MANAGEMENT OF CARDIAC MEDICATION

8.1. Warfarin and heparin anticoagulation

In the absence of significant contraindications, chronic warfarin anticoagulation is indicated in all patients with mechanical prostheses in either the aortic or mitral position, regardless of the cardiac rhythm or prosthetic model used. Chronic anticoagulation is also indicated in patients with a preoperative history of embolism in association with cardiac disease, patients with known left atrial thrombi, and unoperated patients with rheumatic mitral valvular disease who have concomitant atrial fibrillation, depressed ventricular function, or a low cardiac output[65]. Occasionally, patients will receive a short course of warfarin therapy following either native valve repair or implantation of a bioprosthetic valve.

Coumarin-type anticoagulants can usually be safely discontinued 3 days prior to operation[66], but the prothrombin time (PT) should be monitored daily. When the PT drops below 1.5 times the control value, a continuous heparin infusion is started. The heparin should be infused through a dedicated line, with no interruptions due to the infusion of other medications. Thereafter the activated partial thromboplastin time (APTT) or the activated clotting time (ACT) is monitored, initially every 6 hours, and then every 12 hours once these laboratory values have stabilized. The heparin infusion is adjusted to an APTT of 1.8 to 2.5 times the laboratory control, and is discontinued 8 hours prior to operation. Patients not receiving anticoagulants, but who have indications for anticoagulation as listed above, should be similarly treated.

Heparin should be restarted approximately 24 hours postoperatively, after assurance that adequate hemostasis has been accomplished. Heparin anticoagulation is managed as in the preoperative period, and adjusted according to the APTT or the ACT. Bolus heparin therapy is unnecessary unless there is a specific indication (such as a central or peripheral embolus), while subcutaneous heparinization is not recommended for patients requiring long-term anticoagulation. In the absence of specific contraindications, coumadin may be restarted on the night of operation, and anticoagulation be monitored by the prothrombin time. Most patients will require the same maintenance dose of coumadin as was necessary prior to operation.

8.2. Aspirin

Aspirin permanently alters the aggregation of affected platelets, and therefore the half-life of its effect depends on the regeneration of new platelets by the bone marrow. Commonly, six to ten days are required before reversal of abnormal bleeding times can take place. Consideration should be given to delaying all non-urgent operations for this period of time after aspirin or aspirin-containing compounds are withdrawn. In urgent or emergent situations, a platelet transfusion may be used if abnormal bleeding occurs.

8.3. Digoxin

It is often useful to determine the plasma concentration of digoxin in patients receiving the medication, and to delay operation if the digoxin level is excessively high or toxic. Patients with therapeutic plasma concentrations who are receiving digoxin for atrial fibrillation or arrhythmia suppression should receive their usual dose on the morning of operation. Otherwise, it is often acceptable to omit the drug on the morning of operation. Adequate monitoring of cardiac function will give sufficient warning for the institution or reinstitution of digoxin therapy. Postoperatively, patients may resume their usual digoxin dose and schedule as indicated.

8.4. Antiarrhythmic agents

The risk of preoperative arrhythmias relates to the risk of any underlying cardiac abnormalities, as discussed above. The relationship of anesthetic agents to antiarrhythmic agents is complex, but in general, toxic levels of most antiarrhythmic agents are more rapidly reached with the half-life lengthening effects of many of the anesthetic agents. The anesthetic agent may also mask the toxic side effects of the antiarrhythmic agent (e.g., as in the neurologic side effects of lidocaine). For these reasons, antiarrhythmic prophylaxis is generally not recommended in either the pre- or intra-operative period. In patients being treated chronically with an antiarrhythmic agent, adequate preoperative blood levels (if available), or achievement of a therapeutic goal should be attained prior to operation. In the vast majority of cases, the patient's usual antiarrhythmic medication is given in the morning of operation, and intra- or post-operative treatment with intravenous antiarrhythmic agents is reserved for malignant or hemodynamically unstable arrhythmias.

8.5. Calcium-channel and beta-blocking agents

Continuing beta-blocking agents in patients who were receiving beta blockers preoperatively has been shown effective in reducing the incidence of clinically important arrhythmias occurring after both non-cardiac [67] and cardiac [68] operations. Propranolol should be continued up to the morning of operation in those patients who were started on the drug for control of hypertension or angina pectoris [69,70]. This will minimize the risk of propranolol rebound in patients who had been on the drug preoperatively. The preoperative dose of the drug should be instituted as soon as feasible postoperatively.

Similarly, patients receiving calcium channel antagonists should continue on their medication up to the morning of operation. These may be resumed as needed postoperatively in the same dose and schedule.

REFERENCES

1 Greenfield LJ (ed.). Surgery in the Aged. Philadelphia, PA, WB Saunders 1975.
2 Weisfeldt ML. Aging of the cardiovascular system. N Engl J Med 1980; 303: 1172–1174.
3 Gerstenblith G, Lakatta EG, Weisfeldt ML. Age changes in myocardial function and exercise response. Prog Cardiovasc Dis 1976; 19: 1–18.

4 Wells PH, Kaplan JA. Optimal management of patients with ischemic heart disease for noncardiac surgery by complementary anesthesiologist and cardiologist interaction. Am Heart J 1981; 102: 1029–1037.
5 Rao LT, Jacobs KH, El-Etr AA. Reinfarction following anesthesia in patients with myocardial infarction. Anesthesiology 1983; 59: 499–505.
6 Goldman L, Caldera DL, Southwick FS, et al. Cardiac risk factors and complications in noncardiac surgery. Medicine 1978; 57: 357–370.
7 Goldman L. Cardiac risks and complications of noncardiac surgery. Ann Intern Med 1983; 98: 504–513.
8 Driscoll AC, Hobika JH, Etsten BE, Proger S. Clinically unrecognized myocardial infarction following surgery. N Engl J Med 1961; 264: 633–639.
9 Tarhan S, Moffitt EA, Taylor WF, Giuliani ER. Myocardial infarction after general anesthesia. JAMA 1972; 220: 1451–1454.
10 Goldman L, Caldera DL, Nussbaum SR, et al. Multifactorial index of cardiac risk in noncardiac surgical procedures. N Engl J Med 1977; 297: 845–850.
11 Plumlee JE, Boettner, RB. Myocardial infarction during and following anesthesia and operation. South Med J 1972; 65: 886–889.
12 Hertzer NR, Young JR, Kramer JR, et al. Routine coronary angiography prior to elective aortic reconstruction: results of selective myocardial revascularization in patients with peripheral vascular disease. Arch Surg 1979; 114: 1336–1344.
13 Tomatis LA, Fierens EE, Verbrugge GP. Evaluation of surgical risk in peripheral vascular disease by coronary arteriography. Surgery 1972; 71: 429–435.
14 Homma S, Callahan RJ, Ameer B, et al. Usefulness of oral dipyridamole suspension for stress thallium imaging without exercise in the detection of coronary artery disease. Am J Cardiol 1986; 57: 503–508.
15 Leppo J, Plaja J, Gionet M, Tumolo J, Paraskos JA, Cutler BS. Non-invasive evaluation of cardiac risk before elective vascular surgery. J Am Coll Cardiol 1987; 9: 269–276.
16 Goldman L. Assessment of the patient with known or suspected ischaemic heart disease for non-cardiac surgery. Br J Anaesth 1988; 61: 38–43.
17 Jamieson WR, Janusz MT, Miyagishima RT, et al. Influence of ischemic heart disease on early and late mortality after surgery for peripheral occlusive vascular disease. Circulation 1982; 66: 191–197.
18 McPhail N, Calvin JE, Shariatmadar A, Barber GG, Scobie TK. The use of preoperative exercise testing to predict cardiac complications after arterial reconstruction. J Vasc Surg 1988; 7: 60–68.
19 Gage AA, Bhayana JN, Balu V, et al. Assessment of cardiac risk in surgical patients. Arch Surg 1977; 112: 1488–1492.
20 Cooperman M, Pflug B, Martin E, et al. Cardiovascular risk factors in patients with peripheral vascular disease. Surgery 1978; 84: 505–509.
21 Steen PA, Tinker JH, Tarhan S. Myocardial reinfarction after anesthesia and surgery. JAMA 1978; 239: 2566–2570.
22 Carliner NH, Fisher ML, Plotnick GE, et al. Routine preoperative exercise testing in patients undergoing major noncardiac surgery. Am J Cardiol 1985; 56: 51–58.
23 Gerson MC, Hurst JM, Hertzberg VS, et al. Cardiac prognosis in noncardiac geriatric surgery. Ann Intern Med 1985; 103: 832–837.
24 Miller RR, Olson GH, Amsterdam EA, et al. Propranolol withdrawal rebound phenomenon. N Engl J Med 1975; 293: 416–420.
25 Phillips SJ. Percutaneous cardiopulmonary bypass and innovations in clinical counterpulsation. Crit Care Clin 1986; 2: 297–318.
26 Vogel RA, Tommaso CL, Gundry SR. Initial experience with coronary angioplasty and aortic valvuloplasty using elective semipercutaneous cardiopulmonary support. Am J Cardiol 1988; 62: 811–813.
27 Topkins MU, Artusio JF. Myocardial infarction and surgery: A five-year study. Anesth Analg 1964; 43: 716–720.

28 Miller R, Silvay G, Lumb PD. Anesthesia, surgery and myocardial infarction: A review. Anesth Rev 1979; 6: 14–20.
29 Mahar LJ, Steen PA, Tinker JA, Vlietstra RE, Smith HC, Pluth JR. Perioperative myocardial infarction in patients with coronary artery disease with and without aorta-coronary bypass grafts. J Thorac Cardiovasc Surg 1978; 76: 533–537.
30 Skinner JF, Pierce ML. Surgical risk in the cardiac patient. J Chron Dis 1964; 17: 57–72.
31 Arani DT, Carleton RA. The deleterious role of tachycardia in mitral stenosis. Circulation 1967; 36: 511–516.
32 Henry WL, Bonow RO, Borer JS, et al. Observations on the optimal time for operative intervention for aortic regurgitation. I. Evaluation of the results of aortic valve replacement in symptomatic patients. Circulation 1980; 61: 471–483.
33 Cunha CLP, Giuliani ER, Fuster V, et al. Preoperative M-mode echocardiography as a predictor of surgical results in chronic aortic regurgitation. J Thorac Cardiovasc Surg 1980; 79: 256–265.
34 London MJ, Hollenberg M, Wong MG, et al. Intraoperative myocardial ischemia: Localization by continuous 12-lead electrocardiography. Anesthesiology 1988; 69: 232–241.
35 Smith WM, Neutze JM, Barratt-Boyes BG, Lower JB. Open mitral valvotomy: Effect of preoperative factors on result. J Thorac Cardiovasc Surg 1981; 82: 738.
36 Cooperman LH, Price HL. Pulmonary edema in the operative and postoperative period: A review of 40 cases. Ann Surg 1970; 172: 883–891.
37 Zile MR, Gaasch WH, Carroll JD, et al. Chronic mitral regurgitation: Predictive value of preoperative echocardiographic indexes of left ventricular function and wall stress. J Am Coll Cardiol 1984; 3: 235.
38 Schlant RC, Nutter DO. Heart failure in valvular heart disease. Medicine 1971; 50: 421–451.
39 Borow KM, Green LH, Mann T, et al. End-systolic volume as a predictor of postoperative left ventricular performance in volume overload from valvular regurgitation. Am J Med 1980; 68: 655.
40 Miller RR, Awan NA, Maxwell DS, et al. Sustained reduction of cardiac impedance and preload in congestive heart failure with the antihypertensive vasodilator prasozin. N Engl J Med 1977; 297: 303–307.
41 Goodman DJ, Rossen RM, Holloway EL, et al. Effect of nitroprusside on left ventricular dynamics in mitral regurgitation. Circulation 1974; 50: 1025–1032.
42 Lubin MF, Walker HK, Smith III RB. Medical Management of the Surgical Patient, 2nd Ed. London, Butterworths 1988.
43 Rogers WR, Wroblewski F, Ladveps G. Supraventricular tachycardia complicating surgical procedures. Circulation 1952; 7: 192–196.
44 Sapala JA, Ponka JL, Duvernoy WFC. Operative and nonoperative risks in the cardiac patient. J Am Geriatr Soc 1975; 23: 529–534.
45 Finkbeiner JA, Wroblewski F, LaDue JS. The effect of chronic auricular fibrillation on the operative risk. Am J Med Sci 1954; 227: 535–543.
46 DeSilva RA, Graboys TB, Podrid PJ, Lown B. Cardioversion and defibrillation. Am Heart J 1980; 100: 881–895.
47 Lown B, Graboys TB. Management of patients with malignant ventricular arrhythmias. Am J Cardiol 1977; 39: 910–918.
48 Schulze RA Jr, Roulearu J, Rigo P, Bowers S, Strauss HW, Pitt B. Ventricular arrhytthmias in the late hospital phase of acute myocardial infarction: Relation to left ventricular function detected by gated cardiac blood pool scanning. Circulation 1975; 52: 1006–1011.
49 Schulze RA Jr, Strauss HW, Pitt B. Sudden death in the year following myocardial infarction: Relation to ventricular premature contractions in the late hospital phase and left ventricular ejection fraction. Am J Med 1977; 62: 192–199.
50 Fisher FD, Tyroler HA. Relationship between ventricular premature contractions on routine electrocardiography and subsequent death from coronary heart disease. Circulation 1973; 47: 712–719.

51 Kron IL, Lerman B, DiMarco JP. Surgical management of sustained ventricular arrhythmias presenting within eight weeks of acute myocardial infarction. Ann Thorac Surg 1986; 42: 13–16.
52 Nathan AW, Bexton RS, Spurrell RA, Camm AJ. Internal transvenous low energy cardioversion for the treatment of cardiac arrhythmias. Br Heart J 1984; 52: 377–384.
53 Reid PR, Mirowski M, Mower MM, et al. Clinical evaluation of the internal automatic cardioverter–defibrillator in survivors of sudden cardiac death. Am J Cardiol 1983; 51: 1608–1613.
54 Ewy GA. Preoperative evaluation of patients with electrocardiographic conduction defects. Contemp Anesth Pract 1980; 2: 121–136.
55 Lerner SM. Suppression of a demand pacemaker by transurethral electrocautery. Anesth Analg 1973; 52: 703–706.
56 Durack DT, Kaplan EL, Bisno AL. Apparent failures of endocarditis prophylaxis. Analysis of 52 cases submitted to a national registry. JAMA 1983; 250: 2318–2322.
57 Santinga JT, Kirsh M, Fekety R. Factors affecting survival in prosthetic valve endocarditis. Chest 1984; 85: 471–475.
58 Ian EL, Anthony BF, Bisno A, et al. Prevention of bacterial endocarditis. Circulation 1977; 56: 139a–143a.
59 Kaye D. Prophylaxis for infective endocarditis: An update. Ann Intern Med 1986; 104: 419–423.
60 Retchin SM, Fletcher RH, Buescher PC, Waugh RA, Battaglini SW. The application of official policy. Prophylaxis recommendations for patients with mitral valve prolapse. Med Care 1985; 23: 1156–1162.
61 Kaplan EL, Anthony BF, Bisno A, et al. Prevention of bacterial endocarditis. Circulation 1977; 56: 139a–143a.
62 Angaran DM, Dias VC, Arom DV, Northrup WF, et al. The comparative influence of prophylactic antibiotics on the prothrombin response to warfarin in the postoperative prosthetic cardiac valve patient. Cefamandole, cefazolin, vancomycin. Ann Surg 1987; 206: 155–161.
63 Gould IM. Chemoprophylaxis for bacterial endocarditis – a survey of current practice in London. J Antimicrob Chemother 1984; 14: 379–394.
64 Shanson DC. Antibiotic prophylaxis of infective endocarditis in the United Kingdom and Europe. J Antimicrob Chemother 1987; 20 (Suppl A): 119–142.
65 Bodnar AG, Hutter AM Jr. Anticoagulation in valvular heart disease preoperatively and postoperatively. Cardiovasc Clin 1984; 14: 247–264.
66 Tinker JA, Tarhan S. Discontinuing anticoagulant therapy in surgical patients with cardiac valve prostheses. JAMA 1978; 239: 738–739.
67 Ponten J, Biber B, Henriksson BA, et al. Beta-receptor blockade and neurolept anesthesia. Withdrawal vs. continuation of long-term therapy in gall-bladder and carotid artery surgery. Acta Anaesthesiol Scand 1982; 26: 576–588.
68 Matangi MF, Neutze JM, Graham KJ, et al. Arrhythmia prophylaxis after aorta-coronary bypass. The effect of minidose propranolol. J Thorac Cardiovasc Surg 1985; 89: 439–443.
69 Nattel S, Rangno RE, Van Loon G. Mechanism of propranolol withdrawal phenomena. Circulation 1979; 59: 1158–1164.
70 Kopriva CJ, Broun ACD, Pappas G. Hemodynamics during general anesthesia in patients receiving propranolol. Anesthesiology 1978; 48: 28–33.

Current Topics in General Thoracic Surgery: An International Series, Vol. 2
Perioperative Care, edited by R.M. Peters and J. Toledo
Elsevier Science Publishers B.V.

Chapter 3

Simultaneous cardiac and thoracic surgery

Claude Deschamps, Victor F. Trastek and Peter C. Pairolero

1. INTRODUCTION

Patients with simultaneous surgical pathology of the heart and lungs are a therapeutic challenge to the thoracic surgeon. Generally, these patients present with surgically correctable cardiac disease and are found to have a pulmonary process, usually an asymptomatic nodule, for which operative management is also appropriate. Less frequently, these patients present with pulmonary disease and are found to have cardiac disease which, if untreated, would significantly increase the risk of pulmonary surgery. The cardiac and pulmonary lesions could be treated in one combined procedure or alternatively with two procedures in a staged fashion, with the sequence based on clinical priority.

Traditionally, pulmonary resection has not been simultaneously performed with cardiac surgical procedures that require extracorporeal circulation, presumably because of potential intrapulmonary bleeding from altered coagulation mechanisms and of limited pulmonary exposure gained through a median sternotomy approach. Of lesser importance have been concerns of disseminated or local infection following resection of inflammatory nodules, perhaps related to altered immunity associated with cardiopulmonary bypass [1]. Consequently, many thoracic surgeons have advocated staged surgical procedures, usually first correcting the cardiac pathology, as this represents the most immediate threat to the patient. A simultaneous approach to both problems, however, is theoretically advantageous in that all areas of disease are definitively managed without delay and the patient is spared the significant morbidity of a second thoracotomy. Ideally, the decision to perform simultaneous cardiac and pulmonary procedures should be based on a favorable benefit-to-risk ratio. Unfortunately, review of the literature reveals only a few small series of patients treated with a combined approach [2–6], and thus firm conclusions are difficult to obtain.

TABLE 3.1
Type of cardiac surgical procedures in 43 patients undergoing simultaneous cardiac and pulmonary surgery

Procedure	No. of patients
Coronary	26
Aortic valve replacement	4
Mitral valve replacement	4
Mitral valve repair	2
CABG and left ventricular aneurysm repair	1
Mitral valve repair, CABG, and tricuspid annuloplasty	1
Aortic valve and mitral valve replacement	1
Pulmonary atresia and ventricular septal defect repair	1
Atrial septal defect closure	1
Resection of right ventricular tumor	1
Resection of right atrial tumor	1
	+ —
Total	43

2. MAYO CLINIC EXPERIENCE

We have recently reviewed our experience with patients undergoing simultaneous cardiac and pulmonary surgery[6]. Excluded were patients who had: (1) concomitant pulmonary resections required for iatrogenic intraoperative pulmonary complications, (2) pulmonary resections for congenital sequestration at the time of correction of anomalous pulmonary drainage, and (3) pulmonary procedures performed with extracorporeal circulation without a concomitant cardiac procedure.

There were 43 patients (32 male and 11 female). Ages ranged from 12 to 76 years with a mean age of 56.4 years. Over 90% of patients presented with cardiac symptoms, most of which were predominantly related to either coronary artery or valvular heart disease. The pulmonary lesion appeared as a solitary pulmonary nodule in approximately 75% of patients, infiltrate in 10%, multiple nodules in 7%, and other in 10%. Only 7% of patients had signs or symptoms related to their pulmonary lesion. At the time of operation, the pulmonary diagnosis had been established in 5% of patients, was highly suspected in 7%, and was unknown in 88%. All patients required extracorporeal circulation; none had emergency operations.

Coronary artery bypass grafting and valve replacement were the cardiac procedures most commonly performed (Table 3.1). Concomitant pulmonary procedures were performed via median sternotomy in all patients, and included single wedge resection in 32 patients, lobectomy in 7, multiple wedge resections in 3, and pneumonectomy in 1. Standard pulmonary techniques were employed for all resections, the mechanical stapler being utilized for all bronchial closures and for approximately 75% of the wedge excisions. Most resections were performed either before or after cardiopulmonary bypass, during which time anticoagulation with heparin either had not been instituted or had been reversed with protamine

TABLE 3.2
Pulmonary pathology in 43 patients undergoing simultaneous cardiac and pulmonary surgery

Diagnosis	Patients	
	No.	%
Benign	31	72.1
Granuloma	18	41.9
Chronic inflammation	4	9.3
Hamartoma	4	9.3
Pulmonary infarct	3	7.0
Bullae	2	4.6
Malignant	12	27.9
Bronchogenic carcinoma	10	23.3
Metastatic carcinoma	2	4.6
	+ —	+ —
Total	43	100.0

sulfate. Approximately 70% of patients had benign pulmonary disease, 25% had primary lung cancer, and 5% had metastasis from a distant site (Table 3.2). Nearly 25% of patients with undiagnosed pulmonary lesions proved to have malignancy. Pulmonary resection was appropriate for the pathologic condition in 90% of patients in that wedge resections were performed for benign lesions or pulmonary metastases and lobectomies or pneumonectomies for lung cancer.

2.1. Results

There were two 30-day deaths (operative mortality, 4.6%), only one related to the pulmonary resection. Cause of death was acute respiratory insufficiency related to intraparenchymal pulmonary hemorrhage after multiple wedge resections while still on cardiopulmonary bypass in one patient, and acute aorto-coronary graft occlusion and subsequent myocardial infarction in the other. There were also two postoperative complications related to the pulmonary procedure. One patient required re-exploration for pleural space bleeding that originated from the apical chest wall where adhesions had been divided, and a second required ventilatory support for 10 days following pneumonectomy. Except for the latter patient, all the remaining patients were extubated within 36 hours of operation. There were no instances of prolonged pulmonary air leak, excessive chest tube drainage, pleural space infection, wound infection, or other pleural space complications. Follow-up was complete in all patients and averaged 3.8 years, ranging from 1.5 months to 14.8 years. There were no late postoperative sequellae from the pulmonary resections.

2.2. Pulmonary resections for lung cancer

Ten patients underwent pulmonary resection for primary lung cancer (T1N0M0 in 8 patients, T2N1M0 in 2). At the time of our report, six of these patients were still alive, and five had no evidence of disease at postoperative intervals ranging from 3 months to 2.5 years. Three other patients died of metastatic carcinoma from 10 to 30 months postoperatively. Interestingly, two of these patients, one of whom was classified as T1N0M0, had undergone wedge resection as the only surgical treatment for their malignant lesion. The tenth patient died of a late myocardial infarct and at postmortem examination there was no evidence of lung cancer.

2.3. Spared second thoracotomy

Acknowledging the uncertainties of such an analysis, we determined the number of patients who were spared a second staged operation by this combined approach. Two-thirds of our patients had lung lesions that fulfilled currently acceptable criteria for early thoracotomy. Most commonly, such a lesion was a noncalcified indeterminant nodule that was either not present on earlier chest roentgenograms or was increasing in size. Over 40% of this subgroup were found to have malignant tumor. Thus, the combined approach potentially spared a second thoracotomy in all of these patients or two-thirds of our total group. The remaining one-third of patients had pulmonary lesions for which thoracotomy could have been either optional or delayed if the cardiac operation had not been necessary.

3. INDICATIONS

The Mayo Clinic Study suggests that a variety of pulmonary conditions are safely amenable to appropriate resection at the time of elective cardiac surgery that require extracorporeal circulation. In general, intraoperative and postoperative pulmonary complications encountered are few and minor and do not differ significantly from those encountered in isolated routine pulmonary procedures performed through a posterolateral thoracotomy. Moreover, most pulmonary complications are independent of the pulmonary pathology, the location of the lesion, or the use of the mechanical stapler. Local or disseminated infection occurring after resection of inflammatory lung disease is also unlikely, which suggests a less ominous role for altered immunity than has been previously postulated [1]. Exposure for pulmonary resections is usually not difficult, and this fact has been substantiated by others [5,7–10], some of whom advocate the median sternotomy approach for most elective pulmonary operations [8]. Along these same lines, a median sternotomy is associated with less respiratory compromise than is a lateral thoracotomy [5]. Therefore, concomitant procedures would seem to be particularly advantageous in patients with poor pulmonary function.

These observations, however, are based on experience with a very select group of patients. Other patients with combined pathology at our institution have been managed with staged operations, and in these patients the decision to stage is usually based on technical considerations recognized either preoperatively by roentgenographic evaluation such as chest X-ray, computed tomography, and magnetic resonance imaging, or intraoperatively during the cardiac procedure. Reasons for a staged procedure may include those patients with tumors which have parietal fixation or patients with pleural adhesions from a previous thoracotomy. Patients in whom significant postoperative cardiac or pulmonary complications might be anticipated are also probably best managed with staged procedures. Less stringent criteria appear warranted in those patients whose lesion is completely treatable with a simple wedge resection.

Who are candidates for pulmonary resection at the time of cardiac surgery? Assuming that the patient is otherwise in good health and could tolerate any pulmonary resection, we believe that combined procedures, in general, should be reserved for those patients who have limited pulmonary disease which can be excised with a lobectomy or less. Pneumonectomy, radical mediastinal lymphadenectomy and chest wall resections should be avoided. Potential candidates would include patients with benign solitary pulmonary nodules, pulmonary infiltrates limited to a segment or lobe, and clinical stage-I lung cancer (T1 or T2N0M0). If a lung cancer is known or suspected, preoperative computed tomography to evaluate the mediastinum is advised.

What are the safe limits of pulmonary resection in patients who are undergoing simultaneous cardiac and thoracic surgery? In general, the safe limits are defined by three factors: the anatomy of the pulmonary lesion, the cardiopulmonary reserve of the patient, and the experience of the surgeon. Given the large number of permutations and combinations that these factors can pose, specific limits on the extent of pulmonary resection are difficult to define. We would emphasize that the management of these patients must be individualized. There is no question that there are limits to the extent of pulmonary resection that are advisable in any given patient. The fact that limits exist, however, should not deter the use of concomitant procedures in selected situations.

4. TECHNIQUE

Intraoperatively, the anesthetic management of patients undergoing simultaneous cardiac and pulmonary operation does not need to vary significantly from that in routine cardiac and pulmonary cases. Specifically, a double-lumen endotracheal tube is not necessary if a surgeon performs most isolated pulmonary resections without one.

The pulmonary lesion should be visualized immediately after sternotomy. A simple wedge resection utilizing the stapling device can be safely performed either before or after extracorporeal circulation. If knowledge of the pulmonary pathology will alter the conduct of the cardiac surgical procedure, wedge biopsy should be obtained before institution of cardiopulmonary bypass; otherwise, we prefer to biopsy the lung lesion after cessation of bypass when hemodynamics and coagulation are acceptable. The single operative death in our series resulted from intraparenchymal pulmonary hemorrhage which occurred after multiple wedge resections during cardiopulmonary bypass. Although this was clearly a unique clinical situation, the outcome has led to our belief that pulmonary resections performed during systemic anticoagulation are associated with increased risk and should be avoided if possible. This conclusion is supported by the uneventful pulmonary resections performed without anticoagulation in over 85% of our patients.

For pulmonary lesions removed by simple wedge resection that prove to be lung cancer, technical factors regarding potential resection of the lesion need to be assessed. The option of a delayed definitive procedure via a posterolateral thoracotomy could be considered if a simultaneous lobectomy is believed to carry excessive risk. Otherwise, hilar and mediastinal lymph node sampling next should be performed, again preferably before cardiopulmonary bypass, as the discovery of unsuspected nodal metastases might appropriately alter treatment plans and objectives for the proposed operation. If no evidence of lymph node metastases is found, we perform lobectomy after completion of the cardiac procedure and discontinuation of cardiopulmonary bypass. On the other hand, if after cardiac repair either the risk of lobectomy is judged to be increased or hemodynamics are unstable, wedge resection is a reasonable alternative as limited resection is at times adequate treatment for peripheral lung cancer [11–13].

An exception to performing lobectomy after extracorporeal circulation may be those patients who have left lower lobe lesions. While it is entirely possible to safely perform an isolated left lower lobectomy transsternally, such a procedure may not be well tolerated in a patient who has just undergone cardiac repair. The major advantage of performing a left lower lobectomy during cardiopulmonary bypass is the avoidance of unstable hemodynamics which may occur with retraction of the heart medially during exposure of the left hilus. Of lesser importance is the improved visualization of the pulmonary artery that is obtained with a nonventilated lung. These advantages are far less significant with right-sided resections where hemodynamic instability is unlikely and the pulmonary vessels and fissures are more accessible.

We strongly believe that intraoperative staging is crucial to the successful management of lung cancer. This necessitates complete mediastinal lymph node sampling, which should include the paratracheal, subcarinal, and paraesophageal areas. Undoubtedly, mediastinal staging is a major disadvantage of simultaneous transsternal pulmonary resection for lung cancer as exposure is often difficult and frequently not enough time is allowed to adequately assess the anatomic areas. Another disadvantage of the transsternal approach to pulmonary resection during cardiac surgery is the difficulty encountered in performing extended resections such as sleeve lobectomy that may be required if bronchial margins are not free of tumor.

We believe, however, that this latter disadvantage can be minimized by selecting for resection only those cancers that present as solitary pulmonary nodules.

Our experience supports the contention that a curative pulmonary resection for lung cancer can be performed via a median sternotomy and that the concomitant performance of a cardiac procedure does not complicate the pulmonary resection. There is no question, however, that hilar and mediastinal dissections for staging purposes are more easily and completely performed through a posterolateral thoracotomy. Although incomplete lymph node sampling could underestimate the extent of disease and lead to inadequate therapy, there is no reason to believe that the transsternal approach itself compromises the chance of long-term survival.

5. SUMMARY

We conclude that simultaneous cardiac and pulmonary procedures can be safely performed in selected patients. Furthermore, the simultaneous performance of these procedures can define all pathology, accelerate the definitive correction of both problems, and, in many instances, save the patient the expense, potential morbidity, and discomfort of a second operation.

EDITORS' COMMENT

The clinical evaluation of combined cardiac and pulmonary surgery described in this chapter occurred before the advent of videofluoroscopic–thorascopic surgery. The place of this less stressful method of diagnosing and excising pulmonary nodule and infiltrates, mediastinal mass and lymph nodes has not been evaluated for patients requiring cardiac surgery. An early volume in this series will cover videofluoroscopic–thorascopic surgery.

REFERENCES

1 Peters RM, Swain JA. Management of the patient with emphysema, coronary artery disease, and lung cancer. Am J Surg 1982; 143: 701–705.
2 Girardet RE, Masri ZH, Lansing AM. Pulmonary lesions in patients undergoing open heart surgery: Approach and management. J Ky Med Assoc 1981; 79: 645–648.
3 Bricker DL, Parker TM, Dalton ML Jr, Mistrot JJ. Open heart surgery with concomitant pulmonary resection. Cardiovasc Dis, Bull Tex Heart Inst 1980; 7: 411–419.
4 Dalton ML Jr, Parker TM, Mistrot JJ, Bricker DL. Concomitant coronary artery bypass and major noncardiac surgery. J Thorac Cardiovasc Surg 1978; 75: 621–624.
5 Cooper JD, Nelems JM, Pearson FG. Extended indications for median sternotomy in patients requiring pulmonary resection. Ann Thorac Surg 1978; 26: 413–419.
6 Piehler JM, Trastek VF, Pairolero PC, Pluth Jr, Danielson GK, Schaff HV, Orszulak TA, Puga FJ. Concomitant cardiac and pulmonary operations. J Thorac Cardiovasc Surg 1985 90: 662–667 (November).

7 Meng RL, Jensik RJ, Kittle CF, Faber LP. Median sternotomy for synchronous bilateral pulmonary operations. Thorac Cardiovasc Surg 1980; 80: 1–7.
8 Urschel HC Jr, Razzuk MA. Median sternotomy as a standard approach for pulmonary resection. Ann Thorac Surg 1986; 41: 130–134.
9 Asaph JW, Keppel JF. Median sternotomy for the treatment of primary pulmonary neoplasms. Am J Surg 1984; 147: 589–592.
10 Watanabe Y, Ichihashi T, Iwa T. Median sternotomy as an approach for pulmonary surgery. Thorac Cardiovasc Surgeon 1988; 36: 227–231.
11 Peters RM. The role of limited resection in carcinoma of the lung. Am J Surg 1982; 143: 706–710.
12 Hoffmann TH, Ransdell HT. Comparison of lobectomy and wedge resection for carcinoma of the lung. J Thorac Cardiovasc Surg 1980; 79: 211–215.
13 Shields TW, Higgins GA Jr. Minimal pulmonary resection: In treatment of carcinoma of the lung. Arch Surg 1974; 108: 420–422.

Part II

Preoperative preparation for the compromised host

Current Topics in General Thoracic Surgery: An International Series, Vol. 2
Perioperative Care, edited by R.M. Peters and J. Toledo

Chapter 4

Preoperative treatment of chronic obstructive lung disease

V. Schulz

1. INTRODUCTION

Chronic obstructive lung diseases (COLD) are usually found in patients who are meant to undergo thoracic surgery. According to the intensity of symptoms and the extent of pulmonary functional loss, peri- and postoperative complications coupled to the lung will be caused, presenting one decisive factor for the surgical result. Thus, for instance, it is possible to assess the risks of postoperative complications by considering definite threshold values of diagnostic function parameters (Table 4.1). Diseases which affect these parameters therefore ought to be treated preoperatively by all means. To improve an airway disease means to decrease postoperative complications – just as it frequently represents the virtual precondition for surgery.

This chapter is meant to demonstrate the different methods of drug therapy to employ preoperatively in the management of chronic obstructive lung diseases. In accordance with various factors, the treatment of bronchospasm, bronchial inflammation and mucostasis will be discussed. In conclusion a concept will be presented illustrating the combination of the different kinds of treatment.

2. TREATMENT OF BRONCHOSPASM

2.1. Beta-adrenergic agents

Beta-adrenergic agents represent the most efficient group of bronchodilating drugs [1,2]. Their bronchodilating effect results from sluicing the calcium ions stored inside the smooth muscle cells out into extracellular space; as a consequence the bronchial muscle tonus decreases. The process starts by linking the beta-adrenergic agent to specific receptor sites in smooth bronchial muscle, producing stimulation

TABLE 4.1
Postoperative pulmonary complications dependence on preoperative pulmonary function state[a]

Postoperative complications	Preoperative pulmonary function		
	$FEV_1 < 60\%$ of predicted	$FEV_1 < 60\%$ of predicted; $RV > 140\%$ of predicted	$FEV_1 < 60\%$ of predicted; $RV > 140\%$ of predicted; $P_aO_2 < 65$ Torr
atelectasis, pneumonia, therapeutic bronchoscopy, arterial hypoxy ($P_aO_2 < 50$ Torr)	46% (12%)	78% (5%)	73% (7%)
tracheotomy	62% (15%)	69% (12%)	64% (4%)
mechanical ventilation (5 days)	53% (19%)	57% (11%)	86% (9%)

[a]84 patients. Surgical procedures: lobectomy, bilobectomy. Values in parentheses are for patients with function data over/under listed limits

TABLE 4.2
Pulmonary effects of beta-adrenergic agents

- bronchodilation (immediate onset of action)
- activation of tracheobronchial cilia motility (stimulation of mucociliary clearance)
- control of bronchial mucous glands and goblets cells
- increasing contractility of diaphragm and other respiratory muscles
- decrease of pulmonary vascular resistance (precapillary arterioles) and therefore pulmonary hypertension
- prevention of mast cell degranulation (in bronchial mucosa)
- inhibition of histidindecarboxylase (inhibition of intracellular histamine synthesis – mast cell)

of the adenyl cyclase, which results in increasing cyclic adenosine monophosphate and inducing protein kinase into activating CaMW-ANTPa-se, which controls the calcium flow directed towards extracellular space.

In the bronchial treatment of today, the agents isoprenaline and orciprenaline, which stimulate the beta-1- and beta-2-receptors, should no longer be used. It is preferable to employ so-called beta-2-adrenergic agents, which have been developed in increasing numbers since the end of the sixties. As beta-2-receptors are bound to bronchial muscles in an extremely selective way, both cardiac side reactions mediated on beta-1-receptors and any tremorogenic effect on the limb musculature appear far less than with the 'older' drugs, which occupy both receptor groups.

Different efficiencies are reported for the various beta-adrenergic agents, which are related, however, to non-equieffective doses[3]. Considering the proportion of potency to side effects, no advantages of specific beta-adrenergic agents can be

TABLE 4.3
Beta-adrenergics. Generics and their daily dosage

Beta-adrenergic agent (generic name)	Routinely administered puffs of metered aerosol	Daily doses in tablets (retard)
Carbuterol	4×0.10 mg	2×2.0 mg
Clenbuterol	—	2×0.02 mg
Fenoterol	2–4×0.20 mg	2×2.5 mg
Reproterol	4×0.50 mg	2×20.0 mg
Salbutomol	4×0.10 mg	2×8.0 mg
Terbutalin	4×0.25 mg	2×7.5 mg
Tolubuterol	—	1–2×2.0 mg

outlined. It may be postulated that all beta-2-adrenergic agents are comparable for use in clinical applications. Reproterol, tolubuterol and in particular formoterol, however, show longer sustained action than the other beta-adrenergic agents, while the initial bronchodilating effects are comparable. Their dosage can be chosen with wider intervals (Table 4.2).

The decrease in airway resistance, beginning after inhalation, occurs instantaneously and, as a rule reaches its maximum after 5–10 minutes. After a plateau of reduction maintained for up to 3 hours, a gradual rise of airway resistance is seen. Therefore one has to keep to a dosage scheme every 5–6 hours for inhalational administration. The higher the initial value, the more extensive a decrease in airway resistance is found [4]. Airway resistance reduced by more than 90%, the FEV_1-value elevated by more than 30%, can be defined as 'good response'. Decrease in airway resistance by less than 50%, likewise a FEV_1 value not superseding the initial value by 10%, show limited efficacy. In those cases it should be considered that the action pattern of beta-2-adrenergic agents is not confined to bronchodilation. Consistent with the respective basic pathogenetic mechanisms of bronchial obstruction, other effects can be made use of (Table 4.3). If no side reactions occur, the therapy with beta-adrenergic agents can therefore be continued even in patients with 'low response', if required at a reduced dosage. The combination of beta-adrenergic and theophylline agents causes an additive effect, due to the mode of action of the two substrates. Synchronous application of both medications at a lower dose than with single medication may therefore be advantageous to avoid side reactions but obtain sufficient bronchodilating effect. In some patients intensified action of beta-adrenergic agents can also be achieved by means of calcium antagonists (nifedipin).

Because of the immediate onset of action and lower side effect of the inhalational mode compared with oral administration, the former should always be chosen. The patients have to be instructed in the correct use of the metered aerosol. If some patient cannot coordinate dose release with inspiration, various spacer systems attached to the metered dose inhaler can be employed. Breath-actuated inhalers with – environmentally preferable – powder inhalations may be used. Administration with the IPPB-apparatus is advantageous only in patients

TABLE 4.4
Pulmonary effects of theophyllines

- bronchodilation (weaker than beta-adrenergic agents)
- respiration stimulant (increasing alveolar ventilation)
- activation of tracheobronchial cilia motility (stimulation of mucociliary clearance)
- increasing contractility of diaphragma and other respiratory muscles
- decrease of precapillary pulmonary vascular resistance
- synergistic effects with beta-adrenergic agents
- preparation of mast cell degranulation (in bronchial mucosa, stimulation of endogenous catecholamine release)

with extremely low inspiratory flow rates. Such patients are to be deferred from thoracic surgery. In the group of functionally operable patients, however, the bronchodilating effect does not depend on the inhalational method of administration (metered aerosol versus, e.g., IPPB)[5,6].

The oral administration of beta-adrenergic agents, especially in retarded form, has several indications. It may become necessary in patients who are not able to cooperate with the inhalator system, and it will be employed to guarantee a more persistent bronchodilating effect than achieved through inhalation, particularly for evening administration. Occasionally it may also be suitable to use oral and inhalational application side by side, in order to obtain a 'smoothed' course of action.

2.2. Theophylline

The biochemical action mode of theophylline has not yet been explored to its full extent. It seems opportune to doubt the evidently attractive theory that its bronchodilating effect is caused both by the established inhibition of phosphodiesterase with the resulting CAMP-stasis and by the calcium flow of the monofibrils towards the sarcoplasmic reticulum. As a matter of fact, the required theophylline concentrations of 10^{-4} to 10^{-3} mole cannot be obtained therapeutically due to side reactions. Furthermore, the theory of adenosine acting antagonistically at purinergic receptor sites is contestable as well, the more so since theophyllines, without any methyl group to link to that receptor and to mediate adenosine antagonism, block bronchodilating potential.

The bronchodilating effect of theophyllines is lower than that of beta-2-adrenergics[7,8]. Bronchodilation starts to be measurable with a serum level of 8 mg/l. The effect, however, is dose-related, therefore attempts should be made to stabilize the level in the median range (13–16 mg/l) of the therapeutic window between 8 and 20 mg/l. Apart from bronchodilation, several other effects of theophylline are reported, which can be used in the preoperative management of the patients (Table 4.4).

TABLE 4.5
Factors modifying theophylline clearance

Decrease of clearance	Factor	Increase of clearance
premature new-borns; age over 50 (decreasing liver function)	age	adolescence
adipositas (due to steatosis–hepatitis)	body weight	—
carbohydrate-rich diet; methylxanthine-rich diet, alcoholism (decreasing liver function)	diet	protein-rich diet; grilled meat
—	smoking of tobacco and marihuana	induction of P-450-cytochromaxydase (in the liver cell)
macrolid-antibiotics (erythromycin, Vancomycin); H_2-antagonists (cimetidin, ranitidin), allupurinol	drugs	phenobarbital, rifampicin
cirrhosis hepatis, hepatitis/cardiac insufficiency; pneumonias, respiratory viral infections/status febriles; renal insufficiency	diseases	—

From a general viewpoint, the therapeutic range of theophylline is narrow. With a serum level of less than 8 mg/l, some reactions, like the respiratory analeptic effect and an improvement in respiratory muscle contractibility, can certainly be proved by measuring Pi_{max}, although no more bronchodilating effect is found. Side effects, on the other hand, must be reckoned with when values of 20 mg/l are exceeded, and at even lower values in individual cases. At first, symptoms are mostly gastrointestinal pressures over the stomach, nausea and diarrhea; complaints about sleeplessness, headaches and 'heart-hurry' are frequent, too. Most alarming are complications such as tachycardiac arrhythmias and cerebral convulsions which occur at higher serum levels (> 30 mg/l) [9,10].

The metabolism of theophyllines is extremely variable interindividually, or even intraindividually depending on associated disease. 5% of the theophyllines are discharged by the kidney without being metabolized. 90–95% are subject to metabolism in the liver via the microsomal cytochrome-P-450-enzyme system [11]. Factors affecting the hepatic function therefore have to be taken into consideration. Due to their reduced liver function, elder patients show delayed theophylline clearance compared with younger adults and children, so their initial dosage should be chosen in the low range. The same is true for patients at the borderline of right ventricular insufficiency. If it is possible to relieve decompensated cor pulmonale by drug therapy, the congestion of the liver will diminish and its

TABLE 4.6
Pulmonary effects of anticholinergic drugs

- bronchodilation (weaker than beta-adrenergic agents)
- protective effect against vagal mediated reflex bronchoconstriction (cholinergic–muscarinergic receptors)
- mast cell protection

metabolic function will increase. Consequently the dose of theophylline has to be raised to avoid too low serum levels. Smoking intensifies the hepatic metabolism of theophylline through inducing the P-450-enzyme system. On average one may therefore start with higher theophylline dosage in smokers. With the age factor affecting the metabolism the opposite way, it is difficult to find the proper dosage for 'elder smokers'. Several drugs, like chinolone and erythromycin, which are frequently used in patients with obstructive airway diseases, diminish theophylline metabolism. Consequently, this has to be taken into consideration in establishing the dosage regimen (Table 4.5) [10,12].

All insecurities about determining doses and maintaining some serum level within therapeutic range are evaded by determining serum levels during the initial period of treatment. Begin with a daily dose of 10 mg/kg body weight, given in two oral administrations with intervals of 8–12 hours. Level determinations directly before and 3–4 hours after application are suitable to set up some reliable course and thereby adapt the dosage. It has to be kept in mind that steady-state conditions of the theophylline level are not to be expected earlier than three days after the start of the treatment. In most cases in adults, the resulting daily total dose is 12 mg/kg body weight; patients who, due to multiple factors, metabolize slowly need a daily dose of 8 mg/kg. The risk of exceeding the proper dose is generally overestimated: follow-ups in patients who receive strictly the standard doses as quoted in the manufacturers' folders show subtherapeutic theophylline levels in 68%, whereas overdosages could be found in 4% only.

For oral therapy one should use controlled-release preparations, usually one morning and one evening administration. The evening dose is occasionally raised for the purpose of obtaining 'safe' levels, thus avoiding the so-called morning dip. Furthermore this procedure is justified when it is necessary to compensate for delayed intestinal absorption by higher evening administrations. Once an optimal daily dose to be given in the evening, has been established which avoids excessive peak values resulting in sleep disturbances, it is feasable to guarantee therapeutic levels also during the day [13].

2.3. Anticholinergic drugs

The anticholinergics ipratropium-bromide and oxitropium-bromide influence bronchoconstriction induced by vagus nerve [14,15]. When applied by inhalation, they occupy the cholinergic (muscarinergic) receptor sites of the smooth bronchial

TABLE 4.7
Anticholinergics. Generics and their daily dosage

Anticholinergic drug (generic name)	Routinely administered daily doses (puffs of metered aerosol)
ipratropium-bromide	4×2 (one puff 0.02 mg)
oxitropium-bromide	4×2 (one puff 0.10 mg)

muscles, thus initiating bronchodilation competing with the counteracting effect of acetylcholine [16]. Further effects may be used for treatment of obstructive airway diseases, especially the protective action versus bronchoconstrictive stimulants (Table 4.6).

Cholinergic-mediated bronchoconstriction is found uncommonly in patients up to middle age, whereas this pathogenetic factor occurs frequently in elder patients, who consequently profit from the application of anticholinergics.

After inhalation the maximum effect is seen after 20–30 minutes, which is later than with beta-adrenergic agents [16,17]. The bronchodilating potential is generally inferior to that of beta-adrenergics, but this is possibly compensated by more persistent action [14]. Side effects of atropine need not be worried about, as even with exceeded standard doses no essential mucocutaneous resorption (bronchial system, stomach) occurs [14] (Table 4.7).

3. TREATMENT OF BRONCHIAL INFLAMMATION

Bacteriogenic purulent bronchitis, frequently following a respiratory viral infection, must always be treated preoperatively with antibiotics, in order to reduce postoperative complications like bronchopneumonia, empyema, sepsis or disturbed healing of bronchial anastomoses. Most often it is recommended to give (gluco)corticoids at the same time. Their suppressive action on effector cells of the infection and its mediator regeneration will suppress bronchitis. Corticoids, mainly applied topically, have to be employed in cases where smoking, inhaled allergens or occupational noxae might have provoked a bronchial inflammation not related to any infection. Bronchial inflammation contributes to the persistent airway obstruction and particularly promotes bronchial hyperresponsiveness.

3.1. Antibiotics

Any specific antibiotic therapy must be adjusted to pathogens antibiotic sensitivity pattern. Microbiologic investigations show that the acute inflammation of a chronic airway disease is mainly provoked by *Streptococcus pneumoniae* and *Haemophilus influenzae*. Both causative agents colonize by a rate of up to 70% in the healthy oropharynx. Consequently, only quantitative bacteria count of more than 10^5/ml sputum is diagnostic. On the other hand, pathogenic germs might be overgrown

TABLE 4.8
Antibiotic drugs in therapy of chronic obstructive airway disease. Generics and their daily dosage

Antibiotic drug (generic name)	Routinely administered daily doses (orally)
penicillin V	$3\times(5\text{–}10\times10^5$ IE)
tetracyclins	
doxycyclin	$1\text{–}2\times200$ mg
minocyclin	2×100 mg
cotrimoxazol	2×960 mg
aminopenicillins	
ampicillin	3×1000 mg
pivampicillin	3×100 mg
amoxycillin	3×750 mg
makrolids	
erythromycin	3×500 mg

by 'normal' flora, which especially in patients after antibiotic pretreatment leads to false negative findings. This, in addition to faults in collecting and handling the sputum, combined with false assumption of bacterial origin in case of viral etiology, results in pathognomonic germs being diagnosed only in 40–60% of all examined sputa, even by means of Gram staining.

In practice, therapy will be blindly started with penicillin V, tetracyclines, erythromycins, ampicillin or alternatively cotrimoxazol, if *S. pneumoniae* or *H. influenzae* are presumed as causative agents (Table 4.8) [18]. No response of this therapy does not necessarily imply any divergent spectrum of bacteria: resistance of *S. pneumoniae* to tetracycline has to be reckoned with in 10–30%, of *H. influenzae* in 5–10%. Haemophil strains resistent to ampicillin and erythromycin do exist. Penicillins are relatively unfit to penetrate into bronchial secretion, so individual chosen doses might be too low. Therefore one will alternate with some of the specified antibiotics before applying any other chemogroups or even wide-spectrum antibiotics.

In 15–20% of the cases, however, infrequent causative organisms like staphylococci, gramnegative bacteria (pseudomonas, enterobacteriaceae – *Klebsiella*, *Enterobacter*, *Serratia*) and anaerobes have to be assumed from the very first. Besides chronic diseases of the respiratory tract, additional risk factors like alcoholism, gastroesophageal reflux, cardiac insufficiency, or diabetes mellitus may frequently be diagnosed, correlating with the spectrum of those pathogens. Equally, bronchiectasis must be taken into consideration. To be able to initiate a specific therapy, identification of the infectious agents should be done by flexible bronchoscopy and telescopic catheters, if required by transtracheal aspiration. Generally oral treatment with cephalosporins, chinolones or imipenem is sufficient. Only in rare individual cases will parenteral application of ureido penicillins resp. cephalosporins combined with aminoglycosides be used. In case of bronchiectasis, in addition to systemic therapy, inhalation antibiotics should be applied. The

TABLE 4.9
Inhaled corticosteroids. Generics and their daily dosage

Inhaled corticosteroid (generic name)	Routinely administered daily doses
Beclomethasone-dipropionate	1.0–1.5 mg
Budesonid	0.8–1.6 mg
Flunisolonacetonid	1.0–2.0 mg

diffusion of antibiotics via blood circulation into bronchiectatic pus usually is meager. Alternatively, neomycin, gentamycin or acetracin can be recommended.

3.2. Corticosteroids

The effective mechanism of corticosteroids is bound to a series of biochemical reactions which explain the long latency until clinical action starts: after being linked intracytoplasmatically to a receptor protein, this complex is sluiced into the nucleus by means of some still unknown transporting system. In the nucleus the steroid finally acts as zymoinductor, which, by 'unmasking' operating genes and setting free messenger ribonucleinic acid for transcription, causes the synthesis of a polypeptide which procures the specific steroid effect. This polypeptide with the name of lipomodulin or macrocrotin interferes with the metabolism of lipids bound to cell membrane and prevents the formation of mediators (leucotrines, prostaglandins, PAF) causing inflammation and bronchoconstriction, through enzyme inhibition (phospholipase A2).

These effects of corticosteroids on special cell populations of bronchial mucosa, on eosino- and neutrophilic polymorphonuclear granylocytes, lymphocytes, mast cells, smooth bronchial muscles and bronchial glands, may be used above all on bronchial asthma [19], but they are also seen to a varying extent, depending on the respective basic pathogenesis, with other inflammatory conditions of bronchial mucosa. Since inhalation corticoids with low rate of secondary effects are available now, one should generally consider applying these preoperatively in chronic airway diseases [20,21]. Through the anti-inflammatory effect of the steroids the mucosal edema decreases, and the bronchial hypercrinism subsides. Another consequence of the reduced mediator regeneration, diminished bronchial hyperresponsiveness can be established as well. Finally, bronchodilation is additionally induced via 'direct attack' on the smooth bronchial muscles.

Beclomethasone, budesonid and flunisolid can be used as steroids which are effective after inhalation (Table 4.9) [22,23]. Patients accustomed to the immediate action of inhalational beta-adrenergic agents have to be informed that, because of the different mode of action, an immediate effect cannot be expected with steroids. After continued application, however, improvement of the bronchial symptoms, beginning at the 4th or 5th day and increasing from then on, may be related to the steroid inhalation [22,23]. It can be assumed that inhalation administration of corticoid can replace the systemic application of 2.5–7.5 mg prednisone equivalent.

Side reactions of the therapy are sometimes hoarseness, which rapidly disappears after discontinuing the inhalation, and in 10% of the patients an intensifying oropharyngeal candidiasis. If this reaction cannot be avoided by rinsing the mouth after application, and the therapy should still be carried out with inhalation corticoid, application might be done by a spacer, which very sharply lowers the rate of oropharyngeal candidiasis, due to the minor deposition in the affected area. Systemic secondary effects of corticoid need not be worried about if dosage instructions are followed. Compared with beclomethasone and flunisolid, budesonid is additionally metabolized in the liver by some sort of first-pass mechanism, if some aerosol has been 'swallowed'. As to systemic effects, no advantage is derived from the corticosteroids, since none of the three inhalational corticoids, applied in usual dosage, yields a measurable adrenal suppression, judged from the release of cortisol.

Application of systemic corticoids is not presented here, because where such procedures become necessary in the management of airway diseases, a functional inoperability is impossible to overcome. If absolutely necessary, acute systemic administration for a few days might be proposed, in order to 'improve' responsiveness to beta-adrenergic agents. However experience shows that patients who require such permissive effects of corticoids to show sufficient bronchodilating reaction after beta-adrenergic agents, can be brought to the level of functional operability in exceptional cases only.

4. TREATMENT OF MUCOSTASIS

Chronic airway diseases are often accompanied by intensified bronchial secretion. Apart from increased secretion, altered rheologic properties, caused by augmented formation of high-polymeric 'water-deficient' mucines, disturbed ciliary motility and insufficient strength in coughing are responsible for the development of mucostasis, which in turn provokes bronchial obstruction and infections.

According to these various pathogenetic factors, drug therapy has to be started to affect different sites of action: in the form of quantitative and qualitative effects on the secretions at cellular level, diminished viscosity of the secretory product sitting within the lumina, and of improving the ciliary motility [24,25].

Ciliary motility is intensified by beta-adrenergics and theophyllines. Although not proved through experiments, it is postulated from clinical experience that adequate hydration of the patients, while paying attention to cardiac factors, might increase ciliary motility, as that procedure corrects reduced water content of bronchial secretion, thus improving the ciliary kinetics.

Intraluminal adhesive mucus is treated by sulphuric mucolytic drugs (N-acetylcysteine, carbocysteine) (Table 4.10). Due to their unbound SH-group, they disintegrate sulphide bridges, depolymerizing the mucines of the bronchial secretion. Seen from a rheological point of view, viscosity of bronchial secretion decreases, making expectorating easier [26,27]. Sulfuric mucolytics can be applied

TABLE 4.10
Mucolytics. Generics and their daily dosage

Mucolytic drug (generic name)	Routinely administered daily doses
N-acetylcysteine	0.4–0.8 g
Carbocysteine	1.5–2.5 g
Bromhexine	24–48 mg
Ambroxol	60–90 mg

by oral, inhalational or parenteral methods. Inhalational administration is the most efficient, possibly leading, however, to bronchoconstriction as a secondary effect [26]. Equally it has to be taken into consideration that too intensive a decrease in viscosity might easily be accompanied by some deterioration of mucociliary clearance.

There is clear evidence that secretion at the cellular level is affected by corticosteroids, primarily and secondarily through depression of mediator regeneration. Likewise, beta-adrenergic agents interfere with intracellular production of mucus. Bromhexine and its primary metabolite ambroxol increase the rate of liposomal enzymes, which degrade high-polymeric mucines through hydrolysis, thus secretion rheologically returns to normal and mucus is sluiced out (Table 4.10) [28]. Additionally one finds intensified secretion of pneumocytes II and clara-cells; their surface-active secretion through some antiglue effect prevents viscous mucus from adhering to the bronchial mucosa in the area of small airways [28].

5. PRACTICAL PROCEDURES IN PREOPERATIVE TREATMENT

The medicament groups illustrated above are meant to be applied and combined in different ways, according to the primary pathogenous factors of the respective chronic airway disease. Several decisive questions for the choice of drugs have to be clarified through differential diagnosis:

(1) Is any bronchial obstruction measurable by usual methods of functional diagnosis?
(2) Is the predominant nature of an identified limitation in bronchial flow endobronchial or exobronchial? Is there a mixed form of those kinds of obstruction?
(3) Does the bronchial obstruction have to be partly related to bronchospasm? Which bronchodilators definitely cause some response of the bronchospasm?
(4) Can any bronchial hyperresponsiveness be recognized from case history details and functional examinations?
(5) Are there any signs that bronchial asthma had causally existed in the beginning of the chronic airway disease?

(6) Are bronchorrhea and coughing predominating among the signs? Do recurrent infections appear frequently? Is dyspnea rather a receding symptom?

When bronchial obstruction is excluded through the specific spirometric and/or body-plethysmographic studies, the administration of bronchodilators does not seem to be justified. It should, however, be considered, whether one might not use effects of these substances for increasing the ciliary motility, influencing formation and release of mediators, and others. For that purpose beta-adrenergics and theophyllines at low doses can be applied.

In case of measurable bronchial obstruction the endo- and exobronchial ratio in flow limitation must be established after analyzing the functional data in concert with the clinical performance. Patients with mainly endobronchial obstruction, caused to varying extent by edema formations in bronchial mucosa, bronchospasm and hypercrinia, airway resistance, intrathoracic gas volume and dynamic spirometric parameters are pathologically altered. Patients show the clinical picture of blue-bloaters, predominating symptoms are bronchorrhea and cough. Exobronchial obstruction, on the other hand, caused by low static elastic recoil pressure resulting from emphysema, is characterized by the constellation of measured values indicating slightly elevated airway resistance, very high intrathoracic gas volume and extremely low dynamic lung volumes. These patients appear as pink puffers with dyspnea as main symptom. In general mixed pictures occur. Endobronchial obstruction normally can be favorably affected by the named groups of medications, whereas any exobronchial obstruction is impossible to treat by drugs. Prognosis of treatment depends on how both obstruction forms are individually manifest.

In its turn the proportion of endobronchial obstruction related to bronchospasm has to be evaluated before and after application of any bronchodilating agent by spirometric and/or body-plethysmographic tests. If bronchospasm is present, response can be usually obtained to inhalational beta-adrenergic drugs. Bronchodilating therapy is therefore initiated with some beta-adrenergic agent. In case its effect is not sufficient, theophyllines and/or anticholinergic drugs may be added if efficacy is proved through functional diagnosis.

Bronchial inflammation, formation of edema and mucostasis, if diagnosed as pathogenetic factors, have to be tackled additionally by means of topical corticoids, antibiotics and mucolytics. Manifest bronchial hyperresponsiveness as well as case history details on bronchial asthma are always indications for topical administration of corticoids.

With regard to these different pathophysiologic factors, one may follow a therapeutic dosage regimen adjusted to the degree of severity of the airway disease (Table 4.11).

TABLE 4.11
Step-diagram in the treatment of chronic obstructive airway disease

Step 1			
β_2-adrenergics (inhalative)			
Step 2			
β_2-adrenergics	plus theophyllines		
or			
β_2-adrenergics	plus inhalative corticosteroids		
or			
β_2-adrenergics	plus anticholinergics		
Step 3			
β_2-adrenergics (inhalative and orally)	plus theophyllines	plus anticholinergics	plus inhalative corticosteroids
Step 4			
β_2-adrenergics (inhalative and orally)	plus theophyllines	plus anticholinergics	plus inhalative and orally corticosteroids

REFERENCES

1 Popa V. Respiratory Pharmacology, Beta-adrenergic drugs. Clin Chest Med 1986; 7: 313.
2 Svedmyr N. Beta-Adrenergic Agonists. Sweden, National Board of Health and Welfare, Drug Information Committee 1986: No 3.
3 Theodore AC, Beer DJ. Pharmacotherapy of chronic obstructive pulmonary disease. Clin Chest Med 1986; 7: 657.
4 Kaik G. Bronchospasmolytika und ihre klinische Pharmakologie. München, Urban & Schwarzenberg 1980.
5 Larsson S, Svedmayr N. Bronchodilator effects and side effects of beta-2-adrenoceptor stimulants by different modes of administration (tablets, metered aerosol, and combinations thereof). Am Rev Respir Dis 1977; 116: 861.
6 McFadden Jr ER. Inhaled Aerosol Bronchodilators. Baltimore, Williams & Wilkins 1986.
7 Heneles L, Weinberger M. Theophylline. A state-of-the-art review. Pharmacotherapy 1984; 3: 2.
8 Sybrecht G. Theophyllin. In: Schmidt OP (ed.). Mastzellprotektion. München, Dustri 1983.
9 Turner-Warwick M, Levy J (eds.). New Perspectives in Theophylline Therapy. Oxford, Royal Society for Medicine 1984.
10 Weinberger M. The pharmacology and therapeutic use of theophylline. J Allergy Clin Immunol 1984; 73: 525.
11 Morley J. Theophylline in asthma. Bull Eur Physiopathol Respir 1986; 22: 425.
12 Miech RP, Stein M. Respiratory pharmacology. Methylxanthines. Clin Chest Med 1986; 7: 331.
13 Barnes PJ. Therapie des nächtlichen Asthma. In: Nolte D, Kummer F, Dorow P (eds.). Asthma Bronchiale. München, Urban & Schwarzenberg 1986.
14 Gross NJ, Skorodin MS. State of the art: Anticholinergic, antimuscarinic bronchodilatators. Am Rev Respir Dis 1984; 129: 856.
15 Nolte D, Lichterfeld A (eds.). Interaktion von Vagus und Sympathikus bei Bronchialerkrankungen. München, Urban & Schwarzenberg 1980.

16 Brown JG, Chan CS, Kelly CA, Dent AG, Zimmermann PV. Assessment of the clinical usefulness of nebulized ipratropium bromide in patients with chronic airflow limitation. Thorax 1984; 39: 272.
17 Mann JS, Geroge CF. Anticholinergic drugs in the treatment of airways disease. Br J Dis Chest 1985; 79: 209.
18 Lead article. Antimicrobiol treatment of chronic bronchitis. Lancet 1975; 1: 505.
19 Clark TJH, Mygind N, Selroos O (eds.). Corticosteroid treatment in allergic airways diseases. Copenhagen, Munksgaard 1982.
20 Shim C, Stone DE, Williams Jr MH. Response to corticosteroids in chronic bronchitis. J Allergy Clin Immunol 1978; 62: 363.
21 Stokes TC, Shaylor JM, Reilly JFO, Harrison BDW. Assessment of steroid responsiveness in patients with chronic airflow obstruction. Lancet 1982; 2: 345.
22 Harris DM. Clinical Pharmacology of Beclomethasone-Dipropionate Asthma and Rhinitis. London, Bailliere Tind 11, 1980.
23 Johansson SA, Andersson KE, Brattsand R, Gruvstadt E, Hedner P. Topical and systemic glucocorticosteroid potencies of budesonid and beclomethasone-dipropionate in man. Eur J Clin Pharm 1982; 22: 523.
24 Shimura S, Okubo T, Maeda S, Aoki T, Tomioka M, Shiodo Y. Effect of expectorants on relaxation behavior of sputum viscoelasticity in vivo. Biorheology 1983; 20: 677.
25 Olivieri D, Morsico SA, Del Donno M. Improvement of mucociliary transport in smokers by mucolytics. Eur J Respir Dis 1985; 66: 142.
26 British Thoracic Society Research Committee. Oral N-acetylcysteine and exacerbation rates in patients with chronic bronchitis and severe airways obstruction. Thorax 1985; 40: 832.
27 Multicenter Study Group. Long term oral acetylsteine in chronic bronchitis. A double-blind controlled study. Eur J Resp Dis 1980; 61 (Suppl 111): 93.
28 Ericsson CH, Juhasz J, Jonsson E, Mossberg B. Ambroxol therapy in simple chronic bronchitis: effects on subjective symptoms and ventilatory function. Eur J Respir Dis 1986; 69: 248.

Current Topics in General Thoracic Surgery: An International Series, Vol. 2
Perioperative Care, edited by R.M. Peters and J. Toledo

Discussion of "Preoperative treatment of chronic obstructive lung disease" by V. Schulz

F. Hammond Cole Jr. and James W. Pate

Preoperative therapy for the thoracic surgical patient is an integral part of the management of pulmonary lesions. Dr. Schulz has provided a detailed enumeration of the available classes of therapeutic agents available. We shall discuss some personal preferences and emphasize several points.

An adage on our service is that a patient who has abused tobacco enough to develop a lung carcinoma virtually always has accompanying chronic obstructive lung disease. We therefore institute bronchodilator therapy at the initial contact with the patient and continue this treatment throughout the period of diagnostic study and preoperative evaluation. Although the subject of preoperative assessment of pulmonary function is covered elsewhere, several clinical findings are favorable indicators that marginal pulmonary function can be substantially improved by a period of preoperative preparation. These include: improvement following administration of bronchodilators during pulmonary function studies, lack of any current therapy, and most particularly, smoking cessation in an actively abusing patient. In individuals with these factors, substantial improvement can be expected to occur, and a physiologically inoperable patient can occasionally convert to an operable one by preoperative therapy.

The issue of smoking cessation is difficult to evaluate. Sabanathan and associates [1] make the point that in studies of closing volumes in relation to age, smoking has the same effect as adding ten years to the chronological age. Further, although continued improvement in pulmonary function has been reported up to 18 months following smoking cessation, even a short abstention may improve the effectiveness of the mucociliary transport mechanism [1]. All of the studies of therapy detailed below included smoking cessation as an integral and major part of the program. On the other hand, it has proven difficult to clearly ascertain the minimum period of smoking cessation that will decrease complications, with one recent study on abdominal surgical patients suggesting that a period of eight weeks is necessary to produce a diminution in pulmonary complications postoperatively [2]. It would appear reasonable to us to assume that any period off cigarettes prior to thoracic surgery should be beneficial, and that up to a certain point, risks should diminish in proportion to time of abstinence. Cardiac arrhythmic effects and direct irritation of the tracheobronchial tree with excessive secretions are rapid effects which may improve with only a few days of cigarette avoidance.

Several landmark studies have addressed the effects of a vigorous period of preoperative preparation in reducing pulmonary complications. Stein and Cassara [3] reported in 1970 a prospective study in surgical patients. Their patients were randomized and were in a poor risk category so far as pulmonary complications were concerned. The study patients were placed on a regimen of smoking cessation, antibiotics, bronchodilator drugs, ultrasonic nebulizer, and chest physiotherapy; non-study patients received any lung measures deemed necessary by their attending physicians. Complications in these high-risk patients were 60% in the control group compared to 22% in the prophylactically treated group. Gracey et al. [4] reported the results of a 48-hour period of intensive preoperative therapy, and showed a pulmonary complication rate of 19% in a group of 157 patients with chronic obstructive lung disease. Their regimen consisted of an isoproterenol aerosol followed by ultrasonic nebulization and chest physiotherapy, oral theophylline preparation, guaiacol glycerol ether, and hydration. Most patients were able to cease smoking during this period. This study used the historic control of a 43% complication rate in an earlier report from the same institution (Tarhan et al. [5]). A detailed review of all relevant information is beyond the scope of this comment, but a recent critical analysis has questioned both the benefits of preoperative spirometry in the abdominal surgical patient and the methodology of most of the previous studies on preoperative preparation [6].

Our current view is that a period of preoperative preparation is of benefit in the thoracic surgical patient. Such a regimen can be done as an outpatient. We insist on smoking cessation, and feel that even a short period off tobacco is beneficial; we strongly urge patients to plan to remain abstemious postoperatively. We also use nebulized albuterol, either by inhalation therapy or via a multidose inhaler, empiric antibiotics if patient is febrile or sputum is purulent, iodinated glycerol or glycerol quaicholate as an expectorant, oral hydration, and addition of theophylline in refractory cases. As Dr. Schulz, we prefer to avoid systemic steroids, but will add anti-muscarinic agents or topical steroids if the above measures do not result in clinical improvement. In marginal cases, we confirm improvement with repeat spirometry, in addition to ventilation perfusion lung scan to evaluate the contribution of the involved lung to overall pulmonary function. In our opinion, such measures are clearly cost effective when weighed against the expense of even one long-term ventilator patient postoperatively. Despite our efforts, we are occasionally confronted on the eve of thoracotomy by a patient with poor pulmonary function who has been in the hospital for several days of study but who has received no bronchodilator therapy during this time!

Our list of available bronchodilators is considerably shorter than that available outside the United States, but use of the current drugs can improve postoperative morbidity, decrease mortality, and shorten hospital stay following thoracotomy.

REFERENCES

1 Sabanathan S, Eng J, Mearns AJ. Alterations in respiratory mechanics following thoracotomy. J Roy Coll Surg Edinburgh 1989; 35: 144.
2 Jackson CV. Preoperative pulmonary preparation. Arch Int Med 1988; 148: 2120.
3 Stein M, Cassara EL. Preoperative pulmonary evaluation and therapy for surgery patients. JAMA 1970; 211: 787.
4 Gracey DR, Divertie MB, Didier EP. Preoperative pulmonary preparation of patients with chronic obstructive pulmonary disease. Chest 1979; 76: 123.
5 Tarhan S, Moffitt EA, Sessler AD, Douglas WW, Taylor WF. Risk of anesthesia and surgery in patients with chronic bronchitis and chronic obstructive pulmonary disease. Surgery 1973; 74: 720.
6 Lawrence VA, Page CP, Harris GD. Preoperative spirometry before abdominal operations. Arch Int Med 1989; 149: 280.

Current Topics in General Thoracic Surgery: An International Series, Vol. 2
Perioperative Care, edited by R.M. Peters and J. Toledo

Chapter 5

Perioperative nutritional management of thoracic surgical patients

K. Moghissi

1. INTRODUCTION

Throughout the ages those who have had to care for the sick and the wounded have acknowledged the role of nutrition and dietary regimen in the cure of diseases and the healing of wounds. Nevertheless, the scientific basis of nutrition and the practice of artificial feeding particularly in its parenteral aspect is a 20th-century event.

Clearly the development of clinical nutrition could not have taken place without the discovery of a number of scientific principles or in the absence of technical advances. Knowledge of the human anatomy and physiology was essential in order to establish a rational basis for nutritional support in medicine and surgery. However, even before the advancement of scientific knowledge various attempts were made in the practice of artificial feeding. Christopher Wren, better known as the architect of St. Paul's Cathedral in London (1656), attempted the intravenous infusion of ale and wine into the vein of dogs using a goose quill attached to a pig bladder as a delivery system. John Hunter (1793), surgeon to King George III, used eel-skin over a whale bone to feed a patient suffering from "paralysis of the muscle of glutition".

That these and other attempts were made even prior to the description of circulation of blood by Harvey (1578–1657) and ahead of the great physiological discoveries such as those of Claud Bernard (1813–1878) only indicates the state of the searching mind of man in his attempts to find a solution to problems by clinical trials and errors.

Amongst many twentieth-century scientific and technical developments three are particularly relevant to clinical nutrition. First, the understanding of the biochemistry of food and the way in which nutrients are handled by the body, i.e. metabolism, in normal and abnormal situations. Secondly, advances in technology allowing application of scientific and experimental knowledge to therapeutic use.

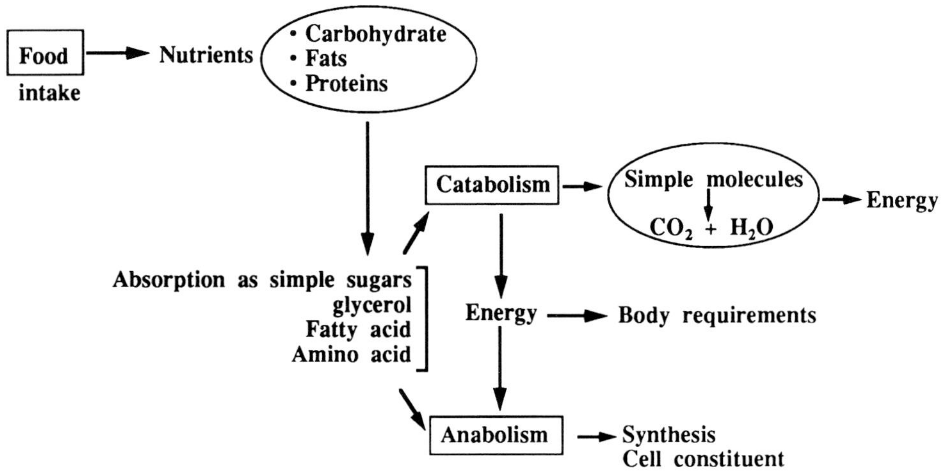

FIGURE 5.1. The phases of metabolism and the role of nutrients.

Thirdly, the manufacture of safe nutrient solution for usage in enteral or parenteral feeding.

It was in this atmosphere of the application of science to medicine and surgery, and in the course of investigation of calcium metabolism in bone, that Cuthbertson [1] in 1933 came to realise that injury resulted in a series of changes in the body constituents and metabolism as a whole. This and subsequent observations by other workers showed that injury in fact affects the whole spectrum of metabolic activity but predominantly that which involves proteins.

Soon after trauma there is an increase in protein breakdown and a decrease in synthesis which promotes the release of energy with increased nitrogen loss in the urine and negative nitrogen balance. The extent and duration of this initial phase, referred to as the catabolic phase, varies according to:

- The severity of trauma and its resultant injury
- The body's ability to overcome the disturbed metabolism
- The therapeutic measures (such as provision of high calorie and protein intake), which are offered to assist the homeostasis.

The catabolic phase is followed by an anabolic phase during which there is synthesis of protein and the resultant positive nitrogen balance.

Whilst there is no room in this chapter to expand fully on all aspects of metabolism and its alteration in the trauma situation, nevertheless several points are worth noting:

Metabolism is essentially concerned with energy transformation and transaction in the body, therefore the key to all metabolic activity is energy. Food is the only source of 'Crude Energy' without continued intake of which the body's reserve will have to be used. The simple scheme shown in Fig. 5.1 illustrates the phases of metabolism and the role of nutrients in the equation.

2. METABOLISM IN HEALTHY INDIVIDUALS

In the normal steady state there is balance between catabolism and anabolism, and food intake maintaining the equilibrium. In healthy individuals, for as long as food intake is sufficient in calorie, protein and other essential requirements and providing that the important food stuffs, that is carbohydrate, fat and protein amino-acid, can be absorbed and utilised, there will be an equilibrium (dynamic equilibrium) between catabolism and anabolism. In starvation, when the diet is deficient in calorie and proteins, the essential metabolic requirements have to be met from the body's reserves. The body's reserve of energy consists of:

2.1. Carbohydrate

Stored as glycogen in the muscle and liver it amounts to no more than a few hundred (500) grams, and with a caloric value of 4 kcal/g. Alone it cannot sustain the body's requirement of energy for any length of time, but it is nevertheless important for the maintenance of blood sugar level.

2.2. Lipids

Fats are stored in adipose tissue and are important sources of energy (caloric values: 9 kcal/g) which can furnish the body requirements for a considerable time. In starvation the body can use lipids and their derived ketone compounds, but the lipids on their own cannot be relied upon to fulfill totally the normal metabolic activities because of their dependence on carbohydrate, without which ketosis and fatty liver will develop. Whilst lack of dietary carbohydrate may not be of importance for a short period, in a state of 'stress' and in cases of prolonged nutritional deficiency the metabolic machinery will become disturbed. Even if energy requirements are fully sustained by mobilisation and breakdown of lipids from the 'fat depot' there is still need for certain amino acids (proteins) to replace those which are broken down as a normal part of the body protein metabolism and its dynamic equilibrium.

2.3. Proteins

These are abundantly present in muscle mass and are an important source of energy in times of need (1 gram of protein provides approximately 4 kcal). The breakdown of muscle protein and degradation of the resulting non-nitrogen residue of amino acid becomes the source of energy when carbohydrate and fat are not available. This occurs in starvation or serious malnutrition when the tissue proteins become

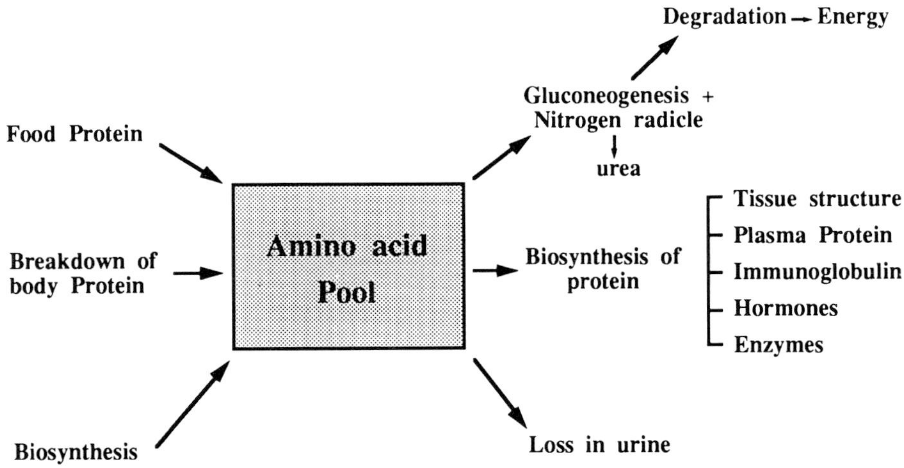

FIGURE 5.2. Diagram to illustrate the metabolism of protein and the amino-acid pool.

catabolised irreversibly with loss of the nitrogen radicle in the urine. The sequence of events in such a situation is:

(a) The breakdown of proteins from the muscle mass produces amino acids which enter the amino-acid pool. The pool is normally, to a great extent, replenished from ingested protein. It is topped up to a lesser extent by biosynthesis (transamination and reamination processes) from non-nitrogenous compounds and through tissue protein catabolism. There is constant change in the amino-acid pool, that is, the pool receives and disposes of amino acids (Fig. 5.2).

(b) In times of need the amino-acid pool contributes to the caloric requirement by a deamination process with production of carbohydrate and ketones which can be used as energy sources. The nitrogen radicle participates in the synthesis of essential cell constituents but is also excreted in the urine, particularly when the non-nitrogenous residues are to be metabolised and used as energy source, i.e. in calorie malnutrition.

There is a state of dynamic equilibrium in the body with respect to the amino-acid pool, this means a balance between the degradation (catabolism) and synthesis (anabolism). This state of equilibrium may be roughly gauged by a ratio between the protein intake expressed as nitrogen (1 gram of nitrogen representing 6.25 grams of protein) and nitrogen output in the urine (normally only small amounts of nitrogen compounds are excreted in the faeces).

(c) When the diet is deficient in energy and/or protein, there is proportionately a higher level of outgoing from the amino-acid pool and a greater need for deamination of the amino acid in order to provide non-nitrogenous compound for use as energy source. The 'surplus' and somewhat redundant nitrogen radicle is eliminated in the urine.

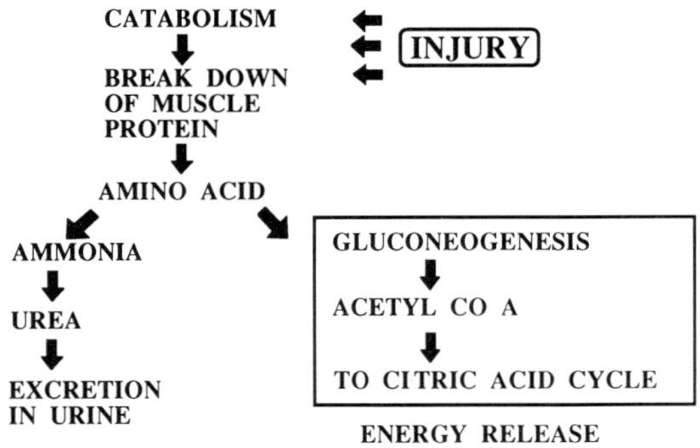

FIGURE 5.3. The influence of injury on protein catabolism.

2.4. Nitrogenous equilibrium

When the nitrogen intake in the food over a period equals the nitrogen output in the urine the individual is said to be in nitrogen balance or in a state of nitrogenous equilibrium. In the normal steady state of metabolism, when calorie and protein provisions are sufficient for metabolic activities, there is no need for the body to withdraw from the amino-acid pool, for biosynthesis of tissue constituents, or for deamination and degradation of non-nitrogenous residue for use as energy. In calorie and protein malnutrition the equilibrium is disturbed, and for the reasons given above there is then a higher nitrogen output than nitrogen intake. The nitrogen balance will therefore become negative. Conversely when intake is over and above the output the individual is in positive nitrogen balance. Nitrogen balance study is one objective way of assessing the state of nutritional intake and gauging the stability of the calorie and protein metabolism.

3. METABOLIC RESPONSE TO TRAUMA, INJURY AND SURGICAL OPERATIONS

Metabolic response to trauma and injury centres around protein turnover which is required to accomplish repair of a wound and recovery from the injury and infection. After serious trauma there is considerable demand on energy and especially on the body's protein. This demand is greater when the intake is deficient, in which case the muscle protein reserves have to be relied upon to provide the metabolic requirement of energy and protein. This results in wasting, loss of weight and a negative nitrogen balance (Fig. 5.3). In individuals with pre-existing malnutrition further strain is placed upon energy and protein reserves of the body.

Metabolic response to major surgical operation is not different from that observed after traumatic injury. Both the magnitude and duration of catabolism parallel the seriousness or extent of the operation. However a major surgical operation affects the metabolism in a number of additional ways:

- For some days after operation, particularly when related to the alimentary tract, the patient does not ingest or cannot absorb nutrients. In this situation there is effectively a state of relative starvation.
- In cases of complication, such as infection, there is yet further metabolic demand and increased catabolism.
- In many patients with malignancy there is preoperative nutritional deficiency.

The metabolic response of a malnourished patient to operation differs from that of one who is well nourished. The malnourished person has already had to make demands on his reserves of energy and proteins and therefore the catabolic effect of an operation, super-imposed onto the effects of malnutrition, will have a greater impact in the depletion of the patient's reserve. Under such circumstances the risk of postoperative complications is much greater. Malnutrition adversely affects the healing of the wound and the resistance to infection[2,3]. It is clear therefore that 'metabolic' care[4] should be an integral part of the overall care of patients undergoing major surgical operation. The corollary of this is that in the period of high metabolic demand nutritional support is mandatory in order to steer the disturbed metabolism back to its normal course. It is important to note that although Moore[4] suggested that postoperative catabolism is an obligatory phenomenon, the negative nitrogen balance can be reversed when the patient is provided with intravenous calorie and amino-acid supplement as has been shown by many, including ourselves, in oesophageal surgical patients[5].

4. NUTRITIONAL MANAGEMENT OF THORACIC SURGICAL PATIENTS

The basic principles of metabolism and nutritional care of patients undergoing thoracic (and oesophageal) surgery do not differ from those having other major surgical operations. In response to the trauma of operation there is an increase in the urinary output of nitrogen reflecting the enhanced catabolism which reaches its peak on the 4–5th postoperative day[5] (Figs. 5.4a,b). Nevertheless there are areas of management which require more specific consideration. These relate to:

- Evaluation of nutritional status by indices most relevant to thoracic surgical patients.
- Planning a dietary scheme suitable to such cases.
- Appropriate delivery route and access.
- Monitoring the progress of artificial feeding and prevention of complications.

4.1. Evaluation of nutritional status in thoracic surgical patients

Most clinicians recognise a severely malnourished individual in the course of simple clinical examination by such findings as oedema, scaling of the skin and decubitus. One has no difficulty in acknowledging the 'cachectic look' of the patient shown in

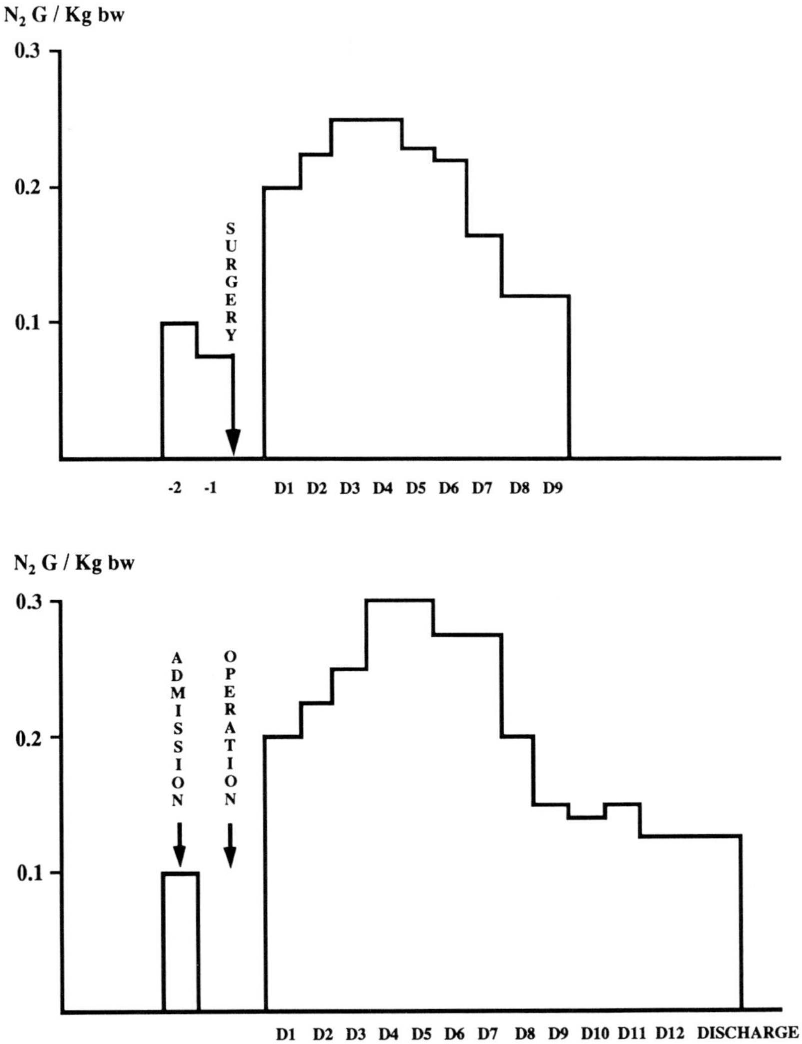

FIGURE 5.4. Mean nitrogen output of (top) 8 patients undergoing major pulmonary operation and (bottom) 10 patients undergoing trans-thoracic oesophagectomy.

Fig. 5.5 and in establishing that the patient is clinically grossly undernourished. It is important though to be able to quantify the degree of calorie–protein malnutrition by objective criteria. There are a battery of anthropometric, biochemical and other laboratory tests which can identify clinical and sub-clinical malnutrition (Table 5.1). However it is relevant to note that: (a) The majority of thoracic surgical patients (except oesophageal neoplastic cases) need simple screening tests and a minority

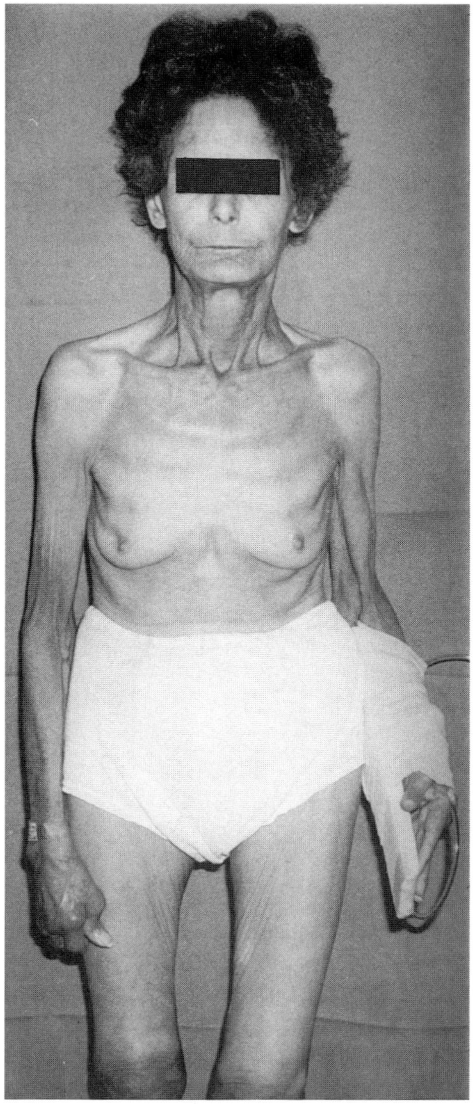

FIGURE 5.5. Patient suffering from extensive tumour involving left main bronchus and oesophagus with marked loss of weight and obvious malnutrition.

may require more elaborate testing to gauge the existence and severity of their nutritional deficiency with a view to corrective measures. (b) Experience shows that only a few selected 'tests' from the existing range of nutritional indicators will have significant relevance in thoracic surgical patients. In short, both the patient and the

TABLE 5.1
Commonly used indicators for assessment of nutritional status

- Percentage of ideal weight
- Weight loss and percentage weight change
- Anthropometric: mid arm circumference (cm) and triceps skin fold thickness (mm)
- Serum albumin
- Serum protein
- Serum Transferrin
- Creatinine/Height index
- Cell-mediated immunity (skin tests to recall antigens)
- Delayed hypersensitivity
- Lymphocyte count
- Nitrogen balance

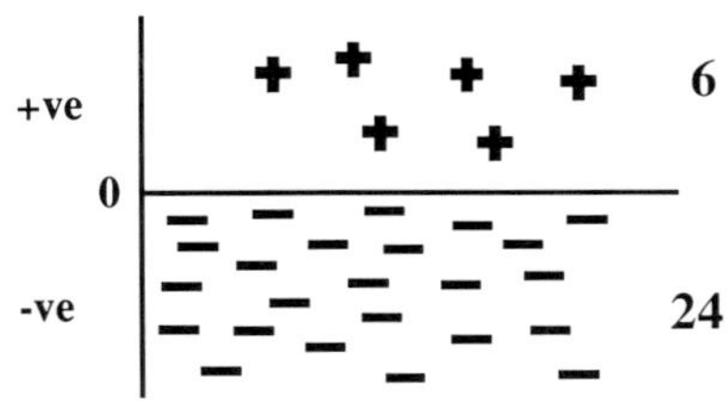

FIGURE 5.6. Nitrogen balance study in 30 patients with extensive bronchial carcinoma: 24 patients were in negative nitrogen balance on admission and there was a 90% correlation between nitrogen balance and the general condition of the patient, scored by 2 independent observers, and the patient's weight loss.

test will have to be selected if time and resources are to be efficiently used. *Screening tests* rely on subjective data obtained by simply interviewing the patient. The history of the illness, pattern of food ingestion, bowel action and weight over the illness period are preliminary indicators. A further simple step would be objective and somewhat quantitative data of the patient's weight, assessed as a percentage of the ideal weight for height and sex, weight loss over a period, and percentual weight loss, expressed as

$$\frac{\text{Weight loss in kg} \times 100}{\text{Usual weight in kg}}.$$

Experience shows that in thoracic and oesophageal surgical patients suffering from malignancies, the extent of dissemination of the tumour correlates closely with general condition (judged by an experienced clinician), loss of weight and nitrogen balance. This is illustrated in Fig. 5.6 and Table 5.2.

TABLE 5.2
Nutritional assessment of 16 patients with oesophageal cancer[a]

ID	%IW	%WL	ST	TSF	MaC	DP	N	Cond
1	72	37.5	+ +	32%	28%	IV	–	Poor
2	81	22.0	– –	60%	84%	IV	–	Poor
3	70	30.0	– –	66%	75%	IV	–	Poor
4	80	13.0	– –	72%	93%	II	+	Fair
5	81	35.0	– –	48%	68%	III	–	Poor
6	85	12.5	– –	85%	91%	III	–	Poor
7	80	13.3	+ –	90%	90%	II	+	Fair
8	80	13.5	– –	45%	85%	II	+	Fair
9	74	15.7	– –	51%	75%	IV	–	Poor
10	73	15.0	+ +	42%	76%	IV	–	Poor
11	59	23.0	+ +	21%	65%	IV	–	Very poor
12	76	30.0	– –	28%	78%	IV	–	Very poor
13	79	12.9	+ –	40%	78%	III–IV	–	Poor
14	60	24.0	+ –	80%	80%	III–IV	–	Poor
15	80	12.0	+ –	40%	71%	III	–	Poor
16	76	45.0	– –		63%	IV	–	Very poor

[a] Abbreviations: ID, patient; %IW, percentage of ideal weight; %WL, percentage weight loss; ST, skin test; TSF, triceps skin fold; MaC, Mid-arm circumference; DP, Dysphagia (see below); N, Nitrogen balance; Cond, General condition.
Dysphagia Grade I–IV, Moghissi K. 1977. I, dysphagia to solid; IV, total dysphagia.

The incidence and the scale of preoperative calorie and protein malnutrition in thoracic surgical patients vary both with respect to the disease and the primary target organ. As may be expected, an obstructive neoplasm of the oesophagus will affect the nutrition and metabolism of the patient in more than one way, whereas an early pulmonary tumour may have negligible metabolic consequences easily compensated by the patient's reserve.

For practical purposes patients who on screening tests are below the normal standard will need to be tested further and the scale of their deficiencies assessed against normal values (Table 5.3 [7,8,9]).

4.2. Planning a nutritional scheme

In planning a nutritional regimen, two important principles will have to be considered: (1) quantitative aspect; (2) composition of the regimen. The quantitative aspect is concerned with the amount of calorie, protein and other essential requirements of diet in specific situations making allowance for:

- basic requirements of a healthy active individual,
- pre-existing nutritional deficiencies,

TABLE 5.3
Indices of calorie and protein malnutrition

Quantity	Index
Weight	$< 60\%$ of ideal
Weight loss (percentual weight change)	$> 10\%$
Triceps skin-fold	< 10 mm in males; < 13 mm in females
Mid-arm circumference	< 23.0 cm in males; < 22.0 cm in females
Serum albumin	< 35 g/l
Serum protein	< 60 g/l
Serum transferrin	< 1.5 g/l
Cell-mediated immunity (skin test to antigens)	Candida skin tests negative and tuberculin skin tests negative
Lymphocyte count	$< 1500/10^{-6}$
Nitrogen balance	negative

TABLE 5.4
Energy and nitrogen requirements for the achievement of nitrogen balance

Nitrogen requirement (g/kg)	Energy requirement (kcal/kg)	Reference
0.20	35	Abbott et al.[10]
0.24	32	Van Larsen and Brockner[11]
0.23	45	Tweedle and Johnston[12]
0.20–0.25	40–45	Moghissi and Teasdale[5]

- catabolism of the operative trauma and the immediate postoperative phase,
- catabolic cost of any serious postoperative complications.

The metabolic requirement of energy recommended for an adult is suggested by Passmore[6] to be 1400 kcal/day for a female and 1700 kcal/day for a male. The recommended daily requirement of energy and protein for adult males in the United Kingdom (by DHSS 1979) is 2150–3350 kcal/day for energy and 54–84 g of protein respectively. For females it is 1680–2500 kcal/day and 42–62 g of protein. The lower ranges are for sedentary individuals and the higher levels for the very active. The daily requirement of a hospital patient is approximately 30 kcal/kg/bw and 0.9 gram protein/kg/bw (or about 0.15 g nitrogen/kg/bw/day). In an uncomplicated major operation the requirement can be considerably higher (Table 5.4), and higher still when complications occur, depending on the level of hyper-catabolism. It is important to have an appropriate ratio of energy to nitrogen allowance. This is suggested to be 150–200 kcal of energy for one gram of nitrogen (Table 5.4)[5,10–12]. The composition of a regimen has to consider the body's needs of:

- energy (calorie),
- protein (nitrogen),
- water,
- electrolytes, minerals,

– non-electrolyte elements (trace elements),
– vitamins.

Composition of a diet must also take into account the quantity and balanced proportion of each constituent of the diet.

4.3. Method of supply – Route of delivery

Total or partial nutritional support can be delivered to patients either by parenteral or enteral routes. The two methods can however be utilised individually, in concert, or sequentially. In practice the parenteral route utilizes the intravenous channel of delivery, when the enteral route is unusable or deficient, to permit ingestion or absorption of food totally or partially adequate to the level of the individual's needs.

In the absence of pre-existing malnutrition the indications for I.V. feeding in an uncomplicated thoracic surgical operation which does not involve the alimentary tract is at least questionable, and in our view is undesirable. This is because, firstly, patients needing such operations are not generally nutritionally deficient. Secondly, in the absence of pre-existing deficiencies or postoperative complications a short spell of surgical catabolism can be covered more than adequately by normal food intake of a high calorie–protein diet postoperatively. The important point is however to assess the patient's nutrition and to adequately compensate for any unexpected complication such as postoperative infection, with its metabolic (catabolic) cost.

Many patients with oesophageal conditions undergoing major resection and reconstruction do require a period of parenteral feeding for at least a few days postoperatively. When there is pre-existing deficiency there is also need for preoperative parenteral nutrition if there is a high grade of dysphagia. Patients in a hyper-catabolic state (e.g. oesophageal rupture) and those with severe postoperative complications (e.g. fistulae, pleuro-pulmonary and mediastinal infection) need more prolonged postoperative I.V. nutritional supply.

There are a variety of techniques to establish I.V. feeding, and the method of access depends on the experience of the team and the individual case [13–16]. It is important however to point out that peripheral lines are unsuitable for parenteral feeding in chest surgery patients, since most patients who need I.V. nutrition require it for more than a short period of a few days and therefore a central venous catheter placement is required. Also, an I.V. infusion catheter placed in a peripheral (limb) vein severely interferes with the patients mobility. In thoracic surgical patients this is often already curtailed because of the presence of intercostal tubes connected to an underwater sealed drainage system. The most suitable central vein is the superior vena cava (or right atrium) which can be approached via a percutaneous sub-clavian or cut-down external jugular vein [14,16].

In both instances it is mandatory to ensure absolute sterility of the catheter and the equipment used for placement of the catheter in order to prevent sepsis. Provision of a subcutaneous tunnel for a short length of the catheter between the point of entry to the vein and its entry through the skin is an added measure to

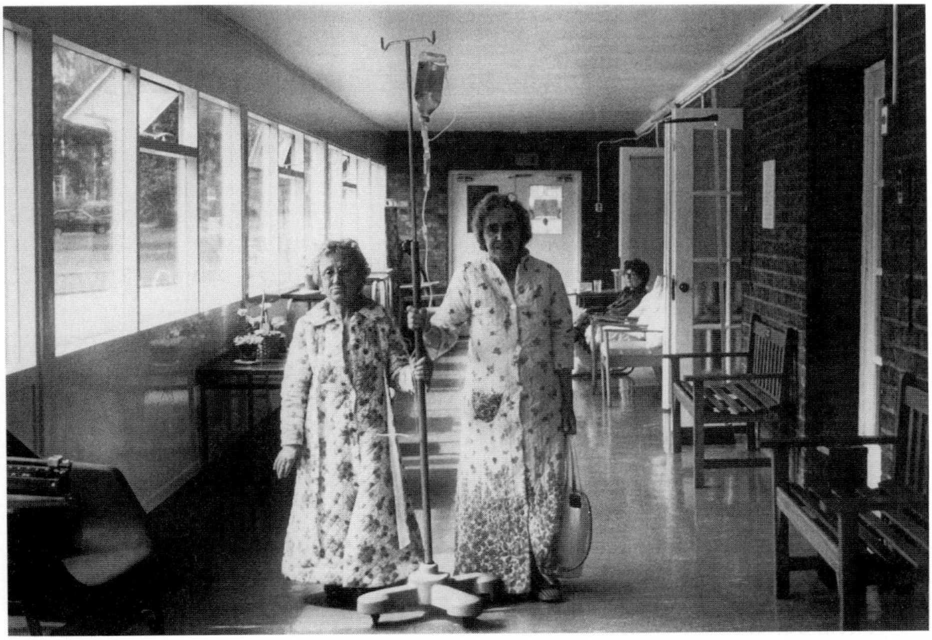

FIGURE 5.7. Patient receiving parenteral nutrition, with chest drain in situ, whilst remaining mobile.

discourage contamination of the catheter at the site of its entry into the vein, as well as being added security towards its remaining safely in place. Fig. 5.7 shows a patient after major thoracic operation receiving supplementary parenteral support whilst still retaining her mobility with the intercostal tube drain in situ.

Enteral nutrition employs the patient's alimentary tract in situations where food or simpler elemental diet can be normally absorbed but ingestion of food by mouth cannot meet full metabolic needs. The simplicity of the method is attractive and accounts for its popularity. It is particularly suitable for many general thoracic surgical patients who may require nutritional support. The commonest routes of access for delivery in enteral feeding are:
- fine-tube naso-gastric,
- gastrostomy (standard or fine tube), and
- fine-tube jejunostomy.

Each of the access methods for enteral feeding has advantages and disadvantages. We do not favour naso-gastric tube feeding since: (a) Many thoracic surgical patients need physiotherapy (breathing, coughing and expectoration exercises); this may either displace the tube or the tube may hamper expectoration. (b) Even the smallest of tubes creates additional secretion and irritation of the oro-pharynx and many cause gastro-oesophageal reflux and oesophagitis. In patients requiring long-term nutritional support, particularly those in whom laparotomy has to be performed, gastrostomy/jejunostomy is preferable.

5. PRACTICAL ASPECTS OF PERIOPERATIVE NUTRITIONAL MANAGEMENT OF THORACIC SURGICAL PATIENTS

Since the functional activities of the body generally, and the regulation of disturbed processes after injury (operation) specifically, are dependent on metabolism, and since the metabolism itself is dependent on energy and the supply of nutrients, nutritional management will have to be considered as an integral part of patient care. This involves the preoperative and immediate and late postoperative periods. It is the author's belief that the terminology 'perioperative' is particularly apt since it refers to the various phases of patients' management before and around the time of operation. It is also more appropriate since it refers to the involvement in the total management of the patient. In this context the nutritional status of every patient who is a candidate for thoracic surgical operation should be evaluated on admission. The questions thereafter should be:

- Which patient requires nutritional support?
- At what stage should this support be given?
- What type of regimen is needed to satisfy the patient's needs, and by what route can the regimen best be provided?

5.1. Which patient requires nutritional support?

As a rule any patient who cannot ingest or absorb nutrients to the level of his metabolic needs will require nutritional support. In disease situations and in the case of a candidate for a major thoracic surgical operation the criteria have to be extended further to include those who by reason of their disease suffer considerable losses of calorie and protein because of postoperative complications and hypercatabolism, and cannot therefore maintain energy and nitrogen equilibrium. The above criteria apply to:

- patients with extensive thoracic neoplasms, particularly but not exclusively of the upper alimentary tract,
- patients with intrathoracic suppuration,
- those with severe postoperative sepsis,
- those with extensive thoracic trauma.

In all of these patients there is frequently an imbalance between food intake and metabolic requirements.

5.2. At what stage should nutritional support commence?

The time to commence nutritional support is when it is considered that food intake cannot cover the patient's requirements of calories and protein. The requirement is assessed from the level of energy expenditure related to metabolic activity and nutritional deficit at the time of assessment. Only a small percentage of thoracic surgical patients need artificial nutritional support preoperatively. Many more need high calorie and protein food intake and the monitoring of nutrition by simple food intake chart and calculation by a dietician of calorie–protein values for a 24 hour intake. Many patients with advanced cancer of the oesophagus and those with suppuration and fistula will require preoperative support via enteral/parenteral routes [2,5,17]. Postoperatively all those undergoing resection and reconstruction of the oesophagus will require a period of parenteral or enteral feeding. Many more patients will require supplementary 'artificial feeding' and support if, by reason of complication, there is an extended catabolic phase.

5.3. What type of regimen and what route of delivery of nutrients?

In planning a nutritional programme for a thoracic surgical patient, both the level of calorie and the composition of the regime need to be considered. It is also important to take into account the ratio of various energy providers in order to achieve a balanced diet. The design of a well-balanced regimen is closely connected with the condition of the patient, the type of operation and the route of delivery of the nutrients. In short, in many cases the choice of treatment, the nutritional regimen and the route of delivery of the nutrients are inter-related. It is therefore important to include the nutritional team in decision-making discussions related to any treatment under consideration.

Experience shows that nutritional requirements for a thoracic surgical patient in a hyper-catabolic state cannot be totally satisfied by an enteral method of feeding. This is even more the case when the alimentary tract is affected by disease or injury. In formulating a nutritional regimen and its route of delivery in a thoracic surgical patient, consideration should be given not only to the principles discussed previously concerning the quantitative aspects and content but also to:

- The importance of caloric density (the amount of calorie/volume of fluid), since overloading with fluid may create serious problems.
- The route of delivery (venous access or upper alimentary tract access).
- The osmolality of the nutrient solution (be it for parenteral or enteral feeding).

In complicated thoracic surgical operations the nutritional scheme, including the method of delivery of nutrient postoperatively, should be incorporated within the plan of operation. In any operation involving the oesophagus, especially those concerned with complicated reconstruction, it is advisable to plan an enteral delivery option which can be utilised postoperatively (Figs. 5.8a,b).

As previously referred to, many thoracic surgical patients may have no need for artificial nutritional support and undergo uncomplicated surgical operation necessitating no more than 24 hours fasting. During this time they receive blood transfusion and a 'low-calorie' (dextrose and saline) solution. Thereafter they have light diet followed by normal food intake. A number of thoracic surgical patients however may be nutritionally deficient on admission. Some others may

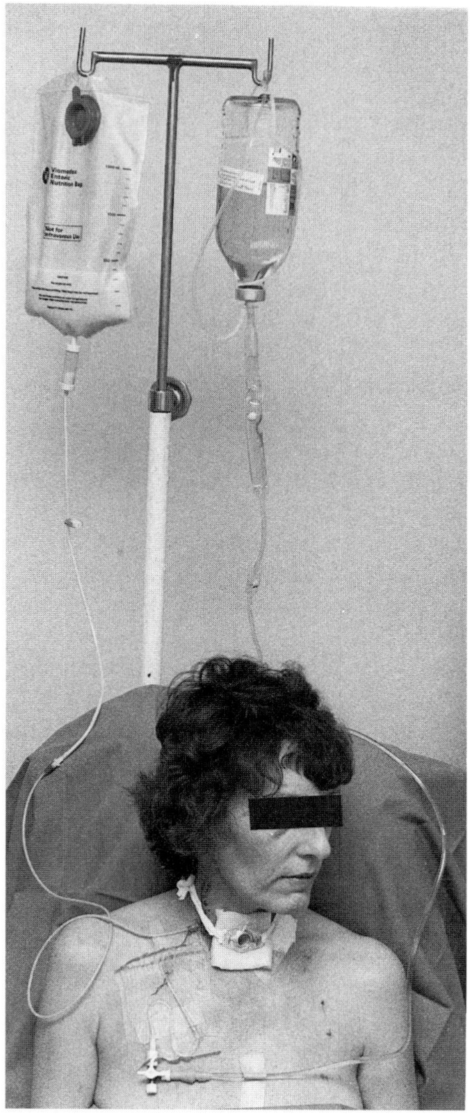

FIGURE 5.8a. A patient with extensive tracheo-oesophageal reconstruction receiving parenteral nutrition through a cut-down external jugular vein with subcutaneous tunnelling through the chest wall, and enteral nutrition through a fine-tube cervical gastrostomy.

have operations which involve their alimentary tract. Yet a third category may be classed as hyper-catabolic. These and a number who develop intractable postoperative septic complications will require to be considered for nutritional

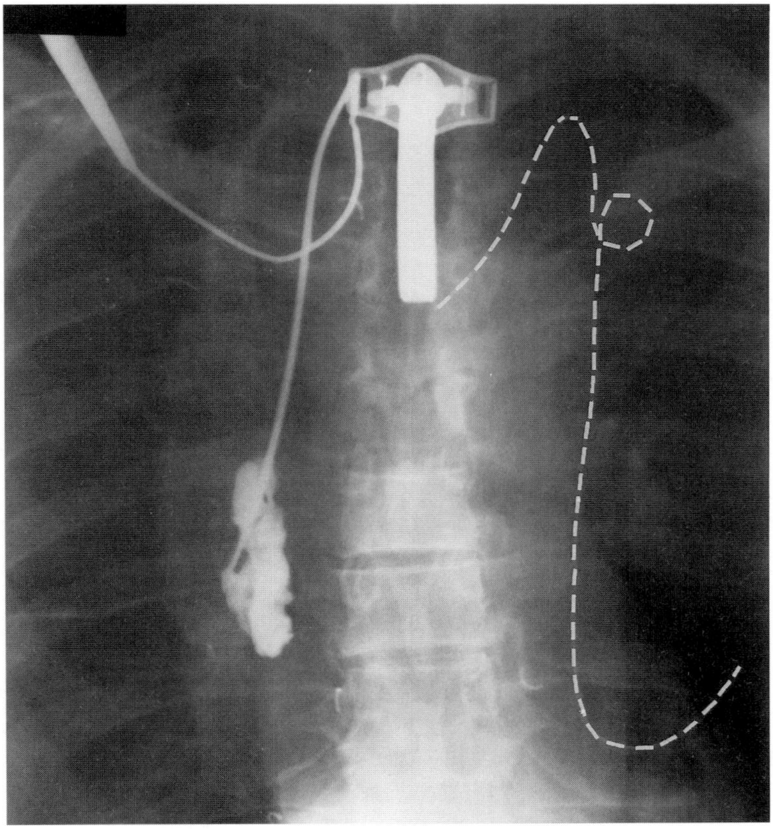

FIGURE 5.8b. Radiograph demonstrating intravenous catheter and fine-tube cervical gastrostomy in situ in a patient as shown in Fig. 5.8a.

support. Our experience shows that patients undergoing complicated thoracic surgical operations who require nutritional planning fall grosso modo into four categories illustrated below by four typical cases:

5.3.1. Case 1. Lung cancer presenting as a pulmonary abscess and empyema, treated by pleuro-pneumonectomy

Patient HD: A man of 56 was admitted to hospital on 7th June 1990 with a febrile illness, cough, copious purulent sputum, anorexia and loss of weight. His chest radiograph showed an opacity in the left lung, pulmonary collapse and pleural fluid. He was originally treated with antibiotics and repeated chest aspiration during which time he continued to lose weight. In spite of treatment he deteriorated and lost a total of 15% of his usual weight. He was referred to the surgical department where his chest was drained and further investigated. A diagnosis

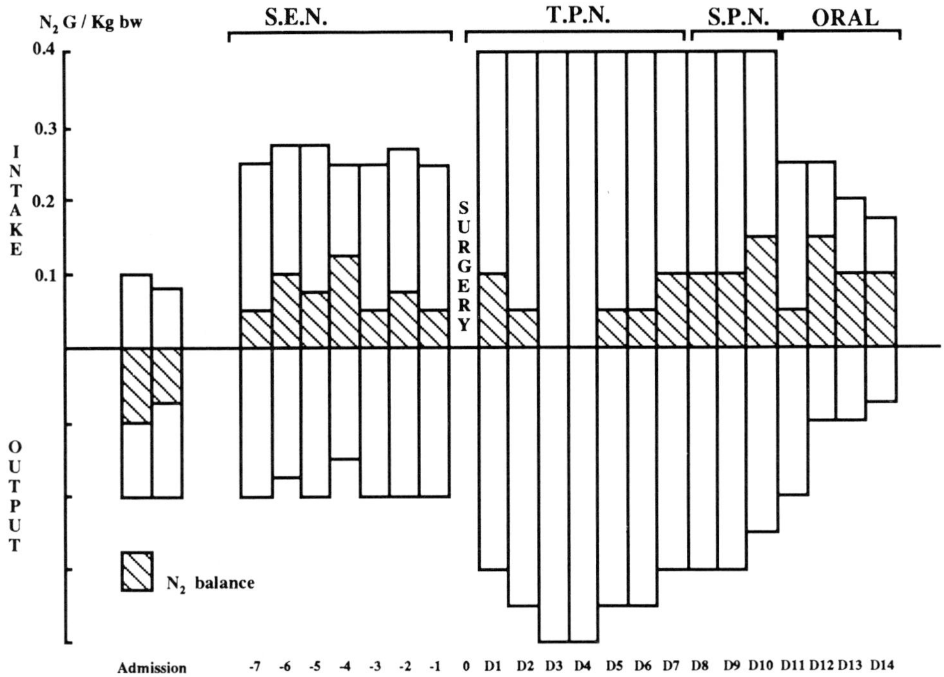

FIGURE 5.9. Nitrogen balance study of patient HD. S.E.N., supplementary enteral nutrition; T.P.N., total parenteral nutrition; S.P.N., supplementary parenteral nutrition.

of carcinoma of the lung, lung abscess and pleural empyema was established. Nutritional assessment at this time showed low blood albumin and anthropometric measurement and negative nitrogen balance. The patient was prepared for thoracotomy and his nutritional intake was supplemented by enteral feeding (fine-tube nasogastric tube). One week later, on 7th July 1990, a pleuropneumonectomy was carried out when the lung containing the tumour and empyema cavity was excised. A temporary elective tracheostomy was also fashioned because of his borderline respiratory function and the presence of copious secretions up to the time of operation. Postoperatively he required ventilatory support for 4 days and he received total and supplementary parenteral nutrition for 10 days, after which time he resumed normal diet. He was discharged on 24th July 1990 when his wound had healed satisfactorily, his tracheostomy was closed and he was fully mobile. Nutritional scheme and nitrogen balance study of this patient is shown in Fig. 5.9. This case illustrates the use of preoperative enteral nutritional support resulting in sufficient improvement in the patient's general condition to allow him to undergo major resectional surgery. The catabolism of surgical trauma

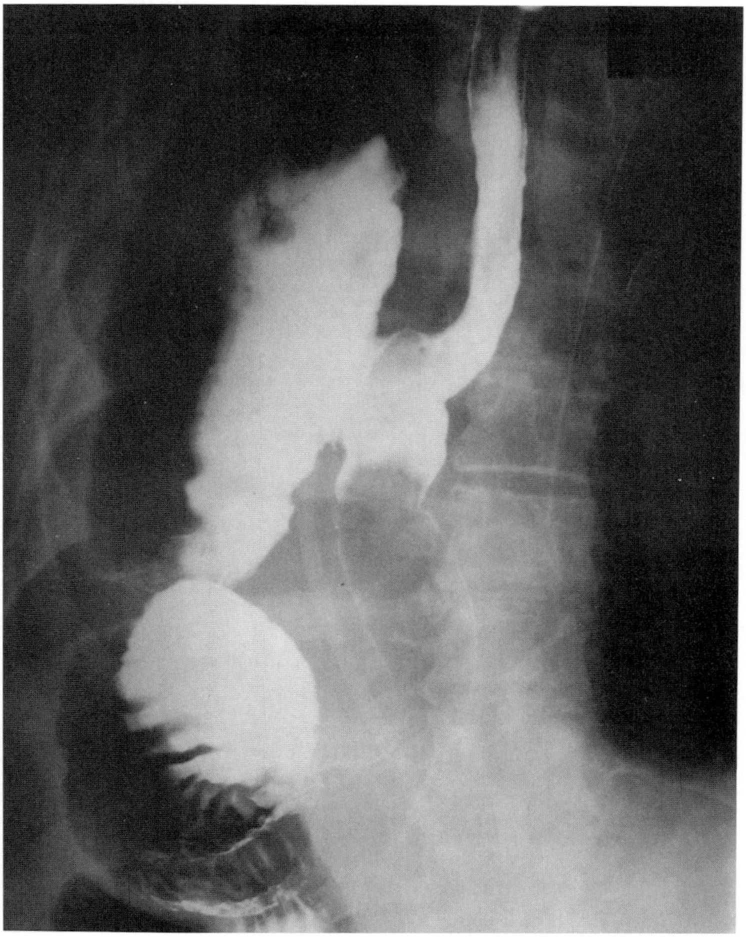

FIGURE 5.10. Oesophagogram of patient RH, clearly demonstrating the entry of barium into the pleural space.

and the assisted ventilation necessitated postoperative nutritional support with satisfactory outcome.

5.3.2. Case 2. Late post-pneumonectomy oesophago-pleural (pneumonectomy space) fistula, treated by oesophageal by-pass operation

Patient RH: A 66-year old man had a left pneumonectomy for bronchial carcinoma in 1982, after which his recovery was uneventful. Early in 1987 he presented with symptoms of infection, loss of weight and dysphagia. Investigations at this time found no evidence of tumour recurrence or metastases, but demonstrated

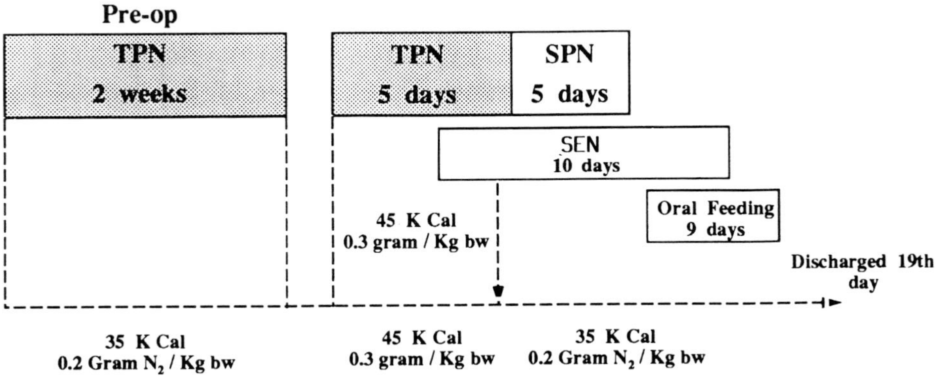

FIGURE 5.11. Nutritional scheme of patient RH. TPN, total parenteral nutrition; SPN, supplementary parenteral nutrition; SEN, supplementary enteral nutrition.

an oesophago-left-pleural fistula (Fig. 5.10). By this time he had lost 12% of his usual weight and was in negative nitrogen balance. It was decided to offer him an oesophageal by-pass operation after clearing of his pleural empyema and improvement in his general and nutritional state. Preoperative preparation lasted 2 weeks during which time he received total parenteral nutrition, using the superior vena cava via access through an external jugular vein cut-down technique. The operation was carried out using upper abdominal and neck incisions. The gastro-oesophageal junction was stapled and severed below the hiatus, a gastric tube was prepared and passed iso-peristaltically and sub-sternally to the left side of the neck. The oesophagus was then stapled and severed proximally to the suture line at the root of the neck. An end-to-side oesophago-gastric anastomosis was performed thus establishing the continuity of the alimentary tract (leaving the isolated oesophagus in situ). A fine tube cervical gastrotomy [15] (below the oesophago-gastric anastomosis) at the root of the neck was also established. Postoperatively the nutritional scheme was as shown in Fig. 5.11. The empyema was cleared by lavage with a disinfectant solution and the patient recovered completely and was discharged 19 days after operation eating normal consistency food. Figs. 5.12a,b show barium swallow a few days prior to discharge.

5.3.3. Case 3. Multiple injuries including the chest and ruptured diaphragm

Patient JP: A woman of 45 years was involved in a road traffic accident in consequence of which she received multiple skeletal and chest injuries. The latter consisted of multiple rib fractures on both sides, contusion and laceration of the left lung and rupture of the left dome of the diaphragm. On admission she required resuscitative measures, chest drainage and positive pressure ventilation. Twelve hours later she was fit to undergo thoracotomy, repair of lacerated lung and repair of ruptured diaphragm. She also had a tracheostomy and fine-tube

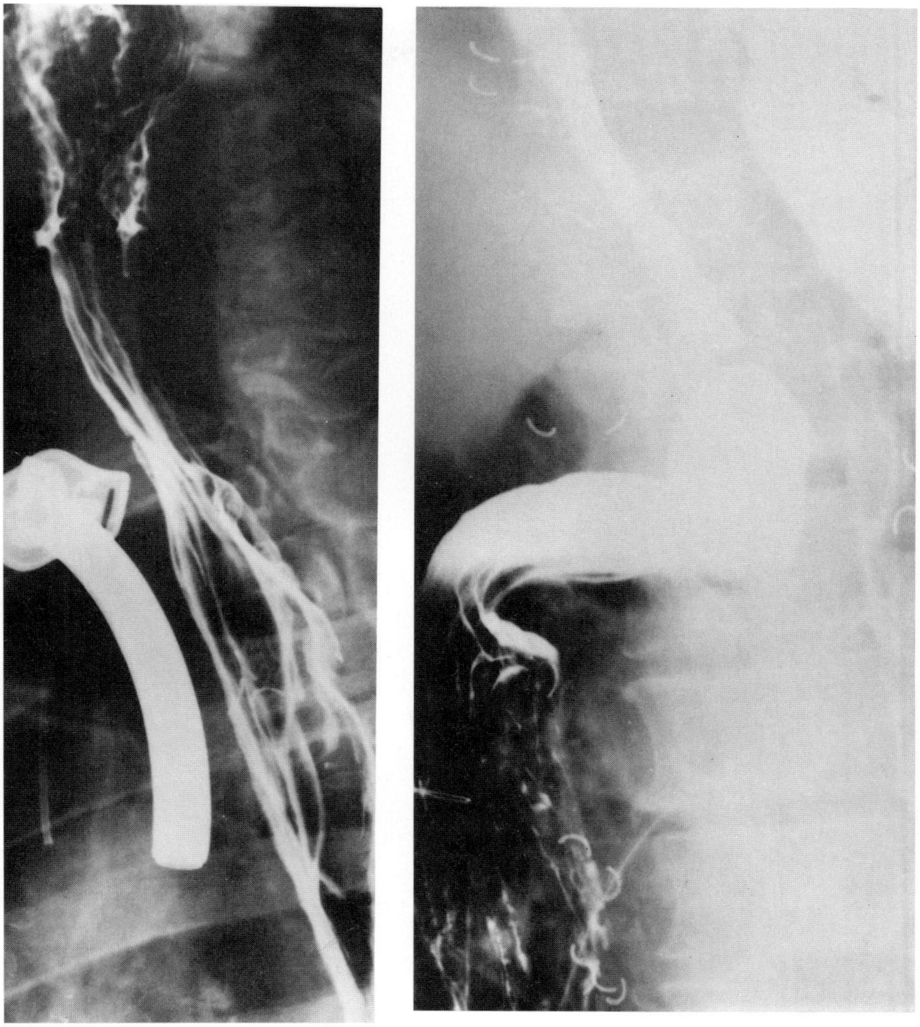

FIGURE 5.12. Contrast studies of patient RH, following oesophageal bypass operation, confirming satisfactory passage of barium.

gastrostomy. During the first week she was unconscious, and developed ileus. Nitrogen excretion on the first 2 days post-accident was 0.30 and 0.35 g/kg of bodyweight of the patient. On the third post-injury day the patient was given TPN to the value of 50–55 kcal/kg of body weight and 0.3 g of nitrogen/kg of body weight for one week. Thereafter enteral feeding via fine-tube gastrostomy was supported by supplementary parenteral nutrition 40 kcal/kg of body weight and 0.20 g of nitrogen/kg of body weight which was maintained for another week, after which

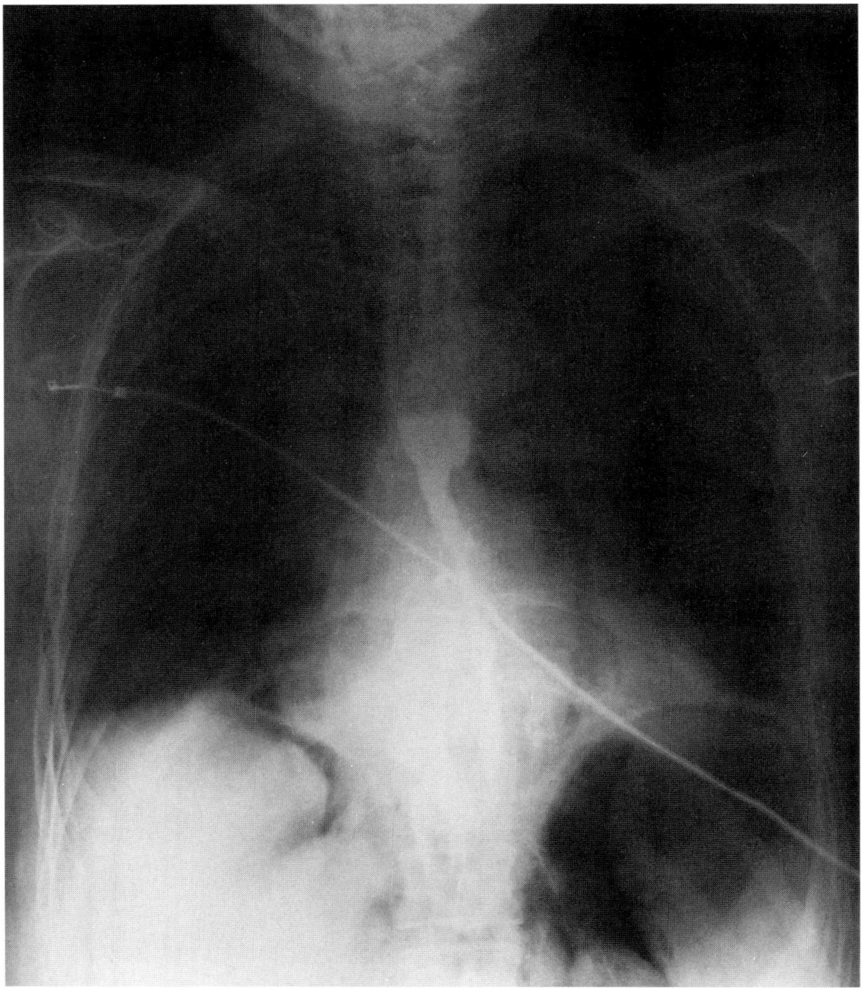

FIGURE 5.13a. Oesophagogram of the patient of case 4, with oesophageal stricture and perforation with leak of contrast medium into the mediastinum and right pleural space, and air in the peritoneum.

time feeding continued first via a fine-tube gastrostomy and oral nutrition until, by one month post accident, the patient was eating normally for her requirements and was transferred into the care of the orthopaedic surgeons.

5.3.4. Case 4. Instrumental perforation of the thoracic oesophagus, mediastinitis and empyema

A 58 year old woman had been known to have chronic benign oesophageal stricture which had been dilated several times previously. At the last occasion 4 days

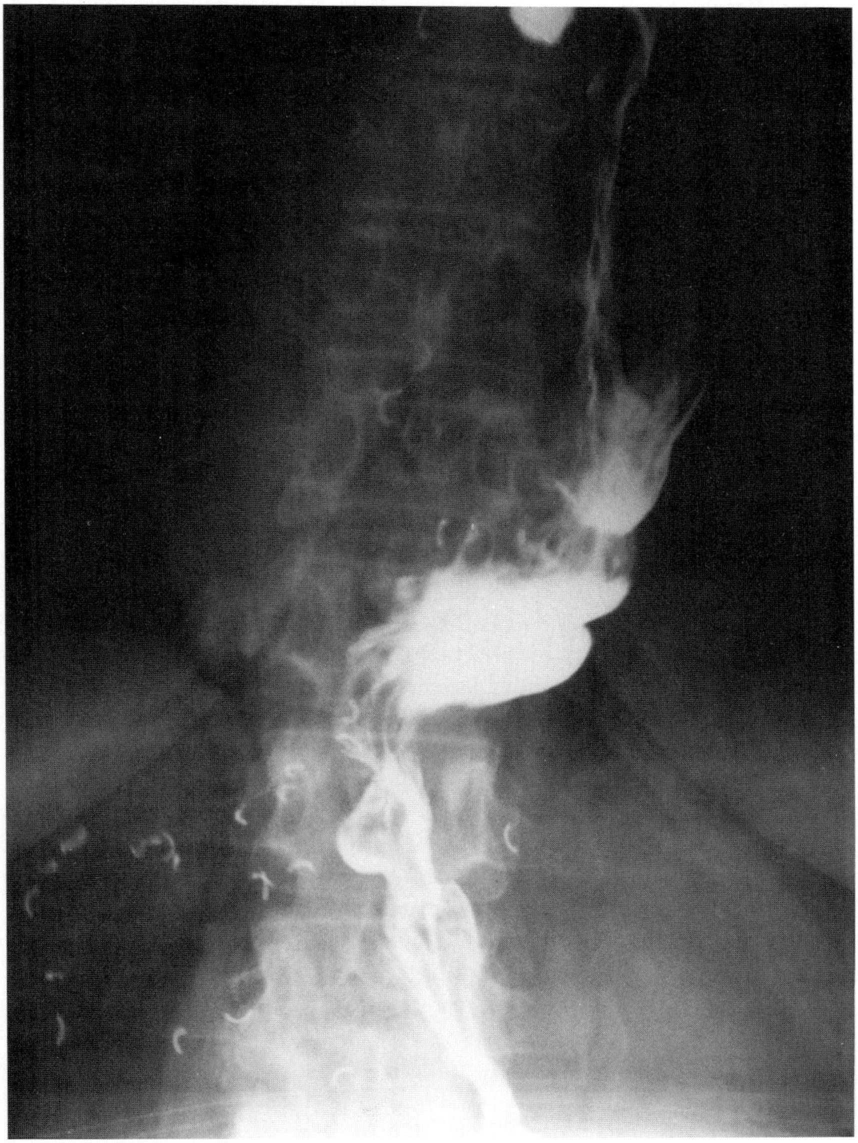

FIGURE 5.13b. Postoperative contrast study of the same patient as in Fig. 5.13a, after oesophageal resection and reconstruction prior to the patient's discharge from hospital.

previously she had oesophagoscopy and dilatation of the oesophageal stricture. Soon after she had pain but was given fluid and soft food which aggravated it. During the next 3 days she had practically no food by mouth but did have some

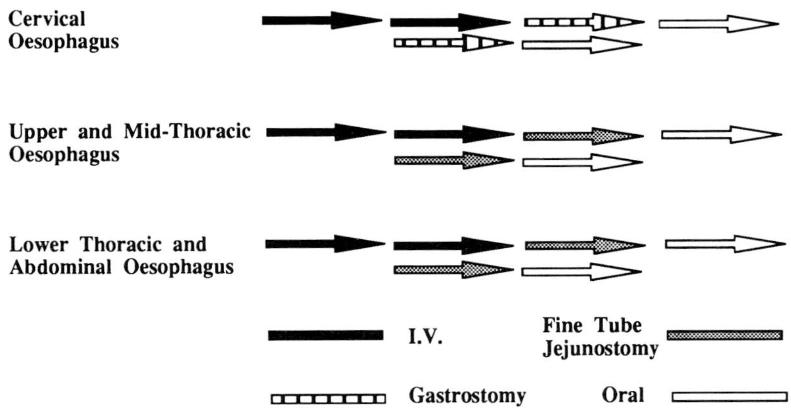

FIGURE 5.14. Nutritional management for a patient with perforations of the oesophagus.

fluid to drink. She remained febrile, in spite of antibiotic administration, and became dehydrated. She was referred to the surgical department and on emergency admission was shown to have oesophageal perforation above a stricture with mediastinitis and pyo-pneumothorax (Fig. 5.13a). The right chest was first drained to relieve the tension pyo-pneumothorax. A partial thoracic oesophagectomy was then carried out through an upper laparotomy and separate right thoracotomy. The oesophagus bearing the perforation and the stricture was resected and the alimentary tract reconstructed by residual oesophago-gastric anastomosis above the azygos vein. Also pulmonary decortication had to be performed. Prior to operation parenteral nutrition commenced (50 kcal/kg of body weight and 0.3 g of nitrogen/kg of body weight), via the external jugular vein into the superior vena cava. At operation a fine-tube jejunostomy was established. The nutritional management followed the scheme shown in Fig. 5.14, with step I, TPN going for 10 days; step II, SPN plus fine-tube jejunostomy feeding for 5 days; step III, fine-tube jejunostomy feeding plus oral intake for 5 days; and finally oral feeding for 5 days. The patient was discharged 22 days later with wounds healed, fine-tube jejunostomy extirpated and eating well (Fig. 5.13b). It is no exaggeration to state that nowhere in thoracic surgery is there a greater need for nutritional planning than in cases of thoracic oesophageal perforation particularly in its late presentation. The treatment of perforation cannot be dissociated from nutritional management and the two should be considered together. Recent experience has shown that aggressive surgical treatment will have to be undertaken in order to reduce the high mortality which is associated with oesophageal perforation in its late presentation. In these cases nutritional planning is crucial since besides the catabolism of the trauma, sepsis, surgical intervention and loss of protein-rich fluid, there is also the problem of the inability to ingest food. Experience based on nutritional study of oesophageal perforation shows that:

(1) There is a considerable metabolic disturbance and catabolism associated with perforated oesophageal cases as judged by an enormous nitrogen loss in the urine.
(2) In late presentation cases both pre- and postoperatively, there is a need for total parenteral nutrition, containing high calorie 55–60 kcal/kg of body weight and 0.35–0.40 g of nitrogen/kg of body weight in order to maintain the calorific and nitrogen equilibrium.
(3) Nutritional schemes should consider the possibility of long-term nutritional support in case of complications, continued presence of sepsis and upper alimentary tract failure. A plan therefore should be made at the outset of treatment planning.

REFERENCES

1 Cuthbertson DP. The disturbance of metabolism produced by bony and non-bony injury, with notes on certain abnormal conditions of bone. Biochem J 1930; 24: 1244–1263.
2 Moghissi K, Hornshaw J, Teasdale PR, Dawes EA. Parenteral nutrition in carcinoma of the oesophagus treated by surgery, nitrogen balance and clinical studies. Br J Surg 1977; 64: 125–128.
3 Heatley RV, Williams RHP, Lewis MH. Preoperative intravenous feeding – a controlled trial. Postgrad Med J 1979; 55: 541–545.
4 Moore F. Metabolic Care of the Surgical Patient. Philadelphia, PA, WB Saunders 1959.
5 Moghissi K, Teasdale PR. Parenteral feeding in patients with carcinoma of the oesophagus treated by surgery: Energy and nitrogen requirements. J Parent Ent Nutr 1980; 4: 371–375.
6 Passmore R. Body size and composition in recommended intake of nutrients for UK. Reports on Public Health and Medical Subjects No 120 (DHSS). London, HMSO 1969.
7 Blackburn GL, Bistrian BR, Maini BS, Schlamm HT, Smith MF. Nutritional and metabolic assessment of the hospitalized patient. J Parent Ent Nutr 1977; 1: 11–22.
8 Hill G, Blacket R, Pickford I, Birkinshaw L, Young G, Warren J, Schorah C, Morgan D. Malnutrition in surgical patients. Lancet 1977; 1: 689–692.
9 Grant JP, Custer PB, Thurlow JL. Current techniques of nutritional assessment. Surg Clin North Am 1981; 6: 437–463.
10 Abbott WE, Levey S, Kriegger H. Metabolic changes in surgical patients in relation to water, electrolyte, nitrogen and calorie intake. Metabolism 1959; 8: 847–861.
11 Van Larsen V, Brockner J. Nitrogen balance and operative stress. Acta Chir Scand 1965 191 (Suppl 343).
12 Tweedle DEF, Johnston IDA. Factor affecting the metabolic expenditure of surgical patients. Br J Surg 1971; 58: 771–774.
13 Page CP, Andrassy RJ, Sandler JT. Techniques in delivery of liquid diets: Short term and long term. In: Dietel M (ed.). Nutrition in Clinical Surgery, 2nd Ed. Baltimore, William and Wilkins 1985: pp 60–85.
14 Steiger E, Grundfest-Broniatowski S, Misny TJ. Intravenous hyper-alimentation: Temporary and permanent vascular access and administration. In: Dietel M (ed.). Nutrition in Clinical Surgery, 2nd Ed. Baltimore, William and Wilkins 1985: pp 88–104.
15 Moghissi K, Dietel M, Taylor GA. Oesophageal problems: Use of nutritional support. In: Dietel M (ed.). Nutrition in Clinical Surgery, 2nd Ed. Baltimore, William and Wilkins 1985: pp 303–319.
16 Moghissi K. A technique of superior vena caval catheterisation for prolonged intravenous feeding. J Roy Coll Surg Edinburgh 1979; 24: 178–179.
17 Fan ST, Lau WY, Wong KK, Chan PM. Preoperative parenteral nutrition in patients with oesophageal cancer: A prospective randomised clinical trial. Clin Nutr 1989; 8: 23–27.

Current Topics in General Thoracic Surgery: An International Series, Vol. 2
Perioperative Care, edited by R.M. Peters and J. Toledo

Discussion of "Perioperative nutritional management of thoracic surgical patients" by K. Moghissi

Arthur E. Baue

The importance of catabolism in surgical patients is well recognized, as is the recognition that total parenteral nutrition (TPN) will support a starving individual indefinitely. Starvation, however, is different from the catabolism of injury. Starvation leading to cachexia stimulates a metabolic adaptation to use fat stores preferentially and minimize protein losses to preserve lean body mass. Thus, in spite of considerable weight loss, the starving patient may maintain normal activity and body strength for some weeks. With the catabolism of injury from operation and/or infection, the drain on lean body mass becomes massive and life-threatening within two weeks. In thoracic surgery patients, the issue is usually not about the amount of weight loss or altered nutritional indices but, rather, how strong is the patient? Can he breathe adequately (adequate pulmonary function)? Can he cough well and ambulate? Thus, preoperative nutritional support is not as important for most thoracic surgical patients. This is certainly true in patients with carcinoma of the lung. If they are so weak and cachectic preoperatively, they will probably not survive an operation, no matter how much nutritional support they are given before, during, or after. Also, their gastrointestinal (G.I.) tracts are intact and should function quickly after operation. A recent patient of mine, who had lost 35 pounds preoperatively, had gastric distention the afternoon after a pneumonectomy for carcinoma of the lung. The next day, after removal of his nasogastric tube, he ate satisfactorily the breakfast he had ordered of scrambled eggs. Some years ago, patients with cardiac cachexia due to valvular heart disease often died postoperatively, because of inability to get off the ventilator, in spite of good postoperative cardiovascular function and nutritional support. In patients with carcinoma of the esophagus, operation and resection should not have a greatly increased hazard because of weight loss alone. Wound infection in a thoracotomy is almost unheard of. Leaking anastomoses are technical, not nutritional errors. Present combined treatment modalities of preoperative chemotherapy and radiation therapy, followed later by resection, will often allow the patient to swallow better and improve his nutrition before the operation. Where there is infection (empyema) in thoracic surgery, or when the gastrointestinal tract is not functional (leaks, perforations, or obstructions), nutritional support is required along with drainage or extirpation of the septic process.

There is now abundant evidence that enteral nutrition is well tolerated and has advantages over TPN. These include prevention of atrophy of the gut, overgrowth of bacterial organisms, and the possibility of translocation of bacterial organisms across the gut wall. Also, enteral nutrition is well-tolerated by the endocrine–hepatic–metabolic system and is associated with few complications, if used appropriately. This is in contrast with TPN, where catheter complications and metabolic problems occur with some frequency. Thus, the important consideration in thoracic surgery is – When is preoperative and perioperative nutritional support necessary and helpful?

Mr. Moghissi has provided a review of the development of knowledge about the metabolic and nutritional problems of surgical patients. He also provides methods of evaluation of nutritional status along with information on planning a nutritional program, which patients require nutritional support, at what stage should it commence, type of regimen and route of delivery, and four clinical examples of where nutritional support was deemed helpful. These are all clear, straightforward, and well understood. The information is available in standard textbooks of surgery.

Although the author cites the contributions of John Hunter, Claude Bernard, and Cuthbertson, he does not bring us up to date with the important contributions of Dudrick and Vars [1], indicating the possibility of TPN; the work of Willmore et al. [2,3] on the use of growth hormone, and other techniques which have led to the modern support of nutrition and altered metabolism. The work of Wretlind [4] and Schuberth [5] in Scandinavia set the stage for modern nutritional support by demonstrating the use of fat in solutions, which eventually became known as Intralipid.

Mr. Moghissi has written a number of papers about nutritional support in esophageal and thoracic surgery. Most of these were published some years ago. There is more information that can be brought to bear on perioperative nutritional support.

The literature on perioperative nutritional support in thoracic surgical patients does not provide clear evidence of benefit. Many studies were not randomized or well-controlled. Many are anecdotal, and the results are not clear cut. It is clear that the routine use of preoperative TPN is not helpful. There may be advantages in patients with severe nutritional deficiencies. In one study, Mr. Moghissi found that many patients with carcinoma of the esophagus were nutritionally deficient (weight loss, negative nitrogen balance, and dysphagia). He defined the postoperative caloric and nitrogen requirements to maintain a positive nitrogen balance [6]. In another study, he treated 15 patients with carcinoma of the esophagus by allocation alternately to receive five to seven days of TPN by central venous catheter preoperatively and six to seven days postoperatively (10 patients), as compared with five patients who received only intravenous dextrose and saline and no nitrogen supplementation[7]. He stated that postoperative progress was not as satisfactory in the patients who received saline alone, as compared with patients receiving TPN. Differences between satisfactory and not satisfactory courses were based on an assessment of general progress and wound healing, but the details of these observations were not provided.

In a study cited by Mr. Moghissi, Heatley et al.[8] in a randomized trial, gave preoperative TPN over a 7–10 day period to patients with gastric or esophageal cancer. There were 38 patients treated and 36 in controls. Most of the operations were total gastric resections. They found a significantly greater number of wound infections in the control group as compared to the treated group (11/3). Since most of the operations were total gastrectomies, I assume that these were abdominal wound infections. We are not told how severe the infections were. They also found that there were more infections in the control group when there were low serum albumin levels (< 35 g/l). They recommended that the routine use of TPN with its attendant hazards was not warranted in preparation of patients with upper G.I. cancer. It should be reserved for patients with severe nutritional deficiencies.

Mr. Moghissi provides four examples of nutritional support in his practice. A man with a carcinoma of the lung and an empyema had a week of enteral feeding with a fine nasogastric tube followed by an extrapleural pneumonectomy. Postoperatively, the patient received total and supplementary TPN for 10 days and did well. We are not told whether the empyema cavity remained closed and uninfected. Did the nutritional support make a difference in this patient? I doubt it.

The second patient had an esophagopleural fistula five years after a pneumonectomy for carcinoma of the lung. He received two weeks of TPN, followed by an abdominal–cervical, total esophagectomy. The patient seemed to do well postoperatively. Here again, nutritional support may have made a difference, but it is not clear cut.

A patient with multiple injuries required repair of a lacerated lung and ruptured diaphragm. A fine-tube gastrostomy was inserted at the time of operation and was used for postoperative feeding until she could be mobilized and take things adequately by mouth. This certainly is an appropriate approach. Whether or not she required supplementary parenteral nutrition, cannot be established.

A fourth patient was treated by the author four days after perforation of the esophagus by dilatation of an esophageal stricture. It is amazing that she was still alive at that time. A very aggressive approach was taken, draining the pyopneumothorax through the right chest. Sometime later, and we are not told how much later, a resection of the stricture and perforation was carried out through a laparotomy and separate right thoracotomy with decortication on the right. TPN was given initially, and then a fine-tube jejunostomy was established at the time of the abdominal procedure. This was appropriate nutritional care, in a patient with prolonged disruption of the G.I. tract. A perforated esophagus with a pyopneumothorax represents a major metabolic insult and requires nutritional support.

In a recent review by Burt and Brennan at Memorial/Sloan Kettering[9] they concluded that malnutrition in patients with esophageal carcinoma is detrimental and probably affects clinical outcome. However, whether nutritional support can positively affect the outcome is questionable. They found that both TPN and enteral feeding can suppress gluconeogenesis, increase protein synthesis, and decrease catabolism – all of which should be biologically favorable. However, data to support the premise that nutritional intervention in all patients with esophageal carcinoma is clinically efficacious, is lacking. Their recommendations for nutritional support for patients with esophageal carcinoma are the standard indications: patients who will not be able to take sufficient calories and nitrogen for one week or more and have lost over 10% of their pre-illness body weight. The enteral route is preferable, since there is no difference between the two in biologic efficacy.

A meta-analysis protocol to evaluate the results of 18 controlled trials of perioperative TPN was reported by Detsky et al.[10]. Their conclusion is that the routine use of perioperative TPN in unselected patients having major surgery is not justified. However, this intervention may be helpful in subgroups who are at high risk. A recent multi-institutional V.A. trial of perioperative TPN was carried out in 395 malnourished surgical patients. They were randomly assigned to receive either TPN for 7–15 days before operation and 3 days afterwards, or no perioperative TPN. Rates of major complications during the first 30 days after operation in the two groups were similar, as was the overall 90-day mortality. There were actually more infectious complications in the TPN group than in the control group. They recommend that preoperative TPN be limited to severely malnourished patients, unless there are other specific indications. They further analyzed several subgroups which were not part of their original protocol. Severely malnourished patients who received TPN had a lower rate of major complications. However, the authors state, "these differences are numerically large, but of marginal statistical significance, presumably because of the small size of the subgroups". In other words, the authors seem to want to have it both ways. There was no statistically significant difference in these patients, with the 95%-confidence intervals being 0.02–0.91 or 0.32–1.24. They defined severely malnourished patients as having a nutrition risk index < 83.5 through various combinations of weight loss and hypoalbuminemia. In an editorial about this study, Detsky[11] states that the study supports the view that only a small portion of patients who undergo elective major surgery ought to receive preoperative TPN. The interpretation of subgroup analysis is always problematic, particularly when the subdivisions of the primary endpoints are done after the fact. They may not yield valid conclusions. The V.A. study does show that poor nutritional status confers a higher risk of major postoperative complications. Unfortunately, the evidence supporting the recommendation that nutritional support be given to severely malnourished patients, is less than conclusive. Readers may be interested in a recent issue of the Surgical Clinics of North America on current strategies in surgical nutrition[13], with Stanley Dudrick as a guest editor.

Ellis et al.[14] state that “despite the generally accepted axiom that perioperative nutritional support decreases morbidity and mortality rates in surgical patients, convincing scientific data are lacking”. Daily et al.[15] indicate that cachexia seems to be related to abnormal changes in host intermediary metabolism induced by host–tumor interactions and indigenous peptides such as tumor necrosis factor. In a chapter that I wrote in this volume[16] on nutrition and metabolism in sepsis and multi-system organ failure, I recommended the G.I. tract be used whenever possible, with a blenderized regular diet containing fiber, glutamine, and short-chain fatty acid supplements to protect and preserve the gut. If TPN is necessary, special solutions may be best for the liver, kidney, or lungs if they are failing. If not, protein with 45% branch chain amino acid[5], medium and short chain triglycerides, glutamine supplementation, and carbohydrates seem best. Other substances are being evaluated that may be helpful in nutrition and organ support such as arginine, xylitol, growth hormone, and anabolic steroid.

A major problem with preoperative nutritional support is the length of time that it takes to correct the problem, get the indices of malnutrition back in order and obtain positive nitrogen balance and improved protein synthesis. If nutrition could be improved and maintained for a number of weeks, many of the metabolic defects would be corrected. Thus, I think the argument is not about whether nutritional support is helpful in severely malnourished patients. Obviously it is. Patients with severe malnutrition are at greater risk for morbidity and mortality after any operative procedure. The difficulty in documenting improvement in morbidity and mortality with preoperative nutrition is related to the time involved. If one would take the time, effort, and expense of two to three weeks or a month to do this, then there should be clinically significant improvement. In that time, a tumor will also be continuing to grow or metastasize. In addition, there is always the question as to whether one is feeding the patient or the tumor. One week of TPN does not do much or enough. Thus, the need for perioperative nutritional support in the thoracic surgical patient is, I believe, limited to patients with septic complication or where the gastrointestinal tract is not functional. In other patients, the gastrointestinal tract can be used, particularly with carcinoma of the esophagus. An improvement in eating follows preoperative chemotherapy and radiation therapy. These and other approaches have recently been reviewed in detail[17].

REFERENCES

1 Dudrick SJ, et al. Long term total parenteral nutrition with growth development and positive nitrogen balance. Surgery 1968; 64: 134–139.

2 Willmore DW, Moyland JA, Briston BF, et al. Anabolic effects of human growth hormone and high caloric feedings following thermal injury. Surg Gynecol Obstet 1974; 138: 875–888.

3 Manson JM, Smith RJ, Willmore DW. Growth hormone stimulates protein synthesis during hypocaloric parenteral nutrition: Role of hormonal substrate environment. Ann Surg 1988; 208: 136–142.

4 Wretlind A. The pharmacological basis for the use of fat in motion in intravenous nutrition. Acta Chir Scand 1964 (Suppl 325): 31–42.
5 Schuberth O. Clinical experience with fat in motion for intravenous use. Acta Chir Scand 1964 (Suppl 325): 43–49.
6 Moghissi K, Teasdale PR. Parenteral feeding in patients with carcinoma of the esophagus treated by surgery: Energy and nitrogen requirements. J Parent Ent Nutr 1980; 4: 371–375.
7 Moghissi K, Hornshaw J, Teasdale PR, Daws EA. Parenteral nutrition in carcinoma of the esophagus treated by surgery: Nitrogen balance in clinical study. Br J Surg 1977; 64: 125–128.
8 Heatley RV, Williams RHP, Lewis MH. Preoperative intravenous feeding – A controlled trial. Postgrad Med J 1979; 55: 541–545.
9 Burt ME, Brennan MF. Nutritional support of the patient with esophageal cancer. Semin Oncol 1984; 11: 127–135.
10 Detsky AS, Baker JP, O'Rourke K, Goel V. Perioperative parenteral nutrition: A meta analysis. Ann Intern Med 1987; 107: 195–203.
11 Veterans Affairs Total Parenteral Nutrition Cooperative Study Group. Perioperative total parenteral nutrition in surgical patients. N Engl J Med 1991; 325: 525–532.
12 Detsky AS. Parenteral nutrition – is it helpful? N Engl J Med 1991; 325: 573–575.
13 Dudrick SJ (ed.). Current Strategies in Surgical Nutrition: Surgical Clinics of North America. Philadelphia, PA, WB Saunders 1991.
14 Ellis LM, Copeland III EM, Suoba WW. Perioperative nutritional support. In: Dudrick SJ (ed.). Current Strategies in Surgical Nutrition. Surgical Clinics of North America. Philadelphia, PA, WB Saunders 1991: pp 493–507.
15 Daily JM, Redman HP, Lieberman MD, Jardines L. Nutritional support of patients with carcinoma of the gastrointestinal tract. In: Dudrick SJ (ed.). Current Strategies in Surgical Nutrition. Surgical Clinics of North America. Philadelphia, PA, WB Saunders 1991: pp 523–536.
16 Baue AE. Nutrition and metabolism in sepsis in multi-system organ failure. In: Dudrick SJ (ed.). Current Strategies in Surgical Nutrition. Surgical Clinics of North America. Philadelphia, PA, WB Saunders 1991: pp 549–565.
17 Baue AE. Multiple Organ Failure: Patient Care and Prevention. St. Louis, Mosby-Year Book 1990.

Current Topics in General Thoracic Surgery: An International Series, Vol. 2
Perioperative Care, edited by R.M. Peters and J. Toledo

Chapter 6

Perioperative management of hemoptysis

John R. Benfield and Daniel P. Link

1. INTRODUCTION

Management of significant airway hemorrhage continues to improve and become more effective. Endoscopy, interventional radiology, and resection all have a place in managing hemoptysis. The selection of patients for the operative or perioperative approach requires a determination of the significance and probable cause of the hemoptysis.

The significance of bleeding is often difficult to access. Traditionally, 600 ml or more in 48 hours is considered massive hemoptysis and the significance of more rapid bleeding has been stressed [1,2].

Amounts ranging from blood-streaked sputum to a single episode of 100 ml are considered small. Often the boundary between small and massive hemoptysis is unclear. When this is the case, it is best to react as if massive hemoptysis is imminent because underestimating the bleeding can lead to disaster [3].

2. DIAGNOSIS AND INITIAL MANAGEMENT

A good clinical history is the crucial first step for diagnosis. As summarized in Table 6.1, over 60% of patients with massive hemoptysis can be expected to have inflammatory lung disease; tuberculosis and bronchiectasis account for nearly 40% of massive bronchial bleeding. Massive hemoptysis is associated with cancer in about 7% of patients [4]. The social history may help to focus upon the probability of diagnosis. Patients from underprivileged socioeconomic groups or survivors of the hardships of wars are prone to have chronic inflammatory or bronchiectatic lesions; well-nourished, working patients are more likely to have bleeding from neoplastic or congenital lesions. Prodromal symptoms may reveal that the probable source of bleeding is the gastrointestinal tract rather than hemoptysis. A history of pulmonary infections, such as tuberculosis, frequent pneumonia during childhood, and cystic fibrosis suggest these etiologies for bleeding. One third of patients with tuberculosis

TABLE 6.1
Causes of massive hemoptysis[a]

Tuberculosis	27	Cystic fibrosis	5
Bronchiectasis	10	Idiopathic	5
Lung abscess	9	After resection	4
Aspergilloma	8	A-V malformation	2
Pneumonia	8	Miscellaneous	15
Carcinoma	7		

[a] Causes among 703 patients, expressed as percentage of total. Pulmonary cysts, foreign bodies and empyema were each causes in four or more of the patients included on the miscellaneous category.

will have hemoptysis during the course of their disease [5]. In such cases, there is often associated bronchiectasis, or localized chronic bronchitis. Patients with tuberculosis cavities colonized by aspergillosis have a propensity for massive hemoptysis [6]. Not infrequently patients can quite accurately localize the source of their bleeding, and most often they can localize the side of the chest from which it originates.

Acute hemoptysis in patients, with normal chest radiographs, and without antecedent history of pulmonary disease, is often caused by endobronchial neoplasm. Carcinoid tumors in major bronchi may present in this way. In our experience, non-small cell cancers uncommonly cause hemoptysis as a first symptom, even when the neoplasms are centrally located in the tracheobronchial tree.

Selection of the proper diagnostic tests, and the sequence of examinations is important. The plain chest X-ray is still the best first diagnostic test. Bronchoscopy is the single most important test for patients with massive hemoptysis. The bronchoscopy should be performed at or near the time of active bleeding to precisely localize the source of bleeding.

How, by whom and where should bronchoscopy for hemoptysis be done?

The response depends upon the extent of the bleeding. Patients with chronic small hemoptysis can safely have flexible fiber-optic bronchoscopy, most often performed in outpatient endoscopy suites – an environment which usually does not offer the recommended contingency equipment and personnel. If an endobronchial lesion is found that is judged to be at risk for significant bleeding upon biopsy, one should insist on preparation to deal with massive hemoptysis.

Under proper conditions, essentially all endobronchial lesions, including carcinoids, can and should be biopsied. One exception to this rule is tortuous blood vessels which may appear at bronchoscopy as either a reddish bulge or an endobronchial mass [7]. In most instances, frozen sections of bronchoscopic biopsies should not be requested because the specimens are too small for optimal evaluation in this way.

Patients with massive hemoptysis should have their bronchoscopies done primarily with rigid instruments because the suction channels of flexible bronchoscopes are inadequate for the management of serious bleeding. It is strongly urged that the surgeon manage the perioperative bronchoscopy personally. The findings will serve as the basis for preoperative discussion and treatment planning with the anesthesiologist; they will dictate whether a tracheal divider, bronchial blocking methodology or jet ventilation methods are most likely to be helpful during operation. Although rigid instruments can be used with topical anesthesia, for the management of massive hemoptysis we recommend general anesthesia for two reasons: (1) to prevent patient motion during the procedures, (2) to be prepared for handling potentially lethal bleeding.

Acute bleeding during bronchoscopy places the patient in danger of drowning. Management requires, first, the establishment of an airway to the lung which is not bleeding. The theoretical choices to accomplishing this include placement of: (a) a ventilating rigid bronchoscope into the appropriate main-stem bronchus, (b) an endotracheal tube into a main-stem bronchus, (c) a bronchial blocking balloon into the bleeding bronchus and an endotracheal tube proximally, (d) a divided endotracheal tube (tracheal divider) of the Carlens or Robertshaw type.

The traditional, and perhaps still the best manner of dealing with the situation is to insert a rigid bronchoscope into the main-stem bronchus of the lung which is not bleeding. An acceptable alternate choice which has become more popular in recent years is placement of a bronchial blocking balloon. If operation is required, it can be accomplished either with the rigid bronchoscope in place, or by waiting until the bleeding has abated enough to place a bronchial blocking balloon and a proximal endotracheal tube. If an endotracheal tube was in place when hemorrhage worsened, it is usually best immediately to advance the endotracheal tube into the appropriate bronchus. Because the endotracheal tube cuff is several centimeters long, it cannot be used for satisfactory prolonged one-lung ventilation. Therefore, at the appropriate time, if possible, a bronchial blocking balloon should be placed. Although we use tracheal dividers regularly for routine operations, we recommend against their use for the management of massive hemoptysis. The lumen of each side of the tube is too small for effective sectioning or for the removal of clotted blood. Accurate and rapid placement of the tube under emergency conditions is likely to be too time consuming or impossible, even for experienced individuals. Nowhere in the practice of thoracic surgery is the help of a trained support team of anesthesiologists and nurses more required than in the management of potentially drowning hemoptysis during bronchoscopy.

Non-invasive diagnostic tests may be helpful. CT can greatly enhance detection of nodules and parenchymal lung disease (Fig. 6.1). V/Q scanning and pulmonary angiograms are applicable to patients with small hemoptysis to evaluate the possibility of pulmonary emboli, and arteriovenous fistula. Although V/Q scanning is the first step in the evaluation for pulmonary emboli on many patients, we recommend pulmonary angiography as the first radiographic test in very ill patients where an immediate definitive answer is required. The risks of selective pulmonary arteriography are very low. In trauma victims, and in patients with pre-existing or diffuse parenchymal lung disease, V/Q mismatching as detected with nuclear medicine methods may be very difficult to interpret. Even on good quality

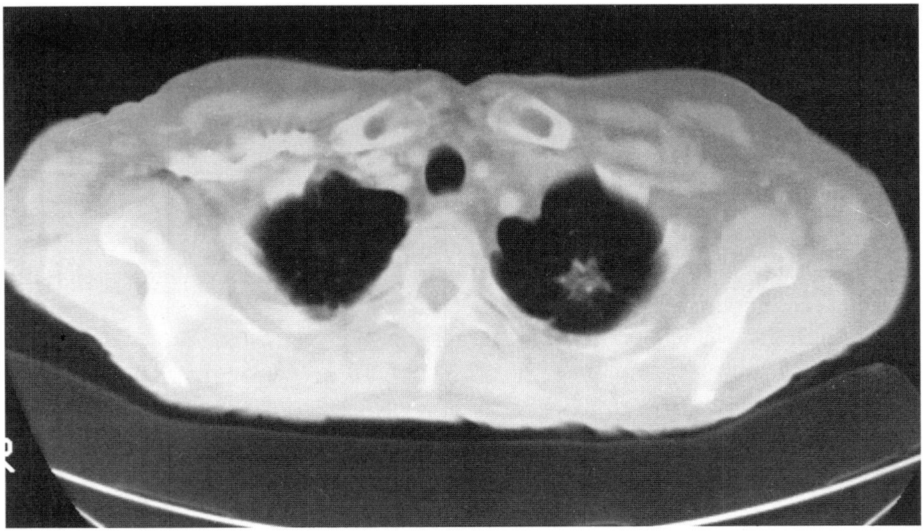

FIGURE 6.1. Classic appearance of apical lung carcinoma which caused hemoptysis; lesion was not well seen on plain radiograph.

pulmonary angiograms, the absence of abnormality does not exclude the diagnosis of pulmonary embolus. Small emboli and blockages which occurred several days prior to angiography may not be visible because the rich pulmonary vasculature has amazing ability to open collaterals and to re-open occluded vessels.

Bronchograms are now rarely done, but they remain important for preoperative evaluation of bronchiectasis. Bronchography yields precise information about which segment(s) of the lungs are involved with disease. Conservative resections, e.g. segmentectomy, are reserved for patients with localized bronchiectasis, and resections need to be conservative. The resection is planned from the bronchogram; thus only the involved bronchial segments are removed sparing the maximum lung parenchyma.

3. TREATMENT

The treatment of small hemoptysis is entirely dependent upon the cause which is found. Full discussion of the nonoperative management of such conditions as bronchiectasis, chronic bronchitis, tuberculosis, other pulmonary granulomatous disease, or lung cancers is not the purpose of this chapter. However, the treatment of carcinoids and benign endobronchial neoplasms justifies commentary. We consider typical carcinoids and atypical carcinoids as part of the Kultschitzsky cell carcinoma (KCC) spectrum which includes small-cell undifferentiated cancers (SCLC). Nearly 10% of carcinoids, followed long-term, may evolve into SCLC, and all carcinoids should be considered as full-thickness bronchial cancers. Therefore, coagulation or endoscopic ablation of carcinoids with laser energy is not recommended. Sleeve resection, not endoscopic ablation, is the treatment of choice for carcinoids.

3.1. Bronchial arteriography with embolization

Bronchial arteriography with embolization to arrest bleeding is most useful for management of massive hemoptysis because acutely exacerbated decreased respiratory reserve is common among such patients. Prior bronchoscopy determines which main-stem bronchus is bleeding. If necessary, a bronchial occlusion balloon for tamponade and protection of the contralateral airway may be placed before angiography.

The bronchial arteries are 1–3 mm in diameter; they originate from the anterior aspect of the aorta, and run to the corresponding bronchus, where they arborize over the tracheo-bronchial tree. In most cases they are easily found because their origin lies at the level of the left main-stem bronchus. The air column of the left main-stem bronchus is easily seen fluoroscopically, and is an excellent reference point for localization of the bronchial artery origin. The anatomy varies from a single artery supplying both main-stem bronchi to bilateral dual arteries. Two arteries on the left and one artery on the right is the most common configuration, seen in 40% of cases. The other common configurations are bilateral single arteries (21%) and bilateral dual bronchial arteries (20%). A single left bronchial artery and two right bronchial arteries occur in approximately 10% of patients, and even less commonly there is a single bronchial artery supplying both main-stem bronchi[8]. Blood supply to the trachea and bronchus can also come from the intercostals, thyrocervical trunk, innominate, or internal thoracic arteries[9]. The variation in bronchial arterial anatomy is species dependent. A single carinal bronchial artery is found in sheep and almost all of the marine mammals, including seals, whales and dolphins. This explains why sheep have been used as a model to study bronchial artery blood flow[9]. Anatomic variations in humans are expected and therefore concentration on identifying the bleeding site(s) and on individual anatomy saves a lot of time.

3.1.1. Technique

The technique of bronchial arteriography begins with a selective catheterization of the bronchial artery on the affected side. A high-quality bronchial angiogram is done, and the findings are analyzed for direct and indirect signs of bleeding. The direct signs of bleeding include visualization of extravasated contrast into the tracheal bronchial tree on the bronchial arteriogram. This is occasionally seen in patients actively bleeding. A second direct sign in chronically bleeding patients is thrombosis in the vessel or an abrupt truncation. Usually the source of bronchial artery bleeding is inferred from indirect signs. These include hypervascularization,

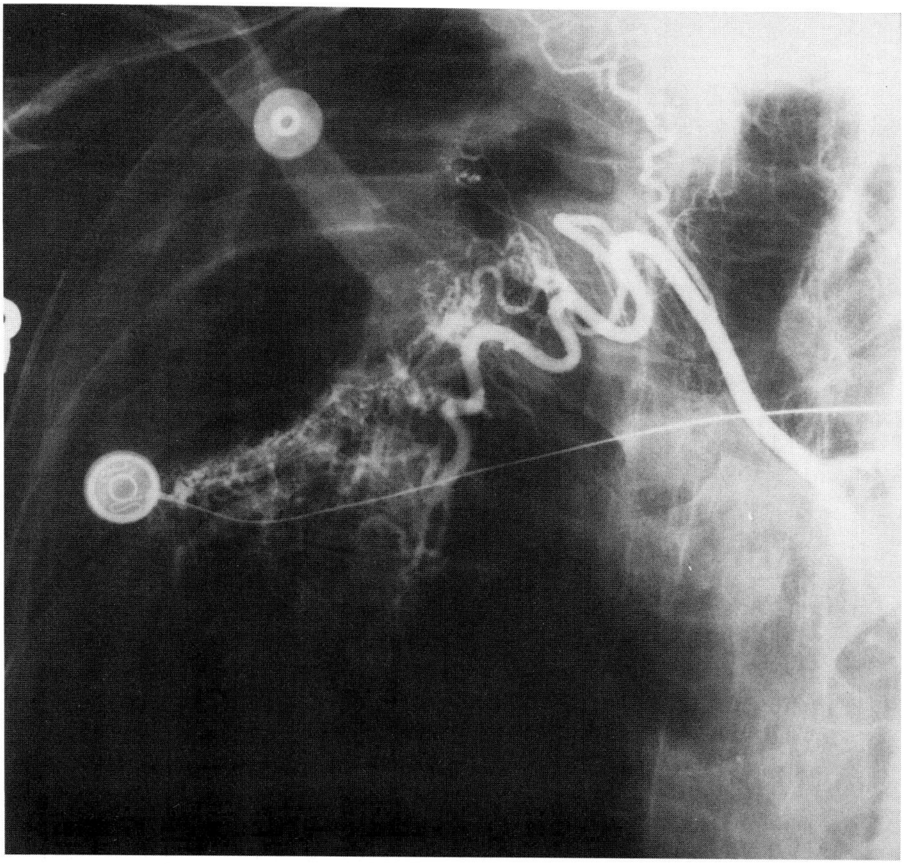

FIGURE 6.2a. Bronchial arteriogram: bronchial bleeding into mass.

irregular capillary stasis, arterial occlusions, and evidence of interarterial bronchopulmonary shunts [10]. Occasionally the bronchial artery can be seen leading into a large mass; such a finding is an indirect sign that the mass may be the source of the bronchial bleeding (Fig. 6.2a).

Following localization of the bronchial artery thought to be causing the bleeding, the artery is embolized with either gel-foam, polyvinyl alcohol, or Gianturco coils. Many angiographers use a combined approach, beginning with gel-foam and ending with the Gianturco coils (Fig. 6.2b). Outside the United States, combinations of macro-aggregated albumin with a particle size of 50–200 μm, as well as sclerosing agents have been used for the control of bronchial hemorrhage. Very small catheters and coils (3 Fr) are now available and greatly enhance our capability to subselect vessels. Microfibrillar collagen particles (Angiostat®, 5×75 μm) might also be useful and pass through the smallest catheters. In patients

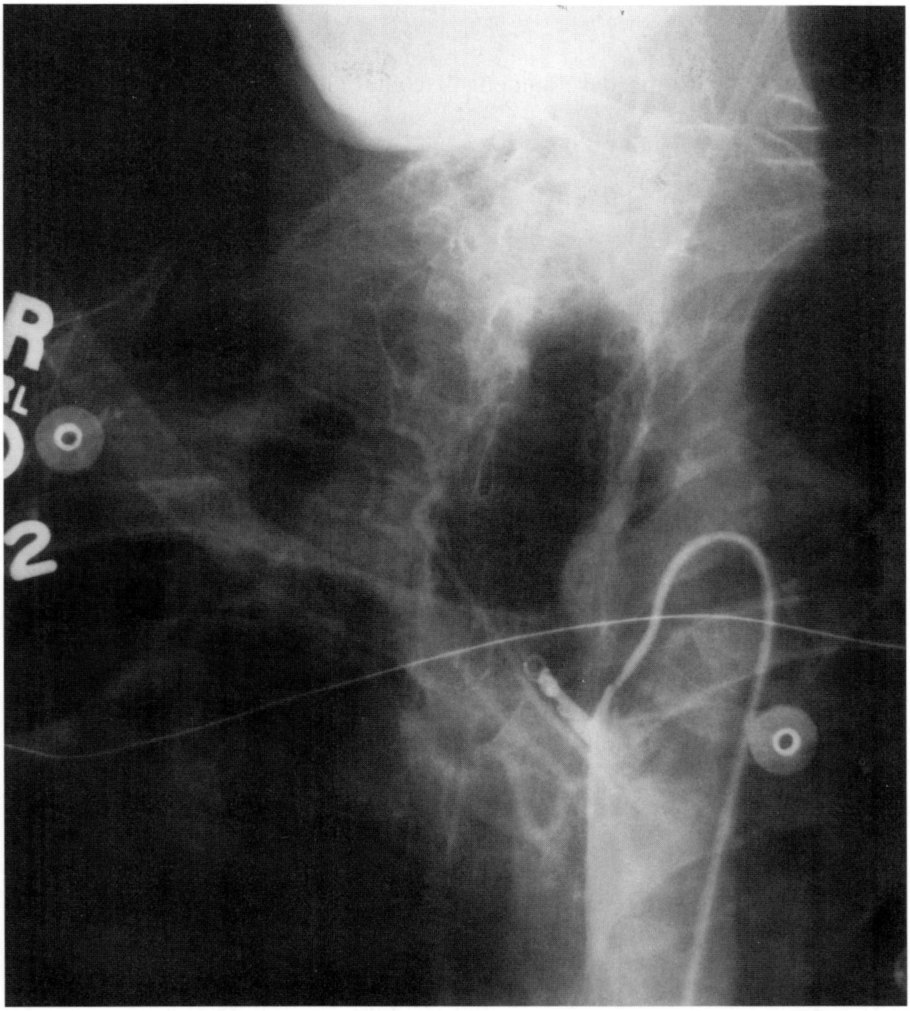

FIGURE 6.2b. Bronchial arteriogram (patient of Fig. 6.2a): occlusion of artery after embolization with gel-foam and Gianturco coils.

with cystic fibrosis who have large ectatic bronchial arteries bilaterally (Fig. 6.3), it is best to perform embolization of all the bronchial arteries during the first sitting [11]. Long-term follow-up of patients with Ivalon embolic show the particles lodged up to the mid-segmental branches. There is chronic inflammation, typical foreign body response and focal recanalization [12].

Embolization of the bronchial arteries for control of hemorrhage is over 90% successful, initially. If hemoptysis is successfully arrested, and an episode of

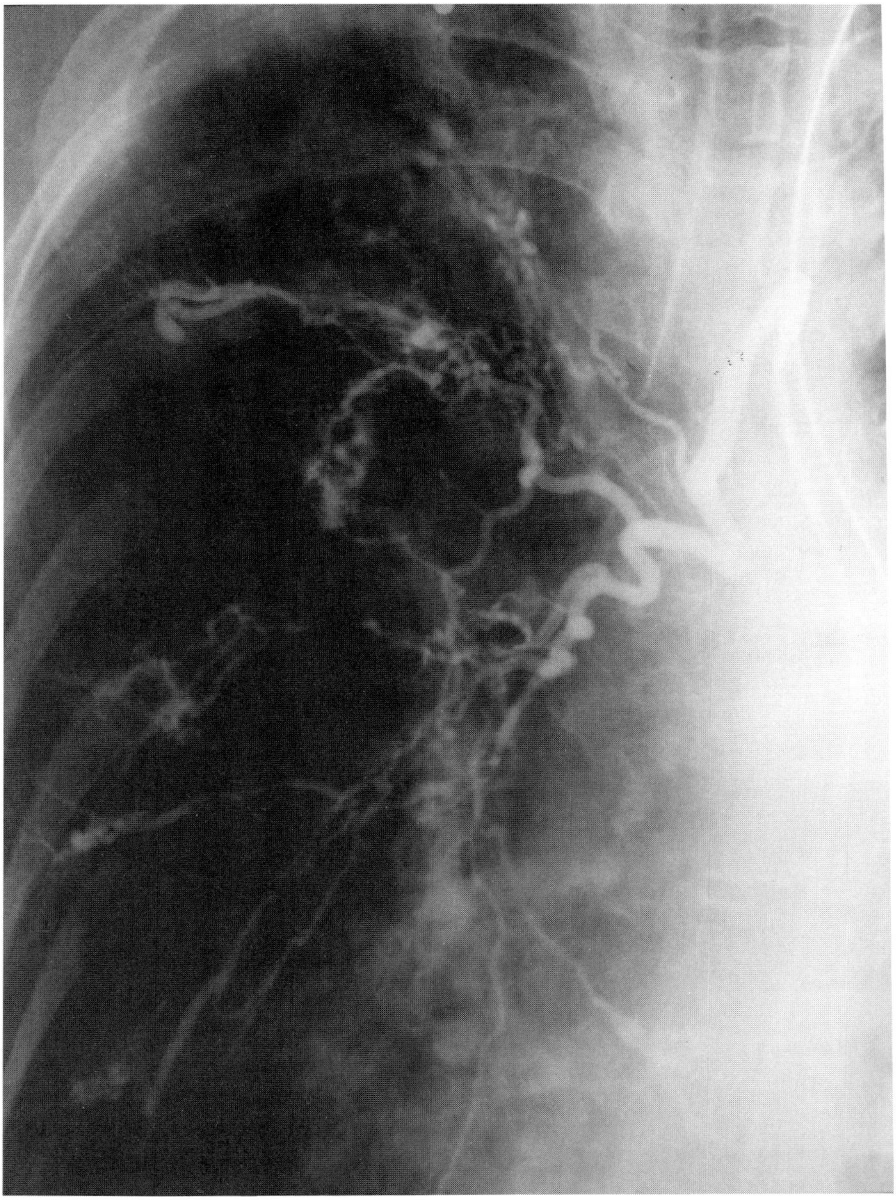

FIGURE 6.3. Arterial changes of cystic fibrosis. Note the irregularity and ectasis of vessels.

rebleeding does not occur immediately, it is highly likely that the patient will be free of hemoptysis for several months to years.

Rebleeding usually results from not finding the involved bronchial artery and from the development of collateral blood supply from the superior intercostal artery or from the internal mammary artery (Fig. 6.4) [13–15]. Bleeding from other feeders including the thyrocervical trunk can also be significant [16]. In these instances, the involved collateral vessels (intercostals) should be embolized. Recurrent bleeding following transcatheter embolization occurs 24–96 hours following the procedure in approximately 14% of patients [10]. Twenty-three percent of patients will develop recurrent hemorrhage months or years after initially successful hemostasis with embolization methods. The source of late recurrent bleeding is either collateral blood supply or recanalization of the bronchial artery [10]. This is least likely to occur when the bronchial artery occlusion has been performed with permanent substances like Ivalon and Gianturco coils.

3.1.2. Complications

Complications following embolization of the bronchial artery include vague chest pain and low-grade fever that is often seen in embolization procedures. The most serious complications involve inadvertent distal embolization [10]. The most dreaded complication of bronchial angiography is paraplegia from infarction of the anterior portion of the spinal cord [7]. The blood supply to the anterior spinal artery is variable and in some cases is supplied by the intercostal branches originating near the bronchial artery origin. In addition, there are anastomotic channels between the bronchial and intercostal vessels. There has been one case of paraplegia from embolization of the spinal artery while embolizing an intercostal, and there have been several reports of spinal complications secondary to the contrast medium injection. Test injection of local anesthetics to evaluate the blood supply [17], or measurement of spinal evoked potentials [18] have been suggested for prevention of spinal cord complications. In practice, we have found there is rarely time for these considerations.

In the management of patients with massive hemoptysis it is critical to have good rapport among the angiographers, pulmonologists, thoracic surgeons and anesthesiologists in order to devise the optimum treatment plan. There has been a recent report of successful hemostasis of massive hemoptysis with Indomethacin in doses equivalent to that used for ductus arteriosus closure [19]. At present, treatment with Indomethacin-type drugs should be considered in the control of massive hemoptysis when no skilled management team is available. Many cases begin with stabilization, followed by embolization, which is then followed by surgical resection of the lesion causing the hemoptysis. Currently, and for the foreseeable future, lung resection remains the court of last resort.

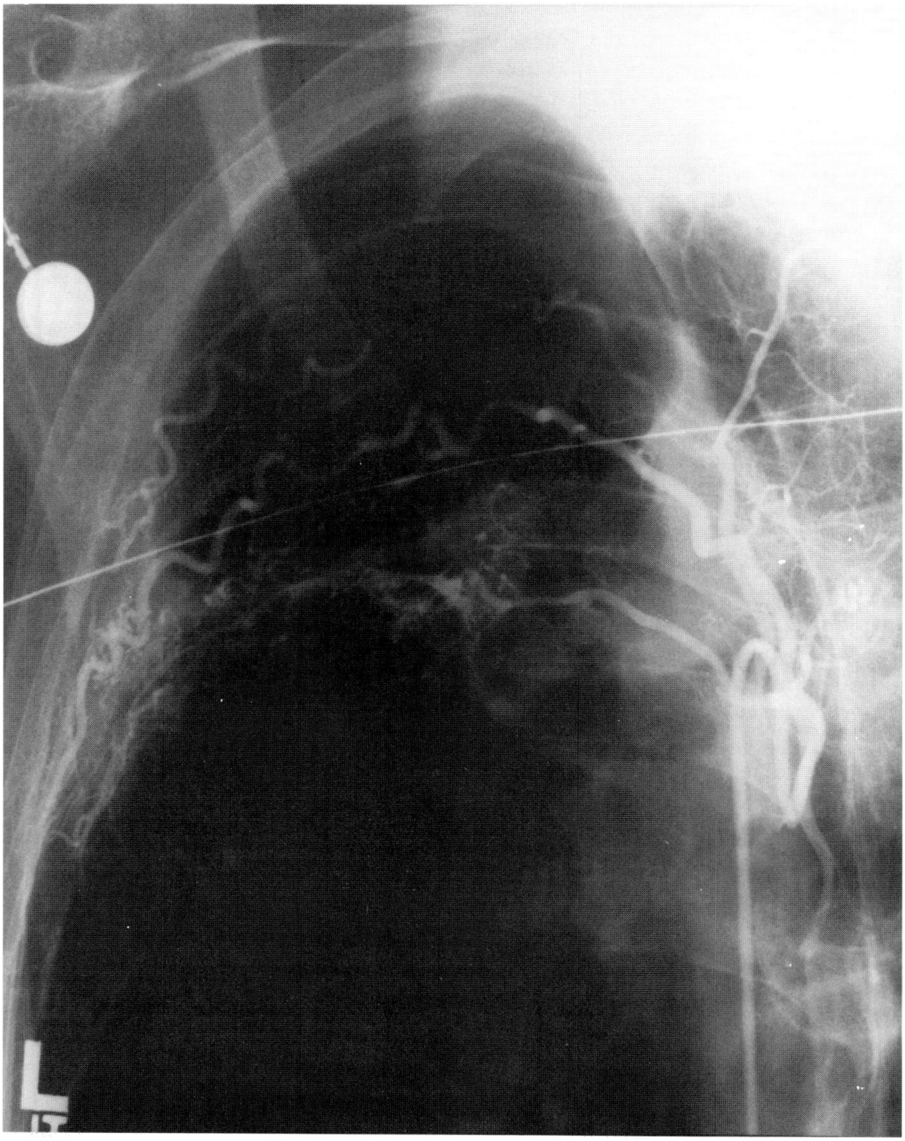

FIGURE 6.4. Re-bleeding several months after the successful embolization shown in Fig. 6.2b. Note the collective vessels from the superior intercostal artery. Repeat embolization stopped the recurrent bleeding.

3.2. Pulmonary resection

Pulmonary resection for the treatment of small hemoptysis is not a special procedure, except insofar as dictated by the underlying disease. For example, segmentectomy is indicated for the treatment of localized bronchiectasis, and bronchial sleeve resection is the treatment of choice for KCC-1 (typical carcinoid) neoplasms. Similarly, for treatment of massive hemoptysis, the extent of resection depends upon classic considerations as to the nature and extent of the underlying lesion. Although it is not the intent of this section to discuss techniques of resections, it is noteworthy that the mortality rate after emergency operations for the treatment of massive hemoptysis has been 20–30%; an early operation decreases the mortality to 12% [14]. Deaths are caused, almost invariably, as the direct or indirect consequence of endobronchial blood leading acutely to asphyxiation, or *in prolonged fashion* to pneumonia or respiratory distress syndrome. The key to success is prompt operation, optimum anesthetic management, and excellent postoperative tracheobronchial hygiene.

4. SUMMARY

Early and prompt diagnosis, including bronchoscopy, is crucial for the management of hemoptysis and prevention of massive hemoptysis. Bronchial arteriography and embolic therapy should be considered early. Resection of localized lesions is the most effective method for control of hemorrhage which fails to cease or to respond to non-invasive management. We have often been called upon too late to operate on patients with airway bleeding. Surgical consultation is recommended early in the course of management, even for patients who may not need operation.

5. Acknowledgement

The assistance of Rana Teresa Tan with the literature review required for the preparation of this manuscript is greatly appreciated.

REFERENCES

1 Garzon AA, Cerruti MM, Gourin A, et al.: Pulmonary resection for massive hemoptysis. Surgery 1970; 67: 633.
2 Garzon AA, Cerruti MM, Golding ME: Exsanguinating hemoptysis. J Thorac Cardiovasc Surg 1982; 84: 829.
3 Rudzinski JP, delCastillo J: Massive hemoptysis. Ann. Emergency Med 1987; 16: 561–564.
4 Tan R, Link D: The radiologic management of hemoptysis – a collective review. Unpublished 1989.

5 Muthuswamy PP, Akbik F, Franklin C, Spigos D, Barker WL: Management of major or massive hemoptysis in active pulmonary tuberculosis by bronchial arterial embolization. Chest 1987; 92: 77–82.
6 Uflacker R, Kaemmerer A, Picon PD, et al.: Bronchial artery embolization in the management of hemoptysis: technical aspects and long-term results. Radiology 1985; 157: 637.
7 Katoh O, Yamada H, Hiura K, Nakanishi Y, Kishikawa T: Bronchoscopic and angiographic comparison of bronchial arterial lesions in patients with hemoptysis. Chest 1987; 91: 486–489.
8 Olson RR, Athanasoulis CA: Hemoptysis: treatment with transcatheter embolization of the bronchial arteries. In: Interventional Radiology. Philadelphia, PA, WB Saunders 1982: pp 196–202.
9 Link DP, Parsons GH, Lantz BMT, et al.: Measurement of bronchial blood flow in the sheep by video dilution technique. Thorax 1985; 40: 143.
10 Rabkin JE, Astafjev VI, Gothman LN, Grigorjec YG: Transcatheter embolization in the management of pulmonary hemorrhage. Radiology 1987; 163: 361.
11 Fellows KE, Khaw KT, Schuster S, Shwachman H: Bronchial artery embolization in cystic fibrosis: technique and long-term results. J Pediatr 1979; 95(6): 959.
12 Tomashefski Jr JF, Cohen AM, Doershuk CF: Long-term histopathologic follow-up of bronchial arteries after therapeutic embolization with polyvinyl alcohol (Ivalon) in patients with cystic fibrosis. Hum Pathol 1988; 19: 555.
13 Jardin M, Remy J: Control of hemoptysis: systemic angiography and anastomoses of the internal mammary artery. Radiology 1988; 168: 377–383.
14 Keller FS, Rosch J, Loflin TG, Nath PH, McElvein RB: Nonbronchial systemic collateral arteries: significance in percutaneous embolotherapy for hemoptysis, Radiology 1987; 164: 687–692.
15 Vujic I, Pyle R, Parker E, Mithoefer J: Control of massive hemoptysis by embolization of intercostal arteries, Radiology 1980; 137: 617.
16 Moore LB, McWey RE, Vujic I: Massive hemoptysis: control by embolization of the thyrocervical trunk. Radiology 1986; 161: 173.
17 Doppman JL, Girton M, Oldfield EH: Spinal wada test. Radiology 1986; 161: 319.
18 Schrodt JF, Becker GJ, Scott JA, et al. Bronchial artery embolization: monitoring with somatosensory evoked potentials. Radiology 1987; 164: 135.
19 Tsukamoto R: Medical bronchial artery embolization [letter], Chest 1988; 93: 1316.
20 Stoll JF, Bettmann MA: Bronchial artery embolization to control hemoptysis: a review. Cardiovasc Intervent Radiol 1988; 11: 263–269.

Current Topics in General Thoracic Surgery: An International Series, Vol. 2
Perioperative Care, edited by R.M. Peters and J. Toledo

Chapter 7

Thoracic surgery in the elderly

Costante Ricci, Erino A. Rendina, Federico Venuta and Renato Guerricchio

1. INTRODUCTION

Much interest has been devoted in recent years to health care problems in the elderly. Individuals over retirement age nowadays constitute an increasingly high percentage of the population in industrialized countries, owing to the increased life expectancy and to the general diminution in birth rate.

The incidence of cardiovascular and neoplastic diseases has grown drastically especially in older age groups. These diseases represent at present the most frequent cause of death in elderly patients. In order to enhance the quality of life and prolong survival, cardiovascular surgery procedures, and even transplantation, have been advocated and successfully performed in patients over 70 or 80 years. The data reported in a number of published series speak for excellent long-term results versus acceptable operative risk and postoperative complication rate [61]. However, general thoracic surgery procedures (Table 7.1), and especially lung operation differ radically from cardiac operations physiopathologically, mostly because they are intended to resect the disease from the affected organ despite the sacrifice of some functioning parenchyma rather than to restore physiological cardiac function. Especially in elderly patients therefore, the surgical team must be prepared to evaluate thoroughly and treat not only complications possibly related to the major impact of the operative trauma on the overall organic functions compromised by age, but also some degree of functional deficit entailed in the parenchymal resection. In addition, patients undergoing general thoracic procedures are usually approached by lateral thoracotomy, while cardiac operations are most often performed via median sternotomy: the extensive trauma on the respiratory musculature caused by the lateral or posterolateral thoracotomy approach represents an additional cause of concern for it may cause marked impairment of the respiratory function, whereas operative trauma is minimized, postoperative pain is reduced and chest wall motility is preserved by the anterior approach.

TABLE 7.1
Thoracic diseases amenable to surgical treatment in elderly patients

- Lung cancer and lung diseases
- Esophageal diseases
- Mediastinal neoplasms
- Myasthenia gravis

TABLE 7.2
Pulmonary resection in elderly patients: operative mortality and 5-year survival[a]

Reference	Year	*N*	Mortality rate (%)				5-Year survival
			mRes	fLob	Pneum	Ovrl	
Golebiowsky [24]	1971	50	0	4	17	8	NA
Evans	1973	114	—	15	27	20	39% (4Y)
Weiss	1974	107	NS	NS	NS	19	NA
Kirsh	1976	58	—	14	16.6	14.4	30%
Harviel	1978	22	NS	NS	NS	18	64% (2Y)
Breyer et al. [8]	1981	175	1.5	5	—	3.5	27%
Ginsberg	1983	453	7.3	—	5.9	7.1	NA
Berggren et al. [5]	1984	82	—	13.6	21	15.9	32%
Yellin et al. [84,85]	1985	58	4.3	4.9	36.4	10.3	40%
Suemasu	1985	252	11	3	13	4.3	36%
Ebner et al. [19]	1985	53	—	—	—	7.5	46%
Present series	1988	72	0	0	25	6.9	28%

[a] Abbreviations:
N, number of patients; mRes, minimal resection; fLob, full lobectomy; Pneum, pneumonectomy; Ovrl, overall mortality rate.

Accurate selection of patients should be undertaken considering the physiologic more than the chronologic age. General surgical procedures in patients over 70 years are associated with a complication rate of about 28%, with cardiocirculatory (45%) and respiratory (38%) complications being the most frequent [7]. Prolonged operations and concomitant diseases also increase the incidence of complications and mortality, as does emergency surgery as opposed to elective surgery duly preceded by thorough preoperative preparation. Also, the derangements in fluid, electrolyte and acid–base balance, often present in the elderly, tend to increase complications and mortality [7].

Almost every thoracic disease can affect elderly patients, but space-occupying masses, and malignant tumors above all, cause special concern to the thoracic surgeon. In fact, they pose as potential or existing threats to patient comfort, function and longevity, and their resection often requires procedures which are stressing for the patient and challenging for the operating team.

Mortality for thoracic surgery procedures has been decreasing consistently over the last two decades (Table 7.2). Reports appearing in the 1970s and referring to elderly patients operated on during the 1950s and 1960s, describe mortality rates of 18 to 20%. In more recent series, operative mortality is reduced to 5 to 10%, and postoperative complication rates have decreased accordingly. This is due to better clinical evaluation and patient selection, enhanced preoperative preparation and intensive postoperative care, and to a change in views concerning the extent of parenchymal resection necessary for the cure of bronchogenic carcinoma.

Cancer in elderly patients presents in many instances as a slow-growing lesion that tends to remain localized for long periods [81]. However, after lung cancer is diagnosed, the 1-year survival rate for non-resected patients is only about 7% [5]. Surgical treatment of bronchogenic carcinoma in the elderly is a controversial issue: the short life expectancy at ages over 70 and the exceedingly high risk for surgery are considered the main contraindications in this age group [84,85]. Reduced life expectancy is however no longer valid as a drawback, because in all industrialized countries the life expectancy is well over 10 years at age 70 and over 8 years at age 80 in men, and even higher in women [8]. In addition, the survival rate at 5 years for patients over 70 years undergoing surgery stands between 27 and 40%. It has been remarked that most late deaths in these patients are due to the original malignancy. This implies that the tumor itself, rather than age per se, is the factor limiting survival, and that a more aggressive approach might be justified even in this high risk group [84,85].

Esophageal procedures, though not implying lung resection, are crucial because of the massive mobilization of intrathoracic organs and because of the risk entailed by the intestinal anastomosis required for reconstruction of the gastro-intestinal pathway. Carcinoma of the esophagus occurs mainly in patients over 60 years. As surgical treatment of this disease is now feasible with a greater margin of safety, elderly patients with esophageal cancer may be candidates for surgery [71].

A great deal of neoplasms and cysts arise from the multiple structures in the mediastinum. However the age distribution of mediastinal masses shows different patterns between children, adults and elderly patients. In fact, most of the lesions seen in childhood are of lymphomatous, neurogenic, teratomatous or vascular nature, while thymoma, pericardial cysts, intrathoracic goiters and primary carcinoma present a higher incidence in middle-aged and elderly patients.

Myasthenia gravis in elderly patients poses difficult therapeutic problems. Controversy exists about the role of thymectomy, plasmapheresis, and administration of steroids or other immunosuppressive agents in the management of these patients. Some authors do not consider thymectomy indicated in older patients and prefer steroid therapy [25,28,76], while others recommend early thymectomy either alone [67] or associated with plasmapheresis [21,49]. According to recent anatomical studies, there is no grossly demonstrable thymic tissue in the mediastinum of patients developing myasthenia gravis in the old age. Therefore, it appears questionable

TABLE 7.3
Surgical staging of 72 patients over 70 years undergoing surgery for lung cancer between 1976 and 1986, in comparison with 717 patients under 70

Patients	Stage I	Stage II	Stage IIIa	Stage IIIb
Over 70	39% (29)	8.2% (6)	45% (33)	6.8% (5)
Under 70	30% (213)	20% (141)	42% (307)	8% (56)

whether attempts to remove or radiate the thymus in elderly myasthenic patients may be rewarding. These data support the clinical finding reported by some authors that the best results with thymectomy are obtained with patients below the age of 40, and that older patients respond poorly to the operation [55,56]. Experiences from the group of Monden [44] and our own group [21] indicate however that thymectomy for thymomatous and non-thymomatous myasthenia gravis may yield marked improvement in elderly patients, and should therefore be considered after careful balancing of all factors.

2. EPIDEMIOLOGY

2.1. Lung cancer

Bronchogenic carcinoma is the most common cancer in men in the USA and is the most common cause of cancer death for both men and women [42]. According to recent epidemiologic data [75], the incidence of lung cancer increases with age, reaching its peak in the eighth decade of life, when 500/100000 men and 91/100000 women are affected. In 1981, lung cancer killed 76764 men in the USA, 17143 (22%) of whom were 75 years or older. Autopsy studies have demonstrated that men over the age of 70 constitute between 8.5 and 11.6% of all patients dying of lung cancer [24]. Overall, documented evidence exists [74] of the age distribution of lung carcinoma patients shifting toward the older age groups. Bronchogenic carcinoma may be anticipated in about 32000 elderly men and 8700 women annually in the United States, and between 10000 and 14000 of them will meet current criteria for thoracotomy [84].

A marked decrease in the degree of histological confirmation of the diagnosis of pulmonary neoplasms occurs with advancing age because of the reluctance to use invasive procedures in these patients [74]. Also, the stage of disease at the time of diagnosis is less advanced in older age groups, and for both men and women squamous cell carcinoma is more frequent in the elderly as compared to younger age groups. It is difficult to draw definitive epidemiological conclusions from these data, because relatively ‘benign’ course of the disease may follow the slow pattern of tumor growth or the lack of detection of more advanced disease because aggressive staging is not always performed in old patients [74]. In our series for example, the stage of disease does not vary between patients over or below 70 years (Table 7.3).

TABLE 7.4
Histological types in 72 patients over 70 years undergoing surgery for lung cancer between 1976 and 1986, in comparison with 717 patients under 70

Patients	Squamous	Adeno	Small cell	Other
Over 70	60%	26%	2%	12%
Under 70	57%	25%	5%	13%

TABLE 7.5
42 mediastinal lesions in patients over 70 years (excluding myasthenia gravis)

Lesion	Number of patients	Percentage
Intrathoracic goiter	9	21.4
Sarcoidosis	6	14.9
Tubercular lympho adenopathy	6	14.9
Thymoma	5	11.9
Neurogenic tumors	5	11.9
Lymphoma	3	7.4
Tubercular mediastinitis	3	7.4
Primary carcinoma	2	4.7
Aspecific mediastinitis	1	2.4
Mediastinal lypomatosis	1	2.4
Pericardial cyst	1	2.4
	—	
Total	42	

The probability of a lung lesion to be carcinoma is about 70% in smokers over 70 years, and increases with age [42]. In our experience, in the past 10 years, a steady increase in the number of patients over 70 years undergoing surgery for lung cancer has been noted, and the stage and histological distribution does not differ significantly from those in younger age groups, as demonstrated in Tables 7.3 and 7.4.

2.2. Esophageal cancer

The incidence of carcinoma of the esophagus is increasing in many areas in Europe, Asia, South Africa and Australia [29,47], but the treatment of this disease remains a subject of controversy [39,79]. It has been demonstrated that there is no difference in incidence of histological type of esophageal cancer between patients below and above 70 years [71].

TABLE 7.6
Surgical approach to 42 patients over 70 years with mediastinal lesions

Technique	Number of patients
Median sternotomy	6
Thoracotomy	6
Sternal split	2
Cervicotomy	9[a]
Anterior mediastinotomy	9
Mediastinoscopy	7
Minor biopsy	3
	—
Total	42

[a] 3 with sternal split.

TABLE 7.7
Functional preoperative evaluation

- Pulmonary function tests
- Blood gas analysis
- ECG
- Renal function tests
- Cerebral blood flow tests

2.3. Mediastinal lesions and myasthenia gravis

Few data have been reported concerning specifically the occurrence of mediastinal lesions in elderly patients. In our experience, 42 patients over 70 years seen at our institution over the last 25 years represent about 7.5% of all patients treated for mediastinal diseases. The majority of lesions treated surgically were benign in nature, while exploratory procedures and simple biopsy were usually performed in malignant tumors or inflammatory diseases (Tables 7.5 and 7.6). The data reported in Table 7.5 are however not totally valid from an epidemiological standpoint, due to the reluctance of general practitioners to refer elderly patients with possibly malignant mediastinal diseases for surgery.

Myasthenia gravis, although more frequent in younger age groups, may have a late onset and myasthenic symptomatology may first present after age 60 in 13.3% of cases [21]. The distribution of patients with non-thymomatous myasthenia gravis according to age at onset of disease is bimodal, with peaks at 10 to 30 years and at 60 to 70 years [44]. The association of myasthenia gravis with other immune diseases is very infrequent in young patients, whereas it is very frequent in elderly patients [14]. Also, the association with thymoma is more frequent in advanced age [21]. In a recent study [58], however, we have demonstrated that thymoma is often benign over age 60, and it may be resected with almost no risk.

3. PREOPERATIVE EVALUATION AND DIAGNOSIS

Physiologic and functional status of the patient is more important than age per se in determining feasibility of thoracic procedures in the elderly. This emphasizes the necessity of individualizing the clinical assessment and of applying thorough clinical judgment to every single case [20] (Table 7.7).

Mental conditions vary a great deal from one patient to another. There are individuals over 70 who look and feel as if whey were 40 and others who present and look much older. Old patients often react unpredictably to physiological and operative trauma and may develop depression. It is wise to consider patients suffering from senile dementia and depression not good candidates for surgery, because they will display a passive attitude in the early postoperative period and therefore be prone to develop serious complications [38].

Careful preoperative evaluation of cellular immunity should be performed in patients over 70 years of age. In fact it has been reported [33] that the OKT-4 activity is reduced in this category of patients, significantly affecting the incidence of postoperative infectious complications.

Postoperative mortality and morbidity are inversely related to the pulmonary reserve in all patients undergoing thoracic surgery; but especially in elderly patients, when the spirometric evaluation of lung function acquires paramount importance. Sex and lifestyle have significant influence on respiratory function, which decays earlier and faster in man than in woman. Male smokers present a decrease in FEV_1 which is double that of women [9]. Central nervous system control over ventilation is also altered in the elderly, as demonstrated by the reduced compensatory increase in the tidal volume in response to hypoxia or hypercapnia [37]. Advancing age causes progressive atrophy of the respiratory musculature, rigidity of the thoracic cage, and decrease in width of diaphragmatic motion [11,16,22]. Changes also occur in the respiratory mucosa, which loses ciliar motility, and in the pulmonary connective tissue, in which the elastic component is decreased [68]. From a physiological standpoint, the vital capacity (VC) decreases between ages 19 and 35 years by 1 ml per year, so that at age 70 the VC is reduced to about 2/3 of that at 20. Forced expiratory volume at 1 second (FEV_1) decreases about 30 ml per year after age 20 [36], and after age 70 the VC/FEV_1 ratio is reduced to 60–65%. Also, a redistribution of lung volumes occurs [45] and the residual volume (FRC) increases at the expense of the inspiratory reserve volume (IRV) and of the expiratory reserve volume (ERV) [11]. As signs of impaired pulmonary elastic performance, the maximum expiratory flow (MEF) and the closing volume (CV) also decay consistently in the elderly [36,40,57]. Alterations of the ventilation/perfusion ratio tend to be increased in the elderly due to diminished cardiac output, and result in a decrement in the P_aO_2 of about 4 mmHg per decade. Consequently, P_aO_2 will not normally exceed 65 or 75 mmHg in patients over age 70 [78], while usually the pH and P_aCO_2 remain within normal limits.

Spirometry and blood gas analysis are most useful and trustworthy in the evaluation of the respiratory function and must be performed in all patients.

Many very learned authors have made attempts to correlate the entity of the pulmonary deficit as demonstrated by spirometry with the actual surgical risk, but no trustworthy figure may be drawn that would per se be an indicator of increased risk. It is generally agreed that the VC, FEV_1 and FEV_1/VC are the most valuable guidelines to assess the pulmonary function, but normal limits are difficult to establish especially if atelectasis due to bronchial obstruction by carcinoma is present. Low P_aO_2 and especially increased P_aCO_2 witness for severely impaired gas exchange through the lung and have a major impact on the incidence of postoperative mortality and morbidity. These data should be evaluated with particular care in elderly patients before thoracotomy is decided.

Ebner and coworkers [19] have reported satisfactorily low postoperative mortality and morbidity rates (7.5 and 17%, respectively) limiting the indication for surgery only to patients with VC > 2.01, $FEV_1 > 1.81$, P_aO_2 at rest > 55 mmHg, P_aO_2 on exercise > 47 mmHg, P_aCO_2 at rest < 45 mmHg. They also performed right cardiac catheterization on borderline cases and considered for lobectomy only patients with PA pressure over 42 mmHg, and for pneumonectomy only patients with PA pressure over 37 mmHg.

History of congestive heart failure increases the surgical risk [8]. In our experience most of the patients had relatively poor pulmonary function and abnormal EKG findings, but the clinical criteria for posing the indication to surgery were not overall different from those employed in younger patients. Xenon 133 scans and perfusion scans with iodine 131 labeled albumine supply data concerning regional pulmonary function and pulmonary vascular resistances which may be important in borderline elderly patients [50,51]. These techniques give information regarding the contribution of each pulmonary area to ventilation and perfusion, and may demonstrate the presence of areas in the lung where right to left shunt occurs (i.e. lobar atelectasis due to bronchogenic carcinoma). These areas might be resected with beneficial effects not only on the primary disease but also on the patient's pulmonary function.

3.1. Lung cancer

Ninety percent of patients over age 70 who undergo thoracotomy will be found to have lung cancer. It is therefore important to evaluate carefully the cost–benefit ratio in these high-risk patients and to assess as precisely as possible the surgical resectability of the tumor and the extent of the resection necessary for this purpose. As a routine, we perform computed tomography on all patients with suspected lung cancer, and in 1986 introduced fine needle percutaneous biopsy in the preoperative work-up of all high-risk patients in whom histological diagnosis had not been obtained by means of bronchoscopic procedures (biopsy, bronchial lavage). This strategy enabled us to achieve positive histological diagnosis in 98.5% of cases. Invasive procedures such as mediastinoscopy and anterior mediastinotomy are controversial in the elderly, because they expose the patient to the additional risk of general anesthesia. They should be reserved to cases where histological diagnosis could not be obtained by lesser procedures, or to cases where irresectability is strongly suspected on the basis of computed tomography. If the tumor is deemed resectable and the patient is expected to tolerate the procedure well, even locally advanced disease (stage IIIa) should not be considered a contraindication for surgery. In our experience 33 patients (45.8%) (Table 7.3) were at stage IIIa and 5 of them had chest wall resection with overall mortality and morbidity rates of 6.9 and 23.6% respectively and a 5-year survival rate of 28%. These rates are in line with the data reported in the literature (Table 7.2).

3.2. Esophageal diseases

Despite modern surgical techniques and the association of radiotherapy and chemotherapy, treatment of carcinoma of the esophagus remains a controversial problem with poor prognosis. In fact, in a worldwide review of about 84000 patients with carcinoma of the esophagus, almost one third (29%) did not survive the operation [17,18]. Thus current therapy for esophageal carcinoma reveals an aura of pessimism, resulting in the attitude among physicians that cure is rarely achieved. This attitude has given rise to different treatment philosophies. The first advocates palliation of dysphagia as the only reasonable therapeutic goal and considers surgical procedures of touted low operative mortality as a means of providing palliation by removal of the primary tumor without regard for the principles of cancer surgery [52]. Proponents of this philosophy cite the high mortality for transthoracic esophagectomy and the miserable death for esophageal obstruction as reasons for this approach [17,52]. The second philosophy considers the operation alone as not radical and the addition of adjuvant radiation or chemotherapy pre- and postoperatively necessary to achieve cure. This approach predestines patients with limited disease to a delay in resection and to the morbidity and mortality of adjuvant therapy without proven benefit [23]. This philosophy exists though postoperative staging has shown that in patients with limited disease the results of surgical resection alone are better than those achieved by any other single or multidisciplinary approach [15,41,72].

We believe that especially in elderly patients the first objective must be to restore normal esophageal transit [82]. Realistically, thoracotomy combined with laparotomy is rarely feasible in the elderly, who are often affected by cardiorespiratory diseases and are malnourished as a consequence of the obstruction. Therefore in old patients the wisest treatment would be palliative, but radiotherapy, chemotherapy, tube insertion, endoscopic dilatation and laser recanalization of the esophagus all have drawbacks and bear the risk of complications [82]. Palliative surgery is indicated in selected cases with non-resectable tumor, and radical surgery may be performed successfully in a limited number of patients.

3.3. Mediastinal tumors

Currently almost all the mediastinal tumors and cysts require surgical procedures. The role of radical and debulking resection or simple biopsy, also as the first

TABLE 7.8
Preoperative management

– Nutritional support
– Fluid and electrolyte balance control
– Bronchial secretion control
– Antibiotic prophylaxis
– Cardiological drug therapy
– Physiokynesis therapy

step of a multidisciplinary approach, should be evaluated in every single case on the basis of the CT data[59] and the nature of the lesion. Less invasive diagnostic procedures should always be performed, if useful, to achieve the exact diagnosis and plan the appropriate treatment (resection vs medical treatment or a combination of both), especially if lymphoma is suspected. In general, if CT data suggest a benign lesion and the general clinical conditions are favorable, we proceed to surgery with radical intent. If malignancy or infiltration is suspected or the general conditions arc critical, we prefer to ascertain the histological nature of the lesion by non-invasive (percutaneous needle biopsy) or invasive (mediastinoscopy, anterior mediastinotomy) means.

3.4. Myasthenia gravis

Several factors should be considered when planning the treatment for elderly myasthenia gravis patients. The severity of symptoms is the main guideline, and the benefits of thymectomy or aggressive pharmacologic treatments such as immunosuppressants or high-dose steroids should be weighted against the risks connected with these therapeutic modalities. Thymectomy may involve some risk in old myasthenic patients, mainly because of the impaired muscular response to general anesthesia, which may result in slower regain of full chest wall motility, longer postoperative incubation and ventilatory assistance, pulmonary infections and respiratory failure. Corticosteroids may also be contraindicated because of the frequent association at this age of other disorders, such as diabetes, cardiovascular diseases or gastrointestinal disorders[56].

4. PREOPERATIVE TREATMENT AND PREPARATION FOR SURGERY (Table 7.8)

4.1. Pneumologic preparation

Pneumologic evaluation is indispensable to assessing cardiopulmonary function and to predicting the overall tolerance to surgery. Evaluation of the patient's ability to perform activities of daily life must be included in the interview phase.

Pertinent questions and observation of performance status allow the physician and the physiotherapist to identify activities wherein the patient utilizes inefficient respiratory or muscle mechanics and to identify specific activities during which the patient is unable to coordinate breathing and gross body movement pattern. The physiotherapist should look at the overall strength, range of motion, posture of the patient and improvement in general fitness; improvement in general fitness and efficiency should be a major goal in the preoperative treatment plan. Preoperative training in chest physiotherapy is therefore most important to enable the patient to cooperate with the nursing staff and the physiotherapist in the postoperative period. The patient must also be instructed in the use of the incentive spirometer and the nebulizer, and the mechanism of proper coughing and deep breathing must be practiced extensively before surgery [42]. Functionally inoperable patients with supposed reversible disorders can be treated medically in order to achieve operability: absolute nicotine abstinence, breathing exercises, inhalations with antibiotics and secretolytics, and administration of bronchodilators may improve the functional status dramatically and bring the patient to meet operability criteria.

4.2. Nutritional support

The nutritional status is as important as the respiratory performance in elderly patients who are candidates for major surgery. Malnutrition is part of the aging process [10,35]: it influences age-related changes, such as osteoporosis and atherosclerosis [46] and a great deal of the increment of the surgical risk in elderly people is due to a deteriorated nutritional status. Aging produces a reduction of total body nitrogen [86] in absolute amounts and as a percentage of body weight [13]. This reduction occurs in muscle more than in visceral proteins [83] but surely it narrows the margin of safety that exists for younger individuals: a further small loss of nitrogen will enhance susceptibility to disease and reduce ability to withstand stress [69]. A potential nutritional risk must be considered for aging patients undergoing surgery. The nutritional status must be carefully evaluated considering that many reference standards of antropometric and laboratory measurement can be misleading for geriatric patients: dietary history, involuntary weight loss and performance status are reliable indexes as well as serial antropometric and laboratory measurements. If nutritional treatment is needed it must be planned carefully. Infusion of 5% glucose is totally inadequate: also, albumin, plasma, and blood infusion must be considered useless from a nutritional point of view. Large amounts of nitrogen and glucose must be infused in the ratio of 1 g of nitrogen for at least 150 calories. Enteral nutrition is the easiest and safest approach when feasible. Otherwise, total parenteral nutrition (TPN) it no longer a heroic measure and must be available in any major hospital [1]. Nutritional treatment is as effective in elderly as in younger patients [31], but nutrients must be administered with caution while monitoring the metabolic equilibrium of the patient. In the young, large amounts of calories and nutrients can be infused, as the kidney will modulate for them. This assumption can be misleading for elderly patients: salt, fluid and energy requirements must be carefully evaluated to prevent overloading of an already compromised cardiorespiratory system [69].

4.3. Preparation of myasthenia gravis patients

The anticholinesterase drug pyridostigmine bromide (Mestinon) is administered to all myasthenia gravis patients adjusting the doses and the intervals between them in order to achieve good control of the symptoms over the 24 hours. It is also crucial to enable the patient to cough satisfactorily and breathe deeply in order to avoid secretion retention in the postoperative period. Corticosteroid therapy is instituted before thymectomy for those patients who had life-threatening signs or incapacitating signs: Prednisone is employed in a single dose of 25 to 100 mg on alternate days [63]. For patients who experienced severe weakness on the 'off' day, a small dose is added on that day for one to six weeks and gradually suspended. A low sodium and low carbonate diet is recommended in addition to an antacid supplement [21].

5. ANESTHESIA

Anesthesia for thoracic operations is crucial in elderly patients. Not only do these subjects display some degree of cardiopulmonary deficit as previously described, but they also undergo progressive decay of overall metabolic activity, affecting pharmacokynetics and pharmacodynamics of the anesthetic drugs [64,66]. In summary, drug metabolism is mainly influenced in the elderly by the different distribution of body fluids, by decreased hepato-biliary and renal clearance, and by the altered binding activity of plasma proteins, which are generally decreased in the old especially if neoplastic diseases or malnutrition coexist [27]. In addition, operative maneuvers such as the lateral decubitus on the operative table, the resection of functioning lung parenchyma and the problems related to single lung ventilation increase anesthesiological risk.

Endobronchial incubation by Carlens, White, Robertshaw or Brice–Smith tubes for single lung ventilation offers a number of advantages to the surgeon [6,53], such as better exposure on the lung and mediastinum, protection of the contralateral lung from blood or infested secretions, safe ventilation even in patients with bronchopleural fistulas or large emphysematous blebs. However, serious disadvantages exist especially in functionally compromised patients. These are the modifications of alveolar ventilation and the impairment of pulmonary blood flow [2,73]. In addition, the mechanism of hypoxic pulmonary vasoconstriction (HPV), which compensates for the functional impairment caused by regional hypoventilation reducing pulmonary blood flow in atelectasic areas of the lung, is partially inhibited by some volatile anesthetics, thus accentuating the V/Q mismatch and increasing the risk of systemic hypoxia. Advanced age also causes decline in the efficacy of the response to stress and complications [26]:

compensation for hemorrage, hypotension and shock will therefore be less effective due to decreased functional reserves.

Patients with a history of myocardial infarction should be carefully monitored intraoperatively [32] in order to identify and treat rapidly episodes of tachyarrhythmias and hypertension. Hemodynamic performance may effectively be checked intraoperatively by EKG monitoring and non-invasive blood pressure control. Invasive hemodynamic monitoring of the cardiac output and pulmonary artery pressure by Swan–Ganz catheter is indicated in selected cases. Monitoring end-tidal CO_2 ($EtCO_2$) allows an approximate estimate of the P_aCO_2, which is important in patients with potentially impaired cerebral blood flow adjustment to CO_2 levels. Percutaneous oximetry and especially oxygen saturation measurement should also be routinely employed [12,64,77]. The administration of myorelaxant drugs must be carefully performed following the data obtained by intraoperative percutaneous monitoring of the neuromuscular transmission, in order to rule out different quantitative responses to the myorelaxant; drug overdose and prolonged curarization after the end of the procedure may thus be avoided. The need for the administration of volatile or intravenous anesthetics tends to decrease progressively during the procedure, because the activity of these drugs is prolonged in elderly patients owing to the modifications in the central nervous system, in the cardiovascular system, in the liver and in the kidney. Awareness of these phenomena will enhance anesthesiological planning on the elderly.

6. SURGICAL STRATEGY

6.1. Pulmonary surgery

Patients with lung cancer or other lung diseases requiring parenchymal resection should be managed as conservatively as possible [20,30]. This does not imply that extensive resections for stage IIIa lesions are always contraindicated, but it emphasizes the opportunity of performing tissue-conserving operations whenever possible. The surgical access to the lung is standard posterolateral thoracotomy, but the extent of the incision must by tailored according to the needs of each procedure. Stage-I lung cancer or lesions requiring limited exposure for resection may be approached via a muscle-sparing lateral thoracotomy, with the advantage of minimizing the trauma on the chest wall and reducing postoperative pain.

Many reports have recently appeared that emphasize the use of limited resections (wedge resection, segmentectomy) over lobectomy for early-stage lung cancer on high-risk patients, stressing the decrease in mortality and morbidity, and the unvaried 5-year survival [5,8,19,20,30,42,48,70,84]. In our experience neither lobectomy nor minor resections were associated with operative deaths, and postoperative complications did not differ significantly between the two procedures (Table 7.9). We have resected stage-IIIa lung cancer with good long-term results, including 5 cases requiring chest wall resection [62] (Figs. 7.1a,b). Due to the high percentage

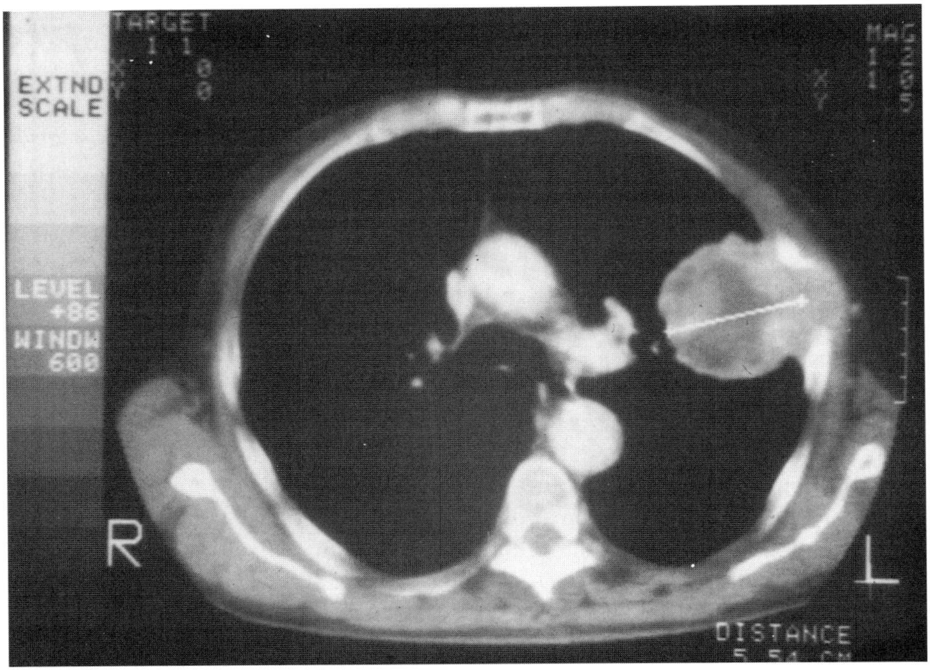

FIGURE 7.1a. CT scan of a 74-year old patient with lung cancer invading the chest wall.

TABLE 7.9
Operative mortality in relation to type of operation

Operation	Number of patients	Number of deaths	Mortality (%)
Pneumonectomy	8	2	25
Bilobectomy	4	2	50
Lobectomy	46	0	—
Explorative	8	1	12.5

of advanced lesions in our series, the number of extended resections is higher in our group than in other reported series (Table 7.10). Our postoperative mortality and morbidity and long term survival, despite 8 exploratory thoracotomies (5 stage-IIIb lesions), does not differ from that recently reported in the literature, indicating that an aggressive approach might be justified in these patients. In the literature, however, evidence exists that far fewer patients over 70 years are subjected to pneumonectomy than younger patients (4% vs. 8%) [42].

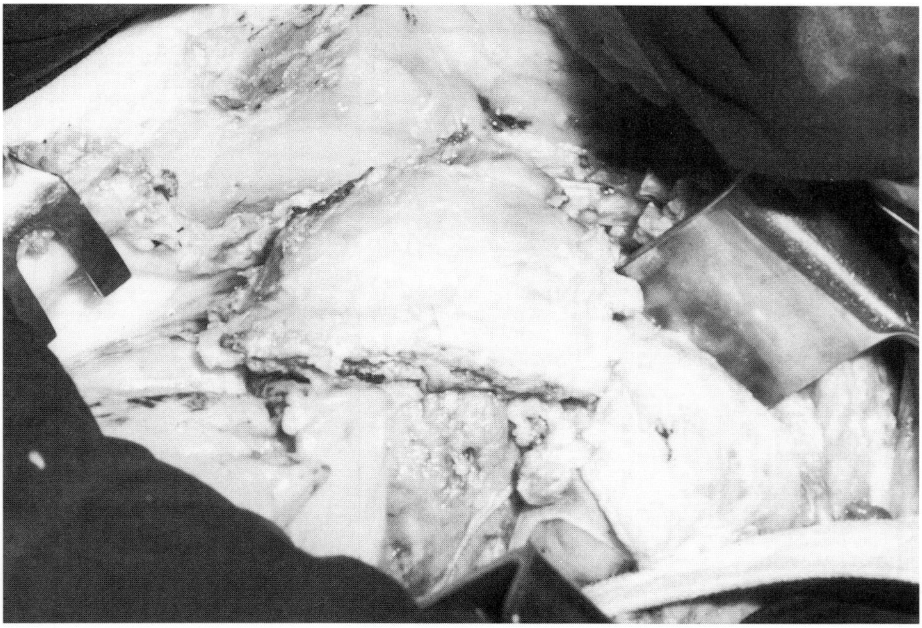

FIGURE 7.1b. Operative view of the patient from Fig. 7.1a, showing en-bloc resection of the tumor and the infiltrated parietes.

TABLE 7.10
Type of operation in 72 patients over 70 years with lung cancer

Operation	Number of patients	Percentage
Pneumonectomy	8[a]	11.1
Lobectomy	46[b]	63.8
Bilobectomy	4[c]	5.6
Wedge or segmental resection	6	8.2
Exploratory thoracotomy	8	11.1

[a] 2 with chest wall resection.
[b] 3 with chest wall resection.
[c] 1 with chest wall resection.

6.2. Esophageal surgery (Table 7.11)

Sugimachi and coworkers[71] operated on 51 patients over 70 years of age with esophageal carcinoma, with a resection rate of 59%. In these patients subtotal esophagectomy, lymph node dissection, and esophageal reconstruction using an antesternal gastric tube were performed. As a routine, we believe that elderly patients with esophageal carcinoma should primarily be considered for palliative

TABLE 7.11
Esophageal diseases in patients over 70 years of age[a]

Disease	Number of patients
Achalasia	7
Hiatal hernia	4
Benign stricture	2
Cancer	48
	—
Total	61

[a] Personal experience.

TABLE 7.12
Operative procedures in patients over 70 years with esophageal cancer

Procedure	Number of patients	Deaths
Celestin tube	12	–
Palliative esophagoplasty	9	–
Gastrostomy	14	–
Jejunostomy	7	–
Transthoracic esophagectomy	2	1
Transhiatal esophagectomy	4[a]	1
	—	—
Total	48	2

[a] 2 anastomotic leaks.

treatment in order to relieve dysphagia and allow normal feeding and swallowing (Table 7.12). Insertion of an endoluminal tube, laser recanalization, palliative esophagogastroplasty or esophago-colonplasty, and gastrostomy may be performed on these patients following thorough clinical evaluation with reasonable risk. In selected cases curative esophagectomy and reconstruction may be performed. Our preference goes to the transhiatal technique because of the reduced operative trauma and because in general we would consider for surgery only elderly patients with disease limited to the esophagus, not requiring mediastinal exploration or dissection. Transabdominal esophagectomy using the EEA stapler to accomplish the end-to-end anastomosis is indicated in patients with cancer of the distal thoracic esophagus at a limited stage [34]. The advantage of this technique is the conversion of a prolonged procedure to a more expeditious one, possibly minimizing the morbidity by not entering the pleural cavity or exploring the neck [3], even though this advantage remains still controversial [54].

6.3. Surgery for mediastinal diseases

As previously reported (Tables 7.5 and 7.6), mediastinal lesions in elderly patients are usually either benign, and therefore resectable with relatively low risk, or

TABLE 7.13
Complications in 72 patients over 70 years with lung cancer

Complication	Number of patients	Percentage
Cardiorespiratory		
Arrhythmia	5	
Persistent air leak	3	
Respiratory failure	2	
Pulmonary edema	1	
Haemothorax	1	
Haemopericardium	1	
Empyema	1	
Total cardiorespiratory:	14	19
General		
Renal failure	2	
Intestinal occlusion	1	
Total general:	3	4
Total	17	23.6

of inflammatory nature where tissue biopsy is the only indicated procedure. Primary carcinoma of the mediastinum or other malignant lesions (Table 7.5) also occurred in our experience, but in these cases biopsy is usually all that can be reasonably done. Our surgical approach to mediastinal lesions in the elderly does not differ from that for younger patients; thymoma and anterior tumor are always approached by total median sternotomy with no difficulty even if limited infiltration is present. We have reported successful resection of thymoma even in an 83-year old patient [60]. Intrathoracic goiter is resected via cervicotomy, and in some cases a sternal split is added to achieve better exposure on the mediastinal vessels.

When the general clinical status permits, thymectomy is indicated in the presence of radiologic signs of thymoma and in all cases of incapacitating myasthenia gravis [21]. We prefer to perform thymectomy by partial median sternotomy from the jugular notch to the II or III intercostal space (sternal split) when there is no evidence of thymoma, and by complete median sternotomy when there is thymoma. Radiotherapy is administered postoperatively in patients with cortical or mixed thymoma at all stages [58].

7. POSTOPERATIVE CARE AND COMPLICATIONS (Tables 7.2, 7.13, 7.14)

7.1. Pulmonary surgery

All authors reporting on the subject (Table 7.2) have emphasized the increased incidence of complications and mortality rates in elderly patients undergoing

TABLE 7.14
Operative mortality in patients over 70 years undergoing surgery for lung cancer[a]

ID	Age	Histological type	Procedure	Fatal complication
1	74	large cell	bilobectomy	haemopericardium
2	76	squamous	bilobectomy + chest resection	respiratory failure
3	79	squamous	pneumonectomy	bleeding
4	71	squamous	pneumonectomy	empyema
5	72	large cell	exploratory	mediastinal syndrome

[a] All patients male, surgical stage III. Overall mortality: 6.9%.

pulmonary surgery as compared to younger age groups. Recent studies reporting on patients operated upon in the 1970s or later display better results because of the better selection of patients, intensive postoperative care and thanks to the widespread acceptance of tissue-conserving operation (wedge resection, segmentectomy) even with curative intent for lung cancer. This conservative approach has been emphasized in recent years [30] for the surgical cure of Stage-I lung cancer, and evidence has been produced that comparable long-term survival may be achieved by wedge resection or lobectomy, with the advantage of decreased mortality and postoperative complications. As reported by Martini [42], elderly patients have a significantly higher major complication rate compared to younger patients (18% vs 9%), and the group treated by pneumonectomy shows a higher morbidity and mortality rate than that treated by lesser procedures. Even when pneumonectomy is deemed indispensable, the procedure is performed with some concern by all authors. In the series reported on by Martini [42], only 4% of patients over 70 years underwent pneumonectomy, versus 8% of patients below this age. In our experience 4 out of 5 postoperative deaths were associated with major resections (Table 7.14); conversely, no patients undergoing lobectomy or minor resections died. According to Yellin and coworkers [84,85] there is statistically significant difference between patients undergoing lobectomy (mortality 4.3%) and pneumonectomy (mortality 36.4%), the overall rate being 10.3%. Moreover, data from the Memorial Sloan-Kettering group points out that all deaths associated with pneumonectomy occurred after right pneumonectomy, thus stressing the importance of the extent of resection on surgical risk [48]. The morbidity rate increases when pulmonary reserve is reduced: while patients with a pulmonary function within normal limits usually do well, a 14% major complication rate was observed in patients with mild restriction and 16% in those with severe restriction [42]. In the series reported on by Martini [42], morbidity is highest in patients with cardiac problems (20%).

The causes of death are varied and often unpredictable after lung surgery (Table 7.14) [84,85], the most frequent being related to cardiorespiratory problems. The sense of 'operative normality' in reference especially to elderly patients and to esophageal surgery is most clearly elucidated by the views of Belsey on the subject [4]: "The operative mortality, as a prestige symbol, is of paramount interest to the surgeon. The limiting of the definition to the 4-week postoperative period is no longer valid: with the help of respiratory and life support systems, the seriously complicated and moribund patient can be kept alive beyond this period; the overall postoperative mortality rate is 30%, considerably higher than the rate confessed to by any individual surgeon."

7.2. Esophageal surgery

According to most reports on the outcome of patients undergoing esophageal surgery, mortality is related to the age of the patient, the type of the operation, the method of suturing and the year of the study [39]. The most frequent causes of death in esophageal surgery are pneumothorax, pleural purulent effusion, visceral and systemic failure, mediastinal abscess, pulmonary infection, myocardial infarction, septic shock and pulmonary embolism [39]. Sugimachi and coworkers [71] demonstrated that complications occurred more frequently in patients over age 70 undergoing esophagectomy for cancer than in younger age groups: mortality was 14% in this group and 4% in younger patients. The most frequent cause of death was pneumonia, occurring always in patients with abnormal preoperative pulmonary functions. According to Launois and coworkers [39], operative mortality differs sensibly between patients younger than 50 years (6.0%) or older than 60 years (20 to 24%). Anastomotic leak is among the most common causes of operative death, but its incidence is not higher in the elderly, although they are more prone to develop general and respiratory complications [43]. Williamson [82] performed transhiatal esophagectomy in 6 patients over 75 years; 2 had major complications, but no deaths occurred. Orringer [52] also performed this operation in 7 elderly patients with satisfactory results. Pneumothorax and pleural effusion are common after transhiatal esophagectomy [82].

7.3. Mediastinal tumors and myasthenia gravis

Median sternotomy is the most frequent way of access for resection of mediastinal tumors, and it encompasses less morbidity than other major surgical approaches to the chest. Therefore, the resection of capsulated mediastinal tumors usually does not present particular postoperative problems [60].

Conversely, the postoperative course of myasthenia gravis patients is delicate at all ages, but in elderly subjects, especially if associated with thymoma, it should be followed even more closely. The impact of myorelaxant drugs used for general anesthesia is greater in the elderly and relatively minor complications like pneumothorax or pleural effusion may interfere dramatically with the unstable muscular and cardiorespiratory balance set in the immediate postoperative period. The incapacity to maintain a sufficient tidal volume, the fear of being weaned from the ventilator, and the impossibility to restore pharmacologically effective breathing ability often leads to respiratory insufficiency and death. Careful administration and dose adjustment of pyridostigmine bromide (Mestinon) and the use of plasmapheresis in life-threatening situations obviates in most cases these complications if the preoperative preparation and the choice of surgery as the treatment modality have been correct.

8. CONCLUSIONS

The risk of general surgery in geriatric patients with cancer is no greater than in younger age groups. A recent review by William [81] reports that 485 patients over 60 years of age underwent surgery for cancer with a mortality of 5.3%, which is comparable with the results obtained in middle-aged patients. The advances in preoperative preparation, combined with anesthesia and postoperative monitoring, have greatly altered the outcome of thoracic surgical procedures in this age group. Therefore there is no reason why elderly patients should not undergo major thoracic surgery procedures after adequate preoperative assessment. Fluid and electrolyte balance and nutritional status is often a major problem, especially in patients with esophageal cancer, but it can effectively be managed by careful preoperative nutritional programs.

Lung cancer in the elderly population is a frequent disease but may be successfully treated surgically with acceptable mortality and morbidity and favorable long term results. Pulmonary resection may be carried out in these patients with reasonable operative risk and should therefore be advocated when curable surgery is deemed possible on the basis of preoperative staging. Also, functional evaluation of the respiratory system is of prime importance, and patients that do not meet strict standards should be excluded as surgical candidates not on the basis of age itself or because of poor results of one test per se, but after complete clinical evaluation. The most important factor determining surgical mortality is the extent of the resection. Pneumonectomy is associated with increased risk and should be performed selectively only in patients with totally favorable preoperative multi-organ function tests. Efforts should be made to perform parenchymal-preserving resections such as wedge resection or segmentectomy and strive to avoid pneumonectomy, especially right pneumonectomy [42,84].

At the present time, operative mortality rates ranging between 4.3% [70] and 15.9% [5], and 5-year survival rates of 32% [5] to 40% [84] may be achieved in patients over the age of 70 undergoing surgery for lung cancer (Table 7.2). When these data are compared to the 1-year survival rate of approximately 7% of untreated cases, it seems evident that surgical treatment is indeed indicated even in elderly patients.

The selection of therapy for esophageal carcinoma in the elderly depends on many factors, especially the stage of disease and the general conditions of these patients. Because cure may only be achieved by surgical treatment, elderly patients might be considered for esophageal surgery after careful selection and clinical investigation [71]. The choice of operation should reflect the patient's physiological status, life expectancy, and associated medical problems [82]. If the functional criteria are fulfilled and the neoplasm is resectable, survival after surgical treatment of carcinoma of the esophagus does not differ much between patients of over and under 60 years [39]. If no overwhelming contraindications exist, radical surgery should be considered the most appropriate approach to esophageal cancer even in advanced age. Nevertheless, palliative surgery may be offered with relatively low risk in order to restore swallowing. The deciding factor for establishing whether or not elderly patients should undergo surgery for benign lesions such as hiatal hernia or achalasia should be the severity of the symptoms as opposed to the increased risk of an operation. Patients with esophageal diseases requiring surgical treatment can tolerate transhiatal esophagectomy and achieve satisfactory swallowing and therefore good quality of life [82].

The mediastinal lesions which are usually considered for surgical treatment in elderly patients are mostly benign or inflammatory in nature. Malignant tumors may also occur but in this case the attempt to perform radical surgery is invariably frustrated by the awareness of the major trauma of an operation (with extensive resection of infiltrated mediastinal organs) and of its scarce oncological effectiveness. Diagnostic biopsy is therefore the most frequently adopted solution in malignant as well as in inflammatory lesions. On the other hand, space occupying benign masses (thymoma, intrathoracic goiter, pericardial cysts, neurogenic tumors) may be resected with relatively low risk.

It has been demonstrated by Monden [42], and our personal experience is in line with his findings, that there is no statistically significant difference between the clinical effect of thymectomy in young versus elderly myasthenic patients. The indications to surgery are however different in the two groups; that is, more restricted in elderly patients. Taking into account clinical contraindications to surgery, thymectomy may be indicated in elderly myasthenia gravis patients.

9. ACKNOWLEDGEMENTS

We wish to thank Dr. G.F. Cappello and Dr. S.J. Steen for their invaluable help in the preparation of this chapter.

REFERENCES

1 Arullani A, Cappello G, Spera E, Tozzo C, Casciani C. Intensive treatment with TON: a true artificial gut. Artific Organs 1977; 1: 120.
2 Bachard R, Audet J. Physiological changes associated with unilateral pulmonary ventilation during operation on lung. Can Anesth Soc J 1975; 22: 659.
3 Bains MS. Transabdominal esophagogastrectomy for the poor-risk patient. In: International Trends in General Thoracic Surgery, Vol 4, Esophageal Cancer. St Louis, MO, Mosby 1988: pp 222–226.
4 Helsey R. Is it possible to talk of cure of carcinoma of the esophagus? In: Giuli R (ed.). Cancer of the Esophagus in 1984: Answers to 135 Questions. Maloine 1984: pp 382–386.

5 Berggren X, Ekroth R, Malmberg R, Naucler J, William-Olsson G. Hospital mortality and long-term survival in relation to preoperative function in elderly patients with bronchogenic carcinoma. Ann Thorac Surg 1984; 38(6): 633–636.
6 Bjork VO, Carlens E, Frieberg O. Endobronchial anesthesia. J Thorac Cardiovasc Surg 1953; 14: 60.
7 Brander P, Kjellberg M, Tammisto T. The effects of anesthesia and general surgery of geriatric patients. Ann Chir Gynaecol Penniae 1970; 59: 138–145.
8 Breyer RH, Zippe C, Pharr WF, Jensik RJ, Kittle CF, Faber LP. Thoracotomy in patients over age seventy years – Ten-years experience. J Thorac Cardiovasc Surg 1981; 81: 187–193.
9 Britt EJ, Shelhamer J, Menkes H, et al. Sex difference in the decline of pulmonary function with age. Chest 1981; 80: 1.
10 Burger M. Altern und Krankheit, 3rd Ed. Leipzig, Georg Thieme Verlag, 1957.
11 Burrows B, Cline MG, Knudson RJ, et al. A descriptive analysis of the growth and decline of the FVC and FEV_1. Chest 1983; 83: 717.
12 Chung M, Lichtory L, Rangachari K. Transcuteneous monitoring of the PaO_2 and $PaCO_2$ during one lung anesthesia. Anesthesiology 1984; 61: A164.
13 Cohn JH, Shock NW. Blood volume in middle age and elderly males. Am J Med Sci 1949; 217: 388.
14 Compston DAS, Vincent A, Newson Davies J, Batchelor JR. Clinical, pathological, HLA antigen and immunological evidence for disease heterogeneity in myasthenia gravis. Brain 1980; 103: 579.
15 DeMeester TR, Zaninotto G, Johnson WE. Selective therapeutic approach to cancer of the lower esophagus and cardia. J Thorac Cardiovasc Surg 1988; 95: 42–54.
16 Dhar B, Saastri SR, Lenora R. Aging and the respiratory system. Med Clin North Am 1976; 60: 1121.
17 Earlam R, Cunha-Melo JR. Esophageal squamous cell carcinoma. I. A critical review of surgery. Br J Surg 1980; 67: 381–390.
18 Earlam R, Cunha-Melo JR. Oesophageal squamous cell carcinoma. II. A critical review of radiotherapy. Br J Surg 1980; 67: 457–461.
19 Ebner H, Sudkamp N, Wex P, Dragojevic D. Election and preoperative treatment of over-seventy-year-old patients undergoing thoracotomy. Thorac Cardiovasc Surgeon 1985; 33: 268–271.
20 Erret LE, Wilson J, Chiu Chu-Jeng, Munro DD. Wedge resection as an alternative procedure for peripheral bronchogenic carcinoma in poor-risk patients. J Thorac Cardiovasc Surg 1985; 90: 656–661.
21 Evoli A, Tonali P, Scoppetta C, David P. Myasthenia gravis in the elderly : Report of 37 cases. J Am Geriatr Soc 1983; 31(6): 352–355.
22 Gaillard J, Glock Y, Dahan M, Eschapasse H. Chirurgie thoracique chez le sujet agé. Ann Chir: Chir Thorac Cardio-Vasc 1984; 38: 545.
23 Giuli R, Sancho-Garnier H. Diagnostic, therapeutic and prognostic features of cancer of esophagus: results of the international prospective study conducted by the OESO group (790 patients). Surgery 1986; 99: 614–622.
24 Golebiowski A. Pulmonary resection in patients over 70 years of age. J Thorac Cardiovasc Surg 1971; 61: 265–270.
25 Herishann Y, Abramsky O, Feldman S. Myasthenia gravis in the elderly. J Am Geriatr Soc 1976; 24: 228.
26 Hilgenberg JC. Inhalation and intravenous drugs in the elderly patients. Semin. Anesth. 1986; 5(1, March).
27 Homer TD, Stansky DR. The effect of increased age on thiopental disposition and anesthetion requirement. Anesthesiology 1983; 62: 74.
28 Howard FM. Myasthenia gravis with onset after 65 years of age: a preliminary report. In: Dan PC (ed.). Plasmapheresis and the Immunobiology of Myasthenia Gravis. Boston, Houghton–Mifflin 1979: p. 281.
29 Huang GJ. Epidemiology of esophageal cancer in China. In: Siewart JR, Halscher AH (eds.). Diseases of the Esophagus. Berlin, Springer: pp 3–5.

30 Jensik RJ, Faber LP, Kittle CF. Segmental resection for bronchogenic carcinoma. Ann Thorac Surg 1979; 28(5, Nov).

31 Kaminsky MV, Nasr NJ, Freed BA. The efficacy of nutritional support in the elderly. J Am Coll Nutr 1982; 1: 35.

32 Keenan RL, Boyanc P. Cardiac arrest due to anesthesia, JAMA 1985; 253: 2373.

33 Kimura M, Kusagawa M, Namikawa S, Tani K. Suppression of cellular immunity affects surgical results of primary lung cancer in patients over 75 years old. Lung Cancer 1988; 4 (Suppl): A86.

34 Kitamura M, Nishimira T, Mirayama K, Kasi M. Surgical treatment for patients 70 years of age or older with carcinoma of the esophagus. In: Siewart JR, Halscher AH (eds.). Diseases of the Esophagus. Berlin, Springer.

35 Kohn RR. Principles of Mammalian Aging. Englewood Cliffs, NJ, Prentice Hall 1971: p 111.

36 Knudson RJ, Slatin RC, Libouritz M, Burrows B. The maximal expiratory flow-volume curve: normal standards, variability and effects of age. Am Rev Respir Dis 1976; 113: 587.

37 Kronenberg RS, Drage CW. Attenuation of the ventilatory and heart rate response to hypoxia and hypercapnia with aging in normal men. J Clin Invest 1972; 52: 1812.

38 LaRue A, Schaefer J. Psychologic reactions of elderly patients to illness and surgery. Semin Anesth 1986; 5 (1, March).

39 Launois B, Paul JL, Lygidakis NJ, Campion JP, Malledant Y, Grossetti D, Delarue D. Results of the surgical treatment of carcinoma of the esophagus. Surg Gynecol Obstet 1983; 156: 753–760.

40 Leblanc P, Ruff F, Milic-Emili J. Effects of age and body position on 'Airway Closure' in men. J Appl Physiol 1970; 28: 448.

41 Lu YK, Yueh ML, Yue ZG. Cancer of the esophagus and esophagogastric junction: an analysis of the results of 1025 resections after 5 to 20 years. Ann Thorac Surg 1987; 43: 176–181.

42 Martini N. Lung cancer in the elderly. Front Radiant Ther Onc 1986; 20; 125–132.

43 Mohansingh MP. Mortality of oesophagal surgery in the elderly. Br J Surg 1976; 63: 579–580.

44 Monden YK, Nakahara Y, Hashimoto K, Ohno A, Masaoka A, Kawashima Y. Myasthenia gravis in elderly patients. Ann Thorac Surg 1985; 39(5): 433–436.

45 Morris JF, Kosky A, Johnson LC. Spirometric standards for healthy non smoking adults. Am Rev Respir Dis 1971; 103: 57.

46 Munro NN. Nutrition and the elderly. Bibl Nutr Dieta 1983; 33.

47 Muir C. Epidemiologie des cancers de l'oesophage en France et dans le monde. Gastrenterol Clin Biol 1981; 5: 239–242.

48 Nagasaky F, Flehinger BJ, Martini N. Complications of surgery in the treatment of carcinoma of the lung. Chest 1982; 82: 25–29.

49 Olanow CW, Lane RJM, Roses AD. Thymectomy in late onset myasthenia gravis. Arch Neurol 1982; 39: 82.

50 Olsen GN, Block AJ, Tobias JA. Prediction of postpneumonectomy function using quantitative microaggregate lung scanning. Chest 1974; 66: 13.

51 Olsen GN, Block AJ, Swensen EW, Castle JR, Wynne JW. Pulmonary function evaluation of the lung resection candidate: a prospective study. Am Rev Respir Dis 1975; 111: 379.

52 Orringer MB. Palliative procedures for esophageal cancer. Surg Clin North Am 1983; 63: 941–950.

53 Pappin JC. The current practice of endobronchial intubation. Anesthesia 1979; 34: 57.

54 Pearson FC. Transabdominal esophagogastrectomy for the poor-risk patient – discussion. In: International Trends in General Thoracic Surgery, Vol 4, Esophageal Cancer. Mosby 1988: p 227.

55 Perlo VP, Poskanzer DL, Schwab RS. Myasthenia gravis: evaluation of treatment in 1355 patients. Neurology 1966; 16: 431.

56 Perlo VP, Arnason B, Castleman B. The thymus gland in elderly patients with myasthenia gravis. Neurology 1975; 25: 294–295.

57 Pierce JA, Ebert RW. The elastic properties of the lung in the aged. J Lab Clin Med 1958; 51: 63.

58 Rendina EA, Venuta F, Pescarmona O, Nardi F, De Rosa G, Martelli M, Ricci C. Thymoma: A clinico-pathologic study based on newly developed morphologic criteria. Tumori 1988; 74: 79–84.

59 Rendina EA, Venuta F, Ceroni L, Martelli M, Gualdi GF, Ceterino M, Ricci C. Computed tomographic staging of anterior mediastinal neoplasms. Thorax 1988; 43: 441–445.
60 Rendina EA, Venuta F, Martelli M, Pescarmona E, Ricci C. Successful resection of a thymoma in an elderly patient. Int J Surg Sci 1988; 18: 79–82.
61 Rich MW, Sandza JG, Kleiger RE, Connors JP. Cardiac operations in patients over 80 years of age. J Thorac Cardiovasc Surg 1985; 90: 56–60.
62 Ricci C, Rendina EA, Venuta F. En bloc resection for T3 bronchogenic with chest wall invasion. Eur J Cardiothorac Surg 1987; 1: 23–28.
63 Scoppetta C, Tonali P, Evoli A, et al. Treatment of myasthenia gravis. Report on 139 patients. J Neurol 1979; 222: 11.
64 Scott JC, Stansky DR. The increased Fentanyl–Alfentanyl requirements with increasing age: a pharmacodynamic basis. Anesthesiology 1985; 63: A374.
65 Shulman MD, Brodsky JB, Mark JBD, Swan M. Non invasive pulse oximetry during one lung ventilation. Anesthesiology 1984; 61: A98.
66 Singleton MA, Rosen JI, Fisher DM. Pharmacokinetics of Fentanyl in the elderly. Anesthesiology 1985; 63: A372.
67 Slater G, Papatestas AE, Genkins G. Thymectomy in patients more than 60 years of age with myasthenia gravis. Surg Gynecol Obstet 1978; 146: 54.
68 Smith TC. Respiratory effects of aging. Semin Anesth. 1986; 5 (1, March).
69 Steffee WP. Nutrition intervention in hospitalized geriatric patients. Bull NY Acad Med 1980; 56: 564.
70 Suemasu K, Yoneyama T, Naruke T, Miyazawa N, Tsuchiya R. Surgical treatment of lung cancer in patients over the age of 70 years. In: Motta G (ed.). Cancer of the lung and pleura. Milan, Masson 1986: pp 87–98.
71 Sugimachi K, Matzuzaki K, Matsuura H, Kuwano H, Ueo K, Inokuchi K. Evaluation of surgical treatment of carcinoma of the oesophagus in the elderly: 20 years' experience. Br J Surg 1985; 72: 28–30.
72 Sweet RH. Late results of surgical treatment of carcinoma of the esophagus. JAMA 1954; 155: 422–425.
73 Tarhan S, Lundborg RO. Blood gas and pH-studies during use of the Carlens catheter. Can Anesth Soc J 1968; 15: 458.
74 Teeter SM, Holmes FF, McFarlane MJ. Lung carcinoma in the elderly population: influence of histology on the inverse relationship of stage to age. Cancer 1987; 60: 1331–1336.
75 The World Almanac. New York, Newspaper Enterprise Association 1983.
76 Tindall RSA. Humoral immunity in myasthenia gravis: effect of steroids and thymectomy. Neurology 1988; 30: 544.
77 Viitanen A, Salmenpera M, Hinonen J. Comparison of transcutaneous oxygenation measurements and pulse oximetry during one lung ventilation. Anesthesiology 1986; 65, A482.
78 Wahaba WM. Influence of aging on lung function – clinical significance of changes from age 20. Anesth Analg 1983; 62: 764.
79 Watson A. Therapeutic options and patient selection in the management of esophageal carcinoma. In: Watson A, Celestin LR (eds.). Disorders of the Esophagus. Advances and Controversies. London, Pitman 1983: pp 167–186.
80 Welch CA. Surgery in the aged. N Engl J Med 1948; 238: 825.
81 William A. Should elderly patients undergo surgery for cancer? Geriatrics 1977; 5: 105.
82 Williamson RCN. Abdominocervical oesophagectomy in the elderly. Ann R Coll Surg Engl 1985; 67: 343–348.
83 Winterer JC, Steffee WP, Perera WD. Whole body protein turnover in aging man. Exp Geront 1976; 11: 79.
84 Yellin A, Benfield JR. Surgery of bronchogenic carcinoma in the elderly. Am Rev Respir Dis 1985; 131: 197.

85 Yellin A, Hill LR, Lieberman Y. Pulmonary resections in patients over 70 years of age. Israel J Med Sci 1985; 21: 833–840.
86 Young VR, Perera WD, Winterer JC, Scrimshaw N. Protein and amino acid requirements of the elderly. In: Winick M (ed.). Nutrition and Aging. New York, Wiley 1976: p 77.

Current Topics in General Thoracic Surgery: An International Series, Vol. 2
Perioperative Care, edited by R.M. Peters and J. Toledo

Pulmonary resection for lung cancer in the elderly

Discussion of "Thoracic surgery in the elderly" by C. Ricci, E.A. Rendina, F. Venuta and R. Guerricchio

G. Varela and J. Toledo

1. INTRODUCTION

The chapter by Dr. Ricci and coworkers is a comprehensive and well documented presentation on a difficult and up to date topic. In fact, in recent years there has been an increase in the number of patients over seventy who are being admitted for thoracotomy in most general hospitals.

We are focusing our discussion on some aspects of surgery for lung cancer in this particular subset of patients. We think that in these cases the surgeon must be specially concerned with a correct evaluation of the risk/benefit ratio of surgical treatment.

In our Centre, patients admitted for lung cancer undergo a staging study[1] and are preoperatively classified as operable or inoperable (for the type of resection needed) and the tumor is judged resectable or unresectable. We include as resectable disease, tumors classified in clinical stages I, II or III-a, except N2. Non-resectable tumors are those having any kind of mediastinal gland extension (N2 or N3) or those classified in stages III-b or IV. Our protocol includes mediastinoscopy as a routine procedure in all cases judged operable and having no other criteria of unresectability.

The data we are presenting are based on a series of 749 mediastinoscopies for lung cancer performed between 1975 and 1988 (operable patients) and on a series of 247 incident cases of lung cancer from our Hospital in 1986 (therefore including operable/inoperable and resectable/non-resectable cases). We also present some data related to all the patients who were 70 years or over at the time of the thoracotomy for lung cancer in a period of 13 years (1976–1989).

TABLE D7.1
Reasons for not selecting patients for surgery

Reason	Percentage of patients[a]		p
	under 70 (n = 186)	70 or over (n = 61)	
Patient inoperable	7.2 (2.9–11.5)	18.7 (7.7–29.8)	< 0.001
Tumor unresectable	89.1 (83.9–94.3)	72.9 (60.3–85.4)	0.159
Patient refused surgery	2.2 (0–4.6)	6.3 (0– 13.1)	0.037

[a] CI95% values shown in parentheses.

2. SURGERY FOR LUNG CANCER IN THE ELDERLY

For some reasons outside the scope of this discussion (interested readers are referred to the excellent review by Lipschitz et al.[2]), prevalence of malignant tumors is higher in oldest people. In a report cited by Fentiman et al.[3], 50% of males diagnosed of lung cancer in Wales are over 70. In our Centre, 61 (25.7%) out of 247 cases of lung carcinoma diagnosed in 1986 were between 70 and 86 years old.

Except in some reported series, where the percentages of elderly people operated on for lung cancer surpass 30%[4], most reports show a small percentage of patients over 70[5,6]. The reason for this can be twofold: (a) elderly patients are usually not referred for surgery, in order to avoid a supposed risky treatment[3], and (b) patients over 70 are more frequently excluded for surgery because of more advanced tumors. The last is not in accord with clinical evidence[7].

Some of our data can be of interest. In 1986, 147 out of 247 lung cancer patients seen in our Centre were not selected for thoracotomy. Table D7.1 lists some of the reasons stated to deny surgery, dividing the patients into two age groups (186 cases under 70 and 61 cases of 70 or over). Eight percent of young and 29% of old patients, respectively, were judged inoperable ($p < 0.001$), while 47% and 53% of patients over 69 and under 70, respectively, had non-resectable tumors. Finally, some patients refused surgery: 5% in the oldest group and 1.6% in the youngest ($p = 0.037$).

Two conclusions can be drawn:

(1) Elderly patients gather more causes of inoperability (poor pulmonary function, other non-treatable concomitant diseases, etc).

(2) Refusing surgical treatment is more common among elderly patients. This appears to be in accord with other published data[8]. Older patients seem to prefer a 'long-term' threat to life (such as a lung carcinoma can be) over an aggressive and dangerous treatment (in this case a pulmonary resection).

We have no data to confirm that clinical stage of lung cancer at the time of diagnosis is lower in older cases, as can be concluded from other reports[2,7]. Our results could be biased by the fact that patients we classified as inoperable are not completely studied for staging the tumor.

TABLE D7.2
Complications of mediastinoscopy in bronchial cancer

Age group	Morbidity	Mortality
Under 70 (n = 617)	1.94% (12)	0.16% (1)
70 and over (n = 93)	1.08% (1)	0

TABLE D7.3
Postoperative course in 62 resections for lung cancer in patients of 70 years and over

Procedure	Postoperative course (%)[a]		
	Uneventful	Morbidity	Death
Pneumonectomy	42.9 (9)	42.9 (9)	14.3 (3)
Lobectomy and minor	68.3 (28)	21.9 (9)	9.8 (4)

[a] Numbers of patients given in parentheses.

3. ROUTINE MEDIASTINOSCOPY: SHOULD IT BE DONE IN THE ELDERLY?

In the preceding chapter, the authors state that mediastinoscopy in the elderly should be reserved for those cases having clinical suspicion of mediastinal spread, according to CT images. By so doing they try to avoid an invasive diagnostic technique in a high-risk population.

In our Hospital (unpublished data) the negative predictive value of CT scan (to assess mediastinal lymph node metastases) is 0.83. Therefore, more than 15% of all patients having lung carcinoma and clinically classified as N0, become N2 after mediastinoscopy. In our experience, in a series of 93 mediastinoscopies in lung cancer cases over 70, we have had one complication (Table D7.2): a patient who suffered an iatrogenic left vocal cord palsy (morbidity of the series, 1.07%). This patient underwent an uneventful lobectomy. As can be seen from Table D7.2, morbidity and mortality due to mediastinoscopy is not higher in older cases. In our series of mediastinoscopy in elderly patients, 19 (20.4%) were classified as N2, N3 or T4. Accordingly, a useless and more dangerous operation was avoided.

4. HOW MUCH LUNG PARENCHYMA CAN BE SAFELY RESECTED?

Dr. Ricci and coworkers support segmental resection in the elderly in order to minimize operative mortality. Although there are other excellent reports on this topic[9,10] there is no definite evidence at the present time that segmentectomy is as good as larger resections in terms of survival.

In Sherman and Guidot's series[4], fewer patients over 70 underwent pneumonectomy (6% vs 27%, $p < 0.01$). In our Centre, around 35% of all patients operated on for lung cancer underwent pneumonectomy. In the series of cases over 70, 28.4% (21 out of 74) were treated by means of a pneumonectomy. There is a significant statistical difference between both percentages ($p < 0.001$) meaning that probably old patients with large or hilar tumors were not referred for surgical evaluation.

Table D7.3 shows postoperative course in 62 elderly patients operated on in which a pneumonectomy or lesser resection was done. In the pneumonectomy group, 3 patients died (14.3%), nine had some kind of relevant complication (42.9%) and nine had no postoperative problems. Operative mortality in the other group is 9.8% (4 of 41 cases), morbidity 21.9%, while 68.3% had an uneventful postoperative period. There are no statistical differences between the groups. In our Centre, operative mortality for pulmonary resection in cases irrespective of age is 5.1% (6.6% in pneumonectomy). Although a 14% operative mortality is a high percentage[5,6,11] we consider it not a prohibitive risk. We are treating selected high-risk cases (77% have some other major concomitant disease). On the other hand, survival in elderly people after pulmonary resection (42% five-year actuarial in our series) is comparable to that of patients in younger age groups.

REFERENCES

1 López-Encuentra A, Martínez J, Cortés H. Protocolo para el estudio y tratamiento del carcinoma broncogénico (I). Med Clin Barcelona 1979; 72: 321–331.

2 Lipschitz DA, Goldstein S, Reis R, Weksler ME, Bressler R, Neilan BA. Cancer in the elderly: Basic science and clinical aspects. Ann Intern Med 1985; 102: 218–228.

3 Fentiman IS, Tirelli U, Monfardini S, et al. Cancer in the elderly: why so badly treated? Lancet 1990; I: 1020–1021.

4 Sherman S, Guidot CE. The feasibility of thoracotomy for lung cancer in the elderly. JAMA 1987; 258: 927–930.

5 Nagasaki F, Flehinger BJ, Martini N. Complications of surgery in the treatment of carcinoma of the lung. Chest 1982; 82: 25–29.

6 Kohman LJ, Meyer JA, Ikins PM, Oates RP. Random versus predictable risks of mortality after thoracotomy for lung cancer. J Thorac Cardiovasc Surg 1986; 91: 551–554.

7 Holmes FF. Clinical evidence for a change in tumor aggressiveness with age. Semin Oncol 1988; 16: 34–40.

8 McNeil BJ, Weichselbaum R, Pauker SG. Fallacy of the five-year survival in lung cancer. N Engl J Med 1978; 299: 1397–1401.

9 Peters RM, Clausen JL, Tisi GM. Extending resectability for carcinoma of the lung in patients with impaired pulmonary function. Ann Thorac Surg 1978; 26: 250–260.

10 Jensik RJ. The extent of resection for localized lung cancer: segmental resection. In: Kittle CF (ed.). Current Controversies in Thoracic Surgery. Philadelphia, PA, WB Saunders 1986: pp 175–182.

11 Ginsberg RJ, Hill LD, Eagan RT, et al. Modern thirty-day operative mortality for surgical resections in lung cancer. J Thorac Cardiovasc Surg 1983; 86: 654–659.

Current Topics in General Thoracic Surgery: An International Series, Vol. 2
Perioperative Care, edited by R.M. Peters and J. Toledo

Chapter 8

The issue of AIDS for thoracic surgeons

J. Allen McCutchan

GLOSSARY

AIDS	acquired immunodeficiency syndrome
ARC	AIDS-related complex
CDC	Center for Disease Control (USA)
CMI	Cell-mediated immunity
CNS	Central nervous system
CMV	Cytomegalovirus pneumonia
EAGA	Expert Advisory Group on AIDS
ELISA test	enzyme-linked immunosorbent assay test
GMS	gomori-methenamine silver
HCW	health-care workers
HIV	human immunodeficiency viruses: HIV-1, HIV-2
MAI	*Mycobacterium avium-intracellulare*
PCP	Pneumocystis pneumonia
PML	progressive multifocal leukoencephalopathy

1. INTRODUCTION

The epidemic of acquired immunodeficiency syndrome (AIDS) has profoundly influenced American medicine over the decade since its recognition in 1981. For the thoracic surgeon practicing in epidemic areas it has created a number of problems, most of which remain unsolved. Rather than attempt a comprehensive review of all the implications of the epidemic, I will attempt to address several major clinical questions after a synopsis of the epidemiology, virology, and clinical evolution of AIDS as understood in 1991.

2. A SYNOPSIS OF HIV INFECTION AND AIDS

2.1. Epidemiology

The human immunodeficiency viruses (HIV-1 and -2), the retroviruses which cause AIDS, probably arose in Africa from closely related primate retroviruses and have spread rapidly there primarily by heterosexual transmission [1]. HIV-1 has been rapidly disseminated by homosexual men in Europe and North America and secondarily via blood to transfusion recipients, hemophiliacs, and intravenous drug users who share needles and syringes. Heterosexual transmission has proceeded relatively slowly in Western countries in contrast to Central Africa where up to 30–40% of sexually active men and women in some cities have been infected [2,3]. Transmission to neonates occurs in about a quarter of live births to infected mothers, although some studies have found lower rates [4]. HIV-2 has not yet become a problem in North America, but could become a problem if it spreads from the current endemic areas of West Africa.

Screening of blood in Western countries by sensitive and relatively inexpensive ELISA tests for HIV-1 has nearly eliminated transfused blood and blood products as a source of infection [5]. Because of the highly variable and prolonged latent period between infection and onset of AIDS (estimated mean of more than five years, and range from one to at least twelve years), large numbers of persons transfused between 1978 and mid-1985 will continue to present with AIDS for many years [6]. Similar considerations imply that a high percentage (more than half by the tenth year) of the 1–1.5 million infected persons in the USA will become ill in the next decade. Antivirals are widely used to extend life in those with AIDS and to prolong the latent period, but these will only marginally decrease the impact of the epidemic in the next five years [7].

The Centers for Disease Control (CDC) report that 100777 persons died of AIDS from 1981 through 1990 in the USA and 31196 died of AIDS in 1990 alone [8]. A substantial percentage of hospital beds in many American cities are now occupied by patients with AIDS, and about 55000 new cases were diagnosed in 1990.

2.2. Evolution of clinical disease

Within a few weeks of infection many people develop a self-limited (3–10 day), *acute, mononucleosis-like illness* with fever, sore throat, lymphadenopathy, malaise, skin rash, headache and a variety of less frequent symptoms [9,10]. In most cases, this is followed by a prolonged asymptomatic or minimally symptomatic period during which variable combinations of generalized lymphadenopathy, fatigue, recurrent low-grade fevers, and other non-specific symptoms may occur. Many infected persons have no physical and few laboratory abnormalities during this period, but most are potentially infectious through sexual activity or blood transfusions. Virtually all have antibody to HIV proteins detectable by ELISA and Western Blot assays. Deterioration of cell-mediated immunity after a variable period is heralded by appearance of a variety of opportunistic infections, tumors, neurological symptoms, or severe non-specific symptoms (fever, diarrhea, and wasting) which progress to death in a few years or less. Immune-mediated cytopenias (especially thrombocytopenia) may precede all other symptoms or complicate AIDS.

Several systems for classifying the progressive stages of HIV infection are in use, but none has yet been adequately validated [11–13]. The most comprehensive

TABLE 8.1
1987 revised case definition of AIDS in adults for surveillance purposes

Without laboratory evidence of HIV infection and in the absence of immunosuppressive drugs or diseases

(A) Candidiasis of esophagus, trachea, bronchi, and lungs
(B) Cryptococcosis outside the lung
(C) Cryptosporidial diarrhea for more than a month
(D) Cytomegalovirus of liver, spleen, or lymph nodes
(E) Herpes simplex causing skin ulcers for more than one month, pneumonia, bronchitis, or esophagitis
(F) Kaposi's sarcoma in patients under 60 years of age
(G) Lymphoma of the brain
(H) Disseminated *Mycobacteria avium*
(I) Pneumocystis pneumonia
(J) Progressive multifocal leukoencephalopathy (PML = parvovirus encephalitis)
(K) Toxoplasmic encephalitis

With laboratory evidence of HIV infection

(A) Disseminated coccidiomycosis
(B) HIV encephalopathy
(C) Disseminated histoplasmosis
(D) Isosporal diarrhea for more than a month
(E) Kaposi's sarcoma at any age
(F) Lymphoma of the brain
(G) B cell, non-Hodgkins' lymphoma
(H) Disseminated mycobacterial infections
(I) Recurrent salmonella (non-typhoidal) septicemia
(J) Severe wasting ('slim disease')

system is that of the Centers for Disease Control (CDC) which has the advantage of subdividing AIDS-Related Complex (ARC) and AIDS patients into subgroups of category IV (Table 8.1), but the disadvantage of grouping asymptomatic patients in categories II or III regardless of their degree of immunosuppression as measured by numbers of circulating CD_4+ lymphocytes [11]. The Walter Reed system stratifies the earlier stages of HIV infection based on the absolute number of CD_4-bearing T lymphocytes and delayed cutaneous hypersensitivity reactions to multiple skin test antigens [12]. The reliability and prognostic significance of the Walter Reed system has been questioned, however, and skin tests are inconvenient and difficult to evaluate reproducibly [13].

The appearance of minor infections (e.g., oral candidiasis, zoster, oral hairy leukoplakia, or frequent recurrences of herpes simplex), non-specific symptoms (fever, weight loss, fatigue, diarrhea, or skin rashes), and laboratory abnormalities (anemia, leukopenia, and profound depletion of helper CD_4+ lymphocytes), is sometimes referred to as AIDS-Related Complex (ARC). The majority of patients with ARC progress to AIDS over the following year. Occurrence of any of the AIDS-defining conditions listed in Table 8.1 establishes the diagnosis of AIDS for epidemiologic purposes.

Despite improvements in prognosis with available antiretroviral therapy (zidovudine, dideoxycytidine, or dideoxyinosine), AIDS remains lethal within three years for the majority ($>80\%$) of patients and for virtually all by five years [7]. During the period following diagnosis of AIDS, many patients return to nearly normal levels of health for months, but most have intermittent illnesses. Prevention of infectious complications with prophylactic drugs increases the length of asymptomatic periods [14]. Kaposi's sarcoma, which occurs much more frequently in homosexual men than in other risk groups, has a slightly better prognosis, probably because it often presents at a less advanced stage of immune deficiency than do the AIDS-defining opportunistic infections [15].

Occasional patients present exclusively or predominantly with neurological problems of cognitive dysfunction caused by HIV without documented opportunistic infections or tumors [16–18]. Most patients die with multiple opportunistic infections involving the lung, gastrointestinal tract, and brain [19–20].

2.3. Virology

Retroviruses are RNA viruses with a unique life cycle involving reverse transcription of their genetic information to form a DNA provirus [21]. The proviral DNA is then integrated into the host cell DNA where it may remain latent or be activated to produce new virus. Intense investigation of the genetics of HIV-1 has revealed a complex network of regulatory genes which control the transcription of the integrated proviral DNA. These elements overlap the major structural genes (*env* for envelope glycoprotein and *gag* for internal structural proteins) and the gene coding for the reverse transcriptase enzyme (*pol* for DNA polymerase).

The comparison of complete genetic sequences of multiple isolates of HIV-1 reveals regions of remarkable variability as well as highly conserved regions which appear necessary for viral functions such as binding to host cell membrane proteins. Conserved regions of particular interest are found in the portion of the envelope gene which projects outside the viral envelope (gp-120) and binds to the CD_4 protein on human lymphocytes, leading to their infection and destruction [22]. Because of their critical functional role and external position, conserved regions of the envelope protein are prime candidates as vaccines, but appear to be relatively inaccessible to antibody because they are surrounded by immunodominant variable regions. Their utility as broadly cross-reactive, protective antigens remains to be demonstrated [23].

The reverse transcriptase enzyme is an inviting target for antiviral chemotherapy because it is unnecessary for human physiology, but crucial to an early step in viral reproduction. The first licensed antiretroviral drug, zidovudine (Retrovir®, azidothymidine, or AZT), interferes with viral replication by terminating the developing DNA chain when utilized by the enzyme in preference to thymidine.

2.4. Pathogenesis and immunology

The striking deficiency of cell-mediated immunity (CMI) in AIDS resembles that of lymphatic neoplasms (lymphomas and Hodgkins' disease) and of the iatrogenic immunosuppression necessary for the maintenance of organ transplants. Certain opportunistic infections (especially pneumocystis pneumonia, disseminated *Mycobacterium avium*, and toxoplasmal encephalitis) and tumors (Kaposi's sarcoma) appear much more frequently than expected from experience with other conditions in which CMI is depressed. The reason for this profound and somewhat selective loss of CMI is the destruction of a crucial subset (helper or CD_4 antigen bearing) of T (thymus-derived) lymphocytes. As mentioned above the CD_4 molecule on the surface of these lymphocytes is used as a receptor by which HIV-1 enters these cells to initiate infection.

During the evolution of HIV infection, a progressive loss of CD_4 cells occurs which predicts the risk of subsequent development of AIDS [24–27]. CD_4 lymphocytes in blood can be enumerated by staining with fluorescent-labeled, monoclonal antibody to the CD_4 protein and counting by microscopy or in a fluorescence-activated cytograph. Most patients with AIDS have less than 20–30% (200–300/mm^3) of the normal number (about 1000/mm^3) of these cells. In addition, the remaining CD_4 cells are functionally impaired. The mechanisms of destruction and functional impairment of CD_4 lymphocytes by HIV-1 are not understood. Since relatively few ($< 1/100$) CD_4+ lymphocytes contain detectable viral DNA or RNA, direct infection of the entire subset of lymphocytes does not seem a likely mechanism [28].

Despite the central importance of infection of CD_4 lymphocytes, cells of monocyte/macrophage lineage in the brain, skin, and lymph nodes and endothelial cells of the brain also contain viral nucleic AIDS or antigens and may contribute to the pathogenesis of HIV infection. Several implications of infection of these cells have been postulated. Either migrating macrophages or infected endothelial cells in the brain may be responsible for the early infection of the central nervous system (CNS) demonstrable in many patients by viral cultures of CSF or the polymerase chain reaction [29]. Neuropsychological tests suggest that mild, asymptomatic neural dysfunction is common in persons who carry the virus asymptomatically [17,18,30]. Histopathology of the brains of persons dying with AIDS may reveal small foci of infected monocytes and microglial cells and atrophy which do not correlate well with the extent of clinical neurological disease [31]. Thus, infected macrophages may be the means by which HIV enters the brain and may cause the functional deficits by mechanisms as yet not understood.

In contrast to its effects on T lymphocytes, HIV-1 infection causes hyperplasia and hypersecretion of antibody by B lymphocytes which are poorly responsive to further stimulation of antibody production [32]. B lymphocyte dysregulation and their reaction to chronic antigenic stimulation by HIV probably contributes to hyperglobulinemia, lymphadenopathy, autoimmune phenomena (e.g., immune thrombocytopenia and lupus-like anticoagulants), and circulating immune complexes found in most HIV-infected patients.

3. IMPLICATIONS OF AIDS FOR THE THORACIC SURGEON

3.1. Care of patients with HIV infection by the thoracic surgeon

The care of patients infected with HIV-1 is complicated by both their unfamiliar clinical problems and the small, but real, risk of HIV infection of health-care providers by penetrating injuries. The latter issue will be dealt with in the following section. Reviews of thoracic surgical experience with AIDS patients have begun to appear in the medical literature [33]. The problems encountered by specialists in abdominal, neurological, head and neck, ophthalmological, cardiovascular, and urological surgery will not be addressed in this chapter.

Diagnostic procedures likely to be referred to thoracic surgeons include (1) biopsies of mediastinal lymph nodes or masses, (2) diagnostic bronchoscopy and (3) open lung biopsy for pulmonary infiltrates and lung nodules or masses. *Supportive procedures* include (1) placement of indwelling catheters for antimicrobial or antitumor therapy or parenteral nutrition, (2) therapeutic bronchoscopy or laser surgery, (3) tracheostomy, (4) chest tube drainage for management of pneumothorax, (5) drainage of abscesses or empyemas, and (6) management of poorly healing chest wounds or fistulas. Major surgical procedures include thoracotomy for esophagogastrectomy or pleurectomy.

3.1.1. Diagnostic procedures

(1) *Lymph node biopsy.* Palpable lymphadenopathy is very common in the anterior and posterior cervical, axillary, inguinal, and femoral chains as well as in less accessible mediastinal and abdominal chains of HIV-infected persons [32]. Extensive experience in biopsying patients with generalized, persistent lymphadenopathy suggests that the pathologist usually finds diffuse, non-specific, follicular hyperplasia [34,35]. The possibility of lymphadenitis caused by sexually transmitted diseases (e.g., lymphogranuloma venereum, syphilis, or primary herpes genitalis) should be entertained when inguinal or femoral nodes are involved. Occasional diagnoses of Kaposi's sarcoma or lymphoma usually do not lead to effective early interventions. Occasionally, *M. avium-intracellulare* (MAI), *M. tuberculosis*, other atypical mycobacteria, *Cryptococcus neoformans, Histoplasma capsulatum, Coccidioides immitis*, the cat scratch bacillus, or *Pneumocystis carinii* are diagnosed from lymph node biopsies. Most clinicians have abandoned biopsy of all but very large (>5 cm), adherent, or peripheral nodes.

Mediastinal nodes are often enlarged by HIV, opportunistic infections such as MAI or tuberculosis, or lymphomas. Because the patient's condition is too poor or because alternative means of diagnosis are available, mediastinal nodes are not frequently biopsied. The indications for mediastinoscopy for biopsy of enlarged nodes in an HIV-infected patient without AIDS have not been established, but a rapidly enlarging node or one impinging on or invading other mediastinal structures probably should be biopsied, if feasible.

(2) *Bronchoscopy* with lavage and trans-bronchial lung biopsy is the standard method to establish the diagnosis of Pneumocystis pneumonia (PCP) [36–38]. Because of the subtle radiographic and clinical presentations of this pneumonia, the value of early treatment, and the persistence of organisms as cysts for weeks despite effective therapy, most clinicians begin therapy based on clinical suspicion of PCP. If patients remain undiagnosed after examination of spontaneously-produced or induced sputum, biopsy is performed within 24–72 hours. Sputum exam for the organism after staining with the gomori-methenamine silver (GMS) or Gram–Weigert techniques has proven to be worthwhile in most centers, but less sensitive than the same stains of bronchial washings or biopsies [39]. Patients with recurrences of clinically-typical PCP or with AIDS diagnosed on other grounds are sometimes treated presumptively without diagnostic biopsies. However, the recent demonstration of the value of adjunctive therapy with corticosteroids during treatment of PCP has increased the need to establish the diagnosis [40–42]. Several studies have demonstrated that corticosteroids reduce respiratory deterioration, need for ventilatory support, and death when administered conjointly at the initiation of standard therapy in patients with moderately to severe hypoxia ($pO_2 < 75$ torr). Although mild and infrequent, side effects of corticosteroids require that they be discontinued in patients without PCP.

Bronchoscopic washing, brushing, and biopsy may also be useful for diagnosis of infections or tumors causing lung nodules, lobar pneumonias, irregular masses, or cavities.

(3) *Open lung biopsy* to establish the causes of diffuse pneumonias or lung masses has been established as safe, but is infrequently necessary [43,44]. A review of early (1983–1986) experience at the National Institutes of Health suggested that open lung biopsy is both safe and diagnostic in about two-thirds of patients who remain undiagnosed after bronchoscopic biopsy [43]. Review of a larger and more recent (1981–1987) experience at St. Vincent's Hospital in New York, supported only very limited use of open biopsy in the same situation [44]. Three major indications each accounted for about one third of 66 patients: (1) patients with respiratory failure too ill for endoscopy, (2) patients with pneumocystis pneumonia unresponsive to therapy, and (3) patients without a diagnosis after transbronchial biopsy. Group 1 patients all died, group 2 patients were not treated differently as a result of the procedure, and in group 3 only 3 of 19 patients had a new, treatable diagnosis established, and only one of these responded.

Patients with Kaposi's sarcoma may have parenchymal lung lesions which are usually, but not always, associated with lesions in the airway and sometimes respond temporarily to chemotherapy [45]. Cytomegalovirus pneumonia (CMV), a common problem in transplantation (especially of bone marrow) is rarely diagnosed in living AIDS patients. Growth of CMV from bronchoscopic washings is paradoxically not a bad prognostic sign in AIDS ([46,47], Bozzette et al., personal communication). Despite the difficulty in establishing its role in pneumonia in AIDS, CMV cells are frequently found in areas of inflammation in post-mortem lungs of AIDS patients [48,49]. Because CMV is treatable, further study of its role in fatal pneumonias in AIDS is needed, but CMV currently does not provide a rationale for open biopsy. Likewise *Mycobacterium avium* often spares the lung despite massive invasion of the blood, bowel wall, and lymph nodes in some AIDS patients [50].

3.1.2. Supportive procedures

(1) *Indwelling catheters* are useful for the prolonged administration of anti-infective therapy (e.g., amphotericin), chemotherapy, or parenteral hydration or nutrition. Despite increased risk of infections with *Candida albicans* or *Staphylococcus aureus*, the majority of these patients have remained remarkably free of catheter-related problems despite their predisposition to other infections [51]. In our experience at UCSD, ease of access and decrease in superficial phlebitis more than compensates for the risk of infection. A prospective study is needed to more carefully assess risks and benefits.

(2) *Kaposi's sarcoma* frequently involves the mucosa of the upper airways, trachea, and bronchi whereas lymphomas do so uncommonly. While most such tumors have been treated with radiation or chemotherapy, the potential for severe mucositis appears to be increased in AIDS patients and calls for new approaches [52,53]. Debulking of such tumors with *endoscopic laser surgery* to preserve swallowing and airway patency is an alternative.

(3) *Tracheostomy* is infrequently indicated in AIDS because of rapid response to early use of appropriate drugs in most cases of PCP and the poor prognosis of patients requiring prolonged intubation [54]. Some centers have abandoned intubation and/or ventilatory support in AIDS because of infrequent survival. A more selective approach to identify persons with a better prognosis should be assessed before dogmatic policies are adopted [55]. Any policy should take into account continuing advances in the management of infections.

(4) *Placement of chest tubes* for spontaneous and ventilator-associated pneumothorax and surgical *closure of air leaks* in patients with persistent leaks are the most common supportive measure required of the thoracic surgeon [33]. The increasing incidence of pneumothorax in AIDS patients results from the continuing high incidence of pneumocystis pneumonia and the use of aerosolized pentamidine as primary and secondary prophylaxis [56]. Although not considered a necrotizing process, pneumocystis was complicated by pneumothorax unrelated to procedures or trauma in 2% of 1030 AIDS patients followed at Memorial Sloan–Kettering Cancer Center in New York between 1980 and 1989. Patients on aerosolized pentamidine were found to be at many-fold (probably > 10) greater risk of this complication. Prolonged, peripheral, destructive infection of poorly ventilated areas may occur in these patients. Delivery of pentamidine to the well-ventilated areas may protect the patient from symptoms without suppressing organisms in these under-ventilated sites. The finding of stainable cysts of *Pneumocystis carinii* in

the pleural fluid of such a patient (McCutchan et al., unpublished) supports such a mechanism. Prophylaxis with systemic drugs (e.g. septra) alone or in combination with aerosolized pentamidine may reduce the incidence of this complication.

Patients with asymptomatic pneumothorax can be observed without intervention. Most patients with spontaneous, symptomatic, PCP-associated pneumothorax respond to closed chest tube drainage. Those patients developing pneumothorax while on mechanical ventilation for respiratory failure during PCP are unlikely to survive (12 of 13 or 92.5% died in one series) [57,58]. Median sternotomy with stapling of blebs or pleurodesis may be necessary.

(6) *Wound management* in AIDS has not been difficult in the majority of patients. Sterile surgical wounds usually heal well and many patients in our experience at UCSD have closed large tissue defects by granulation. A few patients have presented persistent or expanding cutaneous and subcutaneous necrotizing lesions in which no viral, mycobacterial, fungal, or consistent bacterial pathogen could be found by culture or microscopy. Skin grafting has promoted healing in these cases. Because *Herpes simplex* can cause similar lesions (especially in the perirectal skin of homosexual patients), culture should be obtained for this virus in any non-healing wound). If viral cultures are not possible, cytological diagnosis of herpes giant cells or empirical acyclovir therapy may be attempted.

4. RISK OF HIV TO THE SURGICAL STAFF

The risk of infection of medical personnel by penetrating injuries has been demonstrated in a national, multi-institutional study of needle-stick and related injuries conducted by the CDC [59]. Prolonged serological follow-up of 963 persons revealed 4 (0.42%) who appear to have been infected. Other reports have confirmed that the risk is small by finding infections only rarely in workers experiencing multiple needle sticks in hospitals with large AIDS populations [60]. In addition, serological surveys of orthopedic surgeons and dentists attending large, national meetings have revealed very small numbers with positive antibody tests [61]. The low titer of virus in serum and cells may account for the less efficient transmission of HIV than hepatitis B virus which circulates at high titer in the serum of carriers. The best available estimate suggests that less than one in 200 penetrating injuries involving HIV-infected blood will transmit the virus [28].

Reports that HIV can penetrate inflamed skin in the absence of a penetrating wound has increased the concern that blood contacting the hands through torn gloves may also represent a threat [62]. Although transmission via blood exposure to the mouth or eyes remains undocumented, shielding of the eyes and mouth is recommended. Laboratory exposure to high concentrations or purified virus by undetermined routes has also transmitted the virus. There is no evidence that blood or other bodily fluids transmit the virus during ordinary processing in clinical or research laboratories (e.g., centrifugation).

Guidelines for protection of medical staff have been published and widely accepted, if not always practiced[63]. They are based on the assumption that unidentified carriers of HIV are common and all fluids from all patients may be potentially infectious. While this approach has much to recommend it, many surgeons believe that it requires modifications of equipment and techniques which are time-consuming and promote less effective and more expensive surgery in uninfected persons[64]. Slower, but safer, techniques might be utilized for elective surgery on known carriers of HIV or on patients of unknown status. Thus, there is a growing demand for pre-operative screening of either 'high-risk' or of all patients undergoing elective surgery[65]. Before widespread advocacy or adoption of such a practice, the ethical, legal, and economic implications of a program for testing, informing, and counseling large numbers of patients is needed. Surgeons ordering such tests must be prepared to deal with the psychological, social, and legal fall-out[67]. False-negative and false-positive ELISA tests occur at a low, but significant, rate even when tests are repeated[65]. At present, diagnosis of asymptomatic HIV infection can be expected to have severe adverse psychological and social impact. Nevertheless, the intense pressure to reduce risk to health-care providers and minimize the adverse effects on surgical technique mandates that programs be carefully developed and tested.

In the meantime, the value of 'double gloving' needs assessment; impenetrable, but flexible, gloves need to be developed; and techniques to minimize penetrating injuries in and out of the operating room need to be employed. Because recapping needles is a common cause of needle-stick injuries, this practice should be abandoned in favor of immediate disposal in impenetrable bedside containers. 'Body substance' isolation techniques which emphasize treating potentially infectious materials from all patients carefully rather than trying to identify infected patients is the most rational approach outside the operating room[68]. This approach may turn out to be most effective and economical and least disruptive for the operating room as well.

REFERENCES

1 Piot P, Plummer FA, Mhalu FS, et al. AIDS: An international prospective. Science 1988; 239: 573–579.
2 N'Gary B, Ryder, RW. Epidemiology of HIV infection in Africa, J AIDS 1988; 1: 551–558.
3 Piot P, Laea M, Ryder RW, et al. The global epidemiology of HIV infection: Continuity, heterogeneity, and change. J AIDS 1990; 3: 404–412.
4 European Collaborative Study. Children born to women with HIV-1 infection: natural history and risk of transmission. Lancet 1991; 337: 253–260.
5 Ward JW, Holmgren SC, Allen JR, et al. Transmission of human immunodeficiency virus by blood transfusions screened as negative for HIV antibody. NEJM 1988; 318: 473–478.
6 Lagakos SW, De Gruttola V. The conditional latency distribution of AIDS for persons infected by blood transfusion.
7 Moore RD, Hidalgo J, Sugland BW, et al. Zidovudine and the natural history of the acquired immunodeficiency syndrom, NEJM 1991; 324: 1412–1416.

8 Anomymous. Mortality and morbidity weekly reports. Atlanta, GA, Centers for Disease Control 1991; 40 (25 Jan): 41.
9 Cooper DA, Gold J, Maclean P, et al. Acute AIDS retrovirus infection. Lancet 1985, 1: 537.
10 Ho DD, Sarngagharan MG, Resnick L, et al. Primary human T-lymphotropic virus type III infection. Ann Intern Med 1985, 103: 880.
11 Center for Disease Control. Revision of the CDC surveillance case definition for AIDS. Morbid Mortal Wkly Rpts 1987, 36: 15.
12 Redfield RR, Wright DC, Tamont EC. The Walter Reed staging classification for HTLV-III/LAV infection. N Engl J Med 1986, 314: 131.
13 Royce RA, Luckmann RS, Fusaro RE, et al. The Natural History of HIV infection: staging classifications of disease. AIDS 1991; 4: 355–364.
14 Leoung GS, Feigal DW, Montgomery AB, et al. Aerosolized pentamidine for prophylaxis against *Pneumocystis carinii* pneumonia, NEJM 1990; 323: 769–775.
15 Safai B, Johnson KG, Myskawski PL, et al. The Natural History of Kaposi's sarcoma in the acquired immunodeficiency Syndrome. Ann Intern Med 1985; 103: 744–750.
16 Navia BA, Jordon BD, Price RW. The AIDS dementia complex: I. Clinical features. Ann Neurol 1986; 19: 517–524.
17 Grant I, Atkinson H, Hesselink JR. Evidence for early central nervous system involvement in AIDS and other HIV infections. Ann Intern Med 1986; 207: 828–836.
18 Perry KS, Belsky-Barr D, Barr WB, et al. Neuropsychological function in physically asymptomatic, HIV-infected seropositive men. J Neuropsych 1989; 1: 296–302.
19 Reichart CM, O'Leary TJ, Levens DL, et al. Autopsy pathology in the Acquired Immune Deficiency Syndrome. Am J Path 1983; 112: 357–382.
20 Moskowitz L, Hensley GT, Chan JC. Immediate causes of death in Acquired Immunodeficiency Syndrome. Arch Pathol Lab Med 1985; 109: 735–738.
21 Greene WC. The molecular biology of Human Immunodeficiency Virus Type I infection. NEJM 1991; 324: 308–317.
22 Keiber-Emmons T, Jameson BA, Morrow WJW. The GP120-CD_4 interface: structural, immunological, and pathological considerations. Biochim Biophys Acta 1989; 989: 281–300.
23 Fauci AS, Gallo RC, Koenig S, et al. Development and evaluation of a vaccine for Human Immunodeficiency Virus (HIV) infection. Ann Intern Med 1989; 110: 373–384.
24 Polk BF, Fox R, Brookmeyer R, et al. Predictors of the Acquired Immunodeficiency Syndrome developing in a cohort of seropositive homosexual men. N Engl J Med 1987; 316: 61.
25 Goedert JJ, Biggar RJ, Melbye M, et al. Effect of T4 count and cofactors on the incidence of AIDS in homosexual men infected with Human Immunodeficiency Virus. JAMA 1987; 257–331.
26 Kaplan JE, Spira TJ, Fishbein DB, Pinsky PF, Schonberger LB. Lymphadenopathy syndrome in homosexual men: evidence for continuing risk of developing the Acquired Immunodeficiency Syndrome. JAMA 1987; 257: 335.
27 Eyster ME, Gail MH, Ballard JO, Al-Mondhiry H, Goedert JJ. Natural history of Human Immunodeficiency Virus infections in hemophiliacs: effects of T-cell subsets, platelet counts, and age. Ann Intern Med 1987; 107: 1.
28 Ho DD, Mondgic T., Alam M. Quantitation of Human Immunodeficiency Virus Type I in blood of infected persons. NEJM 1989; 321: 1621–1625.
29 Shaunak S, Albright RE, Klotman ME, et al. Amplification of HIV-1 provirus from cerebrospinal fluid and its correlation with neurologic disease. J Infect Dis 1990; 161: 1068–1071.
30 Wilke FL, Eisdorfer C, Morgan R, et al. Cognition in early Human Immunodeficiency Virus infection. Arch Neurol 1990; 47: 433–440.
31 Wiley CA, Schrier RD, Nelson JA, et al. Cellular localization of Human Immunodeficiency Virus infection within the brains of Acquired Immunodeficiency patients. Proc Natl Acad Sci USA 1986; 83: 7089.

32 Jacobson D, McCutchan JA, Spechko PL, Abramson I, et al. The evolution of lymphadenopathy and hypergammaglobulinemia are evidence for early and sustained polyclonal B lymphocyte activation during Human Immunodeficiency Virus infection. J Infect Dis 1991; 163: 240–247.
33 Miller JI, The thoracic surgical spectrum of Acquired Immune Deficiency Syndrome. J Thorac Cardiovasc Surg 1986; 92: 977–980.
34 Levine A, Meyer PR, Gill PS. Results of initial lymph node biopsy in homosexual men with generalized lymphadenopathy. J Clin Oncol 1986; 4: 155–160.
35 Amberson JB, Dicarlo EF, Metroka CE, et al. Diagnostic pathology in the Acquired Immunodeficiency Syndrome. Arch Pathol Lab Med 1985; 109: 345.
36 Kovaks JA, Ng VL, Masur H, et al. Diagnosis of *Pneumocystis carinii* pneumonia: improved detection into sputum with use of monoclonal antibodies. N Engl J Med 1988; 318: 589–593.
37 Hopewell PC, Luce JM. Pulmonary involvement in the Acquired Immmunodeficiency Syndrome. Chest 1985; 87: 104–112.
38 Broaddus C, Dake MD, Stulbarg MS, et al. Bronchoalveolar lavage and transbronchial biopsy for the diagnosis of pulmonary infections in the Acquired Immunedeficiency Syndrome. Ann Intern Med 1985; 102: 745–752.
39 Zaman MK, Wooten OJ, Suprahmanya B. Rapid non-invasive diagnosis of *Pneumocystis carinii* from induced liquified sputum. Ann Intern Med 1988; 109: 7–10.
40 Bozzette S, Sattler F, Chiu J, et al. Controlled trial of early adjunctive treatment with corticosteroids for *Pneumocystis carinii* pneumonia in the Acquired Immunodeficiency Syndrome. N Engl J Med 1990; 323: 1451–1460.
41 Gagnon S, Boota AM, Fischl MA, et al. Corticosteroids as adjunctive therapy for severe *Pneumocystis carinii* pneumonia in the Acquired Immunodeficiency Syndrome: A double-blind, placebo-controlled trial. N Engl J Med 1990; 323: 1444–1450.
42 Masur H, Meier P, McCutchan JA, Feinberg J, Bernard G, Bozzette S, Clement M, Ellenberg S, Feigal D, Gagnon S, Mathews C, Mills J, Montaner J, Nielsen J. Consensus statement on the use of corticosteroids as adjunctive therapy for *Pneumocystis* pneumonia in the Acquired Immunodeficiency Syndrome. N Engl J Med 1990; 323: 1500–1505.
43 Pass HI, Potter D, Shelhammer J, et al. Indications for and diagnostic efficacy of open lung biopsy in patients with Acquired Immunodeficiency Syndrome (AIDS). Ann Thorac Surg 1986; 41: 307–312.
44 Bonfils-Roberts EA, Nickodem A, Nealon TF. Retrospective analysis of the efficacy of open lung biopsy in Acquired Immunodeficiency Syndrome. Ann Thorac Surg 1990; 49: 115–117.
45 Davis SD, Henschke CI, Chamides BK, et al. Intrathoracic Kaposi's sarcoma in AIDS patients: radiographic pathologic correlation. Radiology 1987; 163: 495–500.
46 Millar AB, Patou G, Miller RF, et al. Cytomegalovirus in the lungs of patients with AIDS. Respiratory pathogen or passenger. Am Rev Respir Dis 1990; 141: 1474–1477.
47 Miles PR, Baughman RP, Linnemann CC. Cytomegalovirus in the bronchoalveolar lavage fluid of patients with AIDS. Chest 1990; 97: 1072–1076.
48 Wallace JM, Hannah JB. Pulmonary disease at autopsy in patients with the Acquired Immunodeficiency Syndrome. West J Med 1988; 149: 167–171.
49 Marchevski A, Rosen MJ, Chrystal G, et al. Pulmonary complications of the Acquired Immunodeficiency Syndrome: a clinicopathologic study of 70 cases. Hum Pathol 1985; 16: 659–670.
50 Wallace JM, Hannah JB. *Mycobacterium avium* complex infection in patients with the Acquired Immunodeficiency Syndrome. Chest 1988; 93: 926–932.
51 Jacobson MA, Gellerman H, Chambers H. *Staphylococcus aureus* bacteremia and recurrent Staphylococcus infection in patients with Acquired Immunodeficiency Syndrome and AIDS-Related Complex. Am J Med 1988; 85: 172–176.
52 Chak LY, Gill PS, Levine AM, et al. Radiation therapy for Acquired Immunodeficiency Syndrome-related Kaposi's sarcoma. J Clin Oncol 1988; 6: 863–867.
53 Gill PS, Rarick M, McCutchan JA, et al. Systemic treatment of AIDS-related Kaposi's sarcoma: results of a randomized trial. Am J Med 1991; 90: 427–433.

54 Wachter RM, Luce JM, Hopewell PC, et al. Intensive care for patients with the Acquired Immunodeficiency Syndrome. Am Rev Respir Dis 134: 891–896, 1986.
55 Steinbrook R, Lo B, Tirpack J. Ethical dilemmas in caring for patients with the Acquired Immunodeficiency Syndrome. Ann Intern Med 1985; 103: 787–790.
56 Sepkowitz KA, Telzak EE, Gold JWM, et al. Pneumothorax in AIDS. Ann Intern Med 1991; 114: 455–459.
57 Fleisher AG, McElvaney G, Lawson L, et al. Surgical management of spontaneous pneumothorax in patients with AIDS – acquired Immunodeficiency Syndrome. Ann Thorac Surg 1988; 45: 21–25.
58 Byrnes TA, Brevig JK, Yeoh CB. Pneumothorax in patients with Acquired Immunodeficiency Syndrome. J Thorac Cardiovasc Surg 1989; 98: 546–550.
59 Marcos RA. Surveillance of health care workers exposed to blood from patients infected with the Human Immunodeficiency Virus. N Engl J Med 1988; 319: 118–123.
60 Henderson DK, Fahey BJ, Willy M, et al. Risk for occupational transmission of Human Immunodeficiency Virus Type 1 (HIV-1) associated with clinical exposures. Ann Intern Med 1990; 113: 740–746.
61 Klein RS, Phelan JA, Freeman K, et al. Low occupational risk of Human Immunodeficiency Virus infection among dental professionals. N Engl J Med 1988; 318: 86–90.
62 Centers for Disease Control. Human Immunodeficiency Virus infections in health care workers exposed to blood of infected patients. MMWR 1987, 36: 285.
63 Gerberding JL, Henerson DK. Design of rational infection control policies for Human Immunodeficiency Virus Infection. J Infect Dis 1987; 156: 861.
64 Schiff S. A surgeon's of AIDS. J Neurosurg 1990; 73: 651–660.
65 Day L. The AIDS epidemic from a surgeon's viewpoint. Orthop Rev 1989; 18 (Suppl i): 35–38.
66 Sherer R. Physician use of the HIV antibody test: the need for consent, counseling, confidentiality, and caution. JAMA 1988; 259: 264–265.
67 Schwartz JS, Dans PE, Kingsian BP. Human Immunodeficiency Virus test evaluation, performance, and use. J Am Med Assoc 1988; 259: 2574–2579.
68 Lynch P, Jackson MM, Cummings MJ, et al. Rethinking the role of isolation practices in the prevention of nonsocomial infections. Ann Intern Med 1987; 107: 243–246.

Current Topics in General Thoracic Surgery: An International Series, Vol. 2
Perioperative Care, edited by R.M. Peters and J. Toledo

Discussion of "The issue of AIDS for thoracic surgeons" by J. Allen McCutchan

Martin J. Wood

The epidemic of HIV infection in Europe has not reached (and most projections suggest it will never reach) the level seen in North America but, even so, the problems caused are similar to those outlined by Dr McCutchan. Since reporting began in 1982 a total of about 4500 AIDS cases have been reported in the UK. The principal risk behaviors for HIV transmission are sexual promiscuity (either homosexual or heterosexual) and sharing of contaminated needles and other equipment by intravenous drug users. In most of Northern Europe, although two-thirds or more of AIDS cases and reported HIV infections have followed sexual intercourse between men, a plateau has been reached in the number of new cases of HIV infection in homosexual men. What is giving increasing concern is the number of cases that are being reported following heterosexual exposure. In the UK, for instance, the number of AIDS cases resulting from HIV transmission by sexual intercourse between men and women has increased by 78% in the past year and anonymous screening of women attending antenatal clinics in London confirms that there has been a nine-fold increase in HIV prevalence among heterosexuals over a two-year period [1]. At present, 34% of the total known HIV-infected adults in the UK can be described as heterosexual. In Southern Europe (Italy, Yugoslavia, Spain, Greece, etc.) most cases of AIDS are reported amongst intravenous drug users and here too it is cases in women (and hence the risk of vertical transmission to their children) that is giving great cause for concern. One of the challenges in Europe (and I suspect in the USA) is to increase awareness in heterosexuals of the risks of unprotected sexual intercourse with casual contacts. Europe is also seeing rather more cases of HIV-2 infection than have so far been reported from the USA, probably a result of the historical colonial contacts between the nations of Europe and West Africa where HIV-2 is particularly prevalent [2].

I am in complete agreement with Dr McCutchan's account of the virology, pathogenesis and immunology of HIV infection, although it should also be mentioned that most patients have the highest levels of viraemia (and hence are presumably most infectious) during their primary symptomatic infection (Stage I in the CDC classification) and after the onset of Stage IV disease. During Stages II and III the viraemia drops to much lower levels. When it comes to the time course and clinical disease associated with HIV infection there is again very little difference between the two continents; with the exception of a lower incidence of disease caused by those fungi found chiefly in the USA (histoplasmosis and coccidioidomycosis), the infections and tumours seen in Stage IV of infection are similar on both sides of the Atlantic.

In Europe, the investigation of the HIV-infected patient with respiratory symptoms is chiefly aimed at the early diagnosis of *Pneumocystis carinii* pneumonia (PCP) or mycobacterial infections, and thoracic surgeons are infrequently consulted. The simple measure of pulse oximetry before and after exercise is sensitive and quite specific for PCP [3], and production of a specimen of induced sputum with nebulized saline can often provide the definitive diagnosis (especially with the use of monoclonal antibodies). The adoption of the policy outlined by Dr McCutchan, fibre-optic bronchoscopy with bronchoalveolar lavage and/or transbronchial biopsies, means that almost all patients with respiratory symptoms can be diagnosed without recourse to open lung biopsy. Hence, open lung biopsy is rarely requested in adults (generally for the same indications as those suggested by Dr McCutchan). In children a form of lymphoid interstitial pneumonitis (possibly an Epstein–Barr virus-related infection) is commonly seen and the diagnosis of this *may* require open lung biopsy.

The use of mechanical ventilation for respiratory failure in AIDS is a contentious issue. Occasionally short term incubation may be needed for patients who have deteriorated during bronchoalveolar lavage. Overall, however, there is little evidence of any improved prognosis for most patients developing respiratory failure despite the use of appropriate drugs [4] and, given the relative lack of intensive care facilities (certainly in the UK), mechanical ventilation of AIDS patients is rarely undertaken. Otherwise there is nothing to dispute in Dr McCutchan's account of the therapeutic procedures undertaken by thoracic surgeons in HIV-positive patients.

The debate concerning the best way of reducing the risk of occupational HIV infection among health-care workers (HCW) rages as fiercely in the UK as it does in the USA, and is no nearer being satisfactorily resolved. Surgeons are very concerned even though there is widespread acceptance that the risk to surgical staff is extremely small and there has, indeed, not yet been a proven (by demonstration of seroconversion) occupationally acquired HIV infection in a surgeon. Those infections that have been recorded in other HCWs have principally followed sharps injuries with hollow needles rather than with suture needles. Of course, however low the quantitative risk, everyone on both sides of the Atlantic agrees that efforts should be made to minimize the risks to surgical staff and other HCW and, in an ideal world, guidelines for the protection of HCW would be universally applied and would be simple, cheap and, above all, effective.

Unfortunately, the recommendations made in the UK by the Expert Advisory Group on AIDS (EAGA)[5] (which in essence are the same as the so-called 'universal precautions' of the Centers for Disease Control, and involve routine double-gloving, eye protection and disposable drapes) have not been assessed for efficacy, and the impairments to surgical technique and the increased costs have meant that the recommendations have not been widely adopted. There are vociferous calls for the adoption of the alternative policy – namely the compulsory preoperative screening of patients. This may well improve the medical care and prognosis of the patient with a symptomatic HIV infection, but there are still profound ethical and legal problems to overcome. Furthermore, leaving aside the ethical implications of such a policy, the experience from San Francisco is that staff awareness of a patient's seropositivity or high-risk status does not reduce the rate of perioperative exposure of staff to blood as compared with the rate during operations on noninfected cases[6]. Double-gloving does seem to limit, but not eradicate, the risks of the inoculation injuries that are likely to be the major hazard to the surgeon but it is not clear what additional, more effective, steps could be taken to protect the staff operating upon a patient with proven or suspected HIV infection.

Whatever the merits of the arguments for and against compulsory preoperative screening, my own view is that some surgeons or institutions in the UK will try to implement such a policy and that the ethical and legal implication will then be tested in the law courts. Equally I think the San Francisco experience suggests that it is unlikely that this screening of patients will have any significant effect upon the rate of occupational transmission of HIV. This assessment assumes that necessary surgical treatment would not be withheld merely because of a patient's HIV infection. My own view is that the CDC and EAGA guidelines are the best policies we have and they should be strictly enforced. Essentially I am in agreement with the views expressed in the final sentence of Dr McCutchan's article – rather than identifying high-risk patients it is the risk of blood exposure during various surgical procedures that needs to be assessed and, hopefully, reduced.

There are two related issues that Dr McCutchan does not discuss; what to do if a surgeon is occupationally exposed to a HIV risk, and the possible transmission of HIV from a surgeon to a patient.

However hard we try to minimize the risk, occupational exposure to HIV will continue to occur and there is a need for policies to deal with such incidents. The most favoured approach is to offer prophylactic zidovudine (AZT) to those whose exposure is perceived as most risky[7]. The model policy is that first drawn up at San Francisco General, which defines the types of exposure that warrant prophylaxis[8]. It also emphasises the need for administration to be started as soon as possible (preferably within one hour of exposure) and the need for regular testing for HIV antibodies and for possible toxicity[8]. Although I believe all hospitals need to have a policy offering counseling and prophylactic zidovudine to staff exposed to a genuine risk of HIV transmission, it needs to be stressed that there are no ways of showing that prophylaxis has been successful, and there are at least three published accounts of failure to protect exposed individuals.

Documented transmission of HIV from a health-care worker to patients has now been recorded[9] but as yet there are no legal requirements for infected surgeons to stop operating. In the UK, it is left to the individual to volunteer information concerning his or her HIV infection to appropriate senior medical staff within the institution. Decisions are then made about the advisability of curtailing certain invasive procedures and, if necessary, offering retraining for alternative duties. It is likely, however, that such decisions will need continual review as more becomes known about the degree of risk an infected surgeon poses to patients. Whatever may happen in the USA (where public pressure seems to be much more powerful than in most areas of Europe), in Britain it seems unlikely that, in the foreseeable future, surgeons will be required to undergo compulsory screening for HIV infection.

REFERENCES

1 Ades AE, Parker S, Berry T, et al. Prevalence of maternal HIV-1 infection in Thames Regions: results from anonymous unlinked neonatal testing. Lancet 1991; 337: 1562–1565.

2 Courouce AM, Retrovirus Study Group of the French Society of Blood Transfusion. HIV 2 infection among blood donors and other subjects in France. Transfusion 1989; 38: 368–370.

3 Smith DE, McLuckie A, Wyatt J, Gazzard B. Severe exercise hypoxaemia with normal or near normal X-rays: a feature of *Pneumocystis carinii* infection. Lancet 1988; ii: 1049–1051.

4 El-Sadr W, Simberkoff MS. Survival and prognostic factors in severe *Pneumocystis carinii* pneumonia requiring mechanical ventilation. Am Rev Respir Dis 1988; 137: 1264–1267.

5 Department of Health. Expert Advisory Group on AIDS. Guidance for Clinical Health Care Workers: Protection against Infection with HIV and hepatitis viruses. London, HMSO 1990.

6 Gerberding JL, Littell C, Tarkington A, Brown A, Schecter WP. Risk of exposure of surgical personnel to patients' blood during surgery at San Francisco General Hospital. N Engl J Med 1990; 322: 1788–1793.

7 Anonymous. Zidovudine and needlestick exposure. Lancet 1990; 335: 1271.

8 Henderson DK, Gerberding JL. Prophylactic zidovudine after occupational exposure to the Human Immunodeficiency Virus: an interim analysis. J Infect Dis 1989; 160: 321–327.

9 Centers for Disease Control. Possible transmission of HIV to a patient during an invasive dental procedure. MMWR 1990; 39: 489–493.

Current Topics in General Thoracic Surgery: An International Series, Vol. 2
Perioperative Care, edited by R.M. Peters and J. Toledo

Chapter 9

Nonspecific and specific immune stimulation in lung cancer

James A. Bennett and Martin F. McKneally

GLOSSARY

BCG	Bacillus Calmette–Guerin	IL-2	interleukin-2
CSF	colony-stimulating factors	M-CSF	colony-stimulating factors for macrophages
G-CSF	colony-stimulating factors for granulocytes	TCGF	T-cell growth factor
GM-CSF	colony-stimulating factors for granulocytes and macrophages	TIL	tumor-infiltrating lymphocytes
		TNF	tumor necrosis factor

1. INTRODUCTION

The concept of immune stimulation as a treatment for cancer has enormous appeal because of its potential ability to eliminate micrometastatic cancer with low attendant host toxicity. Since the hallmark of the immune system is its ability to search out and selectively destroy histoincompatible cells, it is completely reasonable to hypothesize that a 'magic bullet' for cancer cells could be found within the immune system. Progress with this approach has been impeded by the low immunogenicity of cancer cells and the tight regulation of the immune system. In the last decade we have learned a great deal about molecules which control the afferent and efferent arms of the immune response. We are in the beginning stages of applying this new knowledge to the immunotherapy of cancer, and promising results have been forthcoming. There has been such an explosion of knowledge in this field that our last review of this topic [1], published six years ago, is virtually obsolete. Three major technical advances have redirected our thinking about immune stimulation as a treatment for cancer: (1) production of monoclonal antibodies through hybridoma technology; (2) production of cytokines through recombinant DNA technology; and (3) identification of oncogenes and oncogene products through several technological advances in protein and nucleic acid sequencing and computerized information storage.

Traditionally, the immunotherapy of cancer has been classified as either *active* or *passive*. *Active* refers to direct stimulation of the host immune system. This can be done either *nonspecifically* with agents like bacterial vaccines or *specifically* with a vaccine that contains tumor-associated antigens. *Active nonspecific stimulation* results in a generalized increase in activation state and quantity of all components within the immune system in the hope that such an environment will interfere with tumor growth.

Active specific stimulation, on the other hand, is more directed to stimulate specific lymphocytes which have receptors for tumor-associated antigens. If the tumor is sufficiently immunogenic, these clones of lymphocytes expand and differentiate, culminating in a coordinated assault of antibodies and killer cells directed against the tumor. *Passive immunotherapy* refers to the transfer of preformed antibodies or effector cells into an inadequately responding immune system. When the transfer of cells is involved, this passive approach is usually referred to as *adoptive immunotherapy.*

Many of the above approaches have been applied to different types of cancer, including lung cancer. There is a data base to support continued exploration of nonspecific and specific immunological reactivity in lung cancer as an approach to understanding the biology and improving the treatment of this disease.

2. NONSPECIFIC STIMULATION

In the nonspecific realm, empyema following surgical resection has long been suspected to improve the prognosis in patients with lung cancer. However, reports from several investigators indicate beneficial [2–4], indifferent [5,6], and even negative effects [7] of empyema on survival. The concept is appealing because activated macrophages are generated during empyema [8], and activated macrophages have been shown to kill cancer cells in vitro [9–11]. We attempted to mimic this natural experiment by deliberately infecting the pleural space with Bacillus Calmette–Guerin (BCG), an attenuated bacterial vaccine for tuberculosis [12]. Significant survival benefit from this treatment was found in patients with Stage I disease, treated with intrapleural BCG followed by oral isoniazid, when compared to control patients treated with oral isoniazid alone [13]. A larger ‘confirmatory’ trial carried out by the North American Lung Cancer Study Group found no survival benefits in patients treated with intrapleural BCG when compared to control patients treated with intrapleural saline [14]. Other studies have reported beneficial [15], indifferent [16], and even negative outcomes [17] from this treatment regimen. The variability in outcome among these studies is difficult to explain. There are several factors that could contribute to this variability, such as, number of patients entered into each trial, extent of disease in the patient population, supportive therapy provided to the patients, dose and schedule of BCG, and biological activity in the BCG preparation. Our conclusion from all of these studies is that nonspecific immune stimulation of lung cancer patients with BCG administered intrapleurally does not reproducibly improve survival.

Several other studies have demonstrated regression of skin cancers [18] including melanoma [19,20] following intratumor injection of BCG or other inflammation-inducing agents. Systemic disease was unaffected. The feasibility of injecting BCG into lung cancer was demonstrated by Holmes et al. [21]. However, Matthay et al. [22] showed that this approach did not improve the survival course of lung cancer patients. In contrast, several studies have shown that intratumoral injection of BCG in superficial bladder cancer markedly reduced tumor recurrence rate and improved survival in this disease [23–26]. This is similar to the outcome in nonmelanomatous skin cancer and suggests a role for intratumoral injection of BCG or other nonspecific inflammation-inducing agents in the less aggressive neoplastic lesions.

Malignant pleural effusions represent a regional manifestation of cancer which has been treated with nonspecific immune stimulants, including living BCG [27], BCG cell wall skeleton [28], *Corynebacterium parvum* [29,30,34], *Nocardia rubra* cell wall skeleton [31], and OK-432 [32,33], a cell lysate prepared from hemolytic streptococcus. The mechanism of action, where studied, appears to be a nonspecific inflammatory reaction and induction of cytotoxic factors [35] leading to pleural fibrosis, rather than a specific immunological attack on cancer cells. The toxicity of some of these preparations may be greater than that of the more commonly used tetracycline [30] and bleomycin preparations, which have been reported to have a mechanism of action similar to that of nonspecific immune stimulants, that is, induction of inflammation and ultimately pleural fibrosis. This similarity in mechanism of action probably accounts for the similarity in clinical response rates to these agents. Casali et al. [29] reported 100% complete responses, as defined by the criterion of no recurrence at one month, in 50 evaluable patients treated with repeated intrapleural injections of *C. parvum* after thoracentesis. Leahy et al. [30] reported slightly greater toxicity (fever and pain) and comparable efficacy in a randomized comparison of *C. parvum* and tetracycline in 32 patients. Reshad et al. [26] reported "55 to 90% success" in 59 cases of malignant pleurisy treated with intrapleural OK-432, though other agents were used in combination with the treatment. Uchida et al. [33] reported favorable results in 8 of 10 patients treated with intrapleural OK-432. Improvement was associated with an increase in natural killer cells in the pleural fluid. There is continued enthusiasm in Japan for these agents, particularly OK-432 for inducing pleural symphysis [37], even in the absence of malignancy (T. Naruke, personal communication). Based on the studies in bladder cancer, which clearly show the value of breaking the integrity of the epithelial barrier [38], it may be appropriate to perform mechanical pleural abrasion, e.g., by thoracoscopy, to allow introduction of the agent into the tissues to derive a maximum effect.

Nonspecific immune stimulants have been injected at sites more distant from the primary lung cancer and have had little or no impact on disease progression [1,39,40].

Thus, other than for resolution of pleural effusion, nonspecific immune stimulation has not reproducibly altered the survival course of lung cancer patients.

3. SPECIFIC STIMULATION

The concept of specific immunological reactivity in lung cancer is supported by the demonstration of tumor-associated antibodies [41–43] and tumor-specific cytotoxic T lymphocytes [42,44,45] in patients with lung cancer. Moreover, tumor-specific [46,47] as well as tumor-associated [48] antigens have been isolated from resected lung cancer specimens, suggesting that intrinsic specific antitumor immunity may be operative in some patients but insufficient to retard disease progression. We carried out a clinical trial designed to augment this specific component of the immune response. Surgically resected Stage II and Stage III lung and esophageal cancer patients were randomized to receive intradermal injections of a placebo (saline) or autologous, mitotically arrested tumor cells admixed with BCG. Patients in the treatment arm received two vaccinations spaced a week apart. In the third week they received a booster injection containing autologous tumor cells alone. Fifty-six patients were randomized into the study. There was no difference in survival between the two groups [49–51]. Two other trials very similar to ours have reported no benefit from a vaccine comprised of autologous tumor cells admixed with BCG [52,53]. In contrast, Hollinshead et al. [54] have reported a significant increase in survival of surgically resected Stage I and Stage II lung cancer patients vaccinated with Freund's complete adjuvant admixed with a purified soluble polypeptide preparation of tumor-associated antigens derived from pooled human lung cancer cell membranes. This very interesting study awaits independent confirmation. Other strategies have been adopted to increase the latent immunogenicity of tumor cells. Treatment of tumor cells with neuraminidase was carried out with the idea of stripping off cell surface sialic acid, leaving putative tumor-associated antigens more exposed [55]. This approach has not improved therapeutic outcome in any of the cancers in which it has been tried, including lung cancer [56]. Deliberate infection of tumor cells with lytic virus such as vaccinia virus and Newcastle disease virus followed by vaccination with the viral oncolysate has been reported. Preliminary studies suggest that this approach may prolong survival of melanoma patients [57], but there are no clinical trials indicating benefit from this treatment in lung cancer.

Thus far the outcome of clinical trials of nonspecific and specific immune stimulation in lung cancer has been disappointing, despite evidence for a detectable level of intrinsic immunological reactivity generated in response to lung cancer. Progress has been curtailed by lack of understanding of this response and what components of it are growth-retardant. The strategies that have been tested until now have stimulated, to varying degrees, multiple components within the immune system. Recently, significant technological advances in two areas, namely, production of monoclonal antibodies through hybridoma technology and production of cytokines through recombinant DNA technology, have enabled new

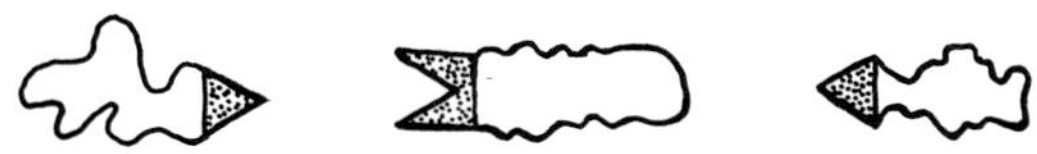

FIGURE 9.1. Model of anti-idiotypic tumor vaccine.

clinical trials with pharmacological levels of purified single components from the immune system.

4. MONOCLONAL ANTIBODIES

Monoclonal antibodies are produced by uniquely engineered homogeneous cell lines called hybridomas [58]. The hybridoma is created by fusing a population of lymphocytes obtained from a host immunized against the antigen of interest with a myeloma tumor cell line adapted to grow in tissue culture. Successfully fused hybrids are selected by transferring all the cells into growth medium that will support only the growth of fused cells and not unfused precursors. The hybrids have the properties of specific antibody production derived from the responding B lymphocyte population of the immunized host and vigorous growth in tissue culture derived from the myeloma tumor cell lines. At this stage in the process there are several different hybrids secreting several different antibodies. Cell cloning (culturing out single cells and expanding the progeny derived from that single parent) is used to isolate the hybrid producing the highest titer of the single (monoclonal) antibody of interest. This homogeneous hybridoma is propagated and is a long-term source of substantial quantities of highly specific antibody. Murine monoclonal antibodies, derived from fusion of mouse spleen cells with mouse myeloma, have been easier to produce than human monoclonal antibodies, which are derived from fusion of human peripheral blood lymphocytes with human myeloma. However, murine monoclonal antibodies have the drawback of being more immunogenic than human monoclonal antibodies when administered to humans.

Monoclonal antibodies have been used in several ways in the treatment of cancer. They have been used to specifically mark tumor cells for killing by complement or by cells (macrophages, granulocytes, and certain lymphocytes) which have receptors on their surface for the Fc portion of antibody molecules [59]. They have been conjugated to cytotoxic drugs (immunoconjugates) and used as a vehicle for guided delivery of drug toxicity [60]. They have been conjugated to isotopes for guided delivery of radiation, which has been used both diagnostically and therapeutically, depending upon the energy emission of the conjugated isotope [60]. Drawbacks to the use of monoclonal antibodies include nonspecific uptake into reticuloendothelial system organs such as the liver, intrinsic tumor heterogeneity in receptor for the antibody (not all tumor cells have receptors for the antibodies), and antigenic modulation induced by exposure to antibodies, which results in endocytosis of surface antigen without immediate regeneration of this receptor. A very recent and promising application of monoclonal antibodies has been their use as a stimulus to produce large quantities of the functional equivalent of tumor-associated antigen [60]. The production process works as follows. Using the lock-and-key analogy, a monoclonal antibody is a key which fits a particular lock or antigen. Since antibodies are large molecules, each having its own unique antigenic configurations, a second monoclonal antibody can be made to the antigen-combining site of the first monoclonal antibody. This second monoclonal antibody is referred to as an anti-idiotype. Since it fits the site of the first antibody that combined with tumor-associated antigen, it has sufficient structural similarity to tumor-associated antigen that it can be immunologically substituted for tumor-associated antigen and used as a tumor vaccine (Fig. 9.1).

Because the production source of such a vaccine is a cloned hybridoma that is propagated in tissue culture, there is a ready availability of large quantities of homogeneous, reproducible, and biochemically defined material. This facilitates clinical testing. Clinical trials of anti-idiotype vaccines have been carried out against B cell and T cell lymphomas [61,62], melanoma [63], and colon carcinoma [64]. Patient responses have included induction of antibodies reactive against tumor, induction of antibodies reactive against non-tumor-associated parts of the vaccine, and in some cases, induction of tumor regression which is rarely complete. Since monoclonal antibodies to lung cancer-associated antigens have been demonstrated [65,66], their application in lung cancer patients can be expected in the near future. Already they are being used for more thorough immunohistochemical characterization of formalin-fixed lung cancer specimens [67] and for detection in sputum samples of cell surface markers that appear to be predictive for subsequent development of lung cancer [68].

5. CYTOKINES

Recombinant DNA technology has enabled the production of large quantities of several different immunoregulatory molecules normally produced in small amounts by cells within the immune system. These molecules are collectively referred to as cytokines. Production has been accomplished by inserting the genome coding for the molecule of interest into bacterial DNA, thereby programming the bacteria to produce that molecule. Cytokines such as interferons, interleukins, tumor necrosis factors and colony-stimulating factors have been mass-produced in this way. The availability of large quantities of purified cytokines has permitted thorough clinical testing of these molecules. Although none of these recombinant immunoregulatory molecules has yet had a direct impact on the treatment of lung cancer, important information has been gained from preclinical and clinical testing of these agents, which will be applied to lung cancer therapy in the future.

Three different *interferons* (*interferon* α, *interferon* β and *interferon* γ) have been purified and characterized. Each interferon is derived from a different cell type; α

from leukocytes, β from fibroblasts, and γ from T lymphocytes. The genes coding for each of these interferons have been identified and used to manufacture the respective recombinant product. *Interferon* α has proved beneficial in the treatment of Kaposi's sarcoma, hairy cell leukemia, low-grade non-Hodgkin's lymphoma, cutaneous T-cell lymphoma, and chronic myelogenous leukemia [69,70]. Biological effects have included inhibition of proliferation, activation of natural killer cells and macrophages, and induction and/or augmentation of gene expression for histocompatibility antigens. *Interferon* α appears to be similar to *interferon* β in its spectrum of antitumor activity. *Interferon* γ has demonstrated very little antitumor activity but has been more potent than interferon α or interferon β in activating macrophages and in augmenting expression of histocompatibility antigens [71,72]. Thus, although interferon is not useful as a single agent in treatment of lung cancer, it may find future use in potentiating lung cancer vaccines by increasing antigenic expression or in sustaining treatment regimens that rely on macrophage activation.

Interleukin-2 (IL-2), formerly referred to as T-cell growth factor (TCGF), is available as a recombinant product. This agent stimulates the growth of T lymphocytes, and it activates less differentiated lymphocytes to become cytolytic for tumor cells. Both of these biological properties have been exploited in recent cancer therapy trials. In these protocols peripheral blood lymphocytes were removed, activated by exposure to IL-2 in culture, and reinfused with IL-2 into patients [73,74]. Similarly, tumor-infiltrating lymphocytes (TIL) have been removed, expanded and further activated by IL-2 in culture, and reinfused into patients [75,76]. This treatment strategy using either IL-2-activated peripheral blood lymphocytes or IL-2-activated tumor-infiltrating lymphocytes has induced significant tumor regression mainly in melanoma and renal cancer but has shown no benefit in lung cancer. The most striking toxicity of IL-2 is a capillary leak syndrome that results in hypotension, tachycardia, oliguria, and sometimes azotemia. This toxicity resolves upon withdrawal of IL-2. It is possible that this effect on capillaries could be exploited to increase the perfusion of solid tumors including lung cancer with chemotherapy or monoclonal antibody therapy following regional treatment with IL-2.

Several *colony-stimulating factors* (CSF) have become available through recombinant DNA technology. Some stimulate growth of macrophages (M-CSF) or granulocytes (G-CSF), while others are more pluripotent, like GM-CSF. Recent studies have shown that GM-CSF accelerates recovery of granulocytes and platelets after chemotherapy [77] and promotes function of autologous bone marrow transplants [78]. This has allowed significant dose escalation in chemotherapy regimens, which may ultimately improve responsiveness of lung cancer to chemotherapy. Also, availability of GM-CSF and M-CSF will permit expansion of monocytes in vitro. This may increase the response rates already reported to be significant in studies in which peripheral blood monocytes are removed, activated with γ interferon, and then reinfused regionally into patients with peritoneal colorectal carcinomatosis [79]. Regional infusion of such activated macrophages may be applicable to patients with Stage II and Stage III lung cancer.

Tumor necrosis factor (TNF) is a recombinant product that has been identified as a primary mediator of septicemic shock in animals and in humans [80]. It has shown significant antitumor activity against rodent tumors in vitro [81,82] and in vivo [81,83] and against human tumors in vitro [84–86]. Significant antitumor activity has not been demonstrated in patients in several different Phase I and Phase II clinical trials of TNF. In preclinical studies, this agent was found to be synergistic with γ interferon as well as with IL-2 in prolonging survival, and in some cases, curing tumor-bearing animals, and may have a future clinical role in cancer therapy in combination with these agents. Apart from its role in cancer therapy, studies with TNF have improved our understanding of septicemic shock [87–89]. This will undoubtedly lead to more effective treatment of this life-threatening disease. Already it has been demonstrated that monoclonal antibody to TNF neutralized the biological activity of TNF and prevented mortality in a preclinical model of septicemic shock [87,90].

6. ONCOGENES

Improved techniques in protein and nucleic acid sequencing and advances in computer technology have led to the identification of several oncogenes and oncogene products. Some of the oncogene products are growth factors or receptors for growth factors. Cancer development and progression may depend in part on deregulated oncogene expression and stimulation of growth by oncogene products. Recent studies using human small cell [91,92] and non-small cell [93] lung cancer cell lines have demonstrated autocrine growth stimulation. This means that these cells produce and secrete growth factors as well as express high affinity receptors on their surface for these same factors. This results in a positive feedback loop which accelerates tumor growth. Administration of monoclonal antibodies made either to the growth factor or to the growth factor receptor interrupted the circuit and significantly inhibited the growth of these cells [93,94]. The utilization of such monoclonal antibodies to antagonize unregulated growth stimulation may become an important strategy in the future treatment of lung cancer.

7. CONCLUSION

Although we began with general nonspecific and specific immune stimulation in lung cancer, we are rapidly evolving to single-component manipulation of natural products in the tumor–host relationship. In all of the examples cited, immunological products were in some way involved in this manipulation. Dissection of the immune system into its component parts and insertion of the required part(s) into a host to neutralize an encroaching tumor is a fruitful avenue for further investigation. Whether it be to boost an insufficiently responding intrinsic immune response, to capitalize on the specificity of tumor-directed antibodies for guided delivery of cytotoxic products, or to utilize newly engineered antibodies to block a molecule that is a driving force behind unregulated tumor growth, immunological products will likely play a role in the multimodality treatment of cancer in the future. After debulking the tumor with the appropriate combination of surgery, radiation, and chemotherapy, the goal will be to then insert the appropriate immunological component(s) to control residual tumor burden and convert the tumor–host relationship from one that is parasitic and pathological to one that is counterbalanced and benign. Based on the substantial progress over the last five years, it appears that we are rapidly developing the tools to achieve this goal.

REFERENCES

1 McKneally MF, Bennett JA. Immunotherapy for lung cancer. In: Choi NC, Grillo HC (eds.). Thoracic Oncology. New York, Raven Press 1983: pp 201–219.
2 Sensenig DM, Rossi NP, Ehrenhaft JL. Results of the surgical treatment of bronchogenic carcinoma. Surg Gynecol Obstet 1963; 116: 279.
3 Takita H. Effect of postoperative empyema on survival of patients with bronchogenic carcinoma. J Thorac Cardiovasc Surg 1970; 59: 642.
4 Ruckdeschel JC, Codish SD, Stranahan A, McKneally MF. Postoperative empyema improves survival in lung cancer. N Engl J Med 1972; 287: 1013.
5 Brohee D, Vanderhoeft P, Smets P. Lung cancer and postoperative empyema. Eur J Cancer 1977; 13: 1429.
6 Minasian H, Lewis CT, Evans SJW. Influence of postoperative empyema on survival after pulmonary resection for bronchial carcinoma. Br Med J 1978; 2: 1329.
7 Cady B, Clifton EE. Empyema and survival following surgery for bronchogenic carcinoma. J Thorac Cardiovasc Surg 1967; 53: 102.
8 Robbins SL, Cotran RS, Kumar V. Pathologic Basis of Disease. Philadelphia, PA, WB Saunders 1984: p 735.
9 Hibbs JB. Hetercytolysis by macrophages activated by Bacillus Calmette–Guérin: lysosome exocytosis into tumor cells. Science 1974; 184: 468.
10 Fidler IJ. Recognition and destruction of target cells by tumoricidal macrophages. Israel J Med Sci 1978; 14: 177.
11 Shimizu H, Wyatt D, Knowles RD, Bucana CD, Stanbridge EJ, Kleinerman ES. Human monocytes selectively bind to cells expressing the tumorigenic phenotype. Cancer Immunol Immunother 1989; 28: 185.
12 McKneally MF, Maver C, Kausel HW. Regional immunotherapy of lung cancer with intrapleural BCG. Lancet 1976; 1: 377.
13 McKneally MF, Maver C, Lininger L, Kausel HW, McIlduff JB, Older TM, Foster ED, Alley RD. Four-year follow-up on the Albany experience with intrapleural BCG in lung cancer. J Thorac Cardiovasc Surg 1981; 81: 485.
14 Mountain CF, Gail MH. Surgical adjuvant intrapleural BCG treatment for Stage I non-small cell lung cancer: Preliminary report of the National Cancer Institute Lung Cancer Study Group. J Thorac Cardiovasc Surg 1981; 82: 649.
15 Jansen HM, The TH, Orie NGM. Adjuvant immunotherapy with BCG in squamous cell bronchial carcinoma. Thorax 1980; 35: 781.
16 Lowe J, Shore DF, Iles PB. Intrapleural BCG in operable lung cancer. Lancet 1980; 1: 11.
17 Bakker W, Nijhuis-Heddes JMA, van der Velde EA. Post-operative intrapleural BCG in lung cancer: A 5-year-follow-up report. Cancer Immunol Immunother 1986; 22: 155.

18 Klein E, Holtermann O, Milgrom H, Case RW, Klein D, Rosner D, Djerassi I. Immunotherapy for accessible tumors utilizing delayed hypersensitivity reactions and separated components of the immune system. Med Clin North Am 1976; 60: 389.
19 Morton DL, Eilber FR, Malmgren RA, Wood WC. Immunological factors which influence response to immunotherapy in malignant melanoma. Surgery 1970; 68: 158.
20 Pinsky CM, Hurshaut Y, Oettgen HF. Treatment of malignant melanoma by intratumoral injection of BCG. Natl Cancer Inst Monogr 1973; 39: 222.
21 Holmes EC, Ramming KP, Bein ME, Coulson WF, Callery CD. Intralesional BCG immunotherapy for pulmonary tumors. J Thorac Cardiovasc Surg 1979; 77: 362.
22 Matthay RA, Mahler DA, Beck GJ, Loke J, Baue AE, Carter DC, Mitchell MS. Intratumoral Bacillus Calmette–Guérin immunotherapy prior to surgery for carcinoma of the lung: Results of a prospective randomized trial. Cancer Res 1986; 46: 5963.
23 Lamm DL. Bacillus Calmette–Guérin immunotherapy for bladder cancer. J Urol 1985; 134: 40.
24 Brosman SA. The use of Bacillus Calmette–Guérin in the therapy of bladder carcinoma in situ. J Urol 1985; 134: 36.
25 Kelley DR, Ratliff TL, Catalona WJ, Shapiro A, Lage JM, Bauer WC, Haaff EO, Dresner SM. Intravesical Bacillus Calmette–Guérin therapy for superficial bladder cancer: Effect of Bacillus Calmette–Guérin viability on treatment results. J Urol 1985; 134: 48.
26 Herr HW, Pinsky CM, Whitmore WF. Long-term effect of intravesical BCG on flat carcinoma in situ of the bladder. J Urol 1986; 135: 265.
27 McKneally MF, Maver C, Civerchia L, Codish S, Kausel HW, Alley RD. Regional immunotherapy for lung cancer using intrapleural BCG. In: Crispen RG (ed.). Neoplasm Immunity: Theory and Application. Chicago, IL, ITR 1975: pp 153–160.
28 Yamamura Y. Immunotherapy of lung cancer with oil-attached cell wall skeleton of BCG. In: Terry WD, Windhorst D (eds.). Immunotherapy of Cancer: Present Status of Trials in Man. New York, Raven Press 1978: pp 173–179.
29 Casali A, Gionfra T, Rinaldi M, Tonachella R, Tropea F, Venturo I, DeMartino C, Curio CG. Treatment of malignant pleural effusions with intracavitary *Corynebacterium parvum*. Cancer 1988; 62: 806.
30 Leahy BC, Honeybourne D, Brear SG, Carroll KB, Thatcher N, Stretton TB. Treatment of malignant pleural effusions with intrapleural *Corynebacterium parvum* or tetracycline. Eur J Respir Dis 1985; 66: 50.
31 Azuma I, Yamawaki M, Yasumoto K, Yamamura Y. Antitumor activity of *Nocardia* cell wall skeleton preparations in transplantable tumors in syngeneic mice and in patients with malignant pleurisy. Cancer Immunol Immunother 1978; 4: 95.
32 Nagao K. Studies on the treatment of pleural carcinomatosis with special reference to effect of OK-432. Chiba Med J 1982; 58: 345.
33 Uchida A, Micksche M, Hoshino T. Intrapleural administration of OK432 in cancer patients: Augmentation of autologous tumor killing activity of tumor-associated large granular lymphocytes. Cancer Immunol Immunother 1984; 18: 5.
34 Rossi GA, Felletti R, Balbi B, Sacco O, Cosulich E, Risso A, Melioli G, Ravazzoni C. Symptomatic treatment of recurrent malignant pleural effusions with intrapleurally administered *Corynebacterium parvum*. Am Rev Respir Dis 1987; 135: 885.
35 Miyai M, Matsuka Y, Tsubota T, Asano K. Induction of human tumor necrosis factor by streptococcal preparation, OK432: A clinical trail in 10 lung cancer patients with pleural fluid. J Jpn Cancer Ther 1986; 21: 1285.
36 Reshad K, Inui K, Takeuchi Y, Takahashi Y, Hitomi S. Treatment of malignant pleural effusion. Chest 1985; 88: 393.
37 Torisu M, Fujimura T, Kato M, Katano M, Yamamoto H, Konomi K, Yoshida T, Sakata M. Successful immunotherapy of carcinomatous pleuritis and peritonitis by intracavitary injection of OK-432. In: Hoshino T, Uchida A (eds.). Clinical and Experimental Studies in Immunotherapy. Amsterdam, Excerpta Medica 1983: pp 99–112.

38 Ratliff TL, Kavoussi LR, Catalona WJ. Role of fibronectin in intravesical BCG therapy for superficial bladder cancer. J Urol 1988; 139: 410.

39 Edwards FR. Use of BCG as an immunostimulant after resection of carcinoma of the lung: A two-year assessment of a trial of 500 patients. Thorax 1979; 34: 801.

40 Miller AB, Taylor HE, Baker MA, Dodds DJ, Falk R, Frappier A, Hill DP, Jindani A, Landi S, Macdonald AS, Thomas JW, Wall C. Oral administration of BCG as an adjuvant to surgical treatment of carcinoma of the bronchus. Can Med Assoc J 1979; 121: 45.

41 Hatzitheofilou C, Kern DH, Gupta RK, Campbell MA, Morton DL. A radioimmunometric assay for the detection and characterization of lung cancer-associated antibodies in sera of lung cancer patients. J Surg Res 1987; 42: 85.

42 Olsen GN, Gangemi JD. Bronchoalveolar lavage and the immunology of primary lung cancer. Chest 1985; 87: 677.

43 Cronin WJ, Dorsett BH, Ioachim HL. Isolation of lung carcinoma-associated antibodies from immune complexes and production of heterologous antisera. Cancer Res 1982; 42: 292.

44 Dean JH, Jerrells TR, Cannon GB, Kibrite A, Baumgardner B, Weese JL. Demonstration of specific cell-mediated antitumor immunity in lung cancer to autologous tissue extracts. Int J Cancer 1978; 22: 367.

45 Vanky F, Peterffy A, Book K, Willems J, Klein E, Klein G. Correlation between lymphocyte-mediated auto-tumor reactivities and the clinical course. II. Evaluation of 69 patients with lung carcinoma. Cancer Immunol Immunother 1983; 16: 17.

46 Yamada T, Iwa T, Kurata Y, Okada S. Extraction and preliminary characterization of tumor antigens in human bronchogenic adenocarcinoma and squamous cell carcinoma. Eur J Cancer 1980; 16: 781.

47 Princler GL, McIntire KR, Braatz JA. Identification and purification of a human lung tumor-associated antigen from a primary lung tumor. Cancer Res 1982; 42: 843.

48 Kelly B, Levy JG. Evidence for a common tumor-associated antigen in extracts of human bronchogenic carcinoma. Br J Cancer 1977; 35: 828.

49 Maver C, McKneally MF. Preparation of autologous tumor cell vaccine from human lung cancer. Cancer Res 1979; 39: 3276.

50 McKneally MF, Maver C, Bennett JA, Lininger L. Treatment of resectable lung and esophageal cancer with adjuvant Bacillus Calmette–Guérin (BCG) and autologous tumor cells. Proc Am Assoc Cancer Res 1981; 22: 198.

51 McKneally MF, Lininger L, Bennett JA. Treatment of lung cancer by surgical excision and adjuvant Bacillus Calmette–Guérin (BCG) stimulation. Proc 13th Intl Cancer Congr (UICC) 1982: p 314.

52 Price-Evans DA, Roberts HL, Hewitt S, Walsh D, Donohoe WT, Lambourne A. A trial of adjuvant immunotherapy for bronchial carcinoma with irradiated autochthonous tumor cells. Int J Immunother 1987; 3: 293.

53 Schulof RS, Mai D, Nelson MA, Paxton HM, Cox JW, Turner ML, Mills M, Hix WR, Nochomovitz LE, Peters LC, Hanna MG. Active specific immunotherapy with an autologous tumor cell vaccine in patients with resected non-small cell lung cancer. Mol Biother 1988; 1: 30.

54 Hollinshead A, Takita H, Stewart T, Raman S. Specific active lung cancer immunotherapy: Immune correlates of clinical responses and an update of immunotherapy trials evaluations. Cancer 1988; 62: 1662.

55 Simmons RL, Aranha GV, Gunnarsson A, Grage TB, McKhann CF. Active specific immunotherapy for advanced melanoma utilizing neuraminidase-treated autochthonous tumor cells. In: Terry WD, Windhorst D (eds.). Immunotherapy of Cancer: Present Status of Trials in Man. New York, Raven Press 1978, pp 123–133.

56 Takita H, Takada M, Minowada J, Han T, Edgerton F. Adjuvant immunotherapy of Stage III lung carcinoma. In: Terry WD, Windhorst D (eds.). Immunotherapy of Cancer: Present Status of Trials in Man. New York, Raven Press 1978, pp 217–223.

57 Hersey P, Edwards A, Coates A, Shaw H, McCarthy W, Milton G. Evidence that treatment with vaccinia melanoma cell lysates (VMCL) may improve survival of patients with Stage III melanoma. Cancer Immunol Immunother 1987; 25: 257.

58 Milstein C. Monoclonal antibodies. Sci Am 1980; 243: 66.
59 Schlom J. Basic principles and applications of monoclonal antibodies in the management of carcinomas. Cancer Res 1986; 46: 3225.
60 Foon KA. Biological response modifiers: The new immunotherapy. Cancer Res 1989; 49: 1621.
61 Miller RA, Maloney DG, Warnke R, Levy R. Treatment of B-cell lymphoma with monoclonal anti-idiotype antibody. N Engl J Med 1982; 306: 517.
62 Bhattacharya-Chatterjee M, Pride MW, Seon BK, Kohler H. Idiotype vaccines against human T cell acute lymphoblastic leukemia. I. Generation and characterization of biologically active monoclonal anti-idiotopes. J Immunol 1987; 139: 1354.
63 Mittelman A, Kageshita T, Kusama K, Kim JW, Arlin Z, Ferrone S. A clinical trial of murine antiidiotype monoclonal antibodies to high molecular weight melanoma associated antigens. Proc Am Soc Clin Oncol 1988; 7: 248.
64 Herlyn D, Wettendorff M, Schmoll E, Iliopoulos D, Schedel I, Dreikhausen U, Raab R, Ross AH, Jaksche H, Scriba M, Koprowski H. Anti-idiotype immunization of cancer patients: Modulation of the immune response. Proc Natl Acad Sci USA 1987; 84: 8055.
65 Fargion S, Carney D, Mulshine J, Rosen S, Bunn P, Jewett P, Cuttita F, Gazdar A, Minna J. Heterogeneity of cell surface antigen expression of human small cell lung cancer detected by monoclonal antibodies. Cancer Res 1986; 46: 2633.
66 Hellström I, Horn D, Linsley P, Brown JP, Brankovan V, Hellström KE. Monoclonal mouse antibodies raised against human lung carcinoma. Cancer Res 1986; 46: 3917.
67 Tong AW, Lee JC, Stone MJ. Discrimination of human small cell and non-small cell lung tumors by a panel of monoclonal antibodies. J Natl Cancer Inst 1986; 77: 1023.
68 Tockman MS, Gupta PK, Myers JD, Frost JK, Baylin SB, Gold EB, Chase AM, Wilkinson PH, Mulshine JL. Sensitive and specific monoclonal antibody recognition of human lung cancer antigen on preserved sputum cells: A new approach to early lung cancer detection. J Clin Oncol 1988; 6: 1685.
69 Roth SM, Foon KA. α-Interferon in the treatment of hematologic malignancies. Am J Med 1986; 81: 871.
70 Kirkwood JM, Ernstoff MS. Interferons in the treatment of human cancer. J Clin Oncol 1984; 2: 336.
71 Nathan CF, Horowitz CR, De La Harpe J. Administration of recombinant interferon gamma to cancer patients enhances monocyte secretion of hydrogen peroxide. Proc Natl Acad Sci USA 1985; 82: 8686.
72 Maluish AE, Urba WJ, Longo DL, Overton WR, Coggin D, Crisp ER, Williams R, Sherwin SA, Gordon K, Steis RG. The determination of an immunologically active dose of interferon-gamma in patients with melanoma. J Clin Oncol 1988; 6: 434.
73 Rosenberg SA, Lotze MT, Muul LM, Chang AE, Avis FP, Leitman S, Linehan M, Robertson CN, Lee RE, Rubin JT, Seipp CA, Simpson CG, White DE. A progress report on the treatment of 157 patients with advanced cancer using lymphokine-activated killer cells and interleukin-2 or high dose interleukin-2 alone. N Engl J Med 1987; 316: 889.
74 Rosenberg SA. The development of new immunotherapies for the treatment of cancer using interleukin-2. Ann Surg 1988; 208: 121.
75 Muul LM, Spiess PJ, Director EP, Rosenberg SA. Identification of specific cytolytic immune responses against autologous tumor in humans bearing malignant melanoma. J Immunol 1987; 138: 989.
76 Belldegrun A, Muul LM, Rosenberg SA. Interleukin 2 expanded tumor infiltrating lymphocytes in human renal cell cancer: Isolation, characterization, and antitumor activity. Cancer Res 1988; 48: 206.
77 Antman KS, Griffin JD, Elias A, Socinski MA, Ryan L, Cannistra SA, Oette D, Whitley M, Frei E, Schnipper LE. Effect of recombinant human granulocyte-macrophage colony-stimulating factor on chemotherapy-induced myelosuppression. N Engl J Med 1988; 319: 593.

78 Brandt SJ, Peters WP, Atwater SK, Kurtzberg J, Borowitz MJ, Jones RB, Shpall EJ, Bast RC, Gilbert CJ, Oette DH. Effect of recombinant human granulocyte-macrophage colony-stimulating factor on hematopoietic reconstitution after high-dose chemotherapy and autologous bone marrow transplantation. N Engl J Med 1988; 318: 869.
79 Lacerna LV, Stevenson GW, Stevenson HC. Adoptive cancer immunotherapy utilizing lymphokine activated killer cells and gamma interferon activated killer monocytes. Pharmacol Ther 1988; 38: 453.
80 Schirmer WJ, Schirmer JM, Fry DM. Recombinant human tumor necrosis factor produces hemodynamic changes characteristic of sepsis and endotoxemia. Arch Surg 1989; 124: 445.
81 Carswell EA, Old LJ, Kassel RL, Green S, Fiore N, Williamson B. An endotoxin-induced serum factor that causes necrosis of tumors. Proc Natl Acad Sci USA 1975; 72: 3666.
82 Matthews N. Production of an antitumor cytotoxin by human monocytes. Immunology 1981; 44: 135.
83 Asher AL, Mule JJ, Rosenberg SA. Recombinant human tumor necrosis factor mediates regression of a murine sarcoma in vivo via Lyt-2^+ cells. Cancer Immunol Immunother 1989; 28: 153.
84 Haranaka K, Satomi N, Sakurai A. Antitumor activity of murine tumor necrosis factor (TNF) against transplanted murine tumors and heterotransplanted human tumors in nude mice. Int J Cancer 1984; 34: 263.
85 Watanabe N, Niitsu Y, Neda H, Sone H, Yamauchi N. Antitumor effect of tumor necrosis factor against various primarily cultured human cancer cells. Jpn J Cancer Res (Gann) 1985; 76: 1115.
86 Wang AM, Creasey AA, Ladner MB, Lin LS, Strickler J, Van Arsdell JN, Yamamoto R, Mark DF. Molecular cloning of the complementary DNA for human tumor necrosis factor. Science 1985; 228: 149.
87 Beutler B, Milsark IW, Cerami AC. Passive immunization against cachectin/tumor necrosis factor protects mice from lethal effect of endotoxin. Science 1985; 229: 869.
88 Michie HR, Spriggs DR, Manogue KR, Sherman ML, Revhaug A, O'Dwyer ST, Arthur K, Dinarello CA, Cerami A, Wolff SM. Tumor necrosis factor and endotoxin induce similar metabolic responses in human beings. Surgery 1988; 104: 280.
89 Michie HR, Kirk MB, Manogue KR, Spriggs DR, Revhaug A, O'Dwyer S, Dinarello CA, Cerami A, Wolff S, Wilmore DW. Detection of circulating tumor necrosis factor after endotoxin administration. N Engl J Med 1988; 318: 1481.
90 Tracey KJ, Fong Y, Hesse DG, Manogue KR, Lee AT, Kuo GC, Lowry SF, Cerami A. Anti-cachectin/TNF monoclonal antibodies prevent septic shock during lethal bacteraemia. Nature 1987; 330: 662.
91 Carney DN, Cuttitta F, Moody TW, Minna JD. Selective stimulation of small cell lung cancer clonal growth by bombesin and gastrin-releasing peptide. Cancer Res 1987; 47: 821.
92 Nakanishi Y, Mulshine JL, Kasprzyk PG, Natale RB, Maneckjee R, Avis I, Treston AM, Gazdar AF, Minna JD, Cuttitta F. Insulin-like growth factor-1 can mediate autocrine proliferation of human small cell lung cancer cell lines in vitro. J Clin Invest 1988; 82: 354.
93 Imanishi K, Yamaguchi K, Kuranami M, Kyo E, Hozumi T, Abe K. Inhibition of growth of human lung adenocarcinoma cell lines by anti-transforming growth factor-α monoclonal antibody. J Natl Cancer Inst 1989; 81: 220.
94 Cuttitta F, Carney DN, Mulshine J, Moody TW, Fedorko J, Fischler A, Minna JD. Bombesin-like peptides can function as autocrine growth factors in human small-cell lung cancer. Nature 1985; 316: 823.

Current Topics in General Thoracic Surgery: An International Series, Vol. 2
Perioperative Care, edited by R.M. Peters and J. Toledo

Chapter 10

Pulmonary resection following chemotherapy

P. Drings and I. Vogt-Moykopf

1. INTRODUCTION

Depending on the clinical stage, lung cancer is treated in accordance with a multimodal concept of therapy. In a few exceptions such as stages I and II of non-small cell lung cancer and the far-advanced extensive disease stage of small-cell lung cancer, primary operation or primary chemotherapy are the sole procedures indicated. In other situations, all three modalities (operation, radiotherapy, chemotherapy) are utilized. The time schedule for use of the various modalities is laid down in an interdisciplinary consultation. Agreement between the specialists is absolutely necessary, since one method of therapy may not only support the effectiveness of another method, but may also impair it.

The very unfavorable overall prognosis of lung cancer (overall survival of all patients less than 10%) requires the development of new concepts of therapy. Clinical studies are an instrument for conceiving new therapies.

This chapter attempts to make an analysis of the results of preoperative chemotherapy in lung cancer which are available. These results are still to be regarded as preliminary.

2. NON-SMALL CELL LUNG CANCER

2.1. Surgical therapy

In operable non-small cell lung cancer up to stage T3N1M0, radical surgical operation is regarded as the first-line form of treatment. It affords the greatest chances of cure, and is thus superior to all other methods of therapy. In a favorable individual constellation, surgical therapy is justifiable even in stage T3N2M0[61]. However, a resection treatment initiated with the objective of cure is feasible in at most 30% of all patients. The five-year actuarial survivals after a potentially curative surgical operation depend on the stage and the histological type of the tumor, the age, sex and functional class of the patient (*Leistungsindex*) as well as the extent of the operation [15,38,49,59]. Clinical studies carried out by various working groups [39,49,61] unequivocally prove that surgical therapy cannot be definitively curative in more than 50% of patients of stages I and II, with the exception of the postsurgical stage pT1N0M0. The five-year actuarial survivals are specified as 50–60% for stage I, 30–35% for stage II and 15% for stage III. The unfavorable late results are to be explained by the pattern of metastatic spread of these tumors. In 65% to 75% of the patients, distant metastases are demonstrated during followup [13,20,39]. This means that the tumor was already present in a disseminated form at the time of the surgical therapy, but had not been diagnosed. Postoperative radiotherapy of the mediastinum may reduce the rate of local recurrences, but has no effect on the actuarial survival of the patients [28].

Besides ruling out distant metastases, it is of crucial importance to know the local tumor extent in order to decide on surgical therapy and possible additional treatment. Massive metastatic spreading into the mediastinum (N3) or an infiltration of the trachea, the bifurcation, large vessels and the heart (T4) require primary radiotherapy. In preoperative suspicion of involvement of mediastinal lymph nodes, which can be detected for example by a diameter over 10 mm in the computer tomogram, meticulous preoperative mediastionoscopy should be carried out in high-risk patients in order to avoid an unnecessary thoracotomy in N3 or multilevel N2 disease. On the other hand, this procedure also ensures that a false positive CT finding does not exclude a patient from potentially curative surgical therapy [28]. Martini and coworkers [34] obtained a three-year actuarial survival of 47% and a five-year actuarial survival of 34% by complete resections carried out in 119 patients with mediastinal lymph node metastases which had not been suspected preoperatively (clinical stages N0 or N1). In the same study, Martini et al. were also able to identify the patients who would not profit from surgical therapy [35]. These were the patients with appreciably enlarged mediastinal lymph nodes or widening of the carina (corresponding to stage N3), which could be discerned in the scout-view thorax X-ray. When tumor resection was attempted, only 14% proved to be completely resectable. Despite the resection, the survival time was unsatisfactory. Only 9 out of 32 patients with complete resection were still alive after three and five years.

The new international staging system for lung cancer is more suitable for establishment of the prognosis, with differentiation of the former stage III into stages IIIa and IIIb [37]. Our own results (Table 10.1) confirm this impressively.

The prognosis is especially unfavorable for all patients treated surgically when the resection is incomplete (corresponding to minimal macroscopically demonstrable residual tumor – R2 – or microscopically demonstrable tumor infiltration – R1). As a rule, these patients do not live for more than 2 years.

TABLE 10.1
Survival of 428 patients after complete resection of lung cancer

Postoperative stage	*n*	Survival rate (%)				Median
		30 days	1 y	2 y	3 y	
I	162	96	86	76	69	NA[a]
II	106	93	78	57	39	817
IIIa	112	95	65	43	34	624
IIIb	48	77	46	28	21	229

[a] Not available.

2.2. Adjuvant chemotherapy

Because the results of resectional surgery often are unsatisfactory even with tumors 'of early stages', it appeared logical to use systemic chemotherapy as an adjuvant form of therapy after operation. In the studies published up to 1980, however, this was unsuccessful. Positive results could be detected only in some retrospective analyses. A significant difference between the treated group and the untreated control group could not be detected either for the disease-free interval or for the median survival time of the patients in randomized studies [24]. This was attributed to the ineffectiveness of the methods of therapy available at that time [20].

With the introduction of new cytostatics, the situation with regard to chemotherapy of non-small cell lung cancers has improved in the course of the last decade. Rates of remission of 25% to 45% were attained in clinical studies [22]. The median survival time of all treated patients (overall survival) is reported to be 8 to 10 months, and that of responders (patients with partial or complete remissions) is reported to be 12 to 15 months. Attainment of complete remissions (5–10%) is regarded as a major advance made in the course of the last decade [19]. Table 10.2 [22] provides an overview of the rates of remission with the modern cytostatic combinations in this tumor. However, it has to be taken into consideration that these results were obtained in tumors with distant metastases. Better results should be expected in only local or regional spread and correspondingly smaller tumor mass.

The use of chemotherapy in later stages of disease led to new attempts to carry out adjuvant treatment after complete tumor resection.

The Lung Cancer Study Group [31] investigated the influence of adjuvant chemotherapy with cyclophosphamide, adriamycin and cisplatinum (CAP) on the survival time and the pattern of recurrences in patients with a raised risk (microscopic and macroscopic detection of tumor at the resection margin or metastatic tumor involvement of the highest para-aortic lymph node). Chemotherapy had a positive effect on the recurrence-free survival of the patients [31,32,18,37]. This effect was especially pronounced in adenocarcinoma and large-cell lung cancer. The difference between the actuarial survivals was 15% in favor of adjuvant chemotherapy. The control group was treated with intrapleural BCG and

TABLE 10.2
Analysis of different polychemotherapy combinations [22], compared with IFO combinations [7]

Treatment[a]	Number of patients	Percentage of patients applied to (%)			
		Squamous-cell	Adeno	Large-cell	Total
MACC	282	20	33	34	29
CAMP	313	30	28	22	26
CAP	718	34	29	26	26
VDS/DDP	329	48	38	40	37
MiViP	358	62	33	45	45
VP/DDP	446	38	24	24	30
IFO/DDP	71	39	29	33	35
IFO/VP	91	26	24	35	27
IFO/VDS	30	29	33	–	30

[a] Abbreviations:
IFO: ifosfamide;
MACC: methotrexate, doxorubicin, cyclophosphamide, lomustine;
CAMP: cyclophosphamide, doxurubicin, methotrexate, procarbacine;
CAP: cyclophosphamide, doxorubicin, cisplatin;
VDS: vindesine;
DDP: cisplatin;
MiViP: mitomycin C, vinca alkaloide, cisplatin;
VP: etoposide.

levamisole, a therapy that proved to be ineffective when compared to untreated patients.

Studies of Ayoub et al.[2] and Kris et al.[26] which are still in progress appear to confirm these results.

2.3. Neoadjuvant and preoperative chemotherapy

Since modern chemotherapy proved its efficacy as a form of adjuvant treatment at least in some studies, it appeared logical that it should be used before operation, i.e. as 'neoadjuvants'. The objective of such a therapy is to increase the rate of resection, to eliminate micrometastases which may be present, and in this way to reduce both the rate of local recurrences and the rate of distant metastatic spreading, thus improving the average survival of the patients.

The possible advantages of a concept of pre-resection chemotherapy would be:

(1) A systemic therapy would be reasonable for the vast majority of patients who may already have systemic spread of disease.
(2) The positive action of the chemotherapy would reduce the spread of the tumor, and the proportion of patients who could receive a potentially curative operation would be increased.
(3) It would also be conceivable that less aggressive methods of surgery might be appropriate.

(4) The blood vessel supplying the tumor would not be impaired by surgical procedures. The cytostatic could reach the tumor tissue at a higher concentration.

However, application of chemotherapy before local treatment also entails undisputable disadvantages:

(1) The tumor stage before the beginning of therapy would only relate to clinical staging and not to the postoperative analysis of the tissue, so that there will automatically be greater uncertainty with regard to its true stage (cTNM versus pTNM).
(2) If chemotherapy is ineffective (this is to be expected in about half of the patients), there would be a delay in the implementation of effective local treatment.
(3) A raised morbidity, more postoperative complications, more pronounced reactions to radiation and the well-known early and late toxicity of chemotherapy is conceivable.
(4) A possible cross-resistance between radiotherapy and chemotherapy is also to be considered.

In the selection of patients for a neoadjuvant chemotherapy, classification in risk groups is recommended. Gail et al.[15] defined a lower risk for patients with stage I squamous epithelial carcinoma, a moderate risk for stage II patients, and a high risk for all patients of stage II with non-small cell carcinomas, with the exception of squamous epithelial carcinoma (the Lung Cancer Study Group). Patients of stage III were not included in this analysis. However, stage III patients should be initially considered in the evaluation of the concept of neoadjuvant chemotherapy, since only a small proportion of these patients may undergo a potentially curative operation. Patients of stage IIIa in accordance with the new classification are to be regarded as the target group for a preoperative chemotherapy[37]. Patients with Pancoast's tumors occupy a special position. In accordance with an international consensus, they receive preoperative irradiation[28]. On the other hand, preoperative radiotherapy is not recommended for patients of stage IIIa with mediastinal lymph node involvement, since it does not improve the late results[28]. Clinical experience shows that an operation is possible after mediastinal radiotherapy if an interval of two months is not exceeded. However, a raised rate of complications (delayed healing, technical difficulties at the operation, development of bronchopleural fistulae, infections, pulmonary fibroses) must be reckoned with. In our experience, arrhythmias and restricted heart function must be reckoned with during the operation and in the early postoperative phase in patients who have been pretreated with cytostatics (this applies in particular to therapy with anthracycline antibiotics). These patients therefore require thorough examination prior to operation with determination of left ventricular ejection fraction (echocardiography, cardiac scintigraphy). If appropriate, a long-term electrocardiogram should also be taken. If a pathological finding is detected, the patient must be digitalized and the arrhythmia must be treated before the operation.

TABLE 10.3
Results of some preoperative chemotherapy trials in patients with non-small cell lung cancer

Regimen[a]	*n*	Resp. rate (%)	Surg. resect.	Median surv. (mo)	Reference	Year
CAP + Rad	41	43	36/37	9 +	Skarin et al.[51]	1985
DDP + FU + Rad	59	61	28/59	25% at 28 mo	Trybula et al.[59]	1985
DDP + VDS + VP-16	20	70	3/3	9	Britan et al.[3]	1986
Various combinations	29	–	29/29	30.5	Takita et al.[58]	1986
DDP + VDS + Rad	22	55	12/13	14 +	Strauss et al.[57]	1986
DDP + BLM resectab.	22	82	22/22	12	Israel et al.[21]	1986
non-resectab.	35	86	33/35	8		
DDP + BLM (+ MIT or FU)	60	64	60/60	45% at 4 yr	Clavier et al.[6]	1986
DDP + MIT + FU	20	60	4/12	21	Bonomi et al.[4]	1986
DDP + VP-16	10	80	8/10	–	Splinter et al.[56]	1986
DDP + BLM + FU	16	71	14/16	–	Zabbè et al.[62]	1986
MIT + VBL or DDP + VDS	20	65	8/19	15 +	Kris et al.[29]	1987
CAP + Rad	42	51		–	Eagan et al.[8]	1987
MIT + DDP + VBL	22	73	5/5	19	Spain et al.[55]	1988
DDP + MIT + FU + Rad	33	74	19/33	15	Pincus et al.[42]	1988
DDP + VDS or VBL + (MIT)	41	73	21/28	34% at 4 yr[b]	Martini et al.[33]	1988
MIT + DDP + VDS	39	70	21/35	–	Burkes et al.[5]	1989
CAP + post- or preop. Rad	39	43	21/32	31	Skarin et al.[52]	1989

[a] Abbreviations:
DDP, cisplatin; BLB, bleomycin; FU, fluoro-uracil; VP-16, etoposide; VDS, vinblastine; MIT, mitomycine; CAP, cyclophosphamide/adriamycin/cisplatin; RAD, irradiation.
[b] 54% for patients with complete resection.

Results of evaluation of neoadjuvant chemotherapy are available from several clinical studies (Table 10.3). However, these are all to be regarded as preliminary. These studies merely document the technical feasibility of this concept of therapy. They do not allow any final appraisals, since five-year actuarial survivals could not yet be calculated. These studies confirm the clinical experience that the rates of remission are higher when the tumor load is lower (Table 10.3).

The cytostatic combinations consisted of two or three drugs. Cisplatinum was chosen most frequently, and was combined either with a vinca alkaloid or etoposide, fluorouracil, adriamycin and bleomycin. In the choice of cytostatics, attention must be paid to good compatibility with a possible subsequent or simultaneous radiotherapy[40].

The high rate of resection after partial or complete remission as a result of chemotherapy is especially noteworthy. For example, Martini et al.[33] attained a rate of remission of 75% compared to only 14% in earlier studies with surgery alone in comparable patients. It is to be especially emphasized that no tumor could be detected in the resectate in eight patients (20% of all patients treated) in this group. These results are still to be confirmed by other research groups. A complete resection is the essential precondition for a long-term survival of the patient. This was indeed attained in the study carried out by Martini et al. [33], since the three-year actuarial survival was 54% with a median follow-up of 44 months. On the other hand, just a 9% three-year actuarial survival could be attained in an earlier study without preoperative chemotherapy [34].

All studies on neoadjuvant chemotherapy presented up to this writing are primarily feasibility studies without comparison with a randomized control group. Consequently, an unequivocal appraisal of the prolongation of patient survival is not feasible. The studies presented up to now are extremely heterogenous. Chemotherapy was very frequently combined with preoperative radiotherapy. In several studies, preoperative adjuvant chemotherapy and/or radiation was administered in addition. There is no doubt that preoperative chemotherapy as well as preoperative radiotherapy diminish the rate of local recurrence. However, there is as yet no proof that this form of treatment also prolongs patient survival. Distant metastases remain the essential problem. It is conceivable that patients require postoperative adjuvant chemotherapy with noncross-resistant drugs even after preoperative chemotherapy in order to eliminate micrometastases which may be present [17]. The preliminary results of these studies are encouraging. However, many questions are still unresolved [16]. The optimal method or duration of therapy is still not known [12]. At present, any form of adjuvant or neoadjuvant chemotherapy still constitutes a therapeutic experiment in non-small cell lung cancer, and should therefore be confined exclusively to clinical studies [29].

3. SMALL-CELL LUNG CANCER

Because of their special biological properties (rapid tendency to systemic spread and high sensitivity to chemotherapy and radiotherapy), treatment of small-cell lung cancers differs in principle from the group of non-small cell lung cancers. Chemotherapy predominates with rates of remission of 80% to 95% (including up to 50% complete remissions). Various polychemotherapy schedules are available. Their effectiveness does not differ significantly in patients not previously treated. The median survival time of the patients in the stage of limited disease extends up to 18 months. About 20% of the patients with complete remission from this stage have chance of surviving without recurrences for two years or more [27,53]. Five-year actuarial survivals of 5% to 10% are found [54,19]. In the stage of limited disease, the late results are significantly improved by radiotherapy of the primary tumor region and the mediastinum [1]. For a small proportion of the patients, surgical resection is considered instead of radiotherapy or as supplemental to radiotherapy. The question is whether surgical therapy should be utilized as the first treatment measure in stage I and II patients and then followed by chemotherapy, or whether a few cycles of chemotherapy should be administered before surgical resection. At present, this question is being investigated in several international studies (e.g. of the EORTC and the Lung Cancer Study Group in the USA).

3.1. Surgery and adjuvant chemotherapy

The results of studies of the combination of operation and chemotherapy in small-cell lung cancer document the major prognostic significance of the tumor stage, as in non-small cell lung cancers [48,23,36].

The relatively favorable late fate of the patients with small-cell lung cancer with primary operation is especially noteworthy, compared to the patients who have received the same chemotherapy without surgical resection. Thus Shepherd et al. [45] reported a median survival of 21 months for the patients who received an operation, as compared to 11 months for the patients without an operation. Friess et al. [14] obtained median survival times of 25 months and 10 months (loc. cit. Ihde [19]). Long-term survival was also especially favorable in the operated group. We were able to confirm this in a retrospective analysis of our own (carried out in 170 patients). Compared to the patients who received radiotherapy, the patients with primary operation had a very low local rate of local recurrences. It is inferred from this that the rate of cure in patients with small-cell lung cancer in the stage of limited disease can be increased by surgery as part of the combined modality treatment concept [47].

However, the question must be raised as to whether the especially favorable result of therapy in the operated patients is due to the operation itself or to an extremely positive selection of patients. In an analysis of the results available up to 1986, this question is raised by Ihde [19]. In his view, the data from Toronto [45] support the argument of the effect of patient selection in favor of surgery. Patients who received primary operation with subsequent chemotherapy and radiotherapy had a median survival time of 21 months and a five-year actuarial survival of 24%. Of the remaining 90% of the patients with limited disease who were merely treated with chemotherapy and radiotherapy, 12% displayed stage 'very limited disease', which is operable. Operability was determined by no detection of mediastinal lymph node metastases in the scout-view X-ray of the thorax and mediastinoscopy. These patients with very limited disease constitute the group of patients who would be most likely to profit from surgical therapy. They had a median survival of 19 months and 23% five-year actuarial survival. These results were very much better than those of the remaining patients in the stage of limited disease, with a median survival time of 11 months and a five-year actuarial survival of 10%. These figures document that the late fate of the patients in the stage of 'very limited disease' was the same irrespective of whether these patients had received surgical treatment or not [45].

3.2. Operation after neoadjuvant chemotherapy

The primary tumor region, the hilus and the mediastinal lymph nodes, are the most frequent location of a recurrence for patients in the stage of 'limited disease'. In a review by Elliott et al.[9], the rate of recurrence in the primary tumor region was 64% and the rate of recurrence in the hilar and mediastinal lymph node stages was 53% even in patients with 'limited disease', who had obtained complete remission under the typical treatment. These data were obtained by autopsy. Radiotherapy is able to reduce the rate of local recurrences, but does not solve the problem. Adjuvant or consolidative radiotherapy reduces the rate of local recurrences and also has a favorable effect on the proportion of patients surviving for a long time without recurrences, but the definitive rates of cure are still unsatisfactory. In this situation, it appears to be conceivable that the tumor could be completely destroyed locally by the adjuvant surgical resection. If the chemotherapy eliminates any distant micrometastases present, the rate of cure may then be increased. The number of possible candidates for adjuvant surgical chemotherapy is determined by the criteria stipulated for a potentially curative operation. If only patients of stages I and II are regarded as suitable, the proportion of these patients will be about 10%. Sheperd et al.[46] have proved that such a prediction is possible. After chemotherapy, 19 out of 20 patients in the stage of 'very limited disease' were indeed resected. This especially high rate of reselection is doubtless due to the inclusion criteria, a negative mediastinoscopy. The proportion of patients who received later resection was very much less at Vanderbilt University. Only 20% of 40 patients in the stage of "limited disease" (which was not further defined) were candidates for surgical resection after two to four cycles of chemotherapy[43].

The results of histological analysis of the tumors with adjuvant resection are interesting. Only tissue of non-small cell lung cancers was found in 13% to 22%, whereas up to 20% of the resectates showed mixed forms of small-cell and non-small cell tumors[19]. 13% to 22% of the surgical preparations contained no tumor tissue[43,11,60]. A differentiation in the sequence of chemotherapy is also under discussion[19].

So far, only preliminary results are available on lung resection after chemotherapy. These are encouraging, but do not allow a final appraisal. At present, only up to 10% to 20% of the patients with limited disease appeared to be candidates for pulmonary resection with primary chemotherapy. The results of the Lung Cancer Study Group comparing the adjuvant resection with adjuvant radiotherapy after primary chemotherapy have to be awaited. There is general agreement that patients with involvement of mediastinal lymph nodes are no longer suitable for surgical therapy.

Of course, the negative effects of primary chemotherapy on surgical therapy must be considered. These include disorders of wound healing and effects on cardiac and pulmonary function.

4. CONCLUSIONS

Neoadjuvant chemotherapy leads to rates of remission of 40% to more than 80% in stage III non-small cell lung cancer. In a portion of the patients, which varies in the different studies, complete surgical resection of the tumor is possible after chemotherapy. These patients may expect a longer survival time compared to patients without curative resection. However, prospectively randomized therapy studies are lacking for ultimate evaluation of this form of therapy. So far, a final appraisal of this form of therapy is not possible. For this reason, combination therapy should be carried out exclusively in the context of clinical studies.

Very much lower numbers are available so far on small-cell lung cancer, since surgical therapy is of less importance in this tumor. However, there is no doubt that surgery has an established place in stages I and II. At present, it is an open question as to whether it should be used as the primary form of therapy or subsequent to chemotherapy. It is expected that this question will be answered by therapy studies which are in progress. Conceivable complications of a neoadjuvant chemotherapy are disorders of wound healing as well as cardiorespiratory complications after the subsequent operation.

REFERENCES

1 Arriagada R, Bertino JR, Bleehen NM, Brodin O, Feld R, Goldie JH, Hansen HH, et al; and Workshop participants. Consensus report on combined radiotherapy and chemotherapy modalities in lung cancer. In: Arriagada R, Le Chevalier T (eds.). Treatment Modalities in Lung Cancer. Basel, Karger-Verlag 1985: Vol 41, pp 232–241.

2 Ayoub J, Duranceau A, Lorange G, Robidoux A, Hanley J, Page A, Joassin A, Doyle D, Lafontaine ER, Delvecchio P, Jean-Francois R, Gauthier J-J, Lemay J, Nutini A-M, Arjane G, Lesage R, Schurch W, Cave N, Dionne J, participating RICUM investigators. Effectiveness of adjuvant chemotherapy in operable non-small-cell lung cancer (NSCLC). In: Salmon SE (ed.). Adjuvant Therapy of Cancer V. Orlando, FL, Grune & Stratton 1987: pp 157–164.

3 Bitran JD, Golomb HM, Hoffmann PC, et al: Protochemotherapy in non-small cell lung carcinoma. An attempt to increase surgical resectability and survival. A preliminary report. Cancer 1986; 57: 44–53.

4 Bonomi P, Trybulla M, Sandler S, Taylor SG, Howard-Ruben J, Busby J, Maffey S, Lee MS, Reddy S, Faber LP. Comparison of neo-adjuvant chemotherapy (Neo-CT) alone to simultaneous chemotherapy (SCT-RT) in locally advanced squamous cell bronchogenic carcinoma (Sq CBS). Neo-adjuvant chemotherapy. Coll. IN-SERM/John Libbey Eurotext 1986; 137: 505–517.

5 Burkes R, Ginsberg R, Shepherd F, Blackstein M, Goldberg M, Waters P, Patterson A, Todd T, Pearson F, Cooper J, Jones D. Neo-adjuvant trial with MVP (mitomycin-c + vindesine + cisplatin) chemotherapy for stage III (T1–3, N2, M0) unresectable non-small cell lung cancer (NSCLC) Proc Am Soc Clin Oncol 1989; 8: 221 (Abstr. 860).

6 Clavier J, Zabbè CL, Raut Y, Bierre J, Larzul JJ, Kerbourc'h JF, Nguyen-Huu N. Chimiothérapie pré-opératoire dans le cancera bronchiques epidermoides. Résultats d'une étude pilote portant sur 60 patients. Neo-adjuvant chemotherapy. Coll. INSERM/John Libbey Eurotext 1986; 137: 473–478.

7 Drings P. European experience with ifosfamide in non-small cell lung cancer. Semin Oncol 1989; 16: 22–30.

8 Eagan RT, Ruud C, Lee R, Pairolero P, Gail M, for the Lung Cancer Study Group: A pilot study of induction therapy with cyclophosphamide, doxorubicin, cis-platinum (CAP) and chest irradiation prior to thoracotomy in initially inoperable stage III M0 non-small cell lung cancer. Cancer Treat Rep 1987; 71: 895–900.

9 Elliot JA, Osterling K, Hirsch FR, Hansen HH. Metastatic patterns in small-cell lung cancer: correlation of autopsy findings with clinical parameters in 537 patients. J Clin Oncol 1987; 5: 246–254.

10 Elliot JA: Is there standard chemotherapy for non-small cell lung cancer? Eur J Cancer Clin Oncol 1986; 22: 369–371.

11 Ettinger DS, Baker RR, Eggleston JC, et al. Prospective evaluation of the role or surgery in limited disease small cell lung cancer: An ECOG pilot study. Proc Am Soc Clin Oncol 1985; 4: 180.

12 Evans WK. Adjuvant therapy for non-small cell lung cancer. Lung Cancer 1988; 4: 64–69.

13 Feld P, Rubinstein LV, Weisenberger TH, Lung Cancer Study Group: Sites of recurrence in resected stage I non-small cell lung cancer: a guide for future studies: J Clin Oncol 1984; 2: 1352–1358.

14 Friess GG, McCracken JD, Troxell ML, et al. Effect of initial resection of small cell carcinoma of the lung: A review of Southwest Oncology Group study 7628. J Clin Oncol 1985; 3: 964–968.

15 Gail MH, Eagan RT, Feld R, Ginsberg R, Coodell B, Hill L, Carmack Holmes E, Lukemann J, Mountain CF, Oldham RK, Pearson FG, Wright PW, Lake WH, Lung Cancer Study Group: Prognostic factors in patients with resected stage I non-small cell lung cancer. Cancer 1984; 54: 1802–1813.

16 Gralla RJ, Kris MG, Martini N, Stampleman LV, Burke MT. Adjuvant chemotherapy approaches in non-small cell lung cancer. In: Salmon SE (ed.). Adjuvant Therapy of Cancer V. Orlando, FL, Grune & Stratton 1987: pp 147–156.

17 Holmes EC. Surgical adjuvant therapy of non-small-cell lung cancer. In: Hansen HH (ed.). Basic and Clinical Concepts of Lung Cancer. Dordrecht, Kluwer Academic Publishers 1989: pp 245–258.

18 Holmes EC. Surgical adjuvant chemotherapy in non-small cell lung cancer. Semin Oncol 1988; 15: 255–260.

19 Ihde DD. Neo-adjuvant chemotherapy of lung cancer: preliminary North-American experience. Neoadjuvant chemotherapy. Coll. INSERM/John Libbey Eurotext 1986; 137: 467–472.

20 Immermann SC, Vanecho RM, Fry WA, Head LR, Shields TW. Site of recurrence in patients with stages I and II carcinomas of the lung resected for cure. Ann Thorac Surg 1981; 32: 3–27.

21 Israel I, Breau JL, Morère JM, Nouvet G, Tcherakian F. Chimiothérapie pré-opératoire dans 57 cas de cancers bronchiques épidermoides. Analyse des responses, des complications et de la survie. Neoadjuvant Chemotherapy. Coll. INSERM/John Libbey Eurotext 1986; 137: 463–465.

22 Joss PA, Brunner KW. Die Chemotherapie der nicht-kleinzelligen Bronchialkarzinome. In: Seeber S, Niederle S (eds.). Interdisziplinäre Therapie des Bronchialkarzinoms. Berlin, Springer 1985: pp 75–94.

23 Karrer K, Shields TW, Denck H, Hrabar B, Vogt-Moykopf I. The importance of surgical and multimodality treatment for small cell bronchial carnoma. J Thorac Cardiovasc Surg 1989; 97: 168–176.

24 Kenis Y. Surgical adjuvant chemotherapy in non-small cell carcinoma of the lung. Radiat Oncol Biol Phys 1980; 6: 1075–1077.

25 Kies MS, Mira JG, Crowley JJ, et al. Multi-modal therapy for limited small-cell lung cancer: a randomized study of induction combination chemotherapy with or without thoracic irradiation in complete responders and with wide-field versus reduced-field radiation in partial responders – a Southwest Oncology Group study. J Clin Oncol 1987; 5: 592–600.

26 Kris MG, Gralla RJ, Wertheim MS. Trial of the combination of mitomycin, vindesin and cisplatin in patients with advanced non-small cell lung cancer. Cancer Treat Rep 1986; 70: 1091–1096.

27 Klastersky J: Therapy of small cell lung cancer: Anything new? Eur J Clin Oncol 1988; 24: 107–112.

28 Klastersky J, Feld R, Kleisbauer JP, Rocmans P. Treatment of N2 non-small cell lung cancer (NSCLC) Chest 1989; 96: 83S–85S.

29 Kris MG, Gralla RJ, Martini N, Stampleman LV, Burke TM. Preoperative and adjuvant chemotherapy in locally advanced non-small cell lung cancer. Surg Clin North Am 1987; 67: 1051–1059.

30 Legha SS, Muggia FM. Adjuvant chemotherapy in lung cancer; an appraisal of past studies. In: Muggia FM, Rozencweig M (eds.). Lung Cancer, Progress in Therapeutic Research. New York, Raven Press 1979: pp 405–410.

31 Lung Cancer Study Group: The benefit of adjuvant treatment for resected locally advanced non-small cell lung cancer. J Clin Oncol 1986; 6: 9–17.

32 Lung Cancer Study Group: Seven years follow up of surgical adjuvant therapy for adenocarcinoma and large cell undifferentiated carcinoma of the lung. Lung Cancer 1988; 4: A119.

33 Martini N, Kris MG, Gralla RJ, Bains MS, McCormack PM, Kaiser LR, Burt ME, Zaman MB. The effects of preoperative chemotherapy on the resectability of non-small cell lung carcinoma with mediastinal lymph node metastases (N2 M0). Ann Thorac Surg 1988; 45: 370–379.

34 Martini N, Flehinger, B. The role of surgery in N2 lung cancer. Surg Clin North Am 1987; 67: 1037.

35 Martini N, Flehinger B, Zaman M, et al. Results of resection in non-small cell carcinoma of the lung with mediastinal lymph node metastases. Ann Surg 1983; 198: 386.

36 Merkle NM, Mickisch GH, Kayser K, Drings P, Vogt-Moykopf I. Surgical resection and adjuvant chemotherapy for small cell carcinoma Thorac Cardiovasc Surg 1986; 34: 39–42.

37 Mountain CF. Prognostic implications of the international staging system for lung cancer. Semin Oncol 1988; 15: 236–245.

38 Mountain CF, Hermes KE. Management implications of surgical staging studies. In: Muggia FM, Rosencweig M (eds.). Lung Cancer: Progress in Therapeutic Research. New York, Raven Press 1979: pp 233–242.

39 Mountain CF, McMurtrey M, Frazier OH, Barkley HT, Valdivieso M. Present status of postoperative adjuvant therapy for lung cancer. Cancer Bull 1980; 32: 108–112.

40 Muggia FM, Blum RH, Cooper JS, McCauley D, Kaplan R, Kaplan Sr H. Chemotherapy for locally advanced lung cancer: Rationale and issues. Primary Chemother Cancer Med (Lissabon) 1985: 119–126.

41 Perez CA, Einhorn L, Oldham RK, et al. Randomized trial of radiotherapy to the thorax in limited small-cell carcinoma of the lung treated with multi-agent chemotherapy and elective brain irradiation: a preliminary report. J Clin Oncol 1984; 42: 1200–1208.

42 Pincus M, Reddy S, Lee MS, Bonomi P, Taylor S, Rowland K, Faber LP, Warren W, Kittle CF, Hendrickson FR. Preoperative combined modality therapy for stage III M0 non-small cell lung carcinoma. Int J Radiat Oncol Biol Phys 1988; 15: 189–195.

43 Prager RL, Foster Jm, Hainswirth JD, et al. The feasibility of adjuvant surgery in limited stage small cell carcinoma: A prospective evaluation. Ann Thorac Surg 1984; 38: 622–626.

44 Sadeghi A, Payne D, Rubinstein L, Lad T, The Lung Cancer Study Group: Combined modality treatment for resected advanced non-small cell lung cancer: Local control and local recurrence. Int.J Radiat Oncol Biol Phys 1988; 15: 89–97.

45 Shepherd FA, Ginsburg R, Evans WK, et al. Reduction in local recurrence and improved survival in surgically treated patients with small cell lung cancer. J Thorac Cardiovasc. Surg. 1983; 86: 498–506.

46 Shepherd FA, Evans WK, Ginsburg R, et al. A prospective study of combined modality therapy including surgery for limited small cell lung cancer. Abstr. World Conf. Lung Cancer 1985; 4: 142.

47 Shepherd FA, Evans WK, Feld R, Young V, Patterson GA, Ginsburg R, Johansen E. Adjuvant chemotherapy following surgical resection for small-cell carcinoma of the lung. J Clin Oncol 1988; 6: 832–838.

48 Shields TW, Higgins GA, Matthews MJ, Keehn RJ. Surgical resection in the management of small cell carcinoma of the lung. J Thorac Cardiovasc Surg 1982; 84: 481–488.

49 Shields TW, Yee J, Conn JH, Robinette CD. Relationship of cell type and lymphnode metastases to survival after resection of bronchial carcinoma. Ann Thorac Surg 1975; 20: 501–510.

50 Shields TW, Humphrey EW, Matthews M, Eastridge CE, Keehn RJ. Pathological stage grouping of patient with resected carcinoma of the lung. J Thorac Cardiovasc Surg 1980; 80: 400–495.

51 Skarin A, Veeder M, Malcolm A, et al. Chemotherapy (CAP) prior to radiotherapy (RT) and surgery in marginally resectable non-small cell lung cancer (NSCLC). Proc Am Soc Clin Oncol 1982; 1: 143.

52 Skarin A, Socinski MA, Kalish L, Frei III E. Neoadjuvant therapy for stage IIIa non-small cell lung cancer (NSCLC). Proc Am Soc Clin Oncol 1989; 8: 241 (Abstr. 941).
53 Seifter EJ, Ihde DC. Therapy of small cell lung cancer: a perspective on two decades of clinical research. Semin Oncol 1988; 15: 278–299.
54 Smyth JF. Chemotherapy of small cell lung cancer. Chest 1989; 96: 61S–62S.
55 Spain R, Anderson P, Speer J, et al. Improved survival with mitomycin-C, cis-platinum and continuous vinblastine infusion plus radiation therapy or surgery over RT alone for stage III limited, initially inoperable, non-small cell lung cancer. Proc IV World Conf on Lung Cancer 1985, p 33 (abstract).
56 Splinter TAW, Kho GS, Frederiksz A, ten Kates FJW. Preoperative chemotherapy in non-small cell lung cancer: a pilot study. Neo-adjuvant chemotherapy. Coll. INSERM/John Libbey Eurotext 1986; 137: 491–499.
57 Strauss G, Sherman D, Schwartz J, et al. Combined modality therapy for regionally advanced stage III non-small cell carcinoma of the lung employing neoadjuvant chemotherapy, radiotherapy, and surgery. Proc Am Soc Clin Oncol 1986; 5: 172.
58 Takita H, Regal AM, Antkowiak JG, et al. Chemotherapy followed by lung resection in inoperable non-small cell lung carcinomas due to locally far-advanced disease. Cancer 1986; 57: 630–635.
59 Trybulla M, Taylor SG, Bonomi P, et al. Preoperative simultaneous cisplatin/5-fluorouracil and radiotherapy in clinical stage III, non-small cell bronchogenic carcinoma. Proc Am Soc Clin Oncol 1985; 4: 182.
60 Valdivieso M, McMurtey MJ, Farha P, et al: Prospective evaualation of adjuvant surgical resection in small cell lung cancer. Proc Am Soc Clin Oncol 1984; 3: 220.
61 Vogt-Moykopf I, Bülzebruck H, Probst G, Merkle N. Chirurgische Therapie des Bronchialkarzinoms. Langenbecks Arch Chir Suppl II 1988: 109–117.
62 Zabbè CL, Khayat D, Gouva S, Kerbourc'h. JF, Jacquillat CL, Clavier J. Cisplatine, bleomycine et 5 fluoro-uracile (CBF) en traitement pré-opératoire du cancer bronchique épidermoide. Neo-adjuvant chemotherapy. Coll. INSERM/John Libbey Eurotext 1986; 137: 501–506.

Current Topics in General Thoracic Surgery: An International Series, Vol. 2
Perioperative Care, edited by R.M. Peters and J. Toledo

Pulmonary resection following chemotherapy – perioperative considerations

Discussion of "Pulmonary resection following chemotherapy" by P. Drings and I. Vogt-Moykopf

Robert J. Ginsberg and Melvyn Goldberg

1. INTRODUCTION

As outlined in the preceding chapter by Drings and Vogt-Moykopf, preoperative chemotherapy (neoadjuvant or, more accurately, induction chemotherapy) is being utilized with increasing frequency in Phase II clinical trials in the management of primary lung cancer with local spread to the mediastinum (stage IIIA, IIIB disease) and in the management of limited stage small cell carcinoma. Until its role is better defined, this treatment should still be considered only in the context of clinical trials.

This type of approach, however, is already part of other solid tumors and of many currently accepted protocols for the treatment of metastases to the lung, especially from testicular and ovarian tumors, and osteogenic sarcomas.

It is possible that such combined modality approaches will become more frequent in the future when treating solid tumors, including primary and secondary lung tumors. Newer chemotherapeutic agents should effect higher response rates, and combined modality treatment with induction chemotherapy may become the rule for even less advanced disease [1].

Induction treatment does have certain theoretical advantages over postoperative therapy. Tumor blood supply is better, allowing increased permeation of the tumor cells with chemotherapeutic agents. The resultant tumor regression may 'downstage' the primary disease allowing resectability where it otherwise could not have been effected, or allowing lesser resections for complete removal of the primary disease. The goals of induction therapy, therefore, include the following: (1) Reduce tumor size. (2) Downgrade the stage. (3) Increase operability.

(4) Destroy micrometastases early, thereby altering the natural history of the disease. (5) Identify patients with chemoresponsive disease.

This latter indication affects postoperative decision making regarding further chemotherapy with similar drugs or non-cross resistant drugs. As well, earlier chemotherapy may decrease the ultimate development of resistant mutant strains by early destruction of malignant cells.

Very frequently, especially in phase II trials for locally advanced lung cancer, radiotherapy has been utilized preoperatively in association with chemotherapy [2,3]. These single or combined modality induction treatments can increase problems in surgical management. It is, therefore, worthwhile to review the more frequent pertinent complications of chemotherapy.

2. COMPLICATIONS OF INDUCTION CHEMOTHERAPY

The various toxicities of chemotherapeutic agents are well known. The most important complications that affect pulmonary resection include the pulmonary and cardiac toxicities that occur with the administration of certain drugs [1].

2.1. Pulmonary toxicity

Bleomycin and mitomycin are frequently used in induction protocols (the former in germ cell tumors and the latter in primary lung carcinoma). Associated with these drugs is significant pulmonary toxicity. Pathologically, diffuse alveolar damage can occur with interstitial pneumonitis and fibrosis. These drugs appear to be toxic for both alveolar endothelium and epithelium. The mechanism of injury is attributed to the production of free radical oxygen formed during the intracellular reductive activation of drug. This free oxygen radical interferes with oxidation of membrane lipids resulting in an inflammatory response. Radiation and exposure to high concentrations of oxygen can be synergistic in the production of these free radicals.

This injury may not be clinically evident, although it has been reported in as high as 25% of patients treated with mitomycin. Despite minimal, if any, clinical manifestations, reduction in carbon monoxide diffusing capacity (DCO) following chemotherapy treatment is commonplace [4,5].

For these reasons, pretreatment investigation mandates prechemotherapy and presurgical DCO estimations. Concomitant administration of steroids may exert some beneficial preventive effect. Intraoperatively, it has been suggested that minimizing the F_IO_2, depending on patient requirements, can also be beneficial. As well, minimizing crystalloid administration perioperatively may help to prevent postoperative pulmonary edema and respiratory failure.

Despite these attempts at prevention, we and others have found the combination of preoperative radiotherapy with bleomycin or mitomycin to have fatal consequences in some patients [6]. A syndrome occurs 24 to 72 hours following surgery, of increasing hypoxemia, sterile pulmonary infiltrates and ultimate respiratory failure and death. Judicious management of the patient during the administration of chemotherapy and in the perioperative period may decrease this type of complication.

2.2. Cardiac toxicity

Cardiac toxicity, manifested by a cardiomyopathy, is particularly important in patients receiving doxorubicin. The recommended limit of 700 mg/M^2 should not be exceeded. Potentiation can occur with concomitant use of radiotherapy or other cardiotoxic agents (e.g. cyclophosphamide). The cardiac changes that occur may be delayed for several weeks after discontinuation of the treatment. Reduction of the ejection fraction is best determined by echocardiography or radionuclide angiography (MUGA scan). If test results indicate a change in cardiac function, one must evaluate the risks of the proposed surgical procedure in light of this change.

2.3. Myelosuppression

Most chemotherapeutic agents do suppress blood elements including precursors of red cells, granulocytes and platelets. The nadir of this suppression is usually 7 to 10 days following administration of the drug, with recovery between 18 and 23 days. During the induction phase, life-threatening pneumonias in the face of profound leukopenia should be avoided by appropriate antibiotic coverage of patients with tumors obstructing the airway. Timing of surgery must take this nadir and recovery into consideration. Frequently, patients develop and continue with an anemia that may have to be corrected prior to surgery (mitomycin).

2.4. Other toxicities

Hepatic, renal, oto- and neurotoxicity all can occur with various chemotherapeutic agents, especially cis-platinum, a frequent induction agent in lung cancer. Although these toxicities have little direct effect on the surgical procedure, renal function must be monitored and a balance must be arrived at such that perioperative fluid administration maintains renal blood flow in compromised patients, but does not embarrass pulmonary function.

Gastrointestinal toxicity usually is short-lived. However, a significant nutritional depletion can occasionally occur and if present, should be corrected prior to surgery.

3. SURGICAL CONDUCT

3.1. Primary lung cancer

Trials involving induction chemotherapy for primary lung cancer have been limited to more locally advanced disease (stage IIIA, IIIB) and very limited small cell carcinoma. Unresectable or barely resectable tumors can be downstaged by such treatment. Five to fifteen percent of such cases will have no viable tumor present at thoracotomy [2,5–7]. Presently this approach is limited to clinical trials since the ultimate benefit of this type of program is yet to be determined. Very accurate pretreatment staging is important, including mediastinoscopy, to assess the mediastinal nodal component of the disease, and computed tomographic organ scanning (lung, liver, adrenal) to ensure an MO status.

The goals of the post-chemotherapy surgical resection are to remove the site of the original primary tumor plus all lymphatics that were involved with the primary disease as identified at the original staging procedures. Only the surgeon is equipped to assess this and therefore **must** be involved in the prechemotherapy evaluation of the patient, including the initial endoscopy.

The surgical resection after a chemotherapy-induced response is often difficult. Lymph nodes that previously contained tumor can be involved in a dense inflammatory reaction such that the dissection can be hazardous and tedious. This will occur especially in the mediastinum and is aggravated by the prior mediastinoscopy. We have found that re-mediastinoscopy just prior to surgery, freeing the fibrotic tissue off the trachea, often will aid in dissection of the superior mediastinal lymph nodes at the time of surgery. Frequently, an intrapericardial dissection is required to completely remove the nodal component of the disease, which can be densely adherent to the pericardium. Where a tumor originally was located within a lobe, lobectomy plus total mediastinal lymph node dissection may be all that is required for complete removal of the primary site and its lymphatic drainage. However, frequently a radical intrapericardial pneumonectomy is necessary.

Postoperative complications due to patient debility and extensive devascularizing dissections are always a concern. Bronchopleural fistulae are a common postoperative complication, especially after right pneumonectomy [6]. For this reason, we believe it important that all bronchial closures be reinforced by vascularized tissue flaps. If radiotherapy has been added to the regimen or a right pneumonectomy is planned, we frequently will utilize pre-mobilized omentum from the abdomen, or well-vascularized pericardial fat, to cover the bronchial stump.

Postoperative infections can be life-threatening and appropriate perioperative prophylactic antibiotics are indicated. Attention to proper placement of chest tubes is important to eliminate potential space problems and resultant infection.

3.2. Metastatic pulmonary tumors

In most instances, especially when multiple metastases are already present, the risk of further occult pulmonary metastases is great. This includes metastatic germ cell tumors, soft tissue tumors and osteogenic sarcomas. For this reason, in most instances we prefer a median sternotomy if multiple pulmonary nodules are present, even if they are unilateral. This allows exploration of both hemithoraces and removal of all metastases simultaneously. Frequently, because of the less than 100% sensitivity of imaging studies, this results in the discovery of additional nodules on either side.

In many instances following chemotherapy, the nodules removed will be sterile or contain mature tissue such as bone or benign teratomas. However, all nodules must be excised to eliminate the risk of microscopic foci of malignancy remaining.

The goal of surgical excision with metastatic pulmonary nodules is to remove as little functioning pulmonary tumor as is necessary for complete excision of the metastatic nodule. In many instances this will require wedge resection. Deep-seated nodules may be excised, conserving pulmonary tissue, by a technique known as ‘precision cautery dissection’. This technique was described by Perelman in Russia and now is being utilized in North America. The precision dissection can be accomplished with electrocautery, CO_2 or argon laser and more recently Nd-YAG laser with contact tips[8]. Wherever possible, segmentectomy is preferred to lobectomy if a larger excision is required in order to preserve pulmonary tissue. One must always be cognizant of the fact that further resections may be required in the future.

Care must be taken to control minor air leaks. This can include the use of staplers, pleural flaps to cover raw surfaces, or fibrin glue to cover leaking large raw surfaces.

As with primary lung carcinoma, meticulous attention to detail will prevent postoperative space problems and resultant infection. Perioperative antibiotic coverage is indicated.

4. ANESTHETIC CONSIDERATIONS

Because of the inherent pulmonary and cardiac toxicities that may occur, attention must be given to proper fluid management. Patients should not be over-hydrated lest pulmonary edema result[9]. Cardiotoxic anaesthetic agents should be avoided since arrhythmias are more prone to develop in the intraoperative or perioperative period.

Since high inspired oxygen concentration can potentiate the pulmonary damage, it has been our practice to use the lowest F_IO_2 necessary to maintain adequate oxygenation for the patient, both in the intraoperative and postoperative periods.

5. POSTOPERATIVE CARE

It has not been our practice to intentionally ventilate patients postoperatively. In all instances, unless indicated for other reasons, patients are extubated at the completion of the surgery and allowed to ventilate spontaneously. As in the intraoperative phase, attention is directed towards optimum fluid management, optimum oxygenation and prevention of postoperative atelectasis and pneumonia.

6. ANALYSIS OF RESULTS

6.1. Neoadjuvant chemotherapy for non-small cancer

Although induction chemotherapy (usually with radiotherapy) for locally advanced stage IIIA and IIIB non-small cell tumors has been employed in phase II clinical trials for almost 10 years, there has never been a random assignment phase III trial to demonstrate its effectiveness compared with standard surgical or non-surgical treatment. To date, most clinical trials reported have used median survival times as an indication of effectiveness. Almost without exception, the median survival following this type of very aggressive treatment is about 12 months. More recently, the MVP regimen (mitomycin, vindesine, cis-platinum) has been reported in 3 clinical trials with more encouraging results [5–7]. The response rate in these clinical trials was about 65% with a complete response rate ranging from 7% to 20%. Median survival times in these reports have been extended to 20 months.

What the ultimate role for neoadjuvant chemotherapy will be in non-small cell carcinoma is yet to be determined. Whether induction chemotherapy in this locally advanced stage of disease alters time to recurrence or survival is still unknown.

In North America, 3 phase III clinical trials examining this question have been proposed. A North American intergroup trial (RTOG, CALGB, ECOG) will randomize stage IIIa patients between induction chemotherapy followed by surgery, and induction chemotherapy followed by radiotherapy. This will answer the question as to whether surgical intervention adds benefit in this stage of disease. A similar trial proposed by The Southwest Oncology Group (SWOG) will use induction chemoradiotherapy, comparing it to non-surgical treatment. As well, SWOG intends to begin a randomized trial in earlier stage (T2N0, T1N1, T2N1) lung cancer, comparing standard surgical treatment to neoadjuvant chemotherapy plus surgery.

We hope that these trials, once completed, will answer some of the questions already posed concerning neoadjuvant treatment of lung cancer.

6.2. Small cell cancer

Whether surgery is ever indicated in locally advanced small cell cancer is still a moot point. In limited small cell cancer, phase II trials have suggested a decreased local recurrence rate using multimodality therapy including surgery [10,11]. However, all of these trials suffer from retrospective non-randomized comparisons. A Lung Cancer Study Group (LCSG) phase III prospective randomized trial comparing induction chemotherapy followed by surgery and standard radiotherapy with chemotherapy plus radiotherapy has been completed. This trial is still being analyzed and results should be forthcoming in the very near future.

6.3. Metastatic germ cell tumors

With combination chemotherapy, radiotherapy and surgery, 80% of males with germ cell tumors can be cured [12]. Patients with stage III testicular cancer have an improved survival expectation (60%–70%). Approximately 25% of patients with non-seminomatous carcinoma of the testes will have pulmonary metastases at the time of diagnosis. Two-thirds of such patients will have persisting nodules following intensive chemotherapy. At pulmonary resection of these residual nodules, in two-thirds of patients, either mature teratoma or fibrosis will be identified with no active disease. Those with persistent carcinoma at the time of surgery require further chemotherapy and have a much diminished chance of ultimate cure (approximately 25%). In contradistinction, most patients with only mature teratoma or fibrosis identified at thoracotomy will be cured of their disease without further therapy.

6.4. Osteogenic sarcoma

As with germ cell tumors, patients presenting with metachronous multiple pulmonary nodules secondary to osteogenic sarcoma are usually treated with induction chemotherapy [13]. Those patients with residual nodules following chemotherapy should undergo resection. Such combined modality treatment will produce up to a 40% four-year survival [14]. However, randomized trials comparing no preoperative chemotherapy to preoperative chemotherapy have never been performed. When patients present with synchronous pulmonary metastases, only 16% survived 4 years despite intensive chemotherapy and surgery to the primary site and lung. With successful chemotherapy, the pulmonary nodules removed may contain no viable tumor or only mature bone.

7. SUMMARY

The role of induction chemotherapy in primary and metastatic pulmonary disease has yet to be completely defined. The role of surgery following this treatment for locally advanced primary lung cancer is still of questionable value, and awaits the results of randomized trials.

Patients undergoing surgery following intensive chemotherapy are at risk for complications related to specific effects of chemotherapy on vital organs as well as those related to the general debilitating effect of chemotherapy (with or without concomitant radiotherapy). The surgeon and anesthetist must be aware of the specific side-effects of the chemotherapy regimens being employed in order to prevent major complications from developing. With the appropriate care in the perioperative period and meticulous technique at the time of surgery, most patients, despite their arduous treatment, can undergo pulmonary resection with few complications.

REFERENCES

1 Klastersky J, Feld R, Leisbauer JP, Rocmans P. Treatment of N2 Nonsmall Cell Cancer of the Lung. Lung Cancer 1988; 4 (Suppl): 62–63 (abstract).

2 Faber LP, Kittle FC, Warren WH, Bonomi PD, Taylor SG IV, Reddy S, Myung-Sook L. Preoperative chemotherapy and irradiation for stage III non-small cell lung cancer. Ann Thorac Surg 1989; 47: 669–677.

3 Trybula M, Taylor SG, Bonomi P, et al. Preoperative simultaneous cisplatin/5-fluorouracil and radiotherapy in clinical stage III, nonsmall cell bronchogenic carcinoma. Proc Amer Soc Clin Oncol 1985; 4: 182.

4 Folman R, Rosman M, Auerbach S. Mitomycin C, vinblastine, cis platinum in the combined treatment of nonsmall cell lung cancer. Proc Amer Soc Clin Oncol 1984; 3: 232.

5 Spain R, Anderson P, Speer J, et al. Improved survival with mitomycin C, cis platinum, and continuous vinblastine infusion plus radiation therapy or surgery over RT alone for stage III limited, initially inoperable, nonsmall cell lung cancer. Proc IV World Conf on Lung Cancer, Toronto, Canada 1985: p 33.

6 Burkes R, Ginsberg R, Shepherd F, et al. Neo-adjuvant trial with MVP (mitomycin-c + vindesine – cisplatin) chemotherapy for stage III (T1–3, N2, M0) unresectable non-small cell lung cancer (NSCLC). Proc Amer Soc Clin Oncol 1989; 8: 221 (Abstr 860).

7 Martini N, Kris MG, Gralla RJ, Bains MS, McCormack PM, Kaiser LR, Burt ME, Zaman MB. The effects of preoperative chemotherapy on the resectability of nonsmall cell lung carcinoma with mediastinal lymph node metastases (N2M0). Ann Thorac Surg 1988; 45: 370–379.

8 Cooper JD, Perelman M, Todd PR, et al. Precision cautery excision of pulmonary lesions. Ann Thorac Surg 1986; 41: 51–53.

9 Zeldin RA, Normandin D, Landtwing D, et al. Postpneumonectomy pulmonary edema. J Thorac Cardiovasc Surg 1984; 87: 359–365.

10 Shepherd FA, Ginsberg RJ, Evans WK, et al. Reduction in local recurrence and improved survival in surgically treated patients with small cell lung cancer. J Thorac Cardiovasc Surg 1983; 86: 498–506.

11 Meyer JA. Indications for surgical treatment in small cell carcinoma of the lung. Surg Clin North Am 1987; 67: 1103–1115.

12 Einhorn, L. Treatment of testicular cancer: A new and improved model. J Clin Oncol 1990; 8: 1777–1781.

13 Rosen G, Huvos AG, Mosende C, et al. Chemotherapy and thoracotomy for metastatic osteogenic sarcoma: A model for adjuvant chemotherapy and the rationale for the timing of thoracic surgery. Cancer 1978; 41: 841.

14 McCormack PM, Bains MS, Martini N. Surgical management of pulmonary metastases. Semin Surg Oncol 1990; 6: 297–302.

Part III

Immediate preparation for thoracotomy

Current Topics in General Thoracic Surgery: An International Series, Vol. 2
Perioperative Care, edited by R.M. Peters and J. Toledo

Chapter 11

Physical condition in preparation for thoracotomy

G. Ramos and Mª.J. Gallo

1. SURGERY AS INJURY

Surgery – whether diagnostic, palliative or therapeutic – means an injury added to the already unfavorable effects that the illness itself has on the individual. However, the response that it induces (triggered by various stimuli acting predominantly through the activation of the hypothalamus–hypophysis–adrenal axis) is actually a biologic process which tends toward recovery of homeostasis and repair of the lesions produced [1]. This hormono-metabolic response which develops in different sequences is proportionate to the magnitude of the injury and in the end permits the restoration of the organism's energy deposits [2].

Thus, after the phase of catabolic hormone activity, once the organism's priority necessities have been taken care of, the anabolic phase begins. Insulin is the key factor in this stage, promoting glycogen deposit in the liver and muscle tissue and inhibiting gluconeogenesis and lipolysis. In this way, protein re-establishment is gradually fostered and, finally, the recovery of lost fats [3].

When this entire process fails, diverse complications can arise, having an influence on the sum total of successive traumas, inadequate therapy or insufficient reaction capacity on the patient's part [1].

In addition, surgical trauma also induces various modifications to the immunologic response, whose negative effect on infections and tumoral evolution is quite well known. The causes of the alterations in immunological response have not yet been completely clarified.

As well as the surgical intrusion, many other overlapping factors affect the patient's immune response: treatment with certain drugs, presence of particular diseases, coexistence of malnutrition, etc. These interactions make the analysis of the problem considerably more difficult, particularly if there are factors that can be simultaneously a cause and a consequence of immunological depression. With this in mind, it is important to point out that the activity of the immune system needs energy to function, which is the reason why anomalies in the defense mechanisms must be expected when the subject is in a catabolic state [4].

The physical status of the person who is to undergo surgery plays an important role in the final outcome of the surgery and in the incidence of possible postoperative complications. This status [5] is a reflection of the patient's cardiorespiratory, muscular and metabolic reserves [6].

2. TYPE OF OPERATION AND PHYSICAL CONDITION, KEY RISK FACTORS

Both the patient's current condition and the proposed surgery must be fully considered in the preparation for the thoracotomy and in the choice of the method to be followed. These elements require the most exacting evaluation possible of risk to permit facing the operation with the minimum discomfort and the maximum security for the desired outcome [7].

In the proposed surgical intervention, it is obvious that the results may be affected by factors as diverse as the type of operation, its length or its possible emergency character. The kind of surgery directly influences the cardiorespiratory mechanics and, logically, the postoperative morbidity and mortality. The length of the procedure, while not having the significance of years ago, seems to be a priori another risk factor, although studies which show its correlation with postoperative mortality perhaps reflect only the gravity of the underlying disease [8]. Finally, emergency treatment clearly worsens the prognosis, since the lack of time precludes a detailed, careful preparation for the surgery.

The risk involved definitely increases with the severity of the operation [7]. Nevertheless, it is often difficult to establish the individual importance of each factor, such as the operating team's experience and the hospital resources available [8].

In the estimation of the individual's condition, physiologic and physical characteristics both influence the illness which is to be treated surgically. One aspect or another can determine the final decision to operate and, particularly, the choice of the most appropriate moment for the intervention.

Together with the prior physiological state, the lesions produced by the surgery itself, the seriousness of possible complications and the effectiveness of the operation or other therapeutic measures also influence the postoperative evolution [9] and the probability that the patient will recover completely.

3. AGING AND PHYSICAL CONDITION

The role of age as a risk factor is not always easy to discern, though it is clear that the aging process determines changes in body structure (Fig. 11.1) and the functioning

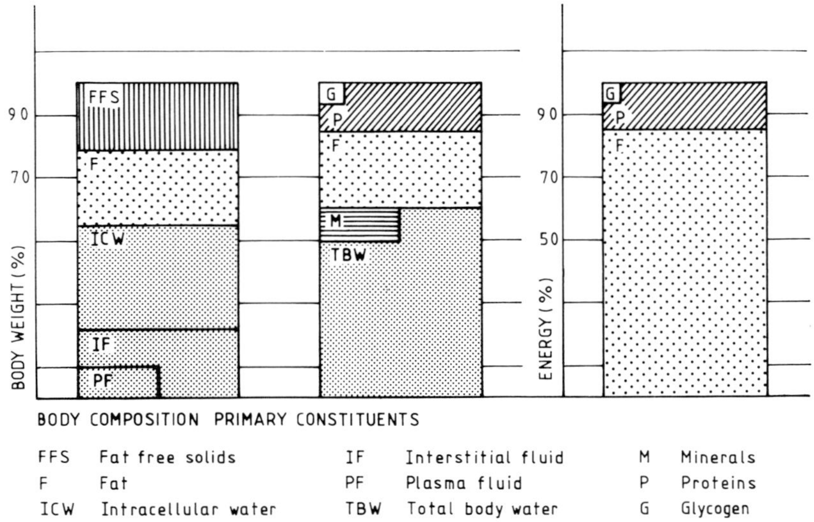

FIGURE 11.1. The approximate normal values for the primary constituents of adult male body composition.

of physiologic systems, which result in a decrease in reserves [10] and in the chances of final recovery [7,8].

As one ages, the proportion of lean body mass to fat diminishes, at the same time as the cellular fraction of the former decreases. The weight loss explains part of the adaptation difficulties of older patients which result from the functional depression of specific organs of vital importance during surgery and in the postoperative period. Thus, the reduction of the cardiac reserve, renal function and pulmonary function, favors the appearance of postoperative complications. One of the compensatory mechanisms for hypovolemia is lowered, so that the risk of postoperative renal insufficiency increases and the necessary tracheobronchial toilette becomes more difficult [7].

The more advanced the age, on the other hand, the greater the number of associated diseases, emergency procedures undergone and malignant tumors, all pejorative circumstances [7,8,10].

The number of pathologic states in fact increases with age, to the point that up to 80% of the geriatric population present multisystemic illness. Cardiopathies, arthritis, visual defects, diabetes, cerebrovascular disturbances, emphysema, psychiatric imbalances, defects of audition, neoplasms, etc., all contribute to limit physical activity in those over 65 [11]. The associated diseases undoubtedly add another risk [12] to a weaker capacity to tolerate complications, sometimes cause delay in recognition of complications, with negative repercussions on the effectiveness of treatment [8].

TABLE 11.1
Classification of physical activities [16]

Type of activity	METs[a]
Light	1.0–2.9
Moderate	3.0–4.9
Hard	5.0–6.9
Very hard	> 7.0

[a] Energy expended by a person at rest = 1 MET

The progressive deterioration seems to be, therefore, a result of the combination of factors such as aging, age-related diseases and atrophies from disuse. All of these mean a loss of capacity to work, think and react in an adequate manner to environmental stimuli: a loss, in summary, of the capacity to perform physical and mental activity necessary to a smooth postoperative recovery [13]. In older patients there is little margin of error [11] and it follows that mortality in major surgery is four to eight times greater in patients who are over 70 years old [14]. Nevertheless, age per se does not constitute an absolute contra-indication for surgery, but it is true that the decision to operate or not requires a careful weighing of the risks and benefits in relation to the natural history of the illness [8].

More extensive knowledge of the biological process of aging and of the response to surgical trauma, together with advances in techniques of anesthesia, surgery and intensive care, currently permit operations on geriatric patients with an acceptable risk. Surgery in these cases obviously demands strict control at all times: appropriate anesthetics, meticulous surgical technique, painstaking postoperative care, etc., elements whose importance is magnified by the weakened functional reserves of this group [11].

4. PHYSICAL CONDITION, ORGAN IMPAIRMENT AND AGE-RELATED DISEASES

Age-associated disease (respiratory, cardiovascular, renal, hepatic, nutritional) has a negative effect on the individual's functional reserves, which is added to any modifications there might be with aging in specific cases.

An exhaustive physical examination and a psychological assessment [15] are obligatory steps in evaluating the patient's global state. Attention should be given to previous diseases and medications and the patient's personal habits. Age-associated disease should be the object of special interest for preparing the patient since age affects the physical condition of the patient who will undergo a thoracotomy.

In this context, the index of the individual's physical activity is an estimation of the metabolic work that takes place in a 24-hour period [5,16] (Table 11.1). The physical fitness describes the limits of the action which the patient is capable of performing [17]. Performance status represents a global appraisal of the patient's own capacity to take care of himself or herself and to undertake daily activities, which has been shown to be a strong prognostic factor in the case of neoplasm [18].

4.1. Respiratory system

Pleural and bronchopulmonary diseases are of the greatest importance, since postoperative pain or complications such as atelectasis, pneumonia or pulmonary embolism make the respiratory reserve a critical factor [8].

Moreover, the number of postoperative complications is elevated in respiratory insufficiency patients, although it is sometimes difficult to determine whether morbidity and mortality increases in proportion to the depression of function [7]. Anamnesis should always be meticulous, in order to detect any respiratory limitations or negative factors [19]. Smoking stands out as a major risk factor. It induces a ciliary paralysis that facilitates the retention of secretions and disturbs the necessary bronchial toilette.

The history and the use of analog scales can quantify the dyspnea, permitting the establishment of useful comparisons in the same patient. Spirometry (Wright, McGavin, Mahler), in contrast, is rarely utilized in clinical practice, particularly when several standard questionnaires enable us to distinguish precisely the intensity of the minimum exercise required to generate the sensation of dyspnea [20]. Alterations of the rib-cage, obesity, etc., also predispose the patient to respiratory complications.

A few simple methods are capable of indicating a functional loss and the difficulty in producing an efficient cough: forced complete expiration time greater than 6 seconds, apnea time less than 30 seconds and problems in blowing out a lighted match 15 cm from the mouth [7]. The stair climbing test is still used as a rough, but efficient and reliable, demonstration of good physical condition for surgery in non-complicated cases [21].

However, in thoracic surgery the habitual clinical examination must be complemented with other tests. A detailed study of respiratory function should be considered above all in patients who present symptoms or signs of acute or chronic pulmonary disease, are smokers or obese, or who are over 60 years old [8]. The more abnormalities found in the functional examination, the greater the percentage of estimated postoperative respiratory insufficiency. It is important to bear in mind that the restriction of the ventilatory function produced by the thoracotomy itself must be added to the initial risk [19].

4.2. Cardiovascular system

The existence of a cardiopathy favors postoperative cardiac complications. The risk in cardiac insufficiency is proportional to the amount of functional limitation; for this reason, the NYHA classification (Table 11.2) is useful. The degree of insufficiency can be taken as an index of myocardial reserve: thus, a patient in

TABLE 11.2
Functional classification of heart disease. Severity of heart failure (New York Heart Association)[7]

Class	Description
I	Patients with cardiac disease but with no limitation of physical activity. Ordinary physical activity causes no undue dyspnea, anginal pain, fatigue or palpitation.
II	Patients with slight limitation of physical activity. They are comfortable at rest and with mild exertion. They experience symptoms only with the more strenuous grades of ordinary activity.
III	Patients with marked limitation of physical activity. They are comfortable at rest, but experience symptoms even with the milder forms of ordinary activity.
IV	Patients with inability to carry on any physical activity without discomfort. Symptoms of cardiac insufficiency or of the anginal syndrome may be present, even at rest, and are intensified by activity.

TABLE 11.3
Goldman and Caldera cardiac risk index

Criteria	Points
(1) History	
(a) Age > 70 yr	5
(b) Myocardial infarction in previous 6 months	10
(2) Physical examination	
(a) S3 gallop or jugular venous distention	11
(b) important valvular aortic stenosis	3
(3) Electrocardiogram	
(a) Rhythm other than sinus or premature atrial contractions on last preoperative ECG	7
(b) more than 5 premature ventricular contractions per minute, documented at any time before operation	7
(4) General status	
$P_aO_2 < 60$ or $P_aCO_2 > 50$ mmHg; K < 3.0 or $HCO_3 < 20$ meq/l; BUN > 50 or Creatinine > 3.0 mg/dl; Abnormal SGOT; Signs of chronic liver disease; Patient bed-ridden from noncardiac causes.	3
(5) Operation	
(a) Intraperitoneal, intrathoracic or aortic operation	3
(b) Emergency operation	4
Total possible score	53

NYHA class 4 will not be able to stand an added demand and, therefore, will not be able to tolerate hypoxia or ischemia[7].

Coronary artery disease, angina at rest, and Prinzmetals angina are among the conditions of highest risk[7]. Patients with a history of prior heart attacks have greater probabilities of cardiac death after surgery. Almost 50% of the individuals who suffer postoperative myocardial infarction die [8]. The location of the previous necroses does not affect the severity of a new attack [11].

Goldman et al. propose a multifactorial index of cardiac risk in non-cardiac surgical operations (Table 11.3), establishing four categories of gravity: Group I, 0–5 points; Group II, 6–12; Group III, 13–25; and Group IV, 26 points or more. They also report a statistically significant increase in the incidence of complications directly proportional to rise in number of points [22].

According to this index, a thoracic operation elevates the risk of cardiac death, though to a lesser extent than a previous myocardial infarction or a congestive heart failure [8].

At any rate, functional deficit is more easily appreciated by a thorough clinical examination, which defines circumstances of the appearance and the intensity of the various symptoms (dyspnea, angina, syncopes, etc.). Without a doubt, the risk grows with the severity of indices [7].

4.2.1. Arterial hypertension

Forty to 50% of individuals over 65 years old suffer from arterial hypertension.

Severe hypertension may represent an unfavorable element per se, while light or moderate hypertension has no influence on the prognosis [23]. The risk thus appears to be more closely related to the visceral effects of a maintained hypertension, although the instability of the blood pressure also favors complications.

4.2.2. Peripheral vascular disease

Peripheral vascular disease is equally important in the evaluation of the patient's physical state. A meticulous physical examination is essential in this definition. The risk factors of arteriosclerosis are arterial hypertension, diabetes, dislipemia, heavy smoking, polycythemia, obesity, alcohol consumption, etc. There are existing clear indicators of generalized illness –chronic ischemia in lower limbs evaluated according to Fontaine–Leriche's clinical states, vascular occlusive disease, ischemic cardiopathy, etc.

The vertebral or carotid artery damage due to arteriosclerotic lesions takes on particular importance because it can lead to severe complications: neurologic sequelae, coma, death.

4.2.3. Thromboembolic disease

Factors which increase the risk of thromboembolic disease can be inherent to the individual or secondary to the type of operation performed. Thus, high-risk patients will require antithrombotic prophylaxis (see Chapter 19, *Prophylaxis and treatment of postoperative thromboembolism*).

4.3. Other systems

4.3.1. Renal impairment

In general, renal impairment elevates surgical risk and morbidity. After a detailed history, edemas, hypertension, nocturia, etc., lead the physician to suspect renal disease alteration, which should be confirmed by preoperative laboratory studies. Obviously, it is essential to study before the operation all of the factors or conditions which can lead to acute renal insufficiency. Chronic renal insufficiency, which modifies the effect of many medications [7], increases the risk even though there may not be a strict relation between morbidity and the decrease in renal function.

4.3.2. Hepatic damage

Different degrees of hepatic damage (acute or chronic) have been shown to be directly related to surgical risk. They are better defined in the case of concomitant portal hypertension, with the clinical manifestations of encephalopathy and ascites. Chronic alcoholism makes the patient sensitive to fluid imbalances and a candidate for delirium tremens in the postoperative stage [7].

With the diagnosis of jaundice, age and sex are sometimes important considerations. However, endocrinometabolic and environmental factors or iatrogenic factors such as the administration of hepatotoxic medication can also cause hepatic disease. Symptomatology, onset of the disease, existence or nonexistence of fever, pain, weight loss or pruritus are all valuable data. An icterus of the skin and mucus membrane, the type and degree of hepatomegaly, the increase in gallbladder size, splenomegaly, etc., all must be assessed [24] by a thorough history and physical examination, together with laboratory tests and complementary studies, including a percutaneous hepatic biopsy if required.

4.3.3. Hiatal hernia and gastroesophageal reflux

The greater incidence of hiatal hernia and gastroesophageal reflux in geriatric patients is also important. Aspiration is associated with diabetic neuropathies or Parkinson's disease and drugs which diminish the tone of the lower esophageal sphincter. A decrease in protective respiratory reflexes facilitates the silent aspiration of gastric contents in the postoperative phase [11].

4.3.4. Endocrinometabolic problems

Among the endocrinometabolic problems, diabetes stands out for its effects and frequent incidence. The deficit in insulin shifts the balance toward the contraregulating hormones with the appearance of hyperglycemia and tendency to ketoacidosis, infections and fluid and electrolyte alterations. Adequate treatment is necessary to forestall serious postoperative complications.

4.4. Nutritional status

Postoperative morbidity and mortality are higher in both obese patients and undernourished patients.

The *obese patients* frequently present signs of hypoventilation, as well as a reduction in vital capacity and tidal volume and an increase in work of breathing [25]. Obesity increases the risk for anesthesia and for surgery. The presence of hypertension, diabetes and arteriosclerosis are common complications of obesity, as are respiratory, infectious, and thromboembolic problems. The obesity can also interfere with the normal action of the liposoluble anesthetic agents [7].

It is essential, therefore, to evaluate the importance of the different comorbid states and to determine whether or not Pickwick's syndrome is present, in which case a loss of weight is necessary to improve the patient's ventilation [7].

Undernourishment has been revealed as a transcendental factor of surgical risk. Weight loss, anemia and protein defect are its most notable elements [7]. Weight loss is not only an expression of the seriousness and development of many diseases, it is an important index of protein–calorie malnutrition [26]. Malnutrition has greater gravity depending on how rapidly it has been established, and has a direct relation to the appearance of complications; among these are a delay in wound healing and a decreased resistance to infections [8].

As a risk factor for infection, malnutrition is of the greatest importance. Other preoperative factors such as neoplasia, prolonged hospitalization, infection or age seem to produce their negative effect by means of the nutritional alteration itself and its associated immune deficit [27].

Infection, in and of itself, can also provoke malnutrition and/or immune deficit [28], although there is no study at the moment which specifies the causal interrelationship. Undernourishment, immune defect, infection can become a truly vicious circle.

Nutritional assessment includes anthropometric, biochemical and immunologic parameters. Mullen's prognostic index (which, in addition to the triceps skinfolds, takes into account the albumin and transferrin count and the response of delayed cutaneous hypersensitivity) appears to be, within certain limits, the best approximation to the quantitative evaluation of nutritional risk. A weight loss above 15%, an albuminemia below 34 g/l and/or an anergia are sound parameters on which to base the initiation of preoperative parenteral nutrition [29].

Undernourishment is accompanied by metabolic and functional abnormalities in the skeletal muscle that favor fatigue [30]. The respiratory muscles decrease in mass [31] and therefore in the force that they are capable of producing. Vital capacity and maximum voluntary ventilation are reduced in direct proportion to the degree of weakness of those muscles [32]; this means a deterioration in the capacity of handling the increased ventilatory loads in thoracopulmonary diseases [33] or in the postoperative period. For all of these reasons, undernourished patients are more prone to presenting respiratory complications [33].

TABLE 11.4
The ASA Physical Status Scale [33]

Class[a]	Description
1	A normally healthy individual.
2	A patient with mild systemic disease.
3	A patient with severe systemic disease that is not incapacitating.
4	A patient with incapacitating systemic disease that is a constant threat to life.
5	A moribund patient who is not expected to survive 24 hours with or without operation.

[a]E is added for a patient in any class with emergency surgery.

5. PHYSICAL CONDITION AND GENERAL RISK IN SURGERY

In 1940, Saklad [34] proposed a classification of surgical patients based on their general status and the severity of their disease. The risk classification of the American Society of Anesthesiologists (ASA) has been and is widely utilized [35], in spite of criticisms voiced at times about the haziness of its definitions and about the fact that a global test of risk only demonstrates that the more seriously ill patients die more often, with or without surgery [8].

According to this scale (Table 11.4), the mortality at six weeks can vary, in extreme cases increasing up to 1400 times [8]. An emergency operation in and of itself causes a doubling of the risk.

Viewed from another perspective, the number of prior medical problems is likewise correlated to operative risk. Specifically, the patients with renal illnesses, diabetes or a history of heart attacks present the highest rates of mortality [36].

In studying the prognostic factors of surgical mortality, Goldman et al. [22] point out that the evaluation of physical condition is the best predictor of non-cardiac death and a clear predictor of cardiac death, although the cardiopathy itself is a more important indicator of risk of cardiac death than the physical state.

In a study from the Massachusetts General Hospital, the frequency of complications which put the individual's life in danger varies from 0.7% in Group I up to 22% in Group IV, while deaths from cardiac causes vary for the same groups from 0.2% to 56% [37]. Based on these results, if the patient presents unstable angina or electrocardiographic alterations which suggest an acute myocardial infarction, all non-urgent operations should be postponed until the cardiac situation stabilizes, while the patients in Group IV (with an index of 26 points or more) should only be operated on in extreme life-or-death circumstances [22].

The ASA physical status classification has been correlated with various hemodynamic data (for example, pulmonary capillary pressure, pulmonary vascular resistance and saturation of mixed venous blood) [38], demonstrating how the latter worsen as the index of risk rises.

It is necessary to focus the greatest attention on the respiratory and the cardiovascular systems [39]. It is beneficial to remember that, independently of the basic disease, a high percentage of the patients over 70 years old present arterial hypertension, renal dysfunction, pulmonary disturbances and/or cardiovascular diseases, too [11].

Prior impairment in vital organ function, the nature and duration of the basic disease, any associated illnesses, age and nutritional condition constitute essential risk factors. Moreover, other factors such as type of anesthesia and operation, a possible emergency situation, the experience of the surgical team and the resources of the hospital itself must not be forgotten [8]. The patient's health status and the type of surgery seem to be more important in predicting short-term mortality than the anesthetic factors [36].

All in all, however, no computerized index can take the place of clinical judgment for a specific patient [11]. As Pettigrew and Hill [40] point out, a meticulous medical study, giving special emphasis to the cardiorespiratory history, the pre-existing sepsis and the nutritional condition, is just as efficient as any other risk indicator commonly used. A weight loss is in itself a basic indicator of severity, given its association with impairment of organic function [15].

The challenge is to identify the problems in time, as well as to prevent and treat postoperative complications, in those patients who suffer from chronic illnesses or who have limited physiological reserves [8]. Furthermore, this identification process gives rise to the frequent necessity for precise nutritional, hemodynamic and functional evaluations, which facilitate the improvement of the patient's physical condition before he or she is submitted to the stress of the anesthesia and of the operation [41].

6. PHYSICAL CONDITION AND PREPARATION FOR THE THORACOTOMY

Although the operation itself is the central act in the surgical therapy, preoperative preparation greatly influences the final result. Preoperative attention, in effect, not only permits a detailed study of the disease affecting the patient's physical state and of the associated medical problems, it also facilitates an adequate control of these defects.

The preoperative period has a triple objective, an opportunity for psychological, functional and therapeutic preparation of major importance for the best surgical result [42].

The initial study should reveal any alteration that requires treatment before the definitive surgery [43]. Only re-establishing the vital organs to a normal functioning for the patient's chronological age can produce optimal conditions for the anesthesia, the planned surgical intervention and the postoperative period [43]. Nevertheless, in urgent cases it may be necessary to limit or even eliminate some preoperative measures.

The respiratory and nutritional preparation is basic in improving the patient's condition [42], apart from, of course, the necessity of specific treatment designed to restore the balance of the primary cardiovascular, digestive and renal function, and to attempt weight loss in the obese when it is required [42].

Respiratory preparation can considerably reduce morbidity and mortality in high-risk patients. These patients must first be identified, so that they can be trained in specific exercises which will be of utmost utility in the postoperative period [8]. Additionally, humidifying the air, the administration of expectorants, bronchodilators and/or selective antibiotics, and the elimination of tobacco use (for at least the last few days before surgery, given its noxious effect on bronchial defense mechanisms) are all measures aimed at improving the patient's physical condition [8,40], to prevent postoperative complications such as atelectasis, pneumonia, and respiratory insufficiencies [43,44].

Ventilatory education and directed ventilation (knowing that its amplitude may be limited by pains, fatigue and the observed volumetric possibilities), diaphragmatic re-education, exercises to facilitate expectoration, corrective exercises to limit or prevent postoperative atelectasis, have all been shown to be fundamental [45].

Measures directed toward alleviating dyspnea and increasing tolerance to exercise can provide clear physiological benefits in patients with COPD after only relatively short periods of 3 to 4 weeks [46]. Such benefits must be viewed in relation to the improvement in strength and endurance of the respiratory musculature [47]. Specific exercises for the upper limbs seem to be especially helpful [48], taking into account that many patients with COPD suffer dyspnea in the course of daily life in activities which require the use of these members [46].

Emphasis on training of the ventilatory muscles improves both their strength and endurance, as well as the parameters of physical activity [49], increasing the tolerance to exertion in COPD patients. This improvement in muscular performance leads to the shifting of the fatigue threshold and perhaps to the avoidance of the need for instrumental ventilation [50].

Well-nourished patients tolerate more easily a surgical intervention than those with a deficient nutritional state [43]. In malnourished cases, the risk is fundamentally metabolic and infectious, though the undernourishment also reduces the strength of the respiratory muscles, which is frequently already diminished by mechanical alterations of the rib cage due to hyperventilation [51].

In severe cases of malnutrition, enteral or parental hyperalimentation reestablishes equilibrium and transforms the patient's physical state. At the same time, the fluid and electrolyte replacement and the restoration of the acid-base balance, when necessary, are indispensable [43].

7. CONCLUSIONS

A meticulous history and a thorough clinical examination continue to be the cornerstone of preoperative evaluation. Such evaluation, which must be adapted to the needs of each patient, should attempt three goals: (1) to assess not only the effect of the illness which indicates the need for operation, but also the theoretical consequences of the planned surgical procedure itself; (2) to recognize any associated disease, as well as the general characteristics of the patient's personality; and (3) to serve as a base, initially, and a confirmation, afterward, that the best possible preparation for the surgery has been achieved [21].

In this way, the surgeon should never consider the performance of an elective operation in conditions that are not ideal, because the preoperative appraisal ought to be accompanied by an adequate preparation for the surgery proposed.

Nevertheless, fixed rules cannot be applied in emergency cases, although there is frequently time even in these circumstances for several studies, which can be of great help in the general therapeutic planning [53]. In that evaluation, the general aspect, the mental state and the conduct of the patient should be carefully observed [54]. The fact is that the individual's general state, which undoubtedly correlates with the final result of the surgery, obviously depends on many factors. Every favorable element assures good operative conditions, while each alteration increases the risks [45]. Taking everything into consideration, the patient's physical condition represents a good indicator of the prognosis after surgery, reaffirming the importance that indexes of this type, synthesis of multiple biological functions have major roles in decisions whether to perform the treatment for a specific patient.

We must emphasize once more the necessity of optimizing cardiovascular function before surgery, and the need to treat whatever hepatic, renal, or endocrinological alteration, etc., which might have negative repercussions on the individual's state. This is basic in the preparation for thoracotomy, as is a rigorous attention to hygiene, including the appropriate buccodental care.

The elimination of all tobacco consumption, as well as that of alcohol, should be considered, explaining to the patient that the complications and risks involved in the surgery increase if he or she does not accept renouncing these habits [42].

Without a doubt, a judicious medical and kinesitherapeutic preparation permits the sick individual to face the operation in optimal condition [52].

REFERENCES

1 Pera C. La respuesta biológica a la agresion accidental y quirúrgica. Cirugía: Fundamentos, indicaciones y opciones técnicas. Barcelona, Salvat Edit. 1983; Vol I, ch 3: pp 55–62.

2 Balibrea JL. Respuesta metabólica a la intervención quirurgica. In: Balibrea JL (ed.). Tratado de Cirugía. Barcelona, Edic. Toray 1988; Vol 1, ch 4: pp 74–84.

3 Drucker WR, Gann DS, McCoy S. Respuesta a la cirugía: alteraciones neuroendocrinas y metabólicas, convalecencia y rehabilitación. In: Hardy JD (ed.). Cirugía. Buenos Aires, Edit. Méd. Panamericana 1985; ch 1: pp 17–41.

4 Abraham E. Mecanismos inmunitarios que explican la sepsis en el paciente quirúrgico en estado crítico. Clín Quir Norte Am 1985; 4: 1019–1032.

5 Caspersen CJ, Powell KE, Christenson GM. Physical activity, exercise, and physical fitness: Definitions and distinctions for health-related research. Public Health Rep 1985; 100: 126–131.

6 Hopkins WG, Walker NP. The meaning of "physical fitness". Prev Med 1988; 17: 764–773.

7 Francois G, Faizende J. Examen pré-opératoire, prémédication et évaluation du risque opératoire. Encycl Méd Chir (Paris), Anesthésie-Réanimation 6–1978; 36375 A05.

8 Feigal DW, Blaisdell FW. The estimation of surgical risk. Med Clin North Am 1979; 63: 1131–1143.

9 Clowes Jr GHA. Cirugía de pulmón, esófago y mediastino. In: Randall HT, Hardy JD, Moore FD (eds.). Tratamiento Pre y Postoperatorio. México, Edit. Interamericana 1969, ch 21: pp 301–316.
10 Shock NW. Aging of physiological systems. J Chron Dis 1983; 36: 137–142.
11 Gilsanz Rodriguez F. El riesgo quirúrgico en el paciente geriátrico. Med Geriat 1989; 2: 102–108.
12 Janis KM. Risk of anesthesia in the geriatric patient. Semin Anesth 1986; 5: 72–80.
13 Rudman D. Nutrition and fitness in elderly people. Am J Clin Nutr 1989; 49: 1090–1098.
14 Cole WH. Medical differences between the young and the aged. J Am Geriat Soc 1970; 18: 589–614.
15 Windsor JA, Hill GL. Weight loss with physiologic impairment. A basic indicator of surgical risk. Ann Surg 1988; 207: 290–296.
16 Wilson PWF, Paffenbarger Jr RS, Morris JN, Havlik RJ. Assessment methods for physical activity and physical fitness in population studies: Report of a NHLBI workshop. Am Heart J 1986; 111: 1177–1192.
17 Powell KE, Caspersen CJ, Koplan JP, Ford ES. Physical activity and chronic diseases. Am J Clin Nutr 1989; 49: 999–1006.
18 Orr ST, Aisner J. Performance status assessment among oncology patients: a review. Cancer Treat Rep 1986; 70: 1423–1429.
19 Coret Coret A. Valoración del riesgo respiratorio. Valoración médica del riesgo quirúrgico. Barcelona, Edit. Jims 1987; ch 3: pp 37–58.
20 Labrune S, Huchon G. Mécanismes et diagnostice des dyspnées. Encycl Med Chir (Paris) 2–1989; Poumon, 6000 C60. 5pp.
21 Gothard JWW, Branthwaite MA. Preoperative considerations. Anesthesia for thoracic surgery. Oxford, Blackwell Scientific Publications 1982, ch 2: pp 8–27.
22 Goldman L, Caldera DL, Nussbaum SR, et al. Multifactorial index of cardiac risk in noncardiac surgical procedures. N Engl J Med 1977; 297: 845–850.
23 Goldman L, Caldera DL. Risk of general anesthesia and elective operation in the hypertensive patient. Anesthesiology 1979; 50: 285–292.
24 Coret Coret A. Valoración del riesgo quirúrgico en las afecciones digestivas, hepatopatías fundamentalmente. Valoración Médica del Riesgo Quirúrgico. Barcelona, Edit. Jims 1987; ch 6: pp 89–115.
25 Wolfe BM, Phillips GJ, Hodges RE. Evaluation and management of nutritional status before surgery. Med Clin North Am 1979; 63: 1257–1269.
26 Morgan DB, Hill GL, Burkinshaw L. The assessment of weight loss from a single measurement of body weight: the problens and limitations. Am J Clin Nutr 1980; 33: 2101–2105.
27 Celaya Perez S, Navarro M, Salinas JC, Salvo L, Pastor C, Sainz M, Lozano R. Factores de riesgo infeccioso en cirugía mayor. Influencia de la desnutrición y de la anergia. Rev Quir Esp 1985; 12: 272–277.
28 Korinek AM. Effets de l'anesthésie et de la chirurgie sur le système immunitaire. Encycl Méd Chir (Paris), Anesthésie–Réanimation 4–1986; 36840 G30. 8pp.
29 Sitges-Serra A, Jaurrieta E. Nutrición del paciente quirúrgico. In: Balibrea JL (ed.). Tratado de Cirugía. Barcelona, Edic. Toray 1988; Vol I, ch 14: pp 251–270.
30 Church JM, Choong SY, Hill GL. Abnormalities of muscle metabolism and histology in malnourished patients awaiting surgery: effects of a course of intravenous nutrition. Br J Surg 1984; 71: 563–569.
31 Arora NS, Rochester DF. Effect of body weight and muscularity on human diaphragm, muscle mass, thickness, and area. J Appl Physiol: Respir Environ Exercise Physiol 1982; 52: 64–70.
32 Wilson DO, Rogers RM, Hoffman RM. Nutrition and chronic lung disease. Am Rev Respir Dis 1985; 132: 1347–1365.
33 Arora NS, Rochester DF. Respiratory muscle strength and maximal voluntary ventilation in undernourished patients. Am Rev Respir Dis 1982; 126: 5–8.
34 Saklad M. Grading of patients for surgical procedures. Anesthesiology 1941; 2: 281–284.
35 Owens WD, Felts JA, Spitznagel Jr EL. ASA physical status classifications: A study of consistency of ratings. Anesthesiology 1978; 49: 239–243.

36 Cohen MM, Duncan PG, Tate RB. Does anesthesia contribute to operative mortality? JAMA 1988; 260: 2859–2863.

37 Bryant LR, Morgan Jr CV. Pared torácica, pleura, pulmón y mediastino. In: Schwartz SI, Shires GT, Spencer FC, Storer EH (eds.). Principios de Cirugía, 3rd Ed. México, McGraw Hill 1987; Vol I, ch 17: pp 601–727.

38 Keating III HJ. Preoperative considerations in the geriatric patient. Med Clin North Am 1987; 71: 569–583.

39 Lewin I, Lerner AG, Green SH, Del Guercio LRH, Siegel JH. Physical class and physiologic status in prediction of operative mortality in the aged sick. Ann Surg 1971; 174: 217–231.

40 Pettigrew RA, Hill GL. Indicators of surgical risk and clinical judgement. Br J Surg 1986; 73: 47–51.

41 Savino JA, Del Guercio LRM. Valoración preoperatoria del individuo con alto riesgo quirúrgico. Clín Quir Norte Am 1985; 4: 779–809.

42 Eschapasse H. L'opéré thoracique. Paris, Masson 1982.

43 Rhoads JE. Preparación preoperatoria del paciente. In: Hardy JD (ed.). Cirugía. Buenos Aires, Edit. Méd. Panamericana 1985; ch 15: pp 344–354.

44 Gaskell DV, Webber BA. Fisioterapia respiratoria. Pamplona, Eunsa 1979.

45 Diziain AM, Plas-Bourey M. Rééducation respiratoire. Bases pratiques et applications thérapeutiques. Paris, Masson 1978.

46 Coll Artes R, Izquierdo Ramirez J. Rehabilitación pulmonar. Arch Bronconeumol 1989; 25: 224–232.

47 Rochester DF, Goldberg SK. Techniques of respiratory physical therapy. Am Rev Respir Dis 1980; 120(Part 2): 133–146.

48 Ries AL, Ellis B, Hawkins RW. Upper extremity exercise training in chronic obstructive pulmonary disease. Chest 1988; 93: 688–692.

49 Belman MJ, Mittman Ch, Weir R. Ventilatory muscle training improves exercise capacity in chronic obstructive pulmonary disease patients. Am Rev Respir Dis 1980; 121: 273–280.

50 Sergysels R. Réadaptation fonctionnelle respiratoire. Encycl Méd Chir (Paris) 7–1985; Poumon, 6000 S10. 8pp.

51 Rochester DF. Body weight and respiratory muscle function in chronic obstructive pulmonary disease. Am Rev Respir Dis 1986; 134: 646–648.

52 Fogliani J, Pons R, Ohresser Ph, Chauvin G, Nicoli M. Anesthésie–réanimation en chirurgie médiastino-broncho-pulmonaire. Encycl Méd Chir (Paris), Anesthésie–Réanimation 9–1977, Fasc 36570, A10.

53 Ballinger II WF. Valoración preoperatoria del paciente quirúrgico. In: Randall HT, Hardy JD, Moore FD (eds.). Tratamiento Pre y Postoperatorio. México, Edit. Interamericana 1969; ch 2: pp 6–14.

54 Johnson J, Kirby ChK. Consideraciones preliminares. Cirugía Torácica, 3rd Ed. México, Edit. Interamericana 1969; ch 1: pp 15–58.

Part IV

Intra- and postoperative management

Current Topics in General Thoracic Surgery: An International Series, Vol. 2
Perioperative Care, edited by R.M. Peters and J. Toledo

Chapter 12

Intraoperative and postoperative fluids

Richard M. Peters

1. INTRODUCTION

To manage intraoperative and postoperative fluids, the physician must have knowledge of the types of fluids available and the basic physiology of fluid distribution and exchange. This knowledge must be applied to the facts about the patient's preoperative cardiopulmonary status and renal function, and the type of operation proposed.

2. TYPES OF FLUIDS

There are five classes of fluids:

(1) Colloids suspended in electrolyte solution with the approximate concentrations and osmolality of extracellular fluid [1].

(2) Electrolyte solutions with electrolyte composition and concentrations that approximate extracellular fluid but with lactate or acetate substituted for bicarbonate (Ringer's lactate solution) or solutions of sodium chloride with osmolality of extracellular fluid [2].

(3) Hypertonic electrolyte solutions – solutions with concentrations of electrolytes of 2 to 3 times the concentration of those in iso-osmolar electrolyte solutions [3,4].

(4) Electrolyte-free glucose solutions in which serum osmolality approximates that of body fluids (5% glucose). When glucose is metabolized, these solutions provide electrolyte-free water.

(5) Red cells. At this time the use of whole blood is rarely justified and components are more appropriate. Red cells are used to treat anemia due to acute loss of blood. If whole blood is used, it provides an amount of plasma equivalent to one-half the volume.

The electrolyte fluids 1–3 are indicated to restore vascular volume resulting from blood loss and any chest drainage or gastrointestinal loss.

3. BLOOD REPLACEMENT

The quantity of fluid required to replace blood loss depends on the type of fluid used. The fluid equivalencies have been derived from numerous animal and clinical studies of hypovolemic shock due to blood loss [1–4].

(1) Colloid: 2 times the amount of blood loss.

(2) Iso-osmolar electrolyte: 3 times the blood loss immediately and over the next 8 hours one more equivalent.

(3) Hypertonic salt: 2 times the blood loss or milliequivalents of sodium equivalent to that with iso-osmolar electrolyte solutions.

(4) 5% glucose solutions do not replace volume deficits due to blood loss. If given for this purpose, they are distributed between intra- and extracellular fluid and lead to hyponatremia and hypo-osmolar state. Five percent glucose solutions are only indicated to replace water loss from respiration and evaporation from skin and open wounds and to provide glucose.

4. PREOPERATIVE PREPARATION

The principles of fluid replacement can best be presented by discussing the management of a patient undergoing pulmonary resection. If the patient has coronary artery disease or other cause for compromise of left ventricular function, insertion of a Swan–Ganz catheter may be indicated to monitor cardiac output and left heart filling pressures. For this discussion I shall assume the state of the patient's cardiopulmonary status is adequate for the type of resection proposed. An often neglected aspect of preoperative preparation is to assure that the patient is not dehydrated at the time anesthesia is induced. The routine preoperative order – nothing by mouth after midnight – usually means nothing by mouth after 8:00 to 9:00 pm, or 20:00 to 21:00 hours. A patient second or third on the operating schedule may thus be denied fluids for 16 to 20 hours. The resultant dehydration may result in hypotension during induction and, if the patient has chronic obstructive airways disease, thickening of the tracheobronchial secretions which will lead to retention of secretions in the postoperative period.

These problems can be avoided by administering a liter of 5% glucose in water at the rate of 100 ml/h starting at 06:00 h the day of operation. This assures that secretions remain thin and the patient is volume replete. The plain water will not hyperexpand the vascular space because it is distributed throughout the entire body fluids, both intra- and extracellular.

If we can assume that patients reach the operating room in normovolemic state, then they can support their circulation during induction and fast infusions of electrolyte to maintain blood pressure are *not* indicated. Fluids should be given to replace losses, not to meet a given filling pressure or blood pressure. The risks of excessive fluids are not uniform but vary with patient, disease and type of operation. If blood pressure falls due to the effects of the drugs used for induction of anesthesia, the more appropriate response is elevation of the legs and dispatch in positioning the patient and initiating surgery to provide the stimulus to reverse the vasodilatory effect of the anesthetic drugs. The practice in the USA of assuming the drop in blood pressure during induction of anesthesia is due to hypovolemia is dangerous. It leads to infusion of excessive amounts of fluid and the risk of postoperative pulmonary congestion and edema.

5. POST LUNG RESECTION PULMONARY CONGESTION AND EDEMA

There is a high risk of post-operative pulmonary congestion and edema if fluid infusion is imprecise during pulmonary resection.

Extra care in perioperative intravenous fluid therapy is needed for patients undergoing pulmonary resection because they are particularly sensitive to both inadequate and excess fluid infusion. Often patients are receiving one lung anesthesia, resulting in an intrapulmonary shunt. If hypovolemia leads to low cardiac output, increased oxygen extraction from blood will decrease mixed venous saturation and the amount of oxygen in the shunted blood which will mix with the saturated blood from the ventilated lung. The admixture of venous blood with a lowered oxygen content with oxygenated blood from ventilated alveoli will drop arterial oxygen saturation and content. Oxygen delivery to tissues is the product of arterial oxygen content and cardiac output. A low cardiac output in a patient with a shunt results in lowering of both factors that control oxygen delivery. The low venous oxygen content associated with low cardiac output combined with an intrapulmonary shunt can result in a critical decrease in the oxygen delivery. These physiologic effects of hypovolemia make it imperative to avoid inadequate volume replacement, but does not warrant excessive fluid infusion.

There is a general misconception about the safety of excessive fluids in comparison to the risks of inadequate fluids. This particular misconception is complicated by the confusion between good and better therapy. It is a sound medical axiom that better is the worst enemy of good and that "more is better" is the trigger that initiates "better therapy". All treatment, and particularly drugs, have toxicity which is altered by the sensitivity of the patient to the drug given. Intravenous fluids are drugs which, when given in inadequate dosage, result in inadequate cardiac output and oxygen delivery and, when given in excessive quantities, manifest their toxicity particularly on the heart and the lungs.

The purpose of fluid infusions to replace lost blood is to maintain an adequate filling pressure for stretching of the myocardial fiber to its optimum length which will result in a cardiac index adequate to support recovery from hemorrhage and operative or traumatic injury. There is no fixed value for the cardiac filling pressures – central venous, pulmonary wedge or left atrial pressure – needed to adequately and not excessively stretch the myofibril. Pressure transducers used for cardiac filling pressures measure the difference between vascular pressure and atmospheric pressure. The stretching force on the myocardial fiber is the difference between end diastolic ventricular pressure and pleural pressure. The same measured end diastolic pressure will result in a smaller transventricular pressure if the pleural pressure is elevated. A spontaneously breathing patient has subatmospheric pleural pressure, while a patient on a ventilator has positive pleural pressure during inspiration. Therefore, a patient on a ventilator has a lower cardiac filling pressure for a given measured wedge pressure. During spontaneous breathing a patient with stiff lungs, less compliant lungs, must create a more subatmospheric pleural pressure to inflate the lungs. In a patient following pneumonectomy where lung compliance is cut in half or a patient with pulmonary edema where compliance may be as low as 20% of normal – the ventricular filling pressure may be much greater than the measured end diastolic pressure.

Other factors that control the level of pressure needed to stretch the myofibril are the stiffness of the heart and its ionotropic state. Since we rarely measure pleural pressure and do not measure cardiac compliance, there is no absolute value for the pulmonary wedge or the central venous pressure that will provide appropriate stretch of the myofibril. This uncertainty is complicated by the fact that the ionotropic state of the heart alters the effect of myofibril length on contractile force and heart rate. Stress and pain increase release of catecholamines and increase contractility of the myocardium, shifting the Starling curve to the left, making a lower filling pressure produce an adequate cardiac output. The heart responds to an increase in filling pressure by increasing its rate and stroke volume, which will result in an elevated cardiac output.

All clinicians are aware that an inadequate filling pressure risks all the well known effects of low cardiac output. The risks of an elevated filling pressure and the resultant increase in cardiac output on the filtration of fluid from the capillaries to the interstitial spaces are not as well recognized. The lung is the organ most vulnerable to excessive fluid filtration. This vulnerability is amplified by pulmonary resection.

When flow rate increases through a given vascular bed, the force to push blood through the capillaries must rise, so the effective capillary hydrostatic pressure rises. Because the lungs must accommodate the entire cardiac output after pulmonary resection, the flow rate through and hydrostatic pressure in the remaining lung capillaries must be elevated. Filtration of fluid depends on the difference between the net hydrostatic transcapillary pressure (the difference between pulmonary hydrostatic capillary pressure and pulmonary interstitial hydrostatic pressure), and net colloidal osmotic pressure (the difference between serum colloidal osmotic pressure and interstitial colloidal osmotic pressure) (Fig. 12.1).

The direct effect of increase in pulmonary capillary pressure on the rate of fluid filtration is well recognized. The effect of hemodilution and increased capillary pressure on transcapillary colloidal osmotic pressure (COP) and the compensating factors controlling accumulation of fluid in the lungs when filtration rises are equally critical. The lung has a high extravascular protein content. When a rise in capillary pressure or fall in serum COP causes increased filtration, the extravascular proteins are diluted, resulting in fall in interstitial COP which results in an increase

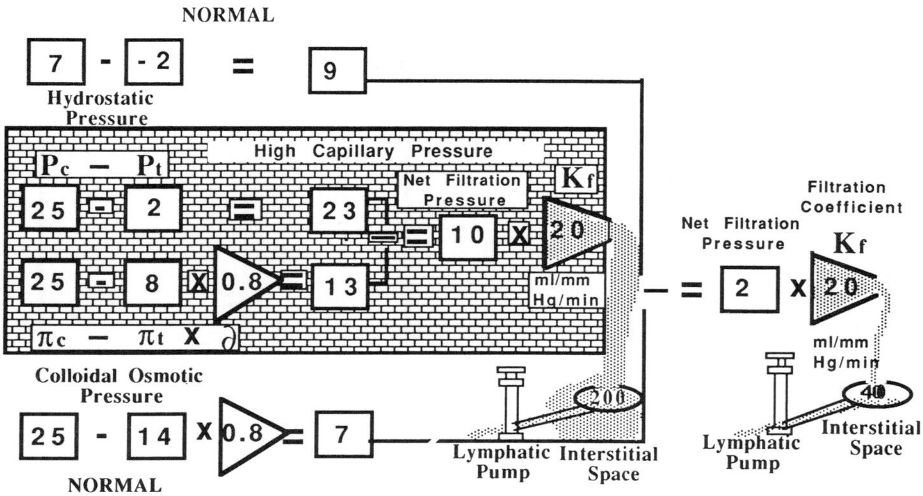

FIGURE 12.1. The normal (unshaded on the top, bottom and left borders of the figure) forces controlling fluid filtration in the lungs. On top, the hydrostatic capillary (P_c) and interstitial (P_t) pressures. The difference between these pressures is the hydrostatic pressure forcing fluid out of the capillaries. On the bottom, the capillary (Π_c) and interstitial (Π_t) colloidal osmotic pressures. The effect of colloidal osmotic pressure is discounted by the filtration fraction (∂), a measure of the protein leak through the capillaries. This fraction is multiplied by the difference between Π_c and Π_t to give the net force of the colloids retaining fluid in the capillaries. The difference between the hydrostatic and the net colloidal osmotic pressures is the net filtration pressure. The pressure multiplied by the filtration coefficient (K_f) gives the amount of fluid filtered per minute. The fluid is filtered into the interstitium of the lung and removed by the lymphatics and probably also by flowing along the perivascular peribronchial space to the mediastinum.

The effects of high capillary pressure are shown in the central portion of the diagram. P_c is raised to 25 mmHg and increase in fluid filtration raises P_t to 2 for a net hydrostatic force of 23 mmHg. Π_t is reduced by increase in filtered protein free water following the rise in P_c. This fall in Π_t partially compensates for the rise in P_c. However, the marked rise in net filtration force overcomes the compensatory effects and the interstitial space is filled and overflows into the alveoli.

in net colloidal osmotic pressure to partially compensate for the rise in pulmonary capillary hydrostatic pressure or fall in serum COP[6,7] (Figs. 12.1, 12.2). At the same time the rate at which the lymphatics (the lymphatic pump [LP]) remove fluid increases. The two compensating factors, fall in extravascular COP and increased lymph removal of filtered fluid, have been calculated by Taylor et al.[5] to be a safety factor preventing pulmonary edema equivalent to 20 mmHg.

Concentration on the role of pressure in controlling capillary fluid filtration has resulted in neglect of two other factors: capillary permeability and capillary surface area[6,7]. The amount of fluid filtered by any given net filtration force (the difference between net hydrostatic and oncotic pressure) is amplified by rises in the permeability of the capillaries and an increase in the capillary surface area.

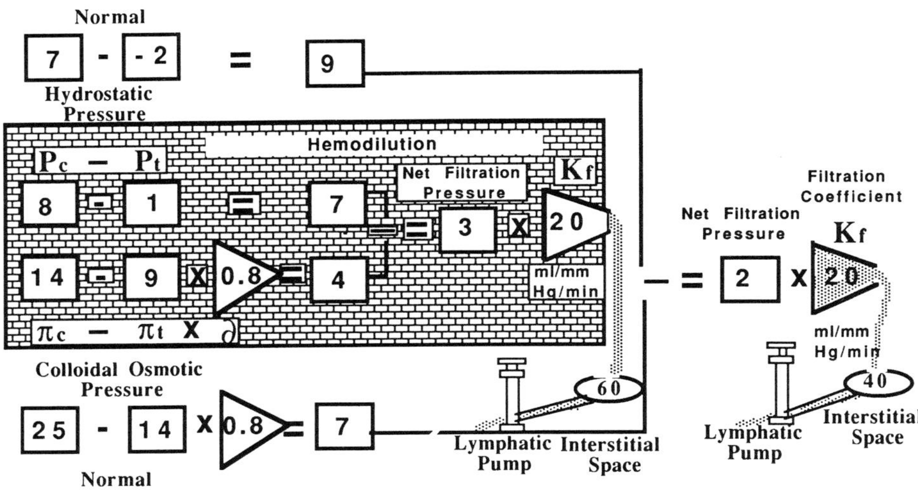

FIGURE 12.2. Normal values as in Fig. 12.1. In the shaded portion in the center Π_c has fallen to 14 and there has been a compensatory fall in Π_t to 9. This diagram shows a modest increase in P_c as a result of infusion of a little too much fluid. The result is an only modest rise in net filtration pressure to 3, and the lymphatic pump is able to keep up with the increase in filtration so that only a modest increase in interstitial fluid in the lung occurs.

Staub[8] has recently emphasized the importance of the lung capillary surface area (Fig. 12.3). The fraction of lung capillaries open and filtering fluid is directly proportional to the cardiac output and inversely proportional to the number of capillaries. For example, following a right pneumonectomy if resting cardiac output is doubled, blood flow through the remaining lung is 4.4 times the preresection resting level, greatly increasing the portion of capillaries open. The increase in capillary surface area for filtration increases the rate of fluid filtration. Right lung resection removes 55% of the capillary bed and 55% of the capacity of the lymphatic pump (if there has been an associated removal of mediastinal lymphatics, a significantly greater decrease in lymph pump capacity may result). The combined factors: (1) increased fraction of open capillary bed; (2) increased capillary pressure due to increased flow; and (3) decreased lymph pump capacity, that result from excessive fluid administration during or after pulmonary resection, can overwhelm the lung safety factors (Fig. 12.4) and lead to pulmonary congestion and edema.

If in addition multiple transfusions, multiple associated injuries, overexpansion of the lungs or sepsis cause capillary injury, the capillary permeability increases and the amount of fluid filtered per mmHg, net filtration force, and per area of lung open, will markedly increase (Fig. 12.4).

Because patients lose compensatory systems which limit lung congestion following lung resection, they need precise replacement of fluids. The greater the amount of lung resected, the more risk of pulmonary edema. The risk with resection

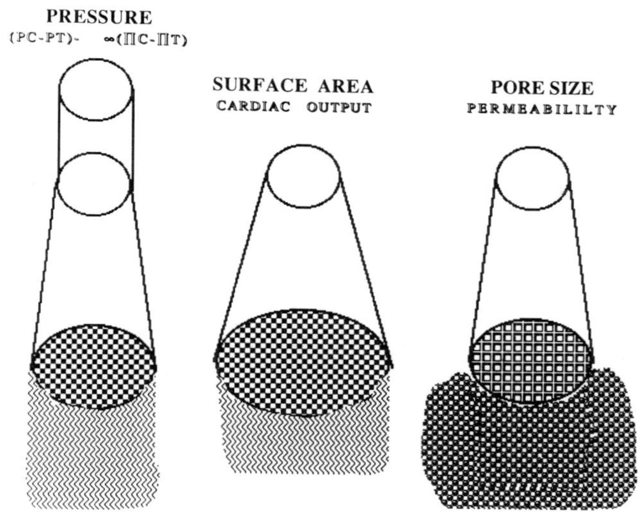

FIGURE 12.3. Comparative effects of rise in capillary pressure, and increase in capillary surface area opened for filtering (capillary surface area open in the lung varies directly as the blood flow [the cardiac output] through a given portion of lung). The third important factor is the size of the pores. As shown in Fig. 12.2, colloidal osmotic pressure has lesser effect because the maximum difference tolerated does not exceed 15 mmHg, and dilution of the normally high interstitial protein concentrations compensates for more than half of such a rise. Note that increase in cardiac output by increasing the surface area can markedly increase filtration without any rise in hydrostatic filtering pressure.

A high cardiac output can be harmful.

of a lobe is greater than a segment, a lung greater than a lobe, and a right lung greater than a left lung [9,10].

One other important basic fact complicates fluid management in patients undergoing a resection of lobe or lung. Pulmonary artery balloon catheters used to measure wedge pressure are for safety reasons placed no farther in the periphery than a lobar bronchus [11]. The result is that following lung resection, particularly following pneumonectomies, balloon inflation blocks a significant portion of the remaining pulmonary vascular bed. The vascular obstruction increases right ventricular afterload and leads to a fall in right heart output and left heart filling. The result is a falsely low wedge pressure reading. Following lung resection it is important to carefully monitor systemic blood pressure during inflation of pulmonary artery balloon catheter. If systemic blood pressure falls, it is likely that the measured wedge pressure is falsely low. Do not control fluid administration by wedge pressure. If circulation is adequate, a low wedge pressure is protective.

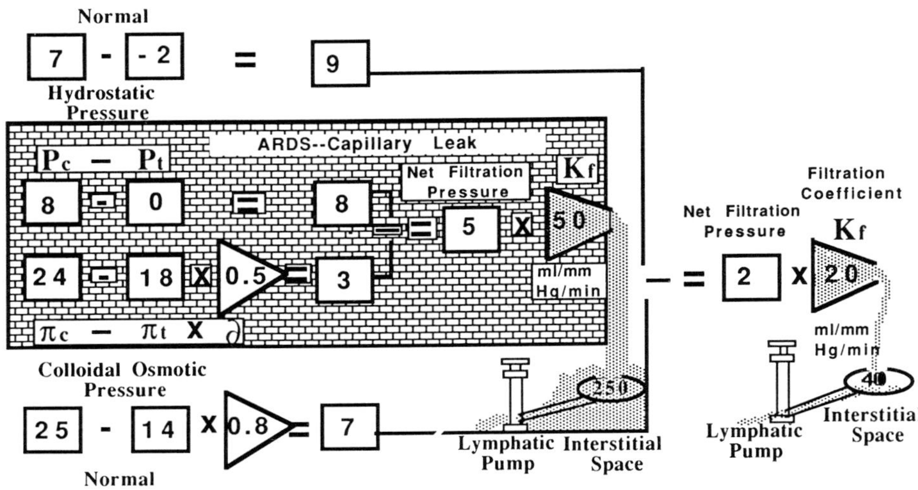

FIGURE 12.4. This figure is similar to Fig. 12.1, normal on the periphery and abnormal in the shaded center. The hydrostatic driving forces are similar to normal. The protein reflectance (∂) falls so protein leaks form the capillary raising interstitial protein content and also the effect of colloidal osmotic pressure has a greater discount from 0.8 to 0.5. The result is a markedly diminished effect of colloidal osmotic pressure in retaining fluid in the capillaries. The net filtration force is elevated. In addition the K_f is increased (ml of water filtered per mmHg/min) and so all the compensatory systems are overwhelmed and pulmonary edema results.

It must be noted that any small rise in P_c in ARDS can cause a marked increase in filtered water.

6. THE PRACTICAL CLINICAL PROBLEM, HYPOVOLEMIA vs. PULMONARY CONGESTION

How can we deal with these complex physiologic conflicting forces when in most instances we have accurate measurement of only a few of the forces controlling filtration? The first and simplest step is to carefully measure blood loss and only infuse the fluids for replacement in direct proportion to losses. It is my practice to use only dry sponges and to weigh the sponges and measure suction drainage to assure accurate estimation of blood loss, which permits precise fluid replacement. At present there is no clear evidence that either colloid, isotonic electrolyte, or hypertonic electrolyte solutions are superior. Non-colloid fluids are 30 to 50 times cheaper, and this is the only significant difference. If colloid or hypertonic saline are used for replacement of blood loss, a volume equal to twice the blood loss is the top limit. With iso-osmolar electrolyte solutions such as Ringer's lactate, the upper limit is 3 times blood loss immediately and slow infusion of another aliquot equal to loss over the next 8 hours. 'Maintenance fluids': non-electrolyte solution (5% glucose in water) should be given at the rate of 50 to 75 cc/h to replace evaporative losses and urine. The maintenance fluid regimen is appropriate for both intra- and postoperative fluid therapy.

Inadequate fluid resuscitation will be manifest by tachycardia, hypotension, low urine output, and low central venous pressure. The acid–base status of the patient is also important to assess. Following significant volume replacement with Ringer's lactate, there will be a moderate 3 to 6 meq base deficit (bicarbonate between 19–22) for a few hours as the excess infused lactate is metabolized to carbon dioxide to form bicarbonate. If tachycardia, acidosis, hypotension, or low cardiac index (C.I.) are present and/or persist, 250 cc aliquots of electrolyte solution or plasma should be administered at 10- to 15-minute intervals to determine the response of central venous pressure (CVP), blood pressure, and heart rate. If there is no response or an inadequate response and no evidence of continued bleeding, then small doses of dopamine starting with 4 μg/kg/min and going up to 10 μg/kg/min are indicated.

Urine output is a useful measure of the volume status of patients but you must factor in the risks of excessive fluids. Patients with cardiac disease decrease urine output during the day and increase it during the night, a reversal of normal diurnal variation. For example, most healthy individuals can sleep 8–10 hours without urinating. At 50 ml/h urine output, they would have 400–500 ml in their bladders, a very full bladder; at 75 ml/h, 600–700 ml. There is no need to be alarmed if urine output falls to 35 ml/h. Fluid infusion is warranted only in the face of vascular instability.

7. PULMONARY EDEMA WARNINGS

We have found that intra- and/or postoperative urine output greater than 50 to 75 ml/h in a patient undergoing lung resection warn of excessive fluid infusion and portend pulmonary edema[9,10]. The important clinical signs of impending pulmonary edema are dyspnea, tachypnea with low tidal volume, and the signs of increased ventilatory effort, retraction and apprehensive facies. The other indicators of impending pulmonary edema are evidence of congestion on chest X-ray and a fall in arterial P_aO_2. These ominous clinical signs may precede other evidence of congestion.

The clinical signs are evidence of increased work of breathing due to fall in lung compliance and must be treated by prompt intubation and ventilatory support together with vigorous diuresis. We also advocate insertion of Swan–Ganz catheter to monitor cardiac output. These patients should be sedated heavily with narcotics to allay apprehension and decrease circulating catecholamines and lower inotropic state.

8. MAINTENANCE FLUIDS

The slang term 'maintenance fluid' has become accepted as an acronym for the amount and kind of fluid needed to replace insensible and renal losses. Gamble [12] during World War II did a beautifully designed simple study on some healthy conscientious objectors to define water needs for fliers downed over the ocean. He found that in fasting normal men the minimum amount of urine to excrete solutes coming from the metabolic processes was 700 ml/24 h if the subjects received 100 g of glucose spread throughout the 24 hours and 1100 to 1200 if no glucose was given. Insensible loss from the lungs and skin is 500 to 700 ml. These studies show that minimal amount of 'maintenance fluids' is 1200 to 1400 ml (50–55 ml/h) if the patient receives 100 g of glucose. The postoperative patient needs some safety factor so we use 75 to 100 ml of 5% dextrose in water per hour. We add 20 meq of KC/L if urine output is adequate. One liter of these fluids can be 5% glucose in 1/4 normal saline to replace any renal sodium losses.

The provision of adequate but not excessive amounts of free water to post-thoracotomy patients is of critical importance, particularly for patients with chronic obstructive lung disease (COLD). If dehydrated, in the postoperative period these patients are more likely to develop thick secretions which cannot be coughed up. A common mistake in postoperative fluid management occurs on the morning of the first or second postoperative day, testing the patient's ability to imbibe enough oral fluid by discontinuing the intravenous infusions. If the patient fails to have an adequate oral intake by the time of evening rounds, they are dehydrated and thick secretions set the stage for atelectasis. It is my practice to provide a liter of 5% glucose in water at the rate of 50–75 cc/h while testing the patient's ability to take oral fluids. If they are able to take adequate oral fluids during the day, intravenous fluids can be discontinued in the evening. If they cannot, dehydration and thick secretions will be avoided.

9. BLOOD REPLACEMENT

I have left red cell replacement until the last because recent knowledge of the risks of transfusion and the safety or perhaps advantages of decreased hematocrit have changed thinking about criteria for blood transfusions. If the surgeon and anesthesiologist have the mind set that transfusion is to be avoided, in most instances this goal is met. Transfusion in association with pulmonary resection should rarely be needed except in patients with many inflammatory adhesions [13]. The indication for red cell infusion is not a given hematocrit but evidence of inadequate oxygen delivery. A young patient with a strong heart that can increase output to compensate for low oxygen-carrying capacity of the blood may tolerate a hematocrit of 20, while a patient with limited cardiac reserve may have 30 as the lower limit. The cardiac surgeons' practice of using hemodilution during perfusion has shown the safety and perhaps advantage of moderate decrease in hematocrit to 25 or 30. The decreased hematocrit lowers blood viscosity so perfusion through stenosed vessels is enhanced. There is also clinical evidence that the incidence of pulmonary embolus has decreased since patients have been carried with hematocrits between 25 and 30 in the postoperative period.

The basic tenet of this method of replacement of blood loss is to separate the correction of volume deficits from red cell deficits [14]. Electrolytes or colloids are used to correct volume deficits and red cells infused only if there is evidence of inadequate red cell mass for oxygen delivery. The major indicator for red cell infusion is lack of rise in cardiac index to compensate for the anemia – decreased oxygen-carrying capacity of the blood. A second indicator is a low venous oxygen. The degrees of rise in cardiac output to compensate for hematocrit drop to 25–30 do not reach levels likely to cause excess lung fluid filtration.

10. SUMMARY

(1) Preoperative fluids: 5% glucose in water at 100 ml/h if the time from cessation of oral intake to induction of anesthesia exceeds 8 to 10 hours.
(2) Intraoperative fluids: Precise measurement of blood loss and replacement with one of the alternatives below.

- (a) colloid solution equal to 2 times blood loss.
- (b) iso-osmolar electrolyte solution equal to 3 times blood loss, and over the first 8 postoperative hours another aliquot equal to blood loss.
- (c) packed red cells to maintain oxygen-carrying capacity at a level consistent with patient's ability to increase cardiac output to compensate for anemia – hematocrit 20 to 30, hemoglobin 7 to 10 μg/100 ml.
- (d) postoperative maintenance fluids of 1500 to 2000 ml of 5% glucose in water with 40 meq of KCl and 500 ml of normal saline until the patient can take an equivalent amount of oral fluids.

REFERENCES

1 Virgilio RW, Rice CL, Smith DE, et al. Crystalloid versus colloid resuscitation: Is one better? A randomized clinical study. Surgery 1979; 85: 129.
2 Virgilio RW, Smith DE, Zarins CK. Balanced electrolyte solutions: Experimental and clinical studies. Crit Care Med 1979; 7: 98.
3 Shackford SR, Fortlage DA, Peters RM, et al. Serum osmolar and electrolyte changes associated with large infusions of hypertonic sodium lactate for intravascular volume expansion of patients underoing aortic reconstruction. Surg Gyne Obst 1987; 164: 127.
4 Shackford SR, Sise MJ, Fridlund PH, et al. Hypertonic sodium lactate versus lactated Ringer's solution for intravenous fluid therapy in operations on the abdominal aorta. Surgery 1983; 94: 41.
5 Taylor AE, Grimbert F, Rutili G, et al. Pulmonary edema: Changes in Starling forces and lymph flow. In: Hargens AR (ed.). Tissue Fluid Pressure and Composition. Baltimore, Williams & Wilkins 1981: p 135.

6 Shires III GT, Peitzman AB, Albert SA, et al. Response of extravascular lung water to intraoperative fluids. Ann Surg 1983; 197: 515.
7 Zarins CK, Rice CL, Peters RM, Virgilio RW. Lymph and pulmonary response to isobaric reduction in plasma oncotic pressure in baboons. Circ Res 1978; 43: 925.
8 Staub NC. New concepts about the pathophysiology of pulmonary edema. J Thorac Imag 1988; 3: 8.
9 Zeldin RA, Normandin D, Landtwing D, Peters RM. Postpneumonectomy pulmonary edema. J Thorac Cardiovasc Surg 1984; 87: 445.
10 Peters RM. Postpneumonectomy pulmonary edema. In: Grillo H, Eschapasse H (eds.). International Trends in General Thoracic Surgery, Vol 2, Major Challenges. Philadelphia, PA, WB Saunders 1986; ch 46: pp 460–464.
11 Wittnich C, Trudel J. Zidulka A, Chiu RC-J. Misleading "pulmonary wedge pressure" after pneumonectomy: Its importance in postoperative fluid therapy. Ann Thorac Surg 1986; 42: 192.
12 Gamble J. Physiological information from studies on the life raft ration. Harvey Lect. 1950; 42: 247.
13 Transfusion Alert. Use of autologous blood. NIH Publication No. 89-3038, September 1989.
14 Martin E, Hansen E, Peter K. Acute limited normovolemic hemodilution: A method for avoiding homologous transfusion. World J Surgery 1987; 11: 53.

Current Topics in General Thoracic Surgery: An International Series, Vol. 2
Perioperative Care, edited by R.M. Peters and J. Toledo

Discussion of "Intraoperative and postoperative fluids" by Richard M. Peters

S.R. Dunn

The administration of fluid is an important aspect of perioperative management of thoracic surgical patients, and Dr. Peters' contribution is unique in bringing together the diverse strands of fluid research. His article reflects greater freedom with crystalloid replacements in thoracic surgery than I am used to. Our unit policy reflects suspicion of large volume clear fluid replacement and greater confidence in the quality of our blood transfusion service. Our practice follows closely that of Twigley and Hillman [1], in a review article entitled 'The End of the Crystalloid Era'. For major thoracic surgery cases I commence with 500 cc of crystalloid (Hartmans solution or 0.9% saline) infused over 10 minutes during monitoring and placement of peripheral lines. We believe that since the patients come to theatre dehydrated and vasodilated from premedication they do not come to detectable harm from this practice. After induction, intubation with a double-lumen tube, placement of subclavian central line on the operated side, a thoracic epidural is inserted. We use a Marcain 0.1% Fentanyl 10 μg/ml solution. There is a possibility of hypotension and hence a fluid load is useful. Until recently the next fluid would have been a further 500 cc of crystalloid run more slowly over approximately 30 minutes, depending on the cardiovascular state. Cook et al. [2] produced an interesting paper in which they showed that different clear fluid infusions, namely Hartmans solution and dextrose 4% saline 0.18%, influenced the recovery of patients from day surgery. So often we are concerned with fluid input, losses and output. They indicated that there is a black box component related to background hormonal changes which may be influenced by different fluid regimes. Since then my second 500 cc has been dextrose 4% saline 0.18%.

Haemacel 500 cc is given next as a temporary colloid plasma expander (if Hb is greater than 12 Gm) to improve tissue perfusion, urine output and contributes to replacement of fluid evaporation at the operation site.

A few years ago Hydroxyethyl Starch (Hespan) was introduced and at this stage 500 cc would have been used to replace the initial blood loss. It also made up the volume of the initial 2 units of packed cells for blood replacement. At this time there was a shortage of blood due to a reduction of donors. We were urged to reduce plasma usage and the majority of blood came in the reduced volume form of packed cells. Around this time, in this Unit, it was noted that a couple of post-thoracotomy patients in the early post-operative period developed slight radiological patchiness suggestive of ARDS. Clinically this did not appear to be detrimental to the progress of recovery but there were similar reports from other thoracic units (personal communication). About this time Lumb [3] published a study using Hydroxyethyl Starch and 25% albumin in cardio-pulmonary pump-prime. He was able to show alterations in extra-vascular lung water (EVLW) with Hespan but not with albumin. He further showed that this change in EVLW with Hespan had returned to normal on the first post-operative day and was not clinically detrimental to the patients. Not every patient in our Unit developed this ARDS-like chest X-ray, but there was sufficient concern among clinicians that Hespan was abandoned. Now only plasma and blood (whole or packed cells) are used to replace operative losses.

Post-operatively 2.5 litres in 24 hours of alternate normal saline and 5% dextrose are given via the subclavian line. Blood loss is replaced through the peripheral cannula which is then capped off. Our intravenous fluid practice does not seem to result in a noticeably higher mortality in thoracic surgery compared with other units.

In the future blood is going to become a scarcer, costlier commodity. Other artificial colloid fluids are going to be developed. Should we be asking the manufacturers to produce studies of the effects on the lung before using them in thoracic surgery?

REFERENCES

1 Twigley AJ, Hillman KM. The end of the Crystalloid era. Anaesthesia 1985; 40: 860–871.
2 Cook R, Anderson S, Riseborough M, Blogg CE. Intravenous fluid load and recovery. Anaesthesia 1990; 45: 826–831.
3 Lumb PD. A comparison between 25% albumin and 6% hydroxyethyl starch solution on lung water accumulation during and immediately after cardio-pulmonary bypass. Annals Surg 1987(August); 206: (2) 210–213.

Current Topics in General Thoracic Surgery: An International Series, Vol. 2
Perioperative Care, edited by R.M. Peters and J. Toledo

Chapter 13

Anesthesia-specific problems for pulmonary resection

Jonathan L. Benumof

GLOSSARY

CPAP	continuous positive airway pressure
FRC	functional residual capacity
F_IO_2	fraction of inspired oxygen
HFJV	high-frequency jet ventilation
HFPPV	high-frequency positive-pressure ventilation
HFOV	high-frequency oscillation ventilation
HFV	high-frequency ventilation
HPV	hypoxic pulmonary vasoconstriction
IPPV	intermittent positive-pressure ventilation
P_aCO_2	arterial partial pressure of carbon dioxide
P_aO_2	arterial partial pressure of oxygen
PEEP	positive end-expiratory pressure
Q_s/Q_t	shunt fraction
V/Q	ventilation perfusion ratio
ZEEP	zero end-expiratory pressure

1. INTRODUCTION

Providing anesthesia for thoracic surgery is a very challenging experience for several reasons. First, the surgery often requires lung separation; this is most commonly done by insertion of a double-lumen tube. Although insertion of a double-lumen tube was a blind haphazard procedure in the past, the advent of fiber-optic bronchoscopy has made it a precise, repeatable, low-risk maneuver. Second, the use of one-lung ventilation to facilitate surgical exposure necessarily creates a large right-to-left shunt through the collapsed operative lung; however, the recent introduction of nondependent lung continuous positive airway pressure (CPAP) into clinical practice has virtually abolished the operative lung shunting. Third, anastomosis of major conducting airways is difficult around large single- or double-lumen tubes. The ability to successfully ventilate and oxygenate patients with high-frequency ventilation now allows a small catheter to pass through the operative field, thereby greatly facilitating anastomosis of airways. Fourth, resection of lung decreases the compliance of the pulmonary vascular bed, which may predispose the patient to pulmonary edema. Consequently, replacement of fluid and blood loss requires extreme care and the need for precise endpoints. Finally, the use of epidural narcotics has greatly aided the treatment of postoperative pain. This chapter discusses the first four of these five anesthesia specific problems for pulmonary resection in the order listed above. The fifth is described in Chapter 17.

2. CORRECT POSITIONING OF THE DOUBLE-LUMEN TUBE

2.1. Introduction

The complete functional separation of the two lungs by a double-lumen tube is often the most important anesthetic consideration for patients undergoing thoracic surgery. The procedure can occasionally be life-saving, and very frequently it greatly facilitates the conduct of surgery. Newly introduced disposable plastic double-lumen tubes, which are relatively non-traumatic and easy to insert, and the advent of fiber-optic bronchoscopy, which makes location of a double-lumen tube under direct vision possible and therefore a precise, repeatable, low-risk maneuver, have greatly increased the efficacy and use of double-lumen tubes. This section sequentially discusses the indications for separation of the two lungs, conventional techniques of double-lumen tube insertion and determination of position, determination of precise double-lumen tube position by fiber-optic bronchoscopy, and finally, use of the fiber-optic bronchoscope to insert a double-lumen tube.

2.2. Indications for double-lumen tube intubation

Double-lumen endotracheal tubes have become the technique of choice for most cases of lung separation and will be discussed here in great detail. Bronchial blockers and endobronchial tubes are not often used today and are only briefly described at the end of the chapter. There are many reasons why double-lumen tubes are favored over bronchial blockers and endobronchial tubes for lung separation. First, double-lumen tubes are relatively easily placed by even inexperienced anesthesiologists, whereas a much higher degree of skill is required to correctly position bronchial blockers and endobronchial tubes correctly. Second, double-lumen tubes allow easy, repeated, and rapid conversion from two-lung ventilation to one-lung ventilation and vice versa at any time during surgery, whereas bronchial blockers and endobronchial tubes preclude two-lung ventilation. Third, double-lumen tubes allow suctioning of both lungs, whereas bronchial blockers and endobronchial tubes preclude suctioning of the collapsed lung. Fourth, double-lumen tubes allow CPAP to be applied to the nonventilated lung

TABLE 13.1
Indications for separation of the two lungs (double- lumen tube intubation) and/or one-lung ventilation

Absolute indications

(1) Isolation of one lung from the other to avoid spillage or contamination
  (a) Infection
  (b) Massive hemorrhage

(2) Control of the distribution of ventilation
  (a) Bronchopleural fistula
  (b) Bronchopleural cutaneous fistula
  (c) Surgical opening of a major conducting airway
  (d) Giant unilateral lung cyst or bulla
  (e) Tracheobronchial tree disruption

(3) Unilateral bronchopulmonary lavage
  (a) Pulmonary alveolar proteinosis

Relative indications

(1) Surgical exposure – high priority
  (a) Thoracic aortic aneurysm
  (b) Pneumonectomy
  (c) Upper lobectomy

(2) Surgical exposure – low priority
  (a) Middle and lower lobectomies and subsegmental resections
  (b) Esophageal resection
  (c) Thoracoscopy
  (d) Procedures on the thoracic spine

(3) Postcardiopulmonary bypass status after removal of totally occluding chronic unilateral pulmonary emboli

(see Next Section) whereas with bronchial blockers and endobronchial tubes no ventilator maneuvers can be used on the lung under operation.

There are several absolute and relative indications for separation of the two lungs during thoracic operations or procedures (Table 13.1).

2.2.1. Absolute indications

Separation of the two lungs for any of the absolute indications discussed here should be considered a life-saving maneuver because failure to separate the two lungs under any of these conditions could result in a life-threatening complication or situation. There are three absolute indications for separating the two lungs (Table 13.1).

First, separation of one lung from the other is absolutely necessary in order to prevent spillage of pus or blood from an infected (abscessed) lung or bleeding lung, respectively, to a non-involved lung. Acute contamination of a lung with either blood or pus from the other lung usually results in severe massive (bilateral) atelectasis, pneumonia, and sepsis.

Second, there are a number of unilateral lung problems that can prevent adequate ventilation of the other non-involved side. A large bronchopleural or bronchopleural cutaneous fistula, or a surgically opened conducting airway, has such a low resistance to gas flow that a tidal inspiration delivered by positive pressure will exit via the low-resistance pathway, and it will become impossible to adequately ventilate the other, more normal, lung adequately. A giant unilateral bulla or cyst may rupture if exposed to positive-pressure ventilation and result in a tension pneumothorax or pneumomediastinum. Third, positive pressure ventilation of a lung with a tracheobronchial tree disruption can result in dissection of gas into the pulmonary interstitial space or mediastinum, resulting in a tension pneumomediastinum.

Fourth, separation of the two lungs is absolutely necessary in order to perform unilateral bronchopulmonary lavage in patients with pulmonary alveolar proteinosis (and rarely, asthma and cystic fibrosis).

2.2.2. Relative indications

There are a large number of relative indications for separation of the two lungs, and they are all for the purpose of facilitating surgical exposure by collapsing the lung in the operative hemithorax. These relative indications can be divided up into high-priority and low-priority categories (Table 13.1).

Of the relative indications, repair of a thoracic aortic aneurysm is usually the highest priority because it requires exposure of the thoracic aorta as it runs the entire length of the left hemithorax. A pneumonectomy, especially if performed through a median sternotomy [1], is greatly aided by the wide exposure of the lung hilum that is afforded by collapse of the operative lung. Similarly, an upper lobectomy, which is technically the most difficult lobectomy, and many mediastinal exposures, may be made much easier by eliminating ventilation to the lung on the side of the procedure.

The surgical items in the low-priority category do not routinely require collapse of the lung on the operative side but still significantly aid surgical exposure and eliminate the need for the surgeon to handle (retract, compress, pack away) the operative lung. Severe intraoperative retraction of the lung on the operated side can traumatize the operative lung and impair gas exchange both intra- and postoperatively [2,3]. The lower priority items consist of middle and lower lobectomies, less extensive pulmonary resections, thoracic spinal procedures that are approached anteriorly through the chest, and esophageal surgery. However, even relatively small operations such as wedge and segmental resections benefit by double-lumen tube insertion because of the ability to alternate easily and quickly between lung collapse and inflation, which is sometimes required to better visualize lung morphology and to facilitate identification and separation of important planes and fissures. Examination of the pleural space (thoracoscopy) is considerably aided by collapse of the ipsilateral lung.

Finally, the separation of the lungs following removal of totally occluding and predominantly unilateral chronic pulmonary emboli (post-cardiopulmonary bypass) can be very helpful because of the possibility of massive transudation of hemorrhagic fluid across the alveolar capillary membrane in the region of the lung supplied by the previously occluded vessel (re-perfusion of a previously and chronically non-perfused vascular bed). Should significant and predominantly unilateral post-thromboembolectomy post-cardiopulmonary bypass pulmonary edema occur, the patient should be returned to cardiopulmonary bypass and a double-lumen endotracheal tube inserted so that differential lung ventilation may be used.

2.3. The conventional double-lumen tube intubation procedure

A left-sided double-lumen endotracheal tube should be used for right thoracotomies requiring collapse of the right lung and ventilation of the left lung. A left- or right-sided tube may be used for left thoracotomies requiring collapse of the left lung and ventilation of the right lung. However, since the right upper lobe ventilation slot of a right-sided tube has to be closely opposed to the right upper lobe orifice in order for unobstructed right upper lobe ventilation to occur, and since there is considerable anatomic variation in the exact position of the right upper lobe orifice and, therefore, length of the right main-stem bronchus (in fact, it is well known that an anomalous right upper lobe can take off from the trachea), use of a right-sided tube for left lung collapse introduces the risk of inadequate right upper lobe ventilation. For this reason, a left-sided tube is preferable for most cases requiring one-lung ventilation; if clamping of the left main-stem bronchus is necessary, the tube can be withdrawn at that time into the trachea and then used in the same manner as a single-lumen endotracheal tube (ventilate the right lung with both lumens). Contraindications to use of a left-sided double-lumen tube are carinal and proximal left main-stem bronchial lesions that could be traumatized by the passage of a left-sided tube. These lesions include strictures, endoluminal tumors, tracheobronchial disruptions, and compression of the airway by an external mass. The largest tube that can comfortably pass the glottis should be used, since a relatively small double-lumen tube may require excessive cuff pressure and volume for an endobronchial cuff seal to be obtained and may cause difficulty with suctioning secretions.

Prior to intubation with a double-lumen endotracheal tube, both cuffs and lumen connections are checked. A 3 ml syringe with stopcock should be placed on the end of the bronchial cuff pilot tube, since proper bronchial cuff inflation rarely requires more than 1–2 ml of air; a 5 or 10 ml syringe with stopcock should be placed on the tracheal cuff pilot tube. Since the high volume/low pressure cuffs can be easily torn by teeth, the distal tube is coated with a lubricating ointment (preferably containing a local anesthetic) in order to minimize this possibility. If a less than optimal view of the larynx is anticipated the stylet that comes packaged with the tube is lubricated, inserted into the left lumen, and appropriately curved. The patient is then anesthetized and paralyzed. A curved open-phalanged blade (MacIntosh) is usually preferred for laryngoscopy, since it approximates the curvature of the tube and therefore provides the largest possible area through which to pass the tube.

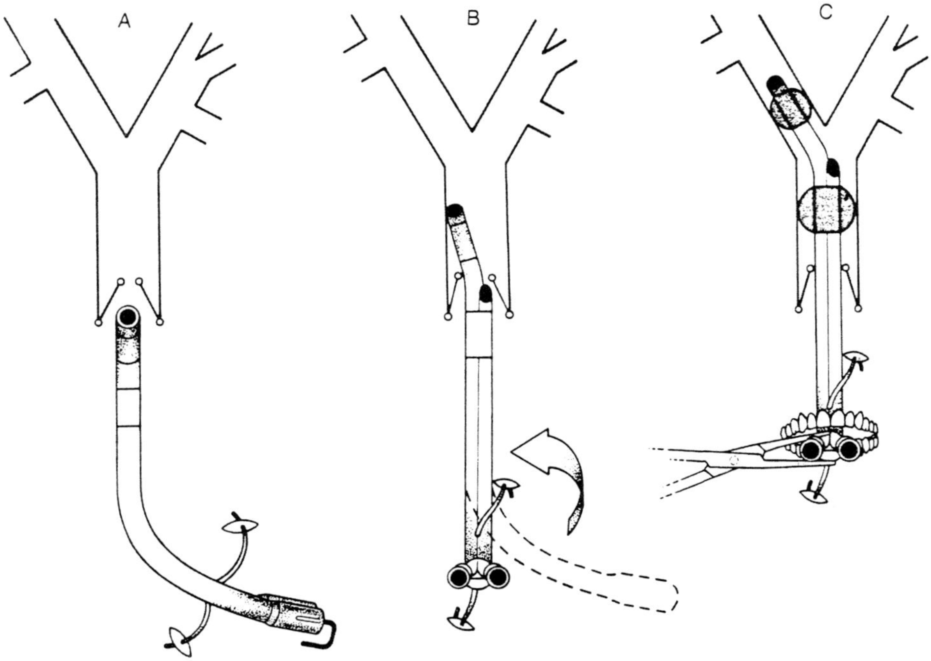

FIGURE 13.1. Passage of the left-sided double lumen tube in a supine patient. (A) The tube is held with the distal curvature concave anteriorly and the proximal curve concave to the right and in a plane parallel to the floor. The tube is then inserted through the vocal cords until the left cuff passes the vocal cords. The stylet is then removed. (B) The tube is rotated 90° counter-clockwise so that the distal curvature is concave anteriorly and the proximal curvature is concave to the left and in a plane parallel to the floor. (C) The tube is inserted until either a moderate resistance to further passage is encountered or the end of the common molding of the two lumens is at the teeth. Both cuffs are then inflated, and both lungs ventilated. Finally, one side is clamped while the other side is ventilated and vice versa (see text for further explanation). (Reproduced with permission from Benumof JL. Anesthesia for Thoracic Surgery. Philadelphia, PA, WB Saunders 1987.)

However, a straight (Miller) blade may be a better choice in patients with overriding teeth or an excessively anterior larynx.

Double-lumen endotracheal tubes with carinal hooks (Carlen's Tube) are first inserted through the vocal cords with the hook facing posteriorly. When the tip of the tube has passed the vocal cords, the tube is rotated 180°, so that the hook passes anteriorly through the glottis. After the tube tip and hook pass the larynx, the tube is rotated 90° so that the tube tip enters the appropriate bronchus.

The Robertshaw double-lumen tube is passed with the distal curvature initially concave anteriorly (Fig. 13.1A). After the tube tip passes the larynx, and while anterior force on the laryngoscope is continued, the stylet (if used) is removed and the tube is carefully rotated 90° (so that the distal curve is now concave towards the appropriate side and the proximal curve is concave anteriorly) to allow endobronchial intubation on the appropriate side (Fig. 13.1B). After rotation, the tube is advanced until most of it is inserted (the proximal end of the common or two-lumen binding mold should be near or at the level of the teeth in a normal-sized person) and/or moderate resistance to further passage is encountered, indicating that the tube tip has been firmly seated in a main-stem bronchus (Fig. 13.1C). Double-lumen endotracheal tubes may also be passed successfully via tracheotomy, although it should be remembered that the tracheal cuff may be at the tracheal stoma or lie partly outside the trachea in this situation [4,5].

Once the tube tip is thought to be in an endobronchial position, the following checklist is carried out to ensure proper functioning of the tube. Inflate the tracheal and endobronchial cuffs until moderate tension is palpated in the external pilot balloons (the endobronchial cuff should not require more than 2–3 ml of air), deliver several positive-pressure ventilations and auscultate and observe the chest bilaterally to determine that the trachea, rather than the esophagus, has been intubated and that both lungs are being ventilated (Fig. 13.1C). In addition to seeing the tube go through the vocal cords, correct intubation position is checked by feeling and observing the anesthesia reservoir bag to make sure it has the appropriate compliance and movement, maintaining normal pulse oximetry and end-tidal CO_2 values, and perhaps palpating the tracheal cuff in the neck. If only unilateral breath sounds or chest movement are present, it is likely that both of the lumens of the tube have entered a main-stem bronchus (if both of the lumens enter the left main-stem bronchus, the findings may mimic an esophageal intubation and vice versa). In this situation, quickly deflate the cuffs, withdraw the tube 1–2 cm at a time, inflate the cuffs, and reassess ventilation until bilateral breath sounds are heard. If bilateral breath sounds are not heard, and the tube has been withdrawn a significant amount, the entire procedure must be repeated, beginning with establishing the airway and oxygen ventilation via mask, laryngoscopy, and reinsertion of the double-lumen tube through the vocal cords. If bilateral breath sounds are present, then one side is clamped and breath sounds and chest movement should disappear on the ipsilateral side and remain on the contralateral side. Next, the clamped side should be unclamped and the breath sounds and chest movement should reappear on that side. During unilateral clamping the breath sounds on the ventilated side should be compared with and calibrated against unilateral chest wall movements and the inspiratory disappearance and expiratory appearance of respiratory gas moisture in the clear tubing of the ventilated side. In addition, the compliance of the lung should be gauged by using hand ventilation. The unilateral clamping and unclamping should then be repeated on the opposite side to assure adequate lung separation and cuff seal.

In summary, when double-lumen endotracheal tube position is correct, the breath sounds are normal and follow the expected unilateral pattern with unilateral clamping, the chest rises and falls in accordance with the breath sounds, the ventilated lung feels reasonably compliant, no leaks are present, and respiratory gas moisture appears and disappears with each tidal ventilation. Conversely, when the double-lumen endotracheal tube is malpositioned, any or all of the following may occur: the breath sounds are poor and correlate poorly with unilateral clamping, the chest movements do not follow the expected pattern, the ventilated lung feels noncompliant, leaks are present, or the respiratory gas moisture in the clear tubing is relatively stationary. It is very important to realize, however, that even if the double-lumen tube is thought to be properly positioned by clinical signs, subsequent fiber-optic bronchoscopy will reveal a 48% incidence of malpositioning [6].

There are several situations in which unilateral clamping, auscultation, and cuff inflation and deflation maneuvers for determining the integrity of lung separation are either unreliable or impossible. First, and most importantly, when the patient is in the lateral decubitus position, has had a skin preparation, and is draped, access to the chest wall is impossible and the anesthesiologist cannot listen to the chest. Second, the presence of unilateral or bilateral lung disease, which either pre-existed before anesthesia and surgery or was induced by anesthesia, may markedly obscure the crispness of the chest auscultation endpoints. Third, the diagnosis of exactly where the double-lumen endotracheal tube has located may be confused when the tube is just slightly malpositioned. Fourth, the tube may have moved due to some event such as coughing, turning into the lateral decubitus position, and tracheal manipulation and hilar retraction by the surgeon. Finally, some combination of the above may culminate in uncertainty as to where the double-lumen tube has located. The solution to any uncertainty as to the exact position of the double-lumen tube is to determine the position by use of fiber-optic bronchoscopy (see next subsection).

2.4. Use of fiber-optic bronchoscope to determine precise double-lumen tube position

As noted previously, even when a double-lumen tube is thought to be in proper position based on clinical signs, subsequent fiber-optic bronchoscopy will reveal a 48% incidence of malpositioning [6]. Indeed, when the position of the double-lumen tube is checked only by clinical signs, 25% of the time there will be intraoperative problems with either deflating the nondependent lung, ventilating the dependent lung, or completely separating the two lungs [7]. The exact position of a left-sided double-lumen endotracheal tube can be ascertained at any time, in less than a minute, by simply passing a pediatric fiber-optic bronchoscope through the tracheal lumen of the double-lumen tube. It is rarely necessary to also have to pass the fiber-optic bronchoscope down the left endobronchial lumen. With reference to a left-sided double-lumen tube, looking down the right (tracheal) lumen the endoscopist should see a clear straight-ahead view of the tracheal carina, the left lumen going off to the left, and the upper surface of the left endobronchial balloon just below the tracheal carina (Fig. 13.2). It is extremely important to be able to visualize the upper surface of the left endobronchial cuff below the tracheal carina because this observation guarantees that the left upper lobe will not be obstructed by the tip of the left lumen. It is important that the volume of air used to fill the left

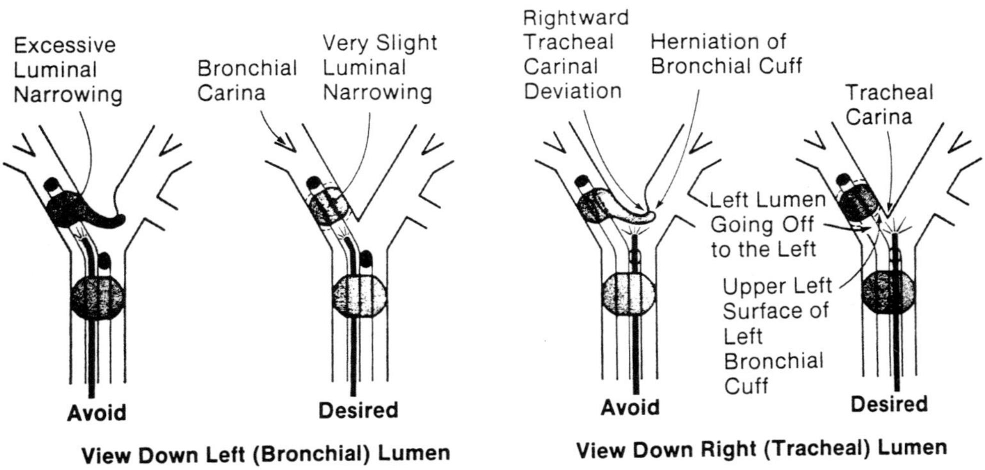

FIGURE 13.2. Use of the fiber-optic bronchoscope to determine the precise position of the left-sided double-lumen tube. When the bronchoscope is passed down the right lumen of the left-sided tube, the endoscopist should see a clear straight-ahead view of the tracheal carina and the upper surface of the blue left endobronchial cuff just below the tracheal carina. Excessive pressure in the endobronchial cuff, as manifested by tracheal carinal deviation to the right and herniation of the endobronchial cuff over the carina, should be avoided. When the bronchoscope is passed down the left lumen of the left-sided tube, the endoscopist should see a very slight left luminal narrowing and a clear straight-ahead view of the bronchial carina off in the distance. Excessive left luminal narrowing should be avoided. (Reproduced with permission from Benumof JL. Anesthesia for Thoracic Surgery. Philadelphia, PA, WB Saunders 1987.)

endobronchial cuff does not cause the endobronchial cuff to herniate over the tracheal carina or cause the tracheal carina to deviate to the right (Fig. 13.2); both cuff herniation and carinal deviation can be readily appreciated looking down the tracheal lumen. Looking down the left lumen [which is sometimes done when inserting a left-sided double-lumen tube with a fiber-optic bronchoscope (see next subsection) and in all cases of bronchopulmonary lavage where perfect tube position and tight cuff seal are extremely critical] the endoscopist should see a very slight narrowing of the left lumen (due to endobronchial cuff pressure) as well as the bronchial carina distal to the end of the tube (Fig. 13.2). The endoscopist should not see excessive left luminal narrowing (due to excessive left cuff pressure) (Fig. 13.2). Thus, aside from gross malposition, important undesirable findings on endoscopy are related to excessive left cuff inflation and pressure and consist of cuff herniation over the tracheal carina, carinal deviation to the right (both of which may block the right main-stem bronchial orifice and impair right lung ventilation), and excessive left lumen constriction (invagination), which may impair

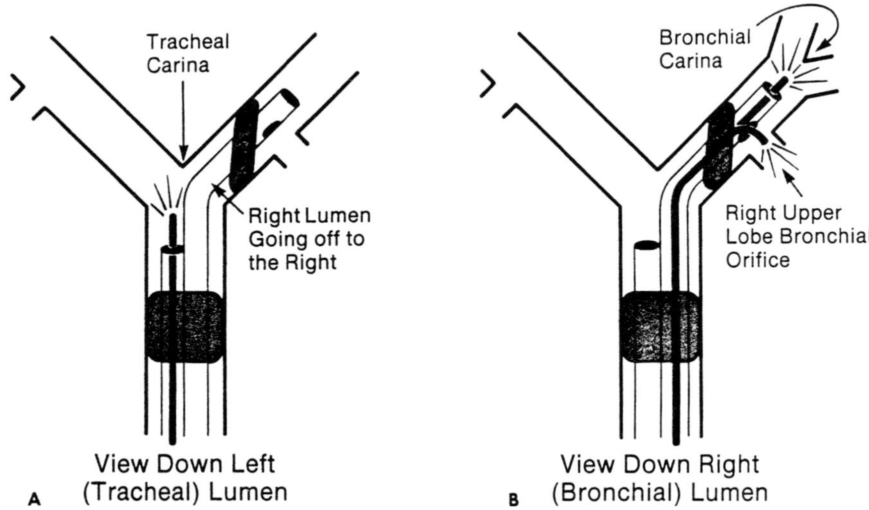

FIGURE 13.3. Use of the fiber-optic bronchoscope to determine the precise position of the right-sided double-lumen tube. (A) When the fiber-optic bronchoscope is passed down the left (tracheal) lumen, the endoscopist should see a clear straight-ahead view of the tracheal carina and the right lumen going off into the right main-stem bronchus. (B) When the fiber-optic bronchoscope is passed down the right (bronchial) lumen, the endoscopist should see the bronchial carina off in the distance; when the fiber-optic bronchoscope is flexed cephalad and passed through the right upper lobe ventilation slot, the right upper lobe bronchial orifice should be visualized. (Reproduced with permission from Benumof JL. Anesthesia for Thoracic Surgery. Philadelphia, PA, WB Saunders 1987.)

left lung ventilation (Fig. 13.2) [8]. In addition, when an inappropriately undersized tube is used, the large endobronchial cuff volume required for endobronchial cuff seal tends to force the entire double-lumen tube cephalad, making a functional bronchial seal more difficult [9].

With reference to a right-sided double-lumen tube, looking down the left (tracheal) lumen, the endoscopist should see a clear straight-ahead view of the tracheal carina and the right lumen going off to the right (Fig. 13.3). The upper surface of the right endobronchial balloon may not be visible below the tracheal carina. Looking down the right lumen, the endoscopist should see a very slight narrowing of the right lumen as well as the right middle-lower lobe bronchial carina distal to the end of the tube. Most importantly, the endoscopist should locate the right upper lobe ventilation slot and be able to look directly into the right upper lobe orifice through the right upper lobe ventilation slot by simply flexing the tip of the fiber-optic bronchoscope superiorly (Fig. 13.3). There should be no overriding of right upper lobe ventilation slot on the bronchial mucosa, and the bronchial mucosa should not be covering any of the right upper lobe ventilation slot. The fact that there is little room for error in aligning the right upper lobe ventilation slot with the right upper lobe orifice will be emphasized in the following section.

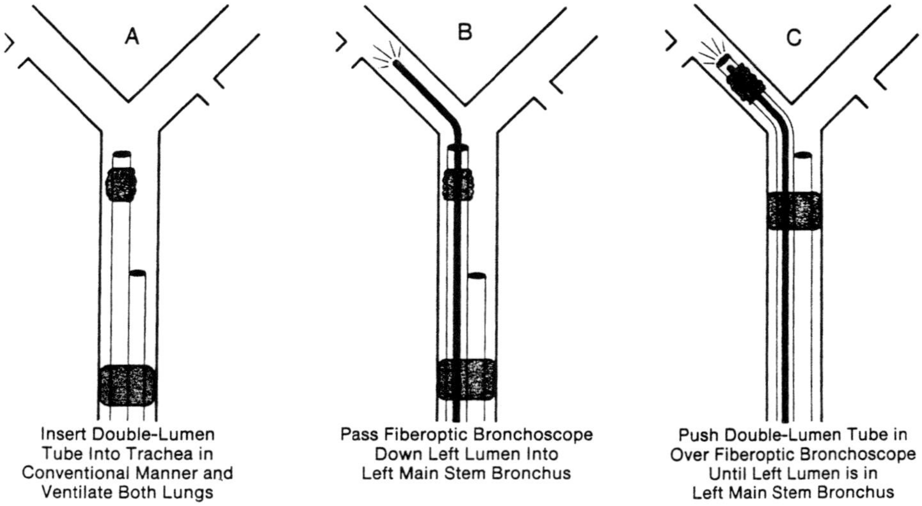

FIGURE 13.4. Use of the fiber-optic bronchoscope to insert a left-sided double-lumen tube. (A) The double-lumen tube can be put into the trachea in a conventional manner, and both lungs can be ventilated by both lumens. The fiber-optic bronchoscope may be inserted into the left lumen of the double-lumen tube through a self-sealing diaphragm in the elbow connector to the left lumen; this allows continued positive pressure ventilation of both lungs through the right lumen without creating a leak. After the fiber-optic bronchoscope has been passed into the left main-stem bronchus (B), it is used as a stylet for the aftercoming left lumen (C). The fiber-optic bronchoscope is then withdrawn. Final precise positioning of the double-lumen tube is performed with the fiber-optic bronchoscope in the right lumen (see Fig. 13.2). (Reproduced with permission from Benumof JL. Anesthesia for Thoracic Surgery. Philadelphia, PA, WB Saunders 1987.)

The right upper lobe ventilation slot may be easily located by first finding the bronchial lumen radiopaque marker. The radiopaque marker appears as either a white or a black line on the inside of the bronchial lumen, which ends at the proximal end of the right upper lobe ventilation slot. If one simply follows the radiopaque line, it will lead the endoscopist to the right upper lobe ventilation slot.

2.5. Use of fiber-optic bronchoscope to insert the bronchial lumen of a double-lumen tube into a main-stem bronchus

The insertion of the bronchial lumen of a double-lumen tube into the appropriate main-stem bronchus may be aided by the use of a fiber-optic bronchoscope (Fig. 13.4). The double-lumen tube is first placed in the trachea in a conventional manner (laryngoscopy, manual tube insertion) until the tracheal cuff just passes the vocal cords, the tracheal cuff is inflated, and both lungs are ventilated with both lumens (use the double-lumen tube as if it were a single-lumen tube). A pediatric fiber-optic bronchoscope can then be inserted into the bronchial lumen through a self-sealing diaphragm in the elbow connector to the bronchial lumen (which permits continued positive-pressure ventilation through that lumen around the fiber-optic bronchoscope) and passed into the appropriate main-stem bronchus. The tracheal cuff is then deflated and the bronchial lumen is passed over the fiber-optic bronchoscope stylet into the appropriate main-stem bronchus. The fiber-optic bronchoscope is then withdrawn from the bronchial lumen and passed down the tracheal lumen to determine the precise double-lumen tube position (see the previous section and Fig. 13.2).

Alternatively, once the double-lumen tube is in the trachea, the fiber-optic bronchoscope can be inserted into the tracheal lumen through a self-sealing diaphragm in the elbow connector to the tracheal lumen (which permits continued positive-pressure ventilation through that lumen around the fiber-optic bronchoscope) and passed just proximal to the tracheal carina. While the carina and the two main-stem bronchial orifices are in view, the double-lumen tube can be advanced and the degree of lateral rotation adjusted so that the left lumen enters the left main-stem bronchus. Final precise positioning (see Previous Section) can be done with the fiber-optic bronchoscope remaining in the tracheal lumen.

3. MANAGEMENT OF ONE-LUNG VENTILATION

3.1. Introduction

The method used to ventilate the dependent lung is especially important in this regard for several reasons. First, if the dependent-lung method of ventilation involves an excessive amount of airway pressure, due either to use of high levels of positive end-expiratory pressure (PEEP) or to very large tidal volumes, then dependent-lung vascular resistance may be increased, which would increase nondependent-lung blood flow. The deleterious effects of increased nondependent-lung blood flow (shunt) may outweigh the beneficial effects of the opening of atelectatic and low ventilation–perfusion areas in the dependent lung. Second, if the dependent lung is hyperventilated (which may require an excessive amount of airway pressure), then the resultant hypocapnia may inhibit hypoxic pulmonary vasoconstriction (HPV). Third, if the dependent lung is ventilated with too small of a tidal volume, then dependent-lung atelectasis may develop. Fourth, a high inspired oxygen concentration to the dependent lung may vasodilate the dependent lung, enhancing nondependent-lung hypoxic pulmonary vasoconstriction [10,11]. On the other hand, a high inspired oxygen concentration to the low ventilation–perfusion dependent lung may promote dependent-lung absorption atelectasis [12,13].

3.2. Conventional management of one-lung ventilation

In view of the fact that one-lung ventilation incurs a high risk of causing systemic hypoxemia (due to shunting through the collapsed operative lung), it is extremely important that dependent-lung ventilation, as outlined above, be optimally managed. This section first considers the usual management of one-lung ventilation in terms of the most appropriate inspired oxygen concentration, tidal volume, respiratory rate, and dependent-lung PEEP level that should be used. The use of differential lung management to treat hypoxemia during one-lung ventilation is then considered. The section concludes with a recommended, combined, conventional and differential lung management of one-lung ventilation.

3.2.1. Inspired oxygen concentration

Although the theoretical possibilities of absorption atelectasis and oxygen toxicity exist, the benefits of ventilating the dependent lung with 100% oxygen far exceed the risks. A high fraction of inspired oxygen (F_IO_2) in the single ventilated lung may critically increase the arterial partial pressure of oxygen (P_aO_2) from arrhythmogenic and life-threatening levels to safer levels. In addition, a high F_IO_2 in the dependent lung will cause vasodilation, thereby increasing the dependent lung capability of accepting blood flow redistribution due to nondependent-lung HPV [11,13,14]. Direct chemical 100% oxygen toxicity will not occur during the time frame of the operative period [15] and absorption atelectasis in the dependent lung [12] is unlikely to occur in view of the remaining one-lung ventilation management characteristics (moderately large tidal volumes with intermittent positive-pressure, low-level PEEP) listed as follows. Although not previously studied during one-lung ventilation, use of a dependent-lung F_IO_2 of 0.8–0.9 may be ideal in view of the fact that a F_IN_2 of 0.1–0.2 greatly reduces the possibility of absorption atelectasis [by allowing some nitrogen to splint open the regions of low ventilation/perfusion ratios (V/Q)] [12], whereas a reduction in F_IO_2 of 0.1–0.2 (from 1.0) will probably cause only a small decrease in P_aO_2.

3.2.2. Tidal volume

The dependent lung should be ventilated with a tidal volume of 10 ml/kg. Use of a tidal volume much less than 10 ml/kg might promote dependent-lung atelectasis. Use of a tidal volume much greater than 10 ml/kg might excessively increase dependent-lung airway pressure and vascular resistance [16], and thereby increase nondependent-lung blood flow (decrease nondependent-lung HPV) [17–19].

A dependent-lung tidal volume of 10 ml/kg represents a volume that is in the middle of a range of tidal volumes (8–15 ml/kg) that have been found to not greatly affect arterial oxygenation during one-lung ventilation [20].

3.2.3. Respiratory rate

The respiratory rate should be set so that the arterial partial pressure of carbon dioxide (P_aCO_2) remains at 40 mmHg. Since a dependent-lung tidal volume of 10 ml/kg represents a 20% decrease from the usual two-lung tidal volume of 12 ml/kg, the respiratory rate usually needs to be increased by 20% in order to maintain carbon dioxide homeostasis. The trade-off between decreased tidal volume and increased respiratory rate is usually a constant minute ventilation; although ventilation and perfusion are considerably mismatched during one-lung ventilation, an unchanged minute ventilation during one-lung ventilation (compared to two-lung ventilation) can continue to eliminate a normal amount of carbon dioxide because of the high diffusibility of carbon dioxide [16,21–23]. In fact, lowering the minute ventilation by approximately one half (tidal volume reduced from 15 to 8 ml/kg while respiratory rate was constant) has little effect on P_aCO_2 [20]. Hypocapnia should be avoided because use of the airway pressure in the dependent lung necessary to produce systemic hypocapnia may excessively increase dependent-lung vascular resistance. Furthermore, hypocapnia may directly inhibit HPV in the nondependent lung [24,25].

3.2.4. Dependent-lung PEEP

No, or just a very low level of, dependent-lung PEEP (less than 5 cm H_2O) should be used initially because of concern of unnecessarily increasing dependent-lung vascular resistance (see Section 3.3.1 below).

In summary, at the commencement of one-lung ventilation, 100% oxygen (although it may be argued on theoretical grounds that 80–90% oxygen decreases the risk of absorption atelectasis and only minimally, or not at all, increases the risk of hypoxemia), a tidal volume of 10 ml/kg, and a 20% increase in respiratory rate are used as initial ventilation settings. Ventilation and arterial oxygenation are monitored by use of frequent arterial blood gases, end-tidal carbon dioxide concentration, and pulse oximetry or transcutaneous tensions. If there is a problem with either ventilation or arterial oxygenation, then one or more of the differential lung management techniques are used.

3.3. Differential lung management of one-lung ventilation

3.3.1. Selective dependent-lung PEEP

Since the ventilated dependent lung often has a decreased lung volume during one-lung ventilation (see Fig. 13.5, upper left-hand panel), it is not surprising that several attempts have been made to improve oxygenation by treating the ventilated lung with PEEP [17–19,26–29]. The most accepted mechanism by which PEEP is thought to be of benefit is that PEEP causes an increase in lung volume at end-expiration (by definition, the functional residual capacity, or FRC). The increase in FRC contributes to the prevention of airway and alveolar closure at end-expiration and to the recruitment of airways and alveoli during inspiration. The increases in lung volume and airway and alveolar openings result in increases in lung compliance, ventilation, and the ventilation-to-perfusion ratio of the single ventilated lung (Fig. 13.5) [30,31]. Consequently, it may be expected that the application of PEEP to the compressed dependent lung would improve dependent-lung volume and ventilation–perfusion relationships.

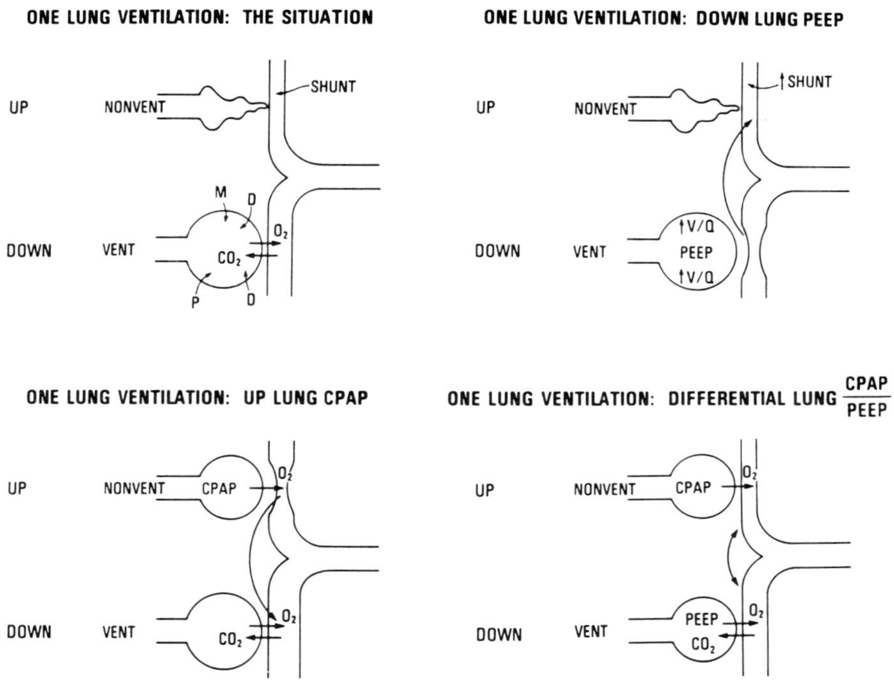

FIGURE 13.5. Schematic diagram of one-lung ventilation situation (upper left panel), selective dependent (down) lung PEEP (upper right panel), selective non-dependent (up) lung CPAP (lower left panel), and differential lung PEEP/CPAP (non-dependent lung/dependent lung, respectively) (lower right panel). Up, non-dependent lung; Down, dependent lung; Nonvent, non-ventilated; Vent, ventilated; M, weight of mediastinum; D, pressure of the abdominal contents pressing cephalad on the diaphragm; P, positioning effects of the supporting roles, packs and shoulder supports. Since the dependent lung is in a low ventilation–perfusion situation (circumferentially compressed by M, D, and P), various authors have sought to rectify this situation by selectively adding PEEP to the dependent lung. However, selective PEEP to the dependent lung may shunt blood flow up to the non-ventilated nondependent lung, thereby increasing the right-to-left shunt through the non-ventilated lung. A far more efficacious remedy to hypoxemia during one-lung ventilation is to CPAP the non-ventilated lung. This creates an oxygen-filled alveolar space which effectively abolishes the shunt through the non-ventilated non-dependent lung. Even if the CPAP to the non-dependent non-ventilated lung shunts blood flow to the dependent lung, the diverted blood flow will still participate in gas exchange in the ventilated dependent lung. Perhaps, the best of all possible situations is to use nondependent lung CPAP along with dependent lung PEEP; in this situation it does not matter where the blood flow goes, for wherever it goes it can participate in gas exchange in either lung. See text for further explanation.

An accepted risk of PEEP is that the PEEP-induced increase in lung volume can cause compression of the small intra-alveolar vessels. If the PEEP-induced intra-alveolar vessel compression is geographically widespread, then total pulmonary vascular resistance increases and cardiac output decreases. If the intra-alveolar vessel compression is limited to the ventilated lung, then the pulmonary vascular resistance of the one lung being ventilated and receiving PEEP will increase, which will divert blood flow away from the ventilated lung to the nonventilated lung (Fig. 13.5, upper right-hand panel), and the shunt will increase, and P_aO_2 will decrease. With regional lung PEEP, pulmonary vascular resistance for the whole lung does not greatly increase and the cardiac output does not decrease [17,19]. The fact that increases in both PEEP and tidal volume in the dependent ventilated lung have an additive effect in decreasing P_aO_2 during one-lung ventilation greatly supports the one-ventilated lung volume versus vascular resistance hypothesis [17]. Consistent with these observations is the fact that the application of 10 cm H_2O PEEP to the dependent lung during one-lung ventilation decreases P_aO_2 in some patients but has had no significant systemic hemodynamic effect in any patient [32,33].

In summary, the effect of dependent-lung PEEP on arterial oxygenation is a trade-off between the positive effect of increasing dependent-lung FRC and ventilation–perfusion ratio and the negative effect of increasing dependent-lung vascular resistance and shunting blood flow to the nonventilated lung. Thus, the various one-lung ventilation-PEEP studies have had patients who have had an increase [18,26,34], no change [18,27,28,34] or a decrease [18,26,29,34] in oxygenation. It may be expected that in patients with a very diseased dependent lung (low lung volume and low ventilation–perfusion ratio), the positive effect of selective dependent-lung PEEP (increased lung volume and increased ventilation–perfusion ratio), might outweigh the negative effects of selective dependent-lung PEEP (shunting of blood flow to the nonventilated, nondependent lung), whereas in patients with a normal dependent lung the negative effects of dependent-lung PEEP would outweigh the benefits. Indeed, in one study in which 10 cm H_2O PEEP was selectively applied to the dependent lung, P_aO_2 increased in those patients with P_aO_2 less than 80 mmHg ($F_IO_2 = 0$–5), whereas P_aO_2 decreased or remained constant in patients with P_aO_2 higher than 80 mmHg ($F_IO_2 = 0.5$) [34]. Presumably, in the patients with P_aO_2 lower than 80 mmHg ($F_IO_2 = 0.5$) the dependent lung had a low functional residual capacity (low ventilation–perfusion ratio and atelectatic regions) and, therefore, the positive effect of increased dependent-lung volume predominated over the negative effect of shunting blood flow to the nonventilated lung. Conversely, the patients with the higher P_aO_2 presumably had a dependent lung with an adequate functional residual capacity and ventilation–perfusion ratio, and the negative effect of shunting blood flow to the nonventilated lung predominated over the positive effect of increased dependent-lung volume.

Although in none of these studies was a dose (ventilated lung PEEP)–response [P_aO_2, shunt fraction (Q_s/Q_t) value] relationship described, it seems reasonable to postulate on the basis of these results that the therapeutic margin of using PEEP to just the ventilated lung to increase P_aO_2 during one-lung ventilation is quite narrow. PEEP to just the dependent ventilated lung may be delivered by the same anesthesia machine apparatus that is ordinarily used to deliver PEEP to the whole lung. Other studies have shown that high tidal volumes [35], variations in the inspiratory-to-expiratory ratio [27], and intermittent manual hyperventilation of the lower lung are not beneficial in increasing P_aO_2 during one-lung ventilation [27].

3.3.2. Selective nondependent-lung CPAP

Positive pressure can be selectively and statically applied to just the nonventilated nondependent lung. Since under these conditions the nonventilated lung is only slightly but constantly distended by oxygen, an appropriate term for this ventilator arrangement is nonventilated lung continuous positive airway pressure (CPAP). Recently, two reports, one in humans [29] and one in dogs [36], have shown that the application of CPAP (without tidal ventilation) to only or just the nonventilated lung significantly increased oxygenation. The latter study was performed with the dogs in the lateral decubitus position and showed that low levels of CPAP (5–10 cm H_2O) to the nonventilated nondependent lung greatly increased P_aO_2 and decreased shunt, while blood flow to the nonventilated lung remained unchanged; presumably, this level of CPAP does not compress the small intra-alveolar vessels in the nondependent lung. Thus, it is not at all surprising to find that the institution of 10 cm H_2O nondependent-lung CPAP in patients has had no significant hemodynamic effect [32,33]. In summary, low levels of CPAP simply maintain the patency of nondependent-lung airways, allowing some oxygen distention of the gas-exchanging alveolar space in the nondependent lung (Fig. 13.5, lower left-hand panel) without significantly affecting the pulmonary vasculature. In all clinical studies [32,33,37] the application of 5–10 cm H_2O CPAP has not interfered with the performance of surgery and may, in fact, facilitate intralobar dissection; this is not surprising in view of the fact that the initial compliance of a collapsed lung is only 10 ml/cm H_2O, and 5–10 cm H_2O CPAP should only create a slightly distended lung that occupies a volume of 50–100 ml, which is hardly or not at all noticed by the surgeon.

On the other hand, in the canine study [36], 15 cm H_2O of nondependent-lung CPAP caused changes in P_aO_2 and shunt similar to those of 5–10 cm H_2O nondependent-lung CPAP, while blood flow to the nonventilated nondependent lung decreased significantly. Therefore, high levels of nonventilated-lung CPAP act by permitting oxygen uptake in the nonventilated lung as well as by causing blood flow diversion to the ventilated lung, where both oxygen and carbon dioxide exchange can take place (Fig. 13.5, lower left-hand panel). Since low levels of nonventilated lung CPAP are as efficacious as high levels of nonventilated lung CPAP and have less surgical interference and hemodynamic implications, it is logical to first use low levels of nonventilated CPAP.

In all patients in all clinical studies to date, 5–10 cm H_2O of nondependent-lung CPAP has significantly increased P_aO_2 during one-lung ventilation [29,33,34,37–40]. It should be concluded that the single most efficacious maneuver to increase P_aO_2 during one-lung ventilation is to apply 5–10 cm H_2O CPAP to the nondependent lung. In my experience, low levels of nonventilated CPAP have corrected severe hypoxemia ($P_aO_2 < 50$ mmHg) greater than 90% of the time, provided the double-lumen tube was correctly positioned. However, the nondependent-lung CPAP must be applied during the deflation phase of a large tidal volume so that the deflating lung can lock into a CPAP level with uniform expansion and avoid the need to overcome critical opening pressures.

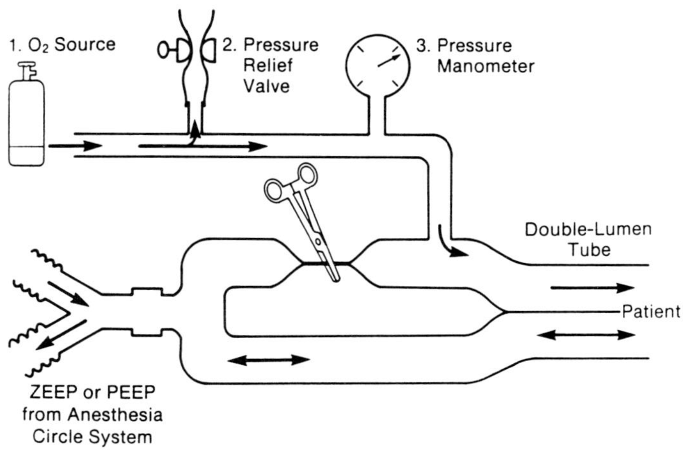

FIGURE 13.6. The three essential components of a non-dependent lung continuous positive airway pressure (CPAP) system consist of (1) an oxygen source, (2) a pressure relief valve, and (3) a pressure manometer to measure the CPAP. The CPAP is created by the free flow of oxygen into the lung versus the restricted outflow of oxygen from the lung by the pressure relief valve. (ZEEP = zero end- expiratory pressure.) It is also highly desirable to have a reservoir bag in-line to provide a tidal volume when desired. (Reproduced with permission from Benumof JL. Anesthesia for Thoracic Surgery. Philadelphia, PA, WB Saunders 1987.)

In both the human [29] and dog [36] studies, oxygen insufflation at zero airway pressure did not significantly improve P_aO_2 and shunt, and this result was probably due to the inability of zero transbronchial airway pressure to maintain airway patency and overcome critical opening pressures. Although one study in patients has concluded that insufflation of O_2 at zero airway pressure does increase P_aO_2, the study is difficult to interpret, since the patients did not serve as their own control [41].

Several selective nondependent-lung CPAP systems that are easy to assemble have been recently described [28,38–40]. All of these nondependent-lung CPAP systems have three features in common (Fig. 13.6). First, there must be a source of oxygen to flow into the nonventilated lung. Second, there must be some sort of restrictive mechanism (hand-screw valve, pop-off valve, weight-loaded valve) to prevent the egress of oxygen out of the nonventilated lung so that the nonventilated lung may become distended. Thus, a free-flowing pressurized source of oxygen flows into a lung, but the escape of the oxygen is restricted; the unrestricted flow in and the restricted flow out creates a constant distending pressure. Third, the distending pressure must be measured by a manometer. In practice it is simplest to keep the restrictive mechanism constant and adjust the distending pressure with a relatively fine sensitivity by changing the oxygen flow rate. If the nondependent-lung CPAP system has a reservoir bag included, which is highly desirable (Fig. 13.6), the nondependent lung may also be ventilated with intermittent positive pressure whenever desired.

3.3.3. Differential lung PEEP, CPAP

In theory, and from the preceding considerations, it appears that the ideal way to improve oxygenation during one-lung ventilation is to apply differential lung CPAP/PEEP (Fig. 13.5, lower right-hand panel) (see Section 3.4 for the step-by-step approach). In this situation, the ventilated (dependent) lung is given PEEP in the usual conventional manner in an effort to improve ventilated-lung volume and ventilation–perfusion relationships. Simultaneously, the nonventilated (nondependent) lung receives CPAP in an attempt to improve oxygenation of the blood perfusing this lung. Therefore, with differential lung PEEP or PEEP/CPAP, it does not matter where the blood flow goes nearly as much as during simple one-lung ventilation, since wherever it goes (to either ventilated or nonventilated lung) it has at least some chance to participate in gas exchange with alveoli that are expanded with oxygen. In indirect support of this contention, arterial oxygenation has been increased significantly in patients during thoracotomy in the lateral decubitus position (utilizing two-lung ventilation) when PEEP has been added to the ventilated dependent lung, while the nondependent lung was also able to participate in gas exchange by virtue of being ventilated at zero end-expiratory pressure (ZEEP)[31]. In direct support of this contention, in patients undergoing thoracotomy and one-lung ventilation, arterial oxygenation was unchanged by the application of 10 cm H_2O dependent-lung PEEP alone (consistent with an equal positive–negative effect tradeoff), was significantly improved by 10 cm H_2O nondependent-lung CPAP alone, and was further and even more significantly increased by use of 10 cm H_2O nondependent-lung CPAP and 10 cm H_2O dependent-lung PEEP together (differential lung ventilation)[32,33]. The use of 10 cm H_2O nondependent-lung CPAP together with 10 cm H_2O dependent-lung PEEP in patients caused only small, clinically insignificant hemodynamic effects[32,33].

3.3.4. Selective nondependent-lung high-frequency ventilation

The studies of selective nondependent-lung CPAP indicate that delivery of any amount of oxygen to the nondependent-lung alveolar space will cause some oxygen uptake from the nondependent lung and decrease the nondependent lung right-to-left shunt. Consequently, it is not surprising that selective high-frequency ventilation of the nondependent lung (see Next Section for extensive discussion of this ventilation modality), while the dependent lung is ventilated with conventional intermittent positive-pressure breathing, increases P_aO_2 compared to simple collapse of the nondependent lung and conventional mechanical ventilation of the dependent lung[42]. However, since the same increase in arterial oxygenation may be obtained by selective nondependent-lung CPAP with much simpler equipment compared with high-frequency ventilation apparatus, it is more logical to use selective nondependent-lung CPAP than high-frequency ventilation to improve arterial oxygenation during 'one-lung ventilation'.

However, there are two relative indications for the combination of nondependent-lung high-frequency ventilation and dependent-lung intermittent positive-pressure breathing [43]. First, if the nondependent lung has a major bronchopleural fistula, high-frequency ventilation may be indicated because it may minimize airway leak. Second, if prolonged surgery has to be performed on a major nondependent-lung conducting airway, high-frequency ventilation may be indicated because it may permit a much smaller catheter to pass through the operating field. This ventilator modality is extensively discussed in the next section.

3.4. Recommended combined conventional and differential lung management of one-lung ventilation

The recommended plan for obtaining satisfactory arterial oxygenation during one-lung ventilation is as follows. Two-lung ventilation is maintained for as long as possible (usually until the pleura is opened). When one-lung ventilation is commenced, a tidal volume of 10 ml/kg is used and the respiratory rate is adjusted so that $P_aCO_2 = 40$ mmHg. A high inspired oxygen concentration ($F_IO_2 = 0.8$–1.0) should be used, and arterial blood gases should be monitored frequently.

If severe hypoxemia is present following this initial conventional approach, then two major causes of hypoxemia, namely malposition of the double-lumen tube and poor hemodynamic status, must be ruled out. If the double-lumen tube is correctly positioned and the hemodynamic status is satisfactory, then simple tidal volume and respiratory rate adjustments should be made [20]. For example, if the tidal ventilation is thought to be too high, it should be decreased, and if the tidal ventilation is thought to be too small, it should be increased. If these simple maneuvers do not quickly resolve the problem, the above studies of selective nondependent-lung CPAP [29,32,33,36–40] and differential lung PEEP [44–56] suggest that the next treatment should be to apply 5–10 cm H_2O of CPAP to the nondependent lung. Nondependent-lung CPAP should be applied during the deflation phase of a large tidal volume breath in order to overcome critical opening pressures in the atelectatic lung. If oxygenation does not improve with nondependent-lung CPAP (which it does in the large majority of cases), 5–10 cm H_2O of PEEP to the ventilated dependent lung should then be applied. If dependent-lung PEEP does not improve oxygenation, nondependent-lung CPAP should be increased to 10–15 cm H_2O while the dependent lung is maintained at 5–10 cm H_2O of CPAP. If arterial oxygenation is still not satisfactory, then the nondependent-lung CPAP level should be matched with an equal amount of dependent-lung PEEP. In this way, a differential lung CPAP/PEEP search for the maximum compliance and a minimum right-to-left transpulmonary shunt is done in an attempt to find the optimal end-expiratory pressure for each lung and the patient as a whole.

If severe hypoxemia is still present following the application of differential lung CPAP/PEEP (which would be extremely rare), it should be remembered that the nondependent lung may be intermittently ventilated with positive pressure with oxygen. Finally, most of the ventilation–perfusion imbalance is eliminated during a pneumonectomy by tightening a ligature around the nonventilated lung pulmonary artery as early as possible, which directly eliminates all shunt flow through the nonventilated lung. Indeed, clamping the pulmonary artery to a collapsed lung functionally resects the entire lung, and the P_aO_2 is restored back to a level not significantly different from a two-lung ventilation or postpneumonectomy one-lung ventilation value.

4. ROLE OF HIGH-FREQUENCY VENTILATION IN THORACIC SURGERY

4.1. Introduction

Conventional positive-pressure breathing can interfere with the performance of thoracic surgery in four ways. First, conventional positive pressure breathing requires large endotracheal tubes (either single- or double-lumen tubes) that can greatly interfere with the performance of surgery on major conducting airways. Second, the expansion and movement of the nondependent lung by intermittent positive-pressure breathing may greatly interfere with access to the surgical field. Third, movement of the dependent lung due to intermittent positive-pressure breathing will cause the mediastinum, and therefore the floor of the surgical field, to move up and down, which may hamper the performance of surgery. Fourth, the airway pressure in the ventilated dependent lung, if too high, can compress the small intra-alveolar vessels in the dependent lung, increase dependent lung pulmonary vascular resistance, and shunt blood flow to the nonventilated nondependent lung.

In theory, high-frequency ventilation (HFV) does not have these disadvantages. HFV requires only a small bore catheter and thereby can potentially facilitate the performance of surgery on major conducting airways. Second, the tidal movements with HFV are very small, thereby minimizing movements of both the nondependent and dependent lungs. In addition, HFV utilizes a low airway pressure so that it is possible to obtain adequate gas exchange whenever airway resistance is extremely low (as it might be in surgery on a major conducting airway or with a large bronchopleural fistula) without a large air leak. Finally, the lower airway pressure associated with HFV [57] and release of vasodilator prostaglandins with HFV [58] can, in theory, lower dependent-lung vascular resistance and improve diversion of blood flow away from an atelectatic nondependent lung. This section reviews clinical experience with HFV during intrathoracic surgery.

4.2. Categories of high frequency ventilation

Conventional intermittent positive-pressure ventilation (IPPV) delivers relatively large tidal volumes (10–15 ml/kg) at respiratory rates usually less than 30 breaths

TABLE 13.2
Characteristics of the three types of high-frequency ventilation

Type of HFV	Rate	Type of ventilator	Gas entrainment	Process of	
				inspiration[a]	exhalation[a]
HFPPV	60–100	Volume	No	Active	Passive
HFJV	100–400	Jet pulsation	Yes	Active	Passive
HFOV	400–2400	Piston pump	Yes	Active	Active

[a] Active: caused by the ventilator,
Passive: caused by elastic recoil of lung.

per minute. With IPPV the basic mechanism of gas transport is by mass movement to the smaller airways and then more distally by mass movement and molecular diffusion[59]. In contrast to IPPV, high-frequency ventilation (HFV) delivers very small tidal volumes (< 2 ml/kg) at rates between 60 and 2400 breaths per minute. Under these circumstances, the proportion of the tidal volume ventilating the dead space increases so that normal alveolar ventilation can be maintained only by the use of high respiratory rates and minute volumes. With HFV, gas transport by mass movement is still important[60], but may be combined with varying degrees of other mechanisms of gas transport such as enhanced molecular diffusion[61], high velocity gas flow[62], coaxial gas flow [bidirectional flow with gases in the center of the airway moving distally (O_2) and gases on the edge of the airway moving proximally (CO_2)][63], asynchronous regional filling and emptying of alveoli ("pendelluft" movement, resulting in smaller gas volumes effectively reaching more respiratory units)[64], and gas trapping[65].

High-frequency ventilation is an umbrella term encompassing different delivery systems and respiratory rate ranges. Current methods used to provide high-frequency ventilation are quite diverse, but by using the criteria of ventilation rate and type of gas delivery mechanism, it is possible to separate high-frequency ventilation into three general categories[60,66] (Table 13.2). The first HFV category, high-frequency positive-pressure ventilation (HFPPV), employs a volume-controlled ventilator with a low internal compressible volume, which delivers small tidal volumes at rates of 60 to 100 breaths per minute (1–1.7 Hz). The negligible internal compliance of the ventilator guarantees that the preset tidal volume [usually approximately equal to the anatomic dead space volume (2 ml/kg)] is the tidal volume that is actually delivered to the patient. The low-compression delivery system enhances gas exchange in the conducting airways by causing a high instantaneous gas flow[62]. There is no gas entrainment so that the delivered tidal volume is all fresh gas and the F_IO_2 is the same as the F_IO_2 of the compressed gas. If a standard endotracheal tube is used for HFPPV, PEEP may be added to maximize P_aO_2[64,67].

The second HFV category, high-frequency jet ventilation (HFJV), employs pulsation of a small jet of fresh gas introduced from a high-pressure source (50–60 psi) into the airway via a small catheter (which can be passed alone or through an endotracheal tube) or via an extra lumen in an endotracheal tube, at rates usually between 100 and 400 breaths per minute (1.7–6.7 Hz). The small catheter tip must be located near the carina (HFJV through catheters located either more distally or proximally do not result in normal CO_2 removal). The jetted fresh gas leaves the narrow injection cannulae at a very high velocity. As it exits from the injection cannulae, the high velocity of the jet flow entrains gas from the endotracheal tube's fresh gas flow or from an injection cannulae side port gas reservoir (Bernoulli effect)[68]. The amount of entrained gas is uncertain and therefore quantification of tidal volume and F_IO_2 is difficult. The jetted and entrained gases (20–40 l/min) impact into the much larger volume of relatively immobile gas in the endotracheal tube and conducting airways and cause the gas to move forward[66,68]. As with HFPPV, oxygenation is enhanced with HFJV when small amounts of PEEP are added (via the endotracheal tube).

The third HFV category, high-frequency oscillation ventilation (HFOV), employs a piston pump or loudspeaker which oscillates gas in the airway back and forth in a sinusoidal fashion at rates of 400 to 2400 breaths per minute (6.7–40 Hz). A fresh gas flow-by (which is entrained) is located between the oscillator and the patient[69]. Delivered tidal volume is very small (50–80 ml) and alveolar gas exchange is obtained by enhanced molecular diffusion and coaxial flow[60,66,69].

One other type of HFV system, the flow interrupter, has features of the HFPPV, HFJV, and HFOV categories. Breaths are generated by using a mechanical valve to interrupt very frequently a continuous flow of gas into a low compression delivery system. Thus, small tidal volumes (HFPPV) with high flow rates (HFJV) at very rapid rates (HFOV) are produced. The interrupters are capable of producing the entire range of HFV respiratory rates, but rates of 100–600 per minute have been found to be most effective[59].

In the last decade, all three types of HFV have been shown to be capable of providing adequate alveolar ventilation and oxygenation in both normal animals and humans and in those with pulmonary disease. In anesthetized animals and in human infants and adults with normal lungs undergoing surgical procedures, arterial blood gases demonstrate adequate alveolar ventilation with high-frequency ventilation[67,70–74]. Studies performed in animals and humans in acute respiratory failure have also shown that HFV can provide adequate gas exchange[75–77]. In some reports of ventilation during acute respiratory failure, HFV was even more effective than IPPV[77,78].

4.3. Use in major conducting airway surgery

The most important thoracic surgery advantage of HFV is that the small rapid tidal volumes may be delivered through small airway tubes; thus if a major conducting airway (trachea, carinal area, main-stem bronchus) has to be divided, the transit of a small airway tube through the surgical field causes much less interference with surgery than the passage of a large standard or double-lumen endotracheal tube. The small airway catheters present the surgeon with an unobstructed, accessible circumference of trachea and bronchus, so that the ends of a divided airway can be properly aligned for the construction of an unstressed and airtight anastomosis. Both HFPPV and HFJV have been successfully used with small airway catheters for three different types of airway surgery [79–84].

The first type of airway surgery that has been aided by HFV is carinal resection (in whole or in part). During sleeve pneumonectomy (which includes part of the carina) a small airway catheter passing through the operative field into the main-stem bronchus of the dependent lung ventilated the dependent lung with either HFJV or, more recently and effectively, with HFPPV [82]. In this author's hands [82], HFV also minimized bronchial and mediastinal movements, and with HFPPV the continuous outflow of gases through the open bronchus minimized soiling of the ventilated lung with blood from the lung under operation, whereas HFJV created a suction effect (entrainment) that drew blood and debris into the open carinal area down into the bronchus of the lung being ventilated [82]. Additionally, when a left sleeve pneumonectomy was being performed, the small catheter inside the right main-stem bronchus eliminated the problem of the right upper lobe collapse associated with the use of right endobronchial tubes. The HFPPV technique described above for sleeve pneumonectomy has also been successfully used for carinal resections with pericardial patch and very low (distal) tracheal resections [82]. In contradistinction to these findings with HFPPV, HFOV delivered through a standard single-lumen tube has been found to cause disturbing changes in the diameter of large airways and a large 'mediastinal bounce' with each oscillation that "made surgery on the major airways and around the hilum and mediastinal structures almost impossible" [85].

At the present time, continued investigation in the use of HFV to facilitate carinal surgery still seems warranted, since older techniques for providing ventilation for major conducting airway surgery leave a great deal to be desired. Previous techniques used with sleeve pneumonectomy after incision of the airway have included use of a conventional double-lumen endotracheal tube, advancing a single-lumen endotracheal tube through the end of the opened trachea into the appropriate main-stem bronchus, or using a separate sterile endobronchial tube through the operative field with a second sterile anesthesia circuit. Since repeated endobronchial intubation and extubation are necessary during construction of the posterior portion of the anastomosis, the technique is cumbersome and requires alternating periods of apnea and ventilation, which may result in poor gas exchange [86–89].

The second type of airway surgery aided by HFV is tracheal reconstruction supported by tracheal Montgomery T-tube. The Montgomery T-tube has two intratracheal limbs (the proximal limb faces the glottis, and the distal limb faces the tracheal carina) and one extratracheal limb which exits from the trachea through a neck incision to the environment. In one approach, the HFPPV catheter passed straight down through the two intratracheal limbs and gas outflow was via the extratracheal limb [83]. Alternatively, the HFPPV catheter can be introduced through the extratracheal limb and gently flexed downward to direct the catheter to lie above the carina.

Previously it was difficult to establish an adequate airway for the administration of conventional IPPV with conventional cuffed tracheotomy tubes using the tracheal Montgomery T-tubes [90,91]. The use of the extratracheal limb as an airway for the delivery of large tidal volume IPPV was associated with a large gas leak through the open proximal intratracheal limb. In order to establish adequate ventilation with conventional IPPV the superior part of the proximal intratracheal limb had to be occluded by a Fogerty embolectomy catheter (introduced through the extratracheal limb) and by a tight pharyngeal pack (introduced through the oral cavity) in order to prevent escape of the tidal volume through the open glottis. IPPV has also been administered to a pediatric patient through the proximal intratracheal limb of the tracheal T-tube; the proximal intratracheal limb was intubated with a Cole tube and then the extratracheal limb was occluded to allow the use of IPPV [92]. These previous conventional IPPV maneuvers and techniques are cumbersome, difficult to apply, and can be dangerous. Blockage of the various T-tube limbs can, for example, occur suddenly and totally obstruct the airway and prevent alveolar ventilation. In addition, use of these IPPV techniques can impair surgical access and complicate the surgery.

The third type of airway surgery aided by HFV is resection of a tracheal stenosis. In one report a small HFPPV insufflating catheter was inserted through a single-lumen endotracheal tube, which lay above the tracheal stenosis, until the distal end of the HFPPV catheter was beyond the tracheal stenosis [84]. Thus, tracheal resection and end-to-end anastomosis could be accomplished easily around the small catheter. This method has the obvious drawback that the relation between the tracheal stenosis and insufflation catheter must permit a sufficiently large passage for exhalation; the passage must be guaranteed at every moment of the surgical procedure [90].

4.4. Use in bronchopleural fistula

The second proposed advantage HFV has for thoracic surgery is that the lower inspiratory pressures and tidal volumes may result in a smaller gas leak through pathologic low-resistance pathways such as bronchopleural fistulae and tracheobronchial disruptions. Consequently, air leaks (loss of tidal volume) and mediastinal and interstitial emphysema may be minimized with this form of ventilatory treatment, and HFJV has been successfully used in the treatment of major bronchopleural fistula [93–98] and tracheobronchial disruptions [79,99,100]. In most cases of bronchopleural fistula, P_aCO_2 was unacceptably high despite a high minute ventilation on volume-controlled IPPV, whereas HFJV restored normocarbia. However, it appears that the reduction in air leak flow through the fistula is directly related to reduced airway pressure with HFV compared to conventional mechanical ventilation; when peak and mean tracheal pressure are decreased by HFV, fistula leak is decreased, and when peak and mean tracheal pressures are increased by HFV, fistula flow increases [96–98]. Thus, in a series of seven consecutive patients with an average bronchopleural fistula leak of greater than 5 l/min, HFJV (125–150/min) caused only two patients to have clinically important decreases in airway pressure and air leak fistula flow, and none had significant improvement in gas exchange [96]. The authors recommend measurement of tracheal pressures to predict what is happening to air leak fistula flow [96]. In one case of bronchopleural-cutaneous fistula [93], intraoperative differential lung ventilation, consisting of conventional IPPV for the normal dependent lung and HFJV for the diseased nondependent lung, was used. HFV has been used prophylactically to prevent the development of a bronchopleural fistula in a patient who had a very friable bronchial stump due to mucormycosis (an opportunistic pulmonary parenchymal infection which occurs in immunocompromised hosts and diabetics, and is associated with a high incidence of postoperative bronchopleural fistula) [101]. HFPPV and HFOV have been successfully used in dogs with bilateral upper lobe bronchopleural fistulas [102], but these two types of HFV have not been used in humans with a bronchopleural fistula. In cases of tracheobronchial disruptions, mediastinal and interstitial emphysema was felt to be minimized by the use of HFV [79,96,100].

The previous methods of trying to make conventional IPPV more effective in the presence of pathologic low-resistance airway pathways (in addition to using a very large tidal volume) all have major drawbacks. Insertion of unidirectional valves in chest tubes, which seat during inspiration, frequently malfunction due to interference by blood and pus within the chest tube [103]. Application of positive counterpressure to the pleural space during inspiration causes hemodynamic interference [103]. Collapse of the diseased lung with the aid of a double-lumen tube for a prolonged period of time requires very careful monitoring, is technically difficult for the non-anesthesia intensive care unit personnel not trained in the use of double-lumen tubes, and predisposes the collapsed lung to infection [103]. Thus, it is likely that investigations in the use of high-frequency ventilation to treat patients with pathologic low-resistance airway pathways will continue.

4.5. Use in minimizing movement of the operative field

The third proposed advantage for HFV for thoracic surgery is to minimize the tidal movement of the operative field; theoretically, the lower peak inspiratory pressures and tidal volumes of HFV should result in much smaller inflation and deflation movements of the lung. Therefore, HFV of the nondependent lung might provide a relatively 'quiet' operative lung field and HFV of the dependent lung could contribute to the 'quiet' lung field by providing a minimally moving mediastinum. In four reports [85,105–107] HFPPV was used to ventilate both the nondependent and the dependent lung during thoracic surgery. With the chest open, the nondependent lung had minimal ventilation-synchronous movements and limited lung expansion, but still had good aeration and no atelectasis. However, hyperinflation of the lungs occurred in some patients with chronic obstructive pulmonary disease, presumably due to air trapping, and resulted in poor operating conditions [107]. In patients who did not experience hyperinflation, operating conditions for peripheral lung procedures were adequate. Arterial blood gases, analyzed frequently in most reports, showed adequate oxygenation and carbon dioxide removal during HFV despite some brief periods of significant nondependent-lung compression by the surgeons. In one report, HFJV was successfully used at 3 Hz to ventilate both lungs, but carbon dioxide retention became a problem at 6 and 12 Hz [108]. During HFPPV the airways could be suctioned without interrupting ventilation. At the conclusion of surgery the nondependent lung fully re-expanded as readily as with conventional techniques. Finally, in one report the dependent lung was selectively ventilated with an HFV flow interrupter (while the operated lung was completely collapsed) [109]. Compared to selective dependent lung IPPV, selective dependent-lung HFV significantly improved arterial oxygenation, presumably because of lower dependent-lung pulmonary vascular resistance (due to either lower dependent-lung airway pressures [57] or release of dependent-lung vasodilator prostaglandins [58]) and enhanced operating conditions (owing to minimal mediastinal movements). In addition, deflation of the dependent-lung endobronchial tube cuff further improved arterial oxygenation owing to overflow of gases from the dependent lung to the nondependent lung, which resulted in recruitment of part of the collapsed lung in gas exchange.

Unfortunately, in none of these reports was the use of HFV compared with conventional one-lung ventilation, with or without nondependent lung CPAP, in terms of operating conditions and efficiency of gas exchange. Since operating conditions and gas exchange are usually excellent with one-lung ventilation and nondependent-lung CPAP, it is unlikely that comparative studies will show much improvement with HFV. In addition, the use of HFV to minimize mediastinal and hilar movements must remain controversial in view of the most recent report describing a mediastinal 'bounce' with each oscillation that made surgery around these structures nearly impossible [85].

In summary, the favorable aspects about HFV for thoracic surgery are adequate pulmonary gas exchange (and, perhaps, increased diversion of blood flow away from the atelectatic lung during ventilation of just the dependent lung) [57,58], good conditions for peripheral lung surgery, possibly good conditions for major airway conducting surgery, possibly improved gas exchange in cases of bronchopleural fistula, and possibly decreased mediastinal and pulmonary interstitial emphysema in cases of tracheobronchial disruption. As previously mentioned, the first two of these favorable aspects, in the context of the availability of one-lung ventilation, seem superfluous and unnecessary. The unfavorable aspects of high-frequency ventilation for thoracic surgery are possibly unsatisfactory surgical conditions for mediastinal and major airway surgery, hyperinflation in patients with chronic obstructive pulmonary disease, use of a new and possibly complicated technology, difficulty in monitoring heart and breath sounds with an esophageal stethoscope, inability to judge the adequacy of ventilation from the motion of the chest wall or lungs, use of high flows of anesthetic gases, and difficulty in assessing lung volume.

Hence, at the present time, the exact role of HFV in thoracic surgery is uncertain. I am certain, however, that the use of HFV as a routine procedure in thoracic surgery cannot be recommended at the present time.

5. REPLACEMENT OF FLUID AND BLOOD LOSS

5.1. Minimal blood loss (< 10% of blood volume): amount of crystalloid fluid infusion

The amount of crystalloid infused during pulmonary resections, particularly during pneumonectomy, requires special consideration. On the one hand, as for any major operation, insensible fluid, nasogastric and urine fluid, extracellular (third space) wound fluid, and blood losses (less than 10% of blood volume) should be replaced by crystalloid infusion. Failure to do so results in unacceptable hemodynamic depression due to anesthetic drugs and positive pressure ventilation, inability to tolerate any further sudden loss of blood, cardiovascular lability with changes in anesthetic depth and surgical stimulation, and oliguria.

However, there are both experimental [110] and clinical [111,112] data suggesting that overinfusion of fluids during pneumonectomy may be particularly hazardous with regard to the development of postpneumonectomy pulmonary edema. There are two inter-related reasons why pneumonectomy may predispose to the formation of pulmonary edema. First, a decreased amount of pulmonary vascular bed has to accommodate all of the cardiac output. On one hand, it has been clearly shown that if the remaining pulmonary vascular bed is normal, then pneumonectomy does not cause an increase in pulmonary extravascular fluid, even if left atrial pressure is deliberately increased to 25 mmHg [113]. If the remaining pulmonary vascular bed is non-distensible (diseased), the cardiac output is greatly increased (as it may be in the early stress-ridden postoperative period), and/or excessive fluids were infused intraoperatively, pulmonary hypertension may occur and cause transmembrane transudation of fluid [112]. Second, pneumonectomy results in removal of half of the lymphatics responsible for clearing pulmonary interstitial fluid. The loss of parenchymal/hilar/mediastinal lymphatic drainage routes, with all other considerations equal, may cause lymphatic clearance thresholds to be more easily exceeded, increasing the risk of pulmonary interstitial fluid accumulation and pulmonary edema.

Postpneumonectomy pulmonary edema has been thought to occur in a few patients [111,112]. The risk factors for this complication appear to be high(er) peri-operative volume of infused fluid, repeat thoracotomy, and right pneumonectomy, leaving a smaller left lung to cope with the entire cardiac output and, perhaps, higher pulmonary vascular pressures. However, as mentioned previously, simple resection of a single lung and minimal to moderate increases in hydrostatic pressure are not likely to be the sole cause of postresection pulmonary edema in patients with relatively normal hearts and remaining lungs [113], and it may be necessary to also have some factor present that disposes the patient toward edema (pre-existing pulmonary vascular disease, very high cardiac outputs, acute injury to the permeability barrier-sepsis, bronchopneumonia or trauma) in order for postpneumonectomy pulmonary edema and the adult respiratory distress syndrome to develop.

In summary, because of the smaller pulmonary vascular bed remaining after resection and the interruption of lymphatic drainage, it is reasonable to consider the possibility that patients undergoing pneumonectomy are at greater risk for the development of pulmonary edema from aggressive intravenous fluid administration than other types of surgery patients, especially if the heart and/or the remaining lung is diseased. A reasonable approach would be to start out with infusing 10 ml/kg during the first hour (mainly to make up insensible losses and minimize cardiovascular depression due to anesthesia) and 5 ml/kg/h thereafter with adjustments made according to the estimated blood loss and cardiovascular responses. If pulmonary edema should develop postoperatively, mechanical ventilation with sufficient PEEP to reduce the F_IO_2 to non-toxic levels should be instituted [114]. Next, a thorough search for a septic focus is warranted; if one is found, it should be promptly removed or drained after appropriate antibiotic therapy has been instituted [114]. Third, and most vital, one should measure pulmonary vascular pressures and examine both right and left ventricles for evidence of failure or overload, which, if present, must be treated with inotropic drugs, diuretics and volume restriction [114]. In cases of extreme right ventricular afterloading, it may be appropriate to assess right ventricular performance by either radioisotopic scanning or thermodilution ejection fractions [115].

5.2. Moderate blood loss (10%–20% of total blood volume): should blood be infused?

The generally accepted safe lower limit of hemoglobin is 10 g/dl. If a patient started out with a normal hemoglobin level of 14 g/dl, a level of 10 g/dl represents a loss of about 28% of the oxygen-carrying capacity of the blood. Thus, blood losses of less than 20% of the blood volume can safely be replaced with non-sanguinous fluids, even with a reasonable margin of error in either the estimation of blood loss or replacement [116]. In addition, in view of the known potentially lethal viral diseases that can be transmitted by blood infusion (hepatitis, acquired immune deficiency syndrome), and the possibility of anaphylactic, hemolytic and febrile reactions [117], it certainly behooves the anesthesiologist to avoid blood transfusion to patients who are initially normal from a cardiovascular point of view when losses are less than 20% of the total blood volume. Concentrations of hemoglobin below 10 g/dl may be accompanied by a progressive increase in the bleeding time [118], and decreases below 9 g/dl require an increased cardiac output to maintain oxygen transport [119]. However, if the cardiac output does not increase, as may be the situation during anesthesia, and the decrease in hemoglobin concentration is large, then anaerobic metabolism and a lactic acidosis may ensue.

Recently, new immunologic and cancer growth data have emerged that reinforce and further support the notion that blood transfusion should be avoided whenever blood loss is less than 20% of the total blood volume and the patient is hemodynamically stable [120–125]. These studies indicate that perioperative blood transfusion is an important immunosuppressant and that immunosuppression may favor growth of cancer [120]. The increased survival of renal allografts following transfusion of whole blood or packed red blood cells indicates that the blood transfusion prior to renal allograft transplant caused immunosuppression. Furthermore, immunosuppressed patients in general are at increased risk for the development of various malignant tumors. For example, it has been found that perioperative blood transfusion is associated with decreased survival of patients undergoing resection for colon and breast cancer due to recurrent or metastatic growths [121–123].

It now appears, based on two new studies, that intraoperative blood transfusion during non-oat cell lung cancer resection is also associated with decreased survival due to cancer recurrence [124,125]. In one study [125], 155 patients undergoing resection for lung carcinoma were analyzed retrospectively, and it was shown that the use of blood transfusion was associated with a significant decrease in survival time in patients undergoing curative resection of lung carcinoma despite multivariate adjustments for age, sex, cell type, right lung versus left lung location, type of operation and stage of cancer. In the other study [124], surgical technique-related variables were minimized by limiting the study to one surgeon. Analysis of age, sex, tumor size, histopathology, admission and discharge hematocrit values, estimated operative blood loss, duration of operation, extent of resection, anesthetic agents, and blood transfusion revealed two significant prognostic factors: extent of resection and use or non-use of transfusions. Transfused patients had lower disease-free rates within five years than non-transfused patients. The results of both of these studies indicate that perioperative blood transfusion of patients with lung cancer undergoing resection accelerates the appearance of recurrent or metastatic cancer. The findings are consistent with the hypothesis that blood transfusion, possibly through an immunosuppressive mechanism, is responsible for a poorer prognosis in patients who undergo resection for carcinoma of the lung.

REFERENCES

1 Urschel Jr HC, Razzuk MA. Median sternotomy as a standard approach for pulmonary resection. Ann Thorac Surg 1986; 41: 130–134.

2 Boysen PG. Pulmonary resection and postoperative pulmonary function. Chest 1980; 77: 718–719.

3 Boysen PG, Block AG, Moulder PV. Relationship between preoperative pulmonary function tests and complications after thoracotomy. Surg Gynecol Obstet 1981; 152: 813–815.

4 Simpson PM. Tracheal intubation with a Robertshaw tube via a tracheotomy. Br J Anaesth 1976; 48: 373–375.

5 Seed RF, Wiley JR. Tracheal intubation with a Robertshaw tube via a tracheotomy [letter]. Br J Anaesth 1977; 49: 639.

6 Smith G, Hirsch N, Ehrenwerth J. Sight and sound: Can double-lumen endotracheal tubes be placed accurately without fiber optic bronchoscopy? Anesth Analg 1986; 65: S1–S170.
7 Read RC, Friday CD, Eason CN. Prospective study of the Robertshaw endobronchial catheter in thoracic surgery. Ann Thorac Surg 1977; 24: 156.
8 Alfery DD, Benumof JL, Spragg RG. Anesthesia for bronchopulmonary lavage. In: Kaplan J (ed.). Thoracic Anesthesia. New York, Churchill-Livingstone 1982: pp 403–419.
9 Sprang RG, Benumof JL, Alfery DD. New methods for performance of unilateral lung lavage. Anesthesiology 1982; 57: 535–538.
10 Benumof JL, Pirlo AF, Trousdale FR. Inhibition of hypoxic pulmonary vasoconstriction by decreased $P_{\bar{v}}O_2$: A new indirect mechanism. J Appl Physiol 1981; 51: 871–874.
11 Johansen I, Benumof JL. Flow distribution in abnormal lung as a function of F_IO_2. Anesthesiology 1979; 51: 369 (abstract).
12 Dantzker DR, Wagner PD, West JB. Instability of lung units with low V/Q ratios during O_2 breathing. J Appl Physiol 1975; 38: 886–895.
13 Lumb TD, Silvay G, Weinreich AI, Shiang W. A comparison of the effects of continuous ketamine infusion and halothane on oxygenation during one lung anesthesia in dogs. Can Anaesth Soc J 1979; 26: 394–401.
14 Scanlon TS, Benumof JL, Wahrenbrock EA, Nelson WL. Hypoxic pulmonary vasoconstriction and the ratio of hypoxic lung to perfused normoxic lung. Anesthesiology 1978; 49: 177–181.
15 Winter PM, Smith G. The toxicity of oxygen. Anesthesiology 1972; 37: 210–241.
16 Kerr JH. Physiological aspects of one lung (endobronchial) anesthesia. Int Anesth Clin 1972; 10(4): 61–78.
17 Benumof JL, Rogers SN, Moyce PR, Berryhill RE, Wahrenbrock EA, Saidman LJ. Hypoxic pulmonary vasoconstriction and whole-lung PEEP in the dog. Anesthesiology 1979; 51: 503–507.
18 Katz JA, Laverne RG, Fairley HB, Thomas AN. Pulmonary oxygen exchange during endobronchial anesthesia: Effects of tidal volume and PEEP, Anesthesiology 1982; 56: 164–171.
19 Finley TN, Hill TR, Bonica JJ. Effect of intrapleural pressure on pulmonary shunt to atelectatic dog lung. Am J Physiol 1963; 205: 1187–1192.
20 Flacke JW, Thompson DS, Read RC. Influence of tidal volume and pulmonary artery occlusion on arterial oxygenation during endobronchial anesthesia. South Med J 1976; 69: 619–626.
21 Bachand RR, Audet J, Meloche R, et al. Physiological changes associated with unilateral pulmonary ventilation during operations on one lung. Can Anaesth Soc J 1975; 22: 659–664.
22 Kerr J, Smith AC, Prys-Roberts C, et al. Observations during endobronchial anesthesia, I. Ventilation and carbon dioxide clearance. Br J Anaesth 1973; 45: 159–267.
23 Hatch D. Ventilation and arterial oxygenation during thoracic surgery. Thorax 1966; 21: 310–314.
24 Benumof JL, Wahrenbrock EA. Blunted hypoxic pulmonary vasoconstriction by increased lung vascular pressures. J Appl Physiol 1975; 38: 846–850.
25 Benumof JL, Mathers JM, Wahrenbrock EA. Cyclic hypoxic pulmonary vasoconstriction induced by concomitant carbon dioxide changes. J Appl Physiol 1976; 41: 466–469.
26 Tarhan S, Lundborg RO. Effects of increased expiratory pressure on blood gas tensions and pulmonary shunting during thoracotomy with use of the Carlens catheter. Can Anaesth Soc J 1970; 17: 4–11.
27 Khanam T, Branthwaite MA. Arterial oxygenation during one-lung anesthesia (2), Anaesthesia 1973; 23: 280–290.
28 Aalto-Setala M, Heinonen J, Salorinne Y: Cardiorespiratory function during thoracic anesthesia: Comparison of two-lung ventilation and one-lung ventilation with and without PEEP. Acta Anaesthesiol Scand 1975; 19: 287–295.
29 Capan LM, Turndorf H, Chandrakant P, Ramanathan S, Acinapura A, Shalon J. Optimization of arterial oxygenation during one-lung anesthesia. Anesth Analg 1980; 59: 847–851.
30 Rehder K, Wenthe FM, Sessler AD. Function of each lung during mechanical ventilation with ZEEP and PEEP in man anesthetized with thiopental-meperidine. Anesthesiology 1973; 39: 597–606.

31 Brown RD, Kafer RED, Roberson VO, Wilcox BR, Murray GF. Improved oxygenation during thoracotomy with selective PEEP to the dependent lung. Anesth Analg 1977; 56: 26–31.
32 Eisenkraft JB, Thys DM, Cohen E, Kaplan JA. Hemodynamic effects of CPAP and PEEP during one-lung anesthesia with isoflurane, Anesthesiology 1984; 61: A520.
33 Cohen E, Thys DM, Eisenkraft JB, Kirschner PA, Kaplan JA. Effect of CPAP and PEEP during one-lung anesthesia: Left versus right thoracotomies. Anesthesiology 1985; 63: A564.
34 Cohen E, Thys DM, Eisenkraft JB, Kaplan JA. PEEP during one-lung anesthesia improves oxygenation in patients with low arterial P_aO_2. Anesth Analg 1985; 64: 201.
35 Khanom T, Branthwaite MA. Arterial oxygenation during one-lung anesthesia (1): A study in man. Anaesthesia 1973; 28: 132–138.
36 Alfery DD, Benumof JL, Trousdale FR. Improving oxygenation during one-lung ventilation: The effects of PEEP and blood flow restriction to the nonventilated lung. Anesthesiology 1981; 55: 381–385.
37 Merridew CG, Jones RDM. Nondependent lung CPAP (5 cm H_2O) with oxygen during ketamine, halothane or isoflurane anesthesia and one-lung ventilation. Anesthesiology 1985; 63: A567.
38 Thiagarajah S, Job C, Rao A. A device for applying CPAP to the nonventilated upper lung during one lung ventilation, I. Anesthesiology 1984; 60: 253–254.
39 Hannenberg AA, Satwicz PR, Pienes Jr RS, O'Brien JC: A device for applying CPAP to the nonventilated upper lung during one lung ventilation, II. Anesthesiology 1984; 60: 254–255.
40 Brown DL, Davis RS. A simple device for oxygen insufflation with continuous positive airway pressure during one-lung ventilation. Anesthesiology 1984; 61: 481–482.
41 Rees DI, Wansbrough SR. One-lung anesthesia: Percent shunt and arterial oxygen tension during continuous insufflation of oxygen to the nonventilated lung. Anesth Analg 1982; 61: 507–512.
42 Wilks D, Schumann T, Riley R, Klain M, Freeman J. Selective high frequency jet ventilation of the operative lung improves oxygenation during thoracic surgery. Anesthesiology 1985; 63: A568.
43 Benjaminsson E, Klain N. Intraoperative dual-mode independent lung ventilation of a patient with bronchopleural fistula. Anesth Analg (Cleveland) 1981; 60: 118–119.
44 Carlon GC, Kahn R, Howland WS, Baron R, Ramaker J. Acute life threatening ventilation–perfusion inequality: An indication for independent lung ventilation. Crit Care Med 1978; 6: 380–383.
45 Venus B, Pratap KS, Op'Tholt T: Treatment of unilateral pulmonary insufficiency by selective administration of continuous positive airway pressure through a double-lumen tube. Anesthesiology 1980; 52: 74–77.
46 Power DJ, Eross B, Grenvik A. Differential lung ventilation with PEEP in the treatment of unilateral lung ventilation. Crit Care Med 1977; 5: 170–172.
47 Gallagher TJ, Banner MJ, Smith RA. A simplified method of independent lung ventilation. Crit Care Med 1980; 8: 396–398.
48 Glass DD, Tonnesen AD, Gabel JC, Arens JF. Therapy of unilateral pulmonary insufficiency with a double-lumen endotracheal tube. Crit Care Med 1976; 4: 323–326.
49 Trew F, Warren BR, Potter WA. Differential lung ventilation in man. Crit Care Med 1976; 4: 112.
50 Rafferty TD, Palma J, Motoyama EK, Schachter N, Ciarcia F. Management of a bronchopleural fistula with differential lung ventilation and positive end-expiratory pressure. Respir Care 1980; 25: 654–657.
51 Rivara D, Bourgaim L, Rieuf P, Harf A, Lemaire F. Differential ventilation in unilateral lung disease: Effects of respiratory mechanics and gas exchange. Intensive Care Med 1979; 5: 189–191.
52 Ray C, Carlon GC, Miodownik S, Glodiner PL. A method of synchronizing two MA-1 ventilators for independent lung ventilation. Crit Care Med 1978; 6: 99.
53 Parish JM, Gracey DR, Southorn PA, Pairolero PA, Wheeler JT. Differential mechanical ventilation in respiratory failure due to severe unilateral lung disease. Mayo Clin Proc 1984; 59: 822.
54 Murray JF. Treatment of acute total atelectasis: Use of a double-lumen tube. Anaesthesia 1985; 40: 158–162.

55 Stow PJ, Grant I. Asynchronous independent lung ventilation: Its use in the treatment of acute unilateral lung disease, Anaesthesia 1985; 40: 163–166.
56 Hillman KM, Barber JD. Asynchronous independent lung ventilation (AILV). Crit Care Med 1980; 8: 390–395.
57 Hall SM, Strawn WB, Levitsky MG. Effect of high-frequency oscillation on blood flow to an atelectatic lung in closed-chested dogs. Crit Care Med 1984; 12: 447–451.
58 Wetzel RC, Gordon JB, Gregory TJ, et al. High-frequency ventilation attenuation of hypoxic pulmonary vasoconstriction. Am Rev Resp Dis 1985; 132: 99–103.
59 Gillespie DJ. High-frequency ventilation: A new concept in mechanical ventilation. Mayo Clin Proc 1983; 58: 187–196.
60 O'Rourke PP, Crone RK: High-frequency ventilation: A new approach to respiratory support. JAMA 1983; 250: 2845–2847.
61 Fredberg JJ. Augmented diffusion in the airways can support pulmonary gas exchange. J Appl Physiol 1980; 49: 232–238.
62 Eriksson I. The role of conducting airways in gas exchange during high frequency ventilation – a clinical and theoretical analysis. Anesth Analg 1982; 61: 483–489.
63 Haselton FR, Scherer PW. Bronchial bifurcations and respiratory mass transport. Science 1980; 208: 69–71.
64 Slutsky AS, Bronw R, Lehr J, et al. High-frequency ventilation: A promising new approach to mechanical ventilation. Med Instrum 1981; 15: 229–233.
65 Kolton M, Cattran CB, Kent G, et al. Oxygenation during high-frequency ventilation compared with conventional mechanical ventilation in two models of lung injury. Anesth Analg 1982; 61: 323–332.
66 Sjostrand UH, Smith RB. Overview of high-frequency ventilation. Int Anesth Clin 1983; 21(3): 1–10.
67 Sjostrand U. High-frequency positive-pressure ventilation (HFPPV): A review. Crit Care Med 1980; 8: 345–364.
68 Carlon GC, Howland WS, Ray C, et al. High frequency jet ventilation: A prospective randomized evaluation. Chest 1983; 84: 551–559.
69 Bohn DJ, Marchak BE, Thompson WK, et al. Ventilation by high-frequency oscillation. J Appl Physiol 1980; 48: 710–716.
70 Lunkenheimer PP, Rafflenbeul W, Keller H, et al. Application of transtracheal pressure oscillations as a modification of diffusion respiration. Brit J Anaesth 1972; 44: 627.
71 Klain M, Smith RB. High frequency percutaneous transtracheal jet ventilation. Crit Care Med 1977; 5: 280–287.
72 Butler WJ, Bohn DJ, Bryan AC, et al. Ventilation by high frequency oscillation in humans. Anesth Analg 1980; 59: 577–584.
73 Heijman K, Heijman L, Jonzon A, et al. High frequency positive pressure ventilation during anesthesia and routine surgery in man. Acta Anaesth Scand 1972; 16: 176–187.
74 Heijman L, Nilsson L, Sjostrand U. High frequency positive pressure ventilation (HFPPV) in neonates and infants during neuroleptal analgesia and routine plastic surgery, and in postoperative management. Acta Anaesth Scand Suppl 1977; 64: 111–121.
75 Carlon GC, Klain M, Kalla R, et al. High frequency positive pressure ventilation in acute respiratory failure. Crit Care Med 1979; 7: 128.
76 Lyrene RK, Wright K, Standaert TA, et al. Rapid oscillation low volume ventilation in oleic acid induced pulmonary disease. Am Rev Respir Dis 1980; 121: 294.
77 Flatau E, Barzilay E, Kaufmann N, et al. Adult respiratory distress syndrome treated with high frequency positive pressure ventilation. Israel J Med Sci 1981; 17: 453–456.
78 Carlon GC, Ray CJ, Pierri MK, et al. High frequency jet ventilation for prolonged respiratory support. Anesthesiology 1979; 51: S189.
79 Carlon GC, Ray Jr C, Pierri MK, et al. High frequency ventilation: Theoretical considerations and clinical observations. Chest 1982; 81: 350–354.

80 Carlon GC, Turnbull AD, Alexander JD, et al. High frequency jet ventilation during tracheal surgery. Crit Care Med 1981; 9: 163.

81 El-Baz N, El-Ganzouri A, Gottschalk W, et al. One-lung high-frequency positive-pressure ventilation for sleeve pneumonectomy: An alternative technique. Anesth Analg 1981; 60: 683–686.

82 El-Baz N, Jensik R, Faber P, et al. One-lung high frequency ventilation for tracheoplasty and bronchoplasty: A new technique. Ann Thorac Surg 1982; 34: 564–572.

83 El-Baz N, Holinger L, El-Ganzouri A, et al. High-frequency positive-pressure ventilation for tracheal reconstruction by tracheal T-tube. Anesth Analg 1982; 61: 796–800.

84 Eriksson I, Nilsson LG, Nordstrom S, et al. High-frequency positive-pressure ventilation (HFPPV) during transthoracic resection of tracheal stenosis and during peroperative bronchoscopic examination. Acta Anaesth Scand 1975; 19: 113–119.

85 Glenski JA, Crawford M, Rehder K. High-frequency, small-volume ventilation during thoracic surgery. Anesthesiology 1986; 64: 211–214.

86 Faber LP, Jensik RJ. The planning of tracheal surgery. Surg Clin North Am 1970; 50: 113–122.

87 Parrish CM, Jones R. Primary tracheal tumors. Am Surg 1960; 26: 95–98.

88 Geffin B, Bland J, Grillo HC. Anesthetic management of tracheal resection and reconstruction. Anesth Analg 1969; 48: 884–894.

89 Theman TE, Kerr JH, Nelems JM, et al. Carinal resection. A report of two cases and a description of the anesthetic technique. J Thorac Cardiovasc Surg 1976; 71: 314–320.

90 Fredrickson JM. Reinforced T-tube tracheal stent. Arch Otolaryngol 1969; 90: 120–123.

91 Montgomery WW. Manual of care of the Montgomery silicone tracheal T-tube. Ann Otol Thinol Laryngol (Suppl 73) 1980; 89: 1–8.

92 Rah KH, Griffith III RL, Jones JR, et al. Anesthetic management of the pediatric patient with a tracheal T-tube. Anesth Analg 1981; 60: 445–447.

93 Benjaminsson E, Klain N. Intraoperative dual-mode independent lung ventilation of a patient with bronchopleural fistula. Anesth Analg 1981; 60: 118–119.

94 Carlon GC, Ray Jr C, Klain M, et al. High frequency positive pressure ventilation in management of a patient with bronchopleural fistula. Anesthesiology 1980; 52: 160–162.

95 Derderian SS, Rajagopal KR, Abbrecht PH, et al. High frequency positive pressure jet ventilation in bilateral bronchopleural fistulae. Crit Care Med 1982; 10: 119–121.

96 Albelda SM, Hanson-Flaschen JH, Taylor E, Lanken PN, Wollman H: Evaluation of high-frequency jet ventilation in patients with bronchopleural fistulas by quantitation of the airleak, Anesthesiology 1985; 63: 551–554.

97 Holzapfel L, Robert D, Lenoir B, Mercatello A, Palmier B, Perrin F, Bertoye A. High-frequency jet ventilation compared with conventional ventilation in patients with acute respiratory failure. Chest 1982; 32: 211 (abstract).

98 Ritz R, Benson M, Bishop MJ. Measuring gas leakage from bronchopleural fistulas during high-frequency jet ventilation. Crit Care Med 1984; 12: 836–837.

99 Carlon GC, Kahn RC, Howland WS, et al. Clinical experience with high frequency jet ventilation. Crit Care Med 1981; 9: 1–6.

100 Turnbull AD, Carlon GC, Howland WS, et al. High frequency jet ventilation in major airways or pulmonary disruption. Ann Thorac Surg 1981; 32: 468–474.

101 Fuhrman T, Reines HD, Kratz J. The use of high frequency jet ventilation in a patient with pulmonary mucormycosis. Anesthesiol Rev 1986; 13: 31–32.

102 Sjostrand UH, Smith B, Hoff BH, et al. Conventional and high-frequency ventilation in dogs with bronchopleural fistula. Crit Care Med 1985; 13: 191–193.

103 Downs JB, Chapman RL. Treatment of bronchopleural fistula during continuous positive pressure ventilation. Chest 1976; 69: 363–366.

104 Kirby RR. Ventilatory support and pulmonary barotrauma, Anesthesiology 1979; 50: 181–182.

105 Malina JF, Nordstrom SG, Sjostrand UH, et al. Clinical evaluation of high-frequency positive-pressure ventilation (HFPPV) in patients scheduled for open-chest surgery. Anesth Analg 1981; 60: 324–330.

106 Smith RB, Hoff BH, Rosen L, et al. High frequency ventilation during pulmonary lobectomy – three cases. Respir Care 1981; 26: 437–441.

107 Sjostrand UH, Wattwil LM, Borg UR, et al. Volume-controlled HFPPV as a useful mode of ventilation during open-chest surgery – a report on three cases. Respir Care 1982; 27: 1380–1385.

108 Seki S, Fukushima Y, Goto K, et al. Facilitation of intrathoracic operations by means of high-frequency ventilation. J Thorac Cardiovasc Surg 1983; 86: 388–392.

109 El-Baz N, Kittle CF, Faber LP, et al. High-frequency ventilation with an uncuffed endobronchial tube. J Thorac Cardiovasc Surg 1982; 84: 823–838.

110 Little AG, Lagmuir VK, Singer AH, Skinner DB. Hemodynamic pulmonary edema in dogs' lungs after contralateral pneumonectomy and mediastinal lymphatic interruption. Lung 1984; 162: 139–145.

111 Zeldin RA, Normandin D, Landtwing D, Peters RM. Postpneumonectomy pulmonary edema. J Thorac Cardiovasc Surg 1984; 87: 359–365.

112 Verheijen-Breemhaar L, et al. Post-pneumonectomy pulmonary edema. Thorax 1988; 43: 323–326.

113 Lee E, Little AG, Hsu WH, Skinner DB. Effect of pneumonectomy on extravascular lung water in dogs. J Surg Res 1985; 38: 568–573.

114 Zapol W. Commentary on postpneumonectomy pulmonary edema, Intellig. Rep. Anesth 1985; 2(4): 15.

115 Sibbald WJ, Driedger AA, Myers ML, Short AIK, Wells GA. Biventricular function in the adult respiratory distress syndrome. Chest 1983; 84: 126–134.

116 Sykes MK. Indications for blood transfusion. Can Anaesth Soc J 1975; 22: 3–11.

117 Pineda AA, Taswell HF, Brzica SM. Delayed hemolytic transfusion reaction; an immunologic hazard of blood transfusion, Transfusion 1978; 18: 1–7.

118 Anonymous. The bleeding time and the hematocrit (Editorial). Lancet 1984; 1: 997–998.

119 Gillies IDS. Anaemia and anesthesia. Br J Anaesth 1974; 46: 589–602.

120 Roth JA, Gollub EA, Grimm BA, Eilber MD, Morton DL. Effects of operation on immune response in cancer patients. Sequential evaluation of in vitro lymphocyte function. Surgery 1976; 79: 46–51.

121 Burrows L, Tartter PI. Effect of blood transfusions on chronic malignancy recurrence rate. Lancet 1982; II: 662.

122 Agarwal M, Blumber N. Colon cancer patients transfused perioperatively have an increased incidence of recurrence. Transfusion 1983; 24: 421 (abstract).

123 Tartter PI, Papatestas AE, Lesnick G, Burrows L, Aufses Jr AH. Perioperative blood transfusion has prognostic significance for breast cancer. Surgery 1985; 97: 225–230.

124 Tartter PI, Burrows L, Kirschner P. Perioperative blood transfusion adversely affects prognosis after resection of stage I (N0) non-oat cell lung cancer. J Thorac Cardiovasc Surg 1984; 88: 659–662.

125 Hyman N, Foster Jr RS, DeMeules JE, Costanza MC. Blood transfusion and survival after lung cancer. Am J Surg 1985; 149: 502–507.

Part V

Postoperative management

Current Topics in General Thoracic Surgery: An International Series, Vol. 2
Perioperative Care, edited by R.M. Peters and J. Toledo

Chapter 14

Chest drainage problems

E. Anyanwu and I. Vogt-Moykopf

1. INTRODUCTION

The basic concept of chest tube drainage is so fundamental that practically every physician should be in the position to handle it. Given the expanding frontiers of medical practice and the facultative increase in the use of chest tubes to solve certain categories of chest disease entities that are not primarily surgical, the problems which chest drainage presents shift from wrong indication to inadequate insertion techniques, traverses inadequate care and finally ends up in complications which compound the chest drainage problem. Ideally, chest drainage, when correctly employed, should cause no problems beyond inconvenience for the patient. If problems arise at all, they should be directly related to the illness requiring chest drainage. However, it is not always possible to avoid drainage problems, but they can be minimized by employing a drainage system one is conversant with. This system should be as basic and simple as possible, so as to enable others to familiarize themselves with it in the shortest possible time. Furthermore, it should have built-in safety devices to prevent a major complication in the chest should the system malfunction. The part of the system in direct contact with the patient should be tissue inert. The basic concept is to have a very effectively functioning system fulfill its mission in the shortest possible time. In this chapter we shall take a close look at the basic principle of closed chest drainage, recall the anatomy of the chest wall relevant for the insertion of chest tubes, the technique of chest tube insertion, indications for chest tube drainage, problems arising from faulty techniques, and problems met frequently in general thoracic surgical practice.

2. PRINCIPLES OF CHEST DRAINAGE

Classically, 'drainage' is understood to mean the guttering off of fluid out of place from a pre-existent or artificially created space. In our context it means the artificial

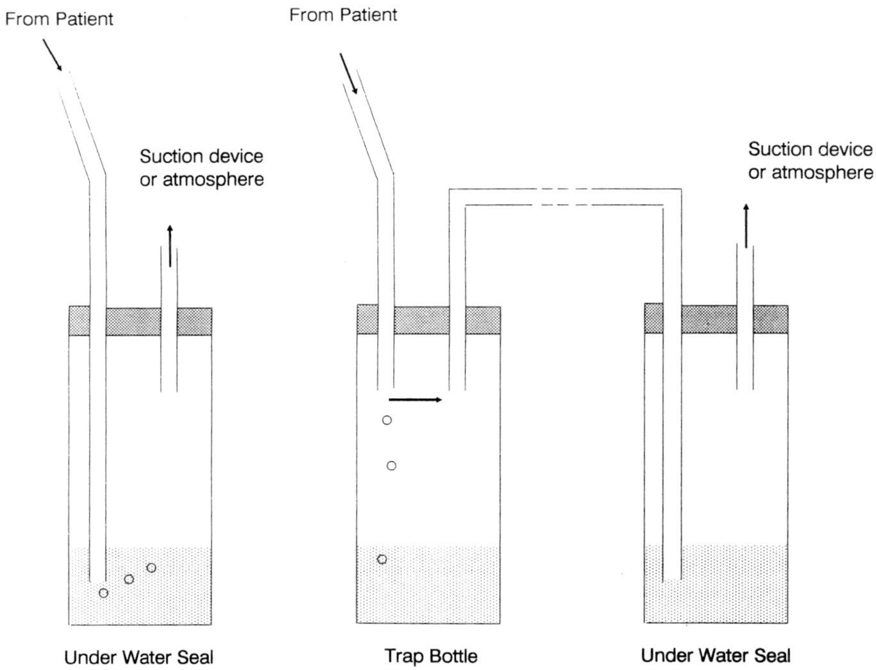

FIGURE 14.1. Chest drainage system for the treatment of pneumothorax without pleural effusion. (left) Air from the pleural cavity escapes with respiratory movements as the lung slowly expands, and bubbles through the water in the bottle. A suction device is always advised when the lung is relatively stiff. (right) A trap bottle is interposed between the patient and the suction device whenever fluid is evacuated from the pleural cavity. More than one bottle can be connected in series.

reintroduction of 'vacuum' in the pleural space – evacuation of matter capable of flowing from this space and reintroduction of negative pressure originally present there, inasmuch as the lung itself cannot take care of it. To achieve this, a rubber or more generally a plastic tubing is introduced into the pleural space and attached to a suction device, which may or may not have a pressure-regulating mechanism. The simplest form is the instantaneous suction of air introduced accidentally into the pleural space during median sternotomy for cardiac surgery or during paravertebral nerve block treatment. This presupposes the absence of concomitant pulmonary injury or pleural laceration and the absence of the pulmonary pathology, which would otherwise maintain the pulmonary collapse. If an instantaneous evacuation is not possible or desirable, the tube is led into an underwater seal, which is either attached to a suction pump or left at atmospheric pressure (Fig. 14.1). As the lung expands, air is dispelled from the pleural space, and this air escapes through the underwater seal. Where fluid is to be drained from the pleural cavity, a bottle trap is introduced between the patient and the underwater seal. This second bottle may be fitted with a manometer having an adjustable vent tube. Depending on the amount

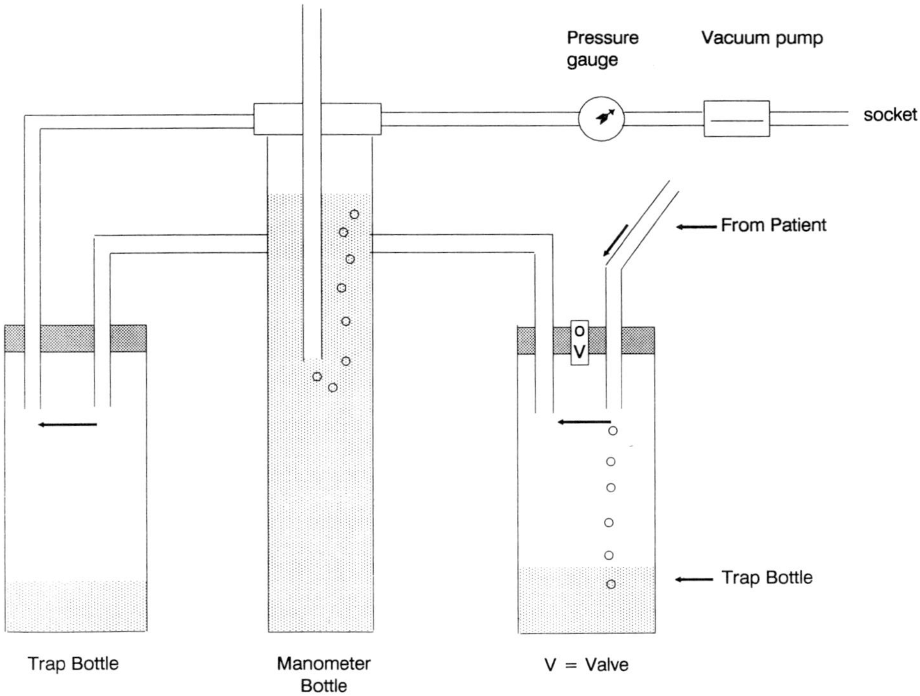

FIGURE 14.2. Chest drainage system. A manometer bottle is introduced between the suction device and the trap bottle(s). We favour this system which allows adjustment of the suction pressure and serves as underwater seal.

of fluid to be evacuated from the thoracic cavity, more than one trap bottle can be connected in series between the patient and thé underwater seal, alternatively between the patient and the suction device (Fig. 14.2).

3. ANATOMIC SITES FOR CHEST TUBE INSERTION

Ordinarily, the chest tube is inserted at the point where it is expected to function optimally. For pneumothorax the second intercostal space in the medioclavicular line is usually selected on the assumption that the air rises to the apex of the thoracic cavity. For a free flowing fluid in the pleural space the theoretically ideal position is the paravertebral gutter, the last opening in the tube flushing with the anticipated lowest fluid level during drainage. However, the anatomy of the chest and the convenience of the patient mostly militate against the placement of the catheter in this ideal position. Anatomically, the ribs run from the spine posterolaterally downwards and turn anteriorly upwards to join the sternum, and ribs 7–10 join at the costal margin before reaching the sternum. As a result of this anatomy the intercostal space is relatively narrow posteriorly and large anteriorly just proximal to the breast bone. While chest tubes placed posteriorly are prone to kinking and compression by the ribs with resultant reduction in effective internal diameter, placement anteriorly carries a higher risk of iatrogenic hemorrhage as a result of injury to the internal thoracic artery. The surgeon is caught between these two extremes in the region between the posterior axillary and the medioclavicular lines. Viewed from the outside, the chest tube must traverse the skin, the subcutaneous tissue, the intercostal musculature and the endothoracic fascia in that order before piercing through the parietal pleura to enter into the pleural space.

4. CHEST DRAINAGE TUBE INSERTION

To insert a chest tube, three techniques are fundamentally used: the trocar method, the method of blunt dissection and intraoperative placement.

4.1. The trocar method

For pneumothorax without pleural effusion a stab incision is made to correspond with the upper margin of the third rib. The trocar, which is usually made of stainless steel, is fitted into an outer cannula, the proximal end of which almost flushes with the tip of the trocar. Both instruments are firmly held in the hand and introduced through the stab incision. While applying light pressure and slightly rotating the instrument alternately clockwise and anticlockwise the pleural cavity is entered into. After withdrawing the trocar, the chest tube is passed through the cannula serving as a guide into the pleural cavity, and the guide is withdrawn over the tube, care being taken not to allow air into the pleural cavity. Before introducing the trocar, mattress sutures are placed to fix the tube in position. Some chest tubes have an integrated trocar serving as an introducer which is withdrawn when the tubes have been introduced into the pleural cavity.

4.2. The method of blunt dissection

In the blunt dissection method the stab incision is bluntly dissected with the scissors or an appropriate instrument, e.g. the Kelly clamp. Withdrawal of instrument is followed by exploration by the finger to control unmistakable entry into the pleural space and to lyse adhesions, should such be present. Finally the chest tube is introduced into the pleural cavity and fixed with a mattress suture placed previously. With the same technique chest tubes are inserted preferably in the fifth and sixth intercostal spaces in the region between the axillary line and medioclavicular line. Tube insertion in this area is also appropriate for the treatment of pneumothorax, pure pleural effusion or a combination of pneumothorax and pleural effusion.

TABLE 14.1
Indications for chest tube drainage

(1)	Non-traumatic spontaneous pneumothorax in the presence of underlying lung disease, e.g. emphysema, bullae, tuberculosis, malignancies
(2)	Traumatic pneumothorax (i) iatrogenic (ii) chest trauma – closed, open penetrating, with or without tension
(3)	Hemothorax: chest trauma, surgery, vascular injuries
(4)	Hematopneumothorax
(5)	Serothorax, e.g., pleural effusion accompanying cardiac disease, kidney failure, liver cirrhosis, malignancies (pleuritis carcinomatosa), mesotheliomas
(6)	Seropneumothorax
(7)	Chylothorax – spontaneous, traumatic, iatrogenic
(8)	Specific and unspecific pulmonary infections: Pneumonias with parapneumonic empyema Bronchopleural fistula
(9)	Tumors with bronchopleural fistulae
(10)	Oesophageal perforation. Boerhaave's syndrome

4.3. Intraoperative placement

In open thoracic surgery, the chest tube can be inserted directly under vision at any desired point on the anterior or posterolateral chest wall. Before close of sternotomies, substernal tubes are guided through stab incisions out of the retrosternal area.

5. INDICATIONS FOR CHEST TUBE DRAINAGE

The classical indications for chest tube drainage are spontaneous pneumothorax in the presence of underlying lung disease and traumatic pneumothorax very often combined with hemothorax. The dominance of cardiothoracic surgery over general thoracic surgery accounts for the high turnover of chest tubes in cardiac surgery. In the course of the invasion of body chambers either for therapeutic or diagnostic purposes pneumo- and hematothoraces arise. The indications for chest tube drainage have been widened to include these iatrogenic cases. Today the indications cover a wide range of thoracic complications of surgical and non-surgical illnesses (Table 14.1).

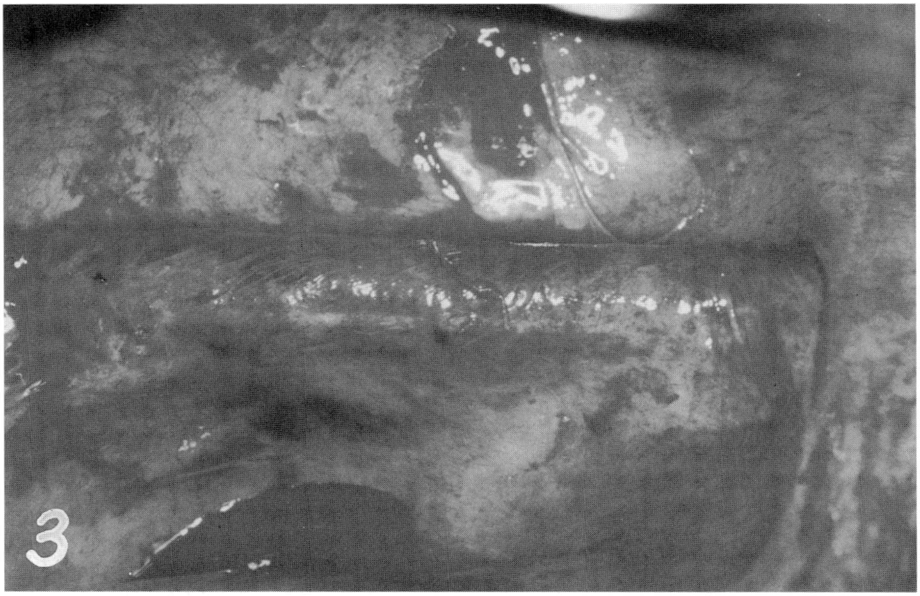

FIGURE 14.3. Placement of tube between the endothoracic fascia and the parietal pleura. Tube inserted in the 2nd intercostal space anteriorly in the medio-clavicular line.

6. COMPLICATIONS AND PROBLEMS ARISING FROM THE PLACEMENT OF CHEST TUBES

The most common problems arising from the insertion of the chest tube may or may not be noted immediately after the operation. Placement of the tube between the endothoracic fascia and the parietal pleura obtains mostly when the trocar method is used. As a result of incomplete perforation of the thoracic wall, the tip of the trocar easily dissects through the space between the endothoracic fascia and the parietal pleura (Fig. 14.3). A chest X-ray will mostly reveal the condition. Either abnormal location of the chest tube is observed or the lung does not expand despite adequate suction. In cases of pleural effusion no fluid is drained from the pleural space. Clinical conditions under which placement of the tube between the endothoracic fascia and the thoracoparietal pleura occur include pleural thickening that would otherwise warrant decortication and mesotheliomas. Anterior–posterior and lateral X-ray view of the chest will mostly delineate this condition from encapsulated effusion or empyema.

One of the most common problems encountered is the placement of the tube in the intrapleural fissure or in the space between the base of the lung and the diaphragm, thus reducing the functional adequacy of the chest tube. This occurs when pleural adhesions prevent proper placement of the tubes.

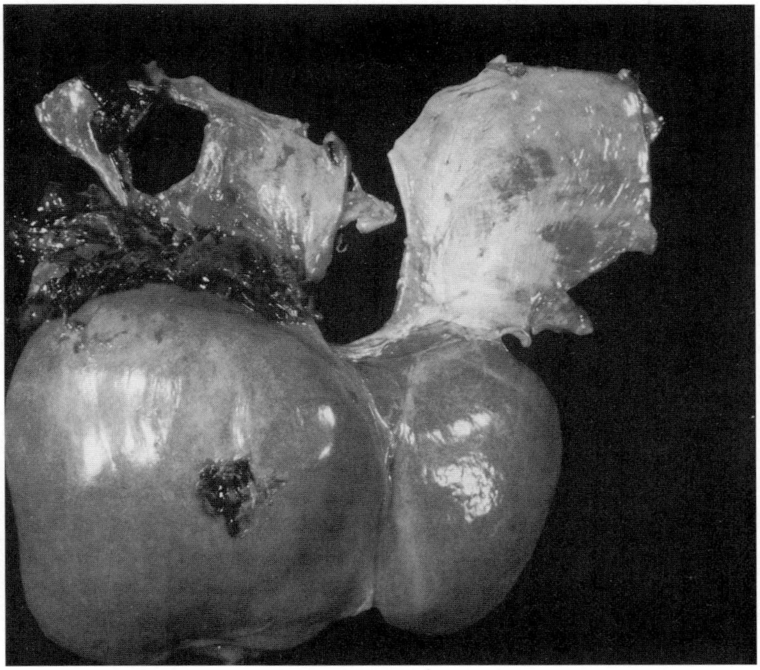

FIGURE 14.4. Referred case of laceration of the liver (below) and of the diaphragm (above) in an 80-year old woman. The contiguous lower lobe of the lung was also injured (not shown in the picture). Trocar method of insertion was used.

Hemorrhages occur occasionally, especially with chest tubes inserted in the parasternal area, where the likelihood of an injury to the internal thoracic artery is increased. In other places hemorrhage results from injury to either the intercostal artery or the intercostal vein, in most cases both.

Some of the typical problems encountered with the use of trocars include laceration of the lung and injuries to the cardiovascular vessels, especially the pulmonary artery and the pulmonary veins. Injuries to the diaphragm and the liver are not as rare as one might like to assume (Fig. 14.4). Independent of the method used to insert the chest tube, cellulitis may occasionally develop at the site of drainage.

7. PROBLEMS ARISING FROM SELECTION OF TUBES

During suction for pneumothorax there is a laminar flow of air through the suction tube. Because of this, the flow of air obeys Poiseuille's law:

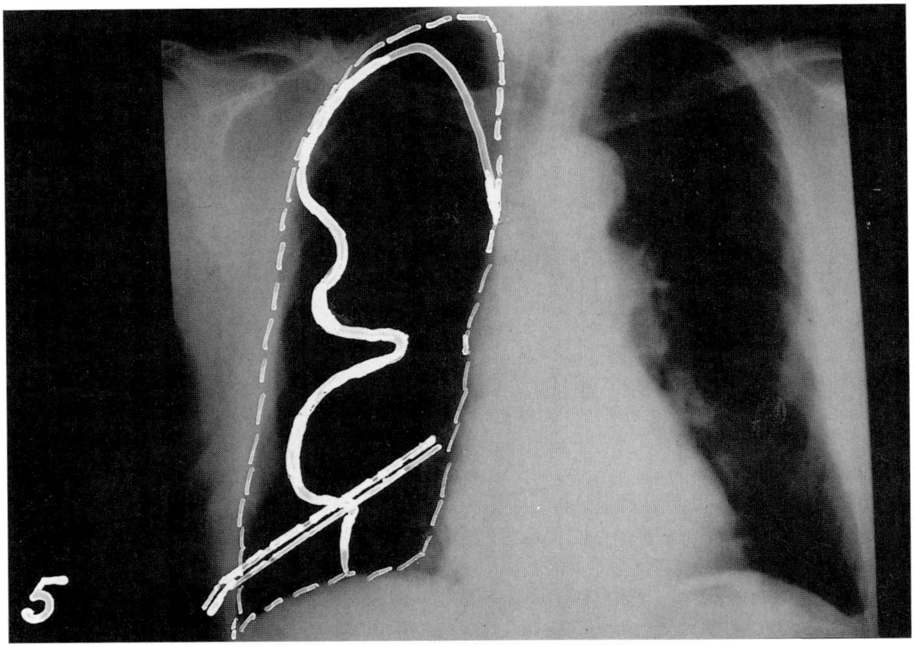

FIGURE 14.5. Inadequate suction. Chest X-ray shows still partially collapsed lung following chest tube drainage for spontaneous pneumothorax in a septuagenerian. Patient had pulmonary to thoracal wall symphysis in several areas as could be seen with the thoracoscope. Thick solid line, contour of partially collapsed lung. Dashed line, parietal pleura.

$$V = \frac{\pi r^4 \sigma p}{8nl}.$$

Accordingly, for any given suction pressure σp, and for a given length of tube l, the amount of flow V increases or decreases exponentially with the change in the radius of the chest tube, the viscosity of air n remaining constant. The treatment of simple pneumothorax generally presents little problem as far as the radius of the chest tube is concerned. If there is continuous leakage into the pleural space, the radius of the tube becomes relevant. The expansion of the lung becomes a function of maintenance of negative pressure in the pleural space. In other words, the flow of air through the chest tube must exceed the inflow of air through the leakage into the pleural space in order to allow for expansion and adhesion of the lung to the thoracic wall. If this is not guaranteed, the result will be apparent tube failure (Fig. 14.5). Tubes with small radius will not function effectively under this condition. Kinks in the course of the chest tube through the thoracic wall, especially for those inserted posteriorly, tend to further reduce the radius and consequently the rate of flow. Another relevant factor is the total length of the tube from the

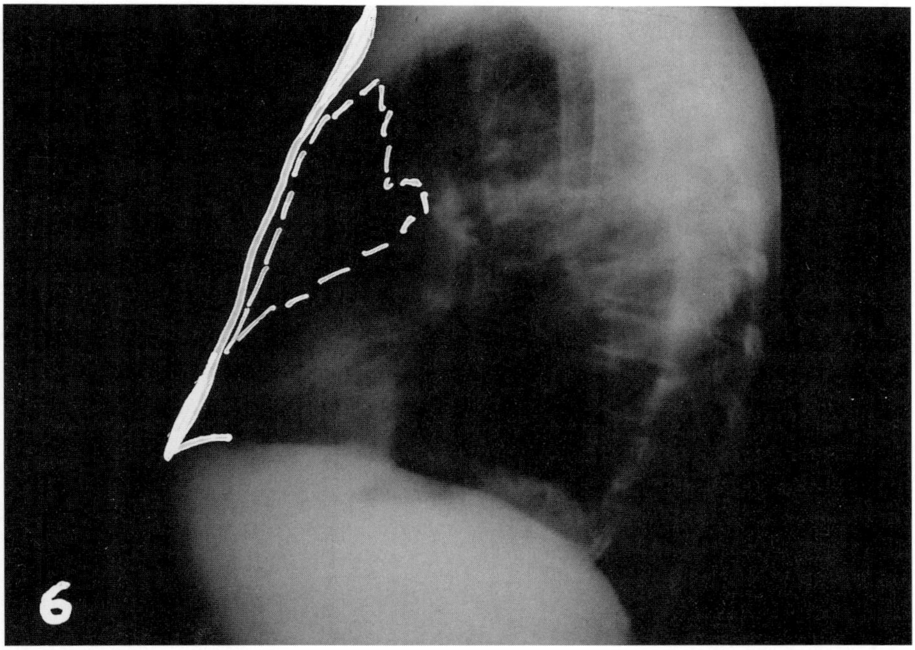

FIGURE 14.6. Lateral chest X-ray. Chronic pneumothorax following anatomical resection of both the lingual and the sixth segment is delineated by the dashed line.

chest to the underwater seal. Since flow is inversely proportional to the length of the tube, long tubes therefore tend to reduce the effectiveness of the suction.

Fundamentally, the flow of fluid through the chest tube in the case of hydrothorax follows the same principle described above. However, the conditions change slightly in turbulent flow, such as obtains in a combination of pneumo-hydro-thorax or pneumo-hematothorax. The radius of the tube becomes more relevant as the flow is directly proportional to r^5 (Fanning equation) [15]. For general and specific purposes of thorax drainage there are chest tubes of various sizes, ranging from French 16 to 36. Most thoracic surgeons use tubes of size French 28 both for evacuation of air and fluid, including hematoma. With fluid of high viscosity such as obtains in empyema, larger sizes, French 32–34 are generally used. The total length of tube up to the underwater seal is approximately two meters.

8. SPECIAL PROBLEMS IN GENERAL THORACIC SURGERY

8.1. Thoracic surgery without reduction in total lung volume

The problems attendant to pulmonary surgery without reduction in the total lung volume could be parenchymal air leakages and leakages from small to medium

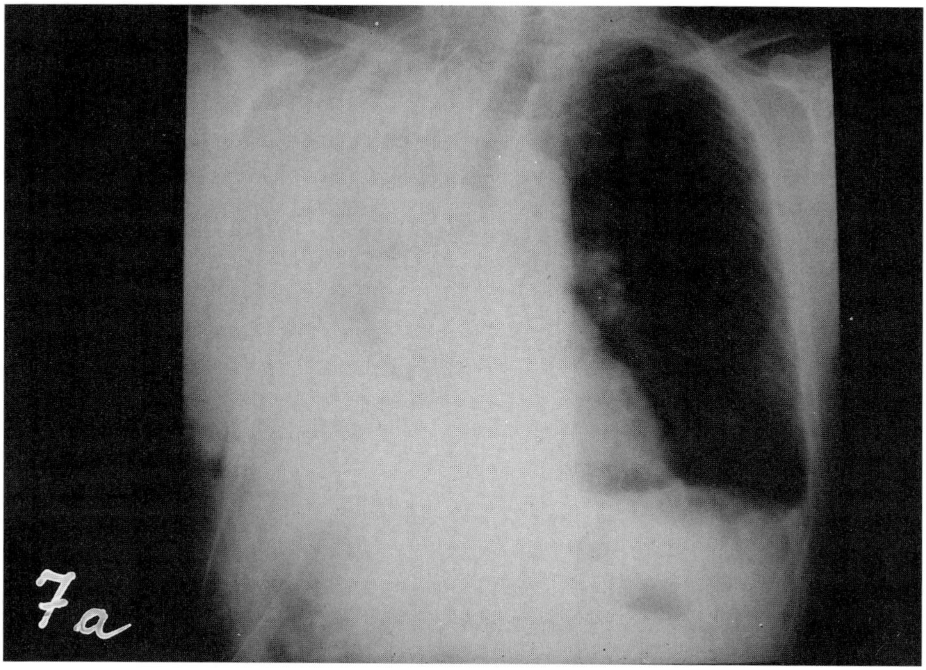

FIGURE 14.7a. Upper bilobectomy with the release of the pulmonary ligament. Two days after operation. (a) Chest X-ray shows complete obliteration of the hemithorax not observed the day before. Patient's circulatory status was stable all the time. At rethoracotomy no source of bleeding was found. Fluid blood minimal. Blood clots mostly parietal and adhesive to the thoracic wall. (b) Two days later, obliteration of the right phrenico-costal sinus and lower chest region by sero-sanguinous blood, and (c) by fibrous tissue 21 days later.

sized bronchopleural fistula. Especially if decortication was performed or the parietal pleura was dissected from the thoracic wall, parenchymal air leakages are mostly accompanied by capillary bleeding, which soon gives way to serosanguinous exudate. Generally, this condition can be managed by the chest tube alone. As long as the tracheobronchial system is not plugged by mucus secretions, the lungs generally expand satisfactorily and align themselves to the thoracic wall. By so doing, the capillary bleeding stops and the bronchopleural fistulae and the parenchymal air leakages cease. The larger bronchopleural fistulae can also be managed effectively if care is taken to select tubes of appropriate size and length. Suction is maintained for 5 to 14 days. If, however, there is no tendency for spontaneous closure of larger bronchopleural fistulae, re-exploration may be considered before infection sets in.

Small parenchymal leakages accompanying wedge resection of the lung usually cause no further problem and are treated as mentioned above.

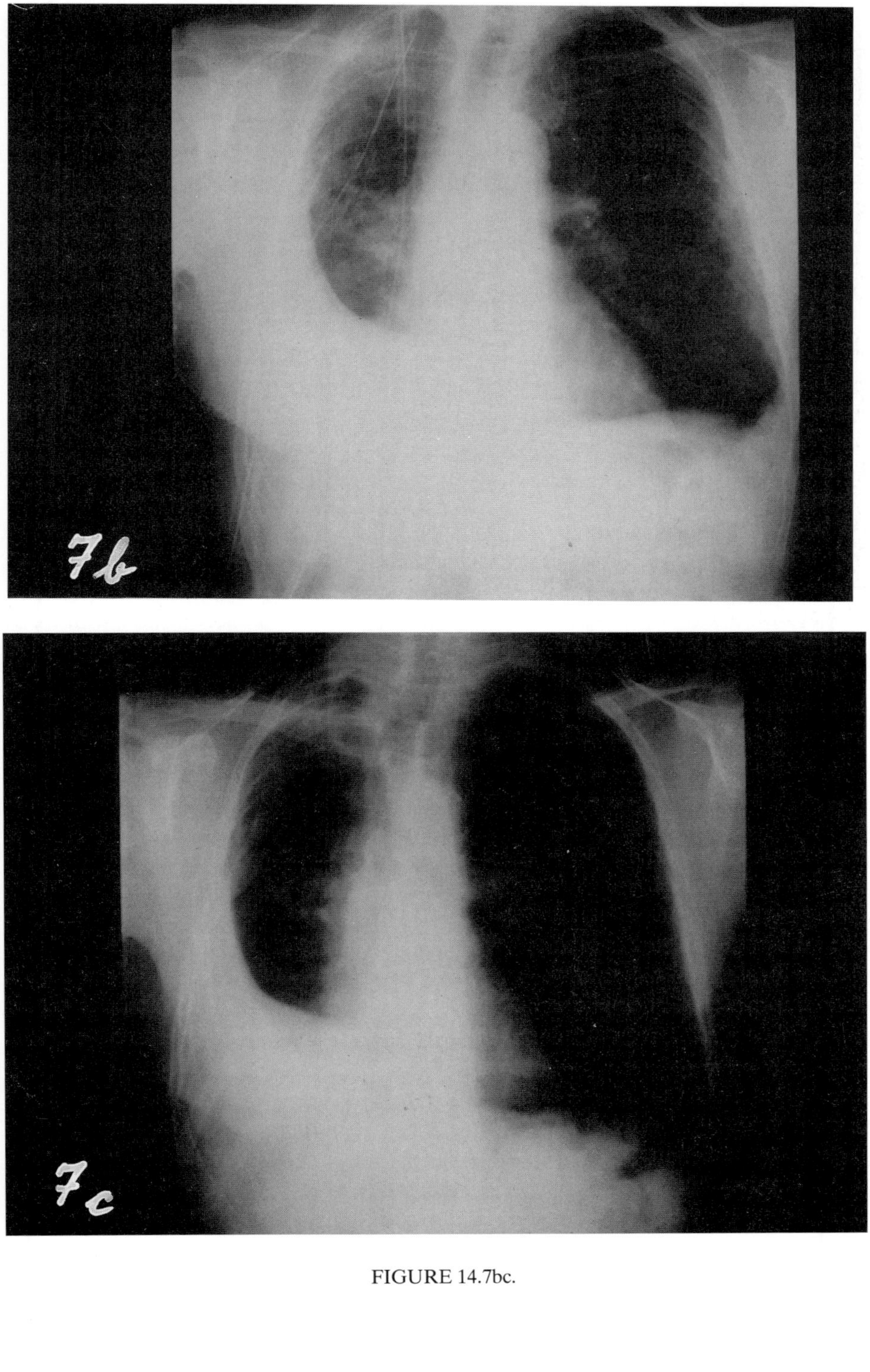

FIGURE 14.7bc.

8.2. Thoracic surgery leading to lobectomies and pneumonectomies

Following a lobectomy the pleural pressure drops slightly because of the reduced mass of lung recoiling in a virtually unchanged thoracic cavity. The negativity is highest following pneumonectomy[6]. The increased negativity facilitates overdistention of the remaining lung. In the left lung the upper lobe re-expands more readily to occupy the remaining space after a lower lobectomy, so that drainage failures are less likely to occur than with the upper lobectomy. In the right lung the middle lobe can be removed without any further consequence, however, upper and lower bilobectomies leave spaces that cannot always be adequately occupied by the overextended remaining lung. Consequently one observes chronic pneumothorax or fibrosis of part of the thoracic cavity (Fig. 14.6). Often a situation arises where the remaining lung fails to fill up the thoracic cavity and at the same time there is continuous postoperative hemorrhage. Blood clots are then likely to plug the chest tube and lead to drainage failure (Fig. 14.7).

8.3. Pneumonectomies

Following a pneumonectomy, a chest tube is left in place for about 24 hours in order to drain the intrathoracic serosanguinous fluid or collecting blood, should significant postoperative blood seepage or frank hemorrhage occur. In the next few days following chest tube removal, fluid rises continuously in the hemithorax and fills up the space. In the process of the organization of the fluid contents and the accompanying fibrosis of the chest cavity, pockets and compartments may be observed which should not be mistaken for encapsulated empyema. Otherwise, a rise in body temperature, increasing leucocytosis and falling fluid levels in serial roentgenograms of the chest and offensive mouth odour are ominous signs of dehiscence of the stump suture line and the obligatory bronchopleural fistula always accompanied by infection. In most cases, bronchoscopy and fistulagrams will clear any doubts.

If a bronchopleural fistula is diagnosed, the first therapeutic measure is usually the insertion of a chest tube, the effective function of which will largely depend on such variables as the presence or absence of multiloculation and the extent of fibrosis in the thoracic cavity.

8.4. Lobectomy and bronchopleural fistula

Early bronchial stump insufficiency following lobectomy in the presence of chest tube drainage follows a fairly predictable course. If infection is not a major problem and the remaining lung can distend to fill the thoracic cavity, the fate of the lung depends on the ability of the chest tube to maintain adequate negative pressure in the chest cavity. If the flow into the pleural cavity exceeds the rate of evacuation of air, the lung will remain collapsed, atelectatic and finally become carnified. The rate of flow of air into the pleural cavity is a function of the diameter of the port of leakage. Ultimately, infection overrides the effect of chest drainage and decides the fate of the chest cavity and remaining lung parenchyma.

8.5. Empyema

Pleural empyemas in the absence of open chest operations always result from non-specific and specific bacterial infections of the lung, parapneumonic empyema being the most common form. Large-bore tube drainage of the pleural space rids it of the pus collection as long as pleural thickening is minimal and loculation of the empyema into multiple cavities has not occurred. However, despite drainage the resolution of the empyema is seldom as fast as it started. Moreover, since the resolution of the primary pulmonary infection itself is not uniform, the pleura is bound to be affected in the same manner. The septation of the empyema cavity by clotting fibrin, which becomes organized as a result of fibroblastic activity, the contraction of the pulmonary parenchyma, as a result of atelectasis and the spatially irregular course of the infective and reparative processes involved, are factors leading to empyema loculation. The problem is further compounded by pleural thickening. Thus, empyema treatment by tube thoracostomy may be unsuccessfull. Not only is one chest tube generally insufficient, but the mandatory drainage of each identified loculation may not lead to a permanent resolution of the empyema. One is left with no other option than a more aggressive therapeutic approach.

8.6. Pulmonary abscess

Subpleural, peripheral abscesses are generally delineated against the rest of the lung and the pleural cavity by a fibrotic wall, making it possible to drain them directly without spillage into the pleural cavity. Centrally located abscesses usually drain via the bronchial system. When an unaffected pulmonary area has to be traversed by the tube to gain access to the abscess, fistula and empyema may be the sequelae. The combination of pulmonary abscess and contiguous pleural empyema generally leads to protracted treatment. Tube thoracostomy alone for the treatment of this condition generally becomes inadequate.

9. DISCUSSION

Chest drainage is the single most regularly applied therapeutic concept in general thoracic and cardiac surgery. Despite the simplicity of its concept and application, it can present with complicated problems ranging from technical application to the therapy of the disease necessitating chest drainage. Consequently, chest drainage treatment can lead from instantaneous success to dejecting failure.

Relatively minor complications accompanying chest tube insertion include hemorrhage as a result of injury either to the intercostal vessels or to the internal mammary vessels and subcutaneous emphysema. Careful selection of the drainage site, placement of the tube just above the lower rib and well below the upper one will avoid injury to the blood vessel. Despite this precaution, it will not always be possible to avoid injury to the intercostal vessels, especially in old people presenting with tortuous blood vessels [5,15]. Inasmuch as injury to the lung can be ruled out, subcutaneous emphysema arises when the space around the tube at its port of entry allows escape of air from the pleural cavity or when the last opening on the tube is very near or at the port of entry. Technical conditions promoting subcutaneous emphysema are entry of the tube into the chest at a near 90° angle, wide incisions, and inadequate fixation of the tube by mattress or similar sutures.

Injuries to the internal organs are not uncommon, however the most serious is the perforation of pulmonary arteries and systemic artery to pulmonary vascular shunts [7]. Lacerations of the liver, the spleen, the stomach, the lungs and the diaphragm have all been described [8,16,18,30]. We have observed combinations of these injuries among patients referred to us for treatment: laceration of the liver together with the contiguous diaphragm and the lung, liver and the diaphragm or diaphragm and lung especially in the elderly whose diaphragm was identified as high up as in the fifth to fourth intercostal space (Fig. 14.4, above). Most cases of pulmonary, liver and diaphragm laceration that came to our hospital occurred with the trocar method. A case of pulmonary artery injury with lethal outcome came to our attention on medico-legal grounds. It was inserted with an introducer. As a result of the awareness of the increased morbidity and perhaps mortality by the use of trocars and introducers, we employ the blunt dissection method. The trocar method may be safe in experienced hands, but we are of the opinion that in teaching hospitals residents and house officers should be groomed in the use of the blunt dissection method and avoid the trocar method. Especially for the treatment of pneumothorax with subtotal to complete collapse of the lung the danger of perforation is negligible. The risk however, increases with parietal pneumothorax, in which only 25% to 35% of the lung is collapsed, in pulmonary emphysema, stiff lung and symphysis of the lung parenchyma with the thoracic wall (Fig. 14.5, above).

The blunt dissection method, while being relatively safe, does not exclude laceration of the lung and the diaphragm, especially if blunt dissection is carried out without alternating digital exploration of the stab incision to identify the depth to which the dissection has been carried and to exclude the presence of pulmonary adhesions with the chest wall. The exploring finger or the tip of the dissecting instrument can penetrate vital structures following inadvertent and uncontrolled movements. Except during open chest operations and in chest trauma with multiple and serial rib fractures, one may consider performing a thoracoscopy before a chest tube is inserted for the treatment of pneumothorax, serothorax, pneumoserothorax, hematothorax and pleural effusions of undefined etiology. This not only enhances diagnostic accuracy but also avoids injuries to the vital structures in the chest and abdomen.

Aside from the combined surgical and endoscopic method of avoiding injuries to the lungs, diaphragm and liver and other extrathoracic structures, other effective methods have been employed. These include fluoroscopy, CT, MRI and ultrasonic scanning [14,23,24,25]. Computed tomograms serve the dual purpose of diagnosis and guidance for tube placement [24,25]. Magnetic resonance imaging and ultrasound serve the same purpose. Ultrasound scanning has the added advantage over all the others of being mobile, handy and economical. The use of these imaging devices makes placement of tubes accurate and avoids gross injuries to the thoracic and extrathoracic structures. MRI is costly and is not readily available on demand, especially in emergency. Fluoroscopy has the disadvantage of increased irradiation both to the patient and to the operator.

With the imaging techniques Stavas et al. [25] preferably use the trocar method to insert chest catheters apparently without complications or injuries. From the point of view of tube insertion and placement, the intraoperative placement under direct vision is the safest method available today.

Parenchymal leakages, and small bronchopleural fistulas following decortication, segmentectomies and minor lung operations can be easily managed, the objective of management being to vent the excess air out of the thoracic cavity and create a negative pressure (subatmospheric) in the pleural space to facilitate pulmonary expansion and to seal off the leakage points [10]. With the submersion of the lung in warm physiologic saline before closure of the thorax the extent and magnitude of the parenchymal leakage is assessed and further therapeutic measures decided upon immediately [28]. Extensive leakages are either closed with automatic suture instruments or with 4–0 monophylic suture material in a continuous double row mattress suture technique. To avoid further injury to the parenchyma, the sutures are made in a collapsed or in a partially collapsed (CPAP) lung. To ensure adequate venting, two chest tubes are inserted.

In closed chest procedures the water probe cannot be carried out. Lateral and P–A chest roentgenograms are used to determine the necessity of additional chest tubes. Re-expansion pulmonary edema occurs occasionally following chest tube drainage but mostly it is not a serious complication.

Bronchopleural fistulae are dreaded complications of both specific infections (e.g. tuberculosis) and of resectional pulmonary surgery. The former generally leads to empyema. The latter arises as a result of dehiscence along the suture line of the bronchial stump. Bronchopleural fistula, in the presence of pleural effusion, usually leads to empyema, although the reverse condition is also true, especially following a pneumonectomy. The outcome of conservative management is not always predictable. If the leak is small, as in lobectomy, increased intrapleural suction may pull the remaining lung over the bronchial stump and seal off the leakage with time [3]. Unfortunately, under the high flow of air the fistula may grow larger to encompass the entire circumference of the stump. The development of this condition is aided by the initial increased negativity of the pleural cavity as a result of increased suction. The problem may be compounded in patients with respiratory insufficiency and atelectasis who have to be ventilated under PEEP. The forces acting on the stump become additive. The insertion of multiple drainage tubes does not often help matters. Rather, it becomes more expedient to consider alternative measures of closing the fistula [4,13,19,27,29,30], while tube management becomes an indispensable component of the overall management both in the short and in the long term, especially in the presence of empyema. However, while ordinarily mechanical ventilation does not seem to increase the incidence of bronchopleural fistula, it does seem to increase the incidence of pleural empyema in resectional pulmonary surgery [9].

Closed tube thoracostomy as initial treatment of pleural empyema can give gratifying results especially in children. In their series, Beg et al. [1] recorded a success rate of 95% in children, whose initial treatment regime consisted of closed tube drainage and parenteral antibiotics. The literature, however, shows that the success rate in adults is considerably lower than in children and differs from one series to another. Lemmer et al. [11] reported a success rate as low as 35% in their series, whereas others presented more optimistic results ranging from 62% to 80% [2,12,22,26].

The varying failure rate of tube drainage is often accounted for by the delay in establishing the diagnosis and treatment of empyema. The earlier tube drainage treatment is instituted in the course of empyema development, the higher the chances of success. On the other hand, delay allows time for multiloculation of the empyema cavity and for pleural thickening, thus leading to drainage failure. The social background of the patients often plays a deciding role. In our hospital the group of empyema patients with tube drainage failure are debilitated patients, chronic alcoholics, drug addicts, diabetics, chronically ill patients and elder citizens living alone. The effect of these social ills seems to be the postponement of the optimal period for the diagnosis and treatment of their empyema. They therefore present with multiloculations, thickened pleura and often lung abscess. In these patients we carry out a more aggressive therapy: rib resection with mechanical breakdown of the multiloculations, decortication and insertion of more than one chest tube. It may become necessary to irrigate the empyema cavity in the long run. In the later stages and in the course of treatment for post-thoracotomy empyema, multiloculations are drained singly and severally by chest tube insertion under imaging guidance, whereby ultrasonography, because of its handling ease is the preferred imaging technique employed.

Finally, chest tube drainage can be frustrating when dealing with multiple complications of an underlying illness, a typical example being the patient with cancer of the lower trachea perforating into the oesophagus and causing pleural empyema. If the course of the illness is not devastatingly fulminant the general thoracic surgeon will have no choice than to leave the draining chest tube indefinitely in place. Similarly, in less dramatic situations, e. g. following thoracoplasties with persistent residual cavities, one will have to accept permanent chest tube drainage.

REFERENCES

1 Beg MH, Ahmad SH, Reyazuddin, Shahab T, Chandra J. Management of empyema thoracis in children – a study of 65 cases. Ann Trop Paediatr 1987; 7: 109–112.

2 Benfield GFA. Recent trends in empyema thoracis. Br J Dis Chest 1981; 75: 358–366.
3 Brewer III LA. Bronchopleural fistula: Management. In: Grillo HC, Eschapasse, H. (eds.). International Trends in General Thoracic Surgery, Vol 2, Major Challenges. Philadelphia, PA, WB Saunders 1987: pp 398–406.
4 Bruni F. Bronchopleural fistula: Treatment of long stump after pneumonectomy. In: Grillo HC, Eschapasse H (eds.). International Trends in General Thoracic Surgery, Vol 2, Major Challenges. Philadelphia, PA, WB Saunders 1987: pp 413–422.
5 Carney M, Ravin CE. Intercostal artery laceration during thoracocentesis: Increased risk in elderly patients. Chest 1979; 75: 520–522.
6 Epstein PE. Effects of pulmonary resection (pneumonectomy). In: Fishman AP (ed.). Pulmonary Diseases and Disorders. New York, McGraw-Hill 1980: pp 1701–1708.
7 Fein AB, Godwin JD, Moore AV, Moran TJ, Young Jr WB. Systemic artery-to-pulmonary vascular shunt: a complication of closed tube thoracostomy. AJR 1983; 140(5): 917–919.
8 Frazer RS. Lung perforation complicating tube thoracostomy: Pathologic description of three cases. Hum Pathol. 1988; 19(5): 518–523.
9 Gaud C. Role of mechanical ventilation in the genesis of empyema and bronchopleural fistula. In: Grillo HC, Eschapasse H (eds.). International Trends in General Thoracic Surgery, Vol 2, Major Challenges. Philadelphia, PA, WB Saunders 1987: pp 447–451.
10 Langston HT, Barker WL. Management of prolonged parenchymal air leaks and residual pleural spaces. In: Grillo HC, Eschapasse H (eds.). International Trends in General Thoracic Surgery, Vol 2, Major Challenges. Philadelphia, PA, WB Saunders 1987: pp 383–391.
11 Lemmer JH, Botham MJ, Orringer MB. Modern management of adult thoracic empyema. J Thorac Cardiovasc Surg 1985; 90: 849–855.
12 Mavroudis C, Symmonds JB, Minagi H, Thomas AN. Improved survival in management of empyema thoracis. J Thorac Cardiovasc Surg 1981; 82: 49–57.
13 McMillan IKR. Bronchopleural fistula: Treatment by space reduction. In: Grillo HC, Eschapasse H (eds.). International Trends in General Thoracic Surgery, Vol 2, Major Challenges. Philadelphia, PA, WB Saunders 1987: 440–446.
14 Merriam MA, Cronan JJ, Dorfman GS, Lambiase RE, Haas RA. Radiographically guided percutaneous catheter drainage of pleural fluid collections. AJR 1988; 151 (6): 1113–1116.
15 Miller KS, Sahn SA. Chest tubes: Indications, technique, management and complications. Chest 1987; 91 (2): 258–264.
16 Millikau JS, Moore EE, Steiner E, Aragon GE, van Way CW. Complications of tube thoracostomy for acute trauma. Am J Surg 1980; 140: 738–741.
17 Montilla PB, Hervas VT. Bronchopleural fistula management with muscle transposition. Discussion. In: Grillo HC, Eschapasse H (eds.). International Trends in General Thoracic Surgery, Vol 2, Major Challenges. Philadelphia, PA, WB Saunders 1987: pp 429–434.
18 Moessinger AC, Driscoll Jr JM, Wigger HJ. High incidence of lung perforation by chest tube in neonatal pneumothorax. J Paediatr 1978; 92: 635–637.
19 Pairolero PC, Arnold PG. Bronchopleural fistula: Management with muscle transposition. In: Grillo HC, Eschapasse H (eds.). International Trends in General Thoracic Surgery, Vol 2, Major Challenges. Philadelphia, PA, WB Saunders 1987: pp 423–428.
20 Perelman MI. Bronchopleural fistula: Treatment of lung stump after pneumonectomy. Discussion. In: Grillo HC, Eschapasse H (eds.). International Trends in General Thoracic Surgery, Vol 2, Major Challenges. Philadelphia, PA, WB Saunders 1987: p 422.
21 Perelman MI, Rymko LP, Ambatiello GP. Bronchopleural fistula: Surgery after pneumonectomy. In: Grillo HC, Eschapasse H (eds.). International Trends in General Thoracic Surgery, Vol 2, Major Challenges. Philadelphia, PA, WB Saunders 1987: pp 407–412.
22 Schachter EN, Kreisman H, Putman C. Diagnostic problems in suppurative lung disease. Arch Intern Med 1976; 136: 167–171.

23 Silverman SG, Mueller PR, Saini S, Hahn PF, Simeone JF, Forman BH, Steiner E, Ferruci JT. Thoracic empyema: Management with image-guided catheter drainage. Radiology 1988; 169(1): 5–9.

24 Stark DD, Federle MP, Gordman PC. CT and radiographic assessment of tube thoracostomy. AJR 1983; 141(2): 253–258.

25 Stavas J, van Sonnenberg E, Casola G, Wittich GR. Percutaneous drainage of infected and non-infected thoracic fluid collections. J Thorac Imag 1987; 2 (3): 80–87.

26 Varkey B, Rose HD, Kutty CPK, Politis J. Empyema thoracis during a 10 year period. Arch Intern Med 1981; 141: 1771–1776.

27 Virkkula L. Bronchopleural fistula: Omental pedicle for treatment. In: Grillo HC, Eschapasse H (eds.). International Trends in General Thoracic Surgery, Vol 2, Major Challenges. Philadelphia, PA, WB Saunders 1987: pp 435–439.

28 Vogt-Moykopf I, Meyer G. Management of prolonged parenchymal air leaks and residual pleural spaces. Discussion. In: Grillo HC, Eschapasse H (eds.). International Trends in General Thoracic Surgery, Vol 2, Major Challenges. Philadelphia, PA, WB Saunders 1987: pp 392–393.

29 Wilkins Jr EW. Bronchopleural fistula: Prophylaxis. In: Grillo HC, Eschapasse H (eds.). International Trends in General Thoracic Surgery, Vol 2, Major Challenges. Philadelphia, PA, WB Saunders 1987: pp 394–397.

30 Wilson AJ, Krous HF. Lung perforation during chest tube placement in the stiff lung syndrom. J Paediatr Surg 1974; 9: 213–216.

Current Topics in General Thoracic Surgery: An International Series, Vol. 2
Perioperative Care, edited by R.M. Peters and J. Toledo

Discussion of "Chest drainage problems" by E. Anyanwu and I. Vogt-Moykopf

Earle W. Wilkins Jr

As the authors state, "chest drainage, when correctly employed, should cause no problems beyond inconvenience for the patient". Indeed, chest drainage is carried out either to relieve an existing problem such as spontaneous pneumothorax or empyema, or to prevent one such as pneumothorax or hydrothorax following resection of the lung. The gold standard, therefore, in the utilization of chest tubes must be freedom from complications.

To this end, it is helpful to think of a check list of possible tube or drainage complications with the goal of anticipating anything that might go wrong and, ideally, preventing it. The categorization employed by the authors, (1) complications and problems arising from the placement of chest tubes, (2) those from the selection of tubes, and (3) special problems, may be restated in such a check list: see Table D14.1.

The intraoperative placement of chest tubes obviates the likelihood of most of these complications, particularly in the first three categories. Bleeding at the tube site, if it occurs, can be controlled under direct vision. Accurate placement of the tube is easily achieved without inadvertent trauma to underlying lung or other viscera. The tip of the tube can be loosely anchored in planned position with an absorbable suture around it and its point of egress through the skin securely fixed with double suture ligatures of heavy non-absorbable material.

The greatest frequency of chest drainage tube problems occur with the so-called closed tube thoracostomy method. It has been very thoroughly and accurately assessed by the authors. At the Massachusetts General Hospital we advocated their "method of blunt dissection". We consider it a modified open thoracostomy, actually an ultra-minithoracotomy involving digital palpation of both the tract for the tube and the space into which it is to be placed. The technique is sufficiently important to warrant its illustration (Figs. D14.1A–E).

Citing its particular merit as a teaching or training exercise, we emphasize its preference over the closed trochar method. The principal complication of the

TABLE D14.1
Checklist of possible tube or drainage complications

(1) Bleeding
  (a) laceration of an intercostal vessel
  (b) trauma to an intrathoracic vessel or viscus
  (c) compromised coagulation of the patient

(2) Air leakage
  (a) injury to underlying lung parenchyma
  (b) inadequacy of a solitary tube
  (c) subcutaneous emphysema

(3) Improper placement
  (a) extrapleural
  (b) within a fissure
  (c) failure to locate the space or collection to be drained

(4) Mechanical
  (a) failure to anchor the tube appropriately
  (b) kinking of the tube
  (c) disconnection from the closed drainage system
  (d) improper connection to the system
  (e) inadequate calibre of the tube

(5) Uncooperative patient
  (a) pulling on the tube

trochar technique is damage to intrathoracic structures. When a trochar is utilized for placement of a chest tube, its sheath must be phlanged so that when the pressure 'give' of pleural entry occurs, the distance traversed by the sharp point of the trochar is limited. United States medical officers returning from duty in the Vietnam war described impalement of literally every intrathoracic structure, and some subdiaphragmatic, during use of a non-phlanged trochar introducer of a plastic tube. (It was ultimately removed from the medical supply table.)

The trochar method is therefore better reserved for the experienced physician and then, perhaps, only for pneumothorax of a major degree when the target space for the chest tube is sizeable.

This leaves a number of general principles which should be observed. Recalling the philosophy that anything that may go wrong will, the physician is cautioned to observe the following guidelines in placement of chest tubes:

(1) If the tube is being inserted at the patient's bedside, have the X-ray at hand. Tubes have been placed into the wrong hemithorax. Does the patient have situs inversus? Don't forget the principles of physical examination: inspection, percussion, auscultation.

(2) Use an appropriate tube. A number of siliconized plastic tubes are available; blood coagulation is less of a problem. Size is important. The authors cite the little-known Poiseuille law; a minimum calibre tube of 20F is essential for evacuation of a continuing air leak. A No. 28F tube is suggested for drainage of fluid. Larger tubes are often necessary for drainage of an empyema; in this

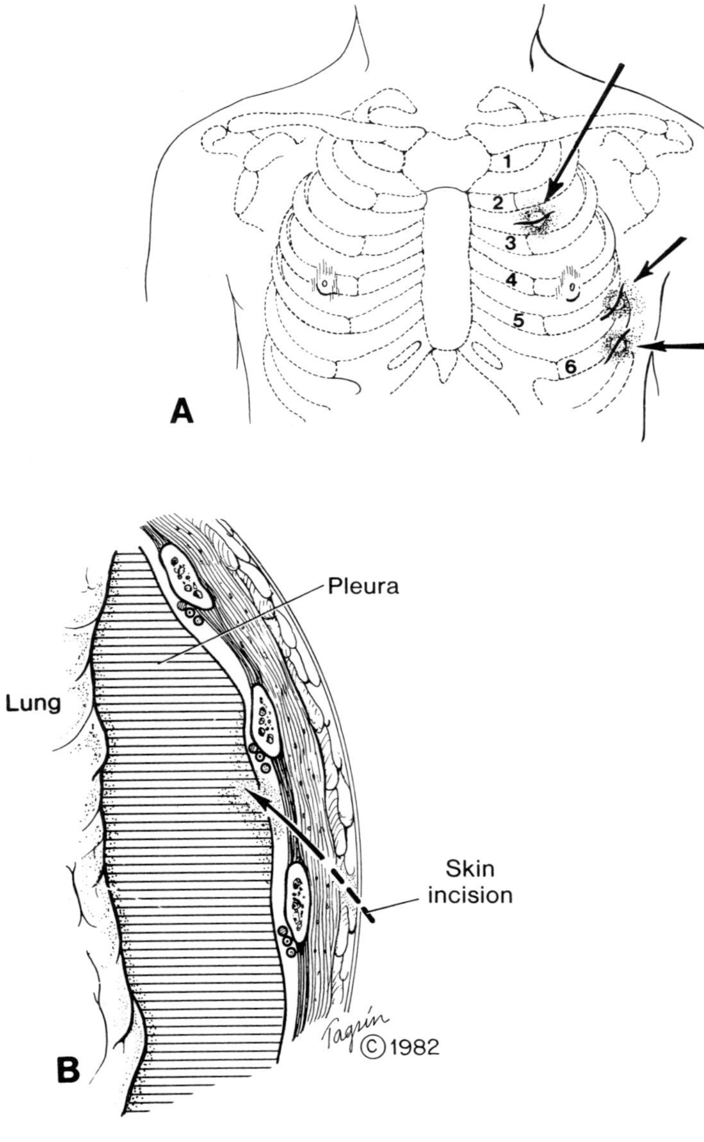

FIGURE D14.1AB. Chest tube insertion. (A) The site of insertion is usually the second intercostal space at the midclavicular line or the fifth or sixth interspace at the midaxillary line. A linear incision is made over the area of insertion after local anesthesia with 1% lidocaine (Xylocaine). Liberal use of lidocaine is recommended to provide anesthesia to the pleural level. (B) The skin incision is made 2–3 cm below the interspace through which the chest tube will be inserted. This allows for a skin and subcutaneous flap to develop with insertion. The neurovascular bundle that runs along the under surface of the rib is avoided.

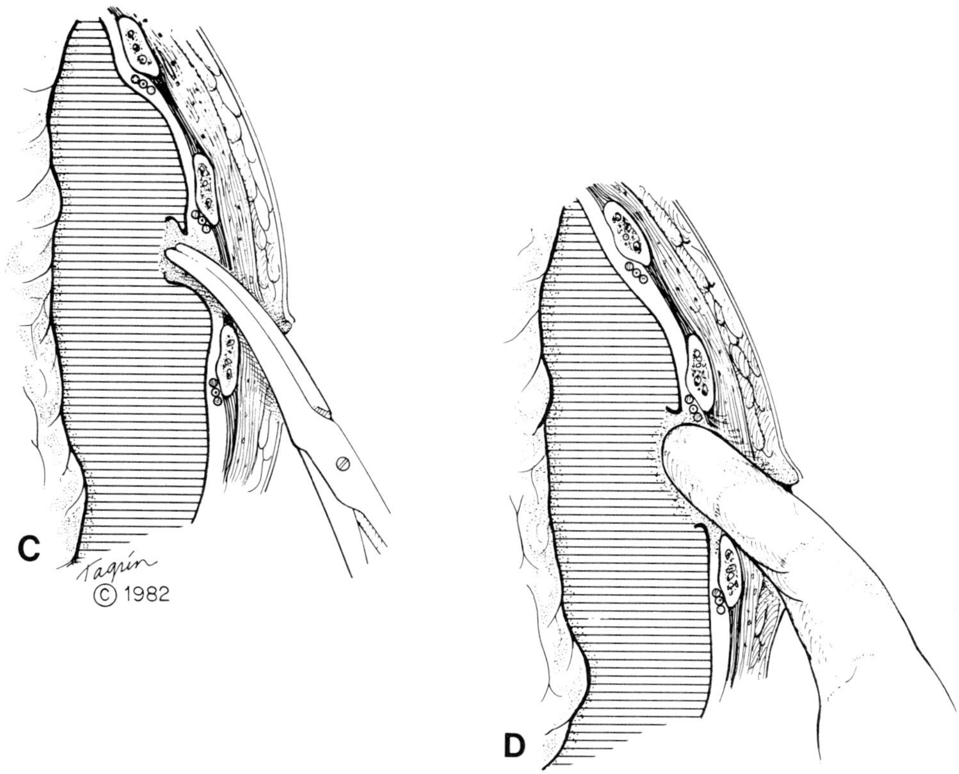

FIGURE D14.1CD. (C) A Kelly clamp is used to spread the subcutaneous tissue and muscle fibers to allow penetration of the intercostal muscle. (D) Once the intercostal muscles have been spread, the digit is inserted through the intercostal space and muscle so that no damage to the underlying lung will occur. This allows digital exploration of a limited portion of the pleural space.

case, ligation of the intercostal artery and vein or excision of a segment of rib must be considered.

(3) Avoid obstruction of the tube by kinking or the patient's lying on it. In a patient with a continuing parenchyma air leak, this is the leading cause of subcutaneous emphysema.

(4) Anchor the tube by two sutures to the skin and with tape to the dressing – to minimize the likelihood of inadvertent withdrawal of the tube, or the patient's intentional pulling on it.

(5) Tape the connecting tubes together to minimize disconnection during patient care and/or ambulation.

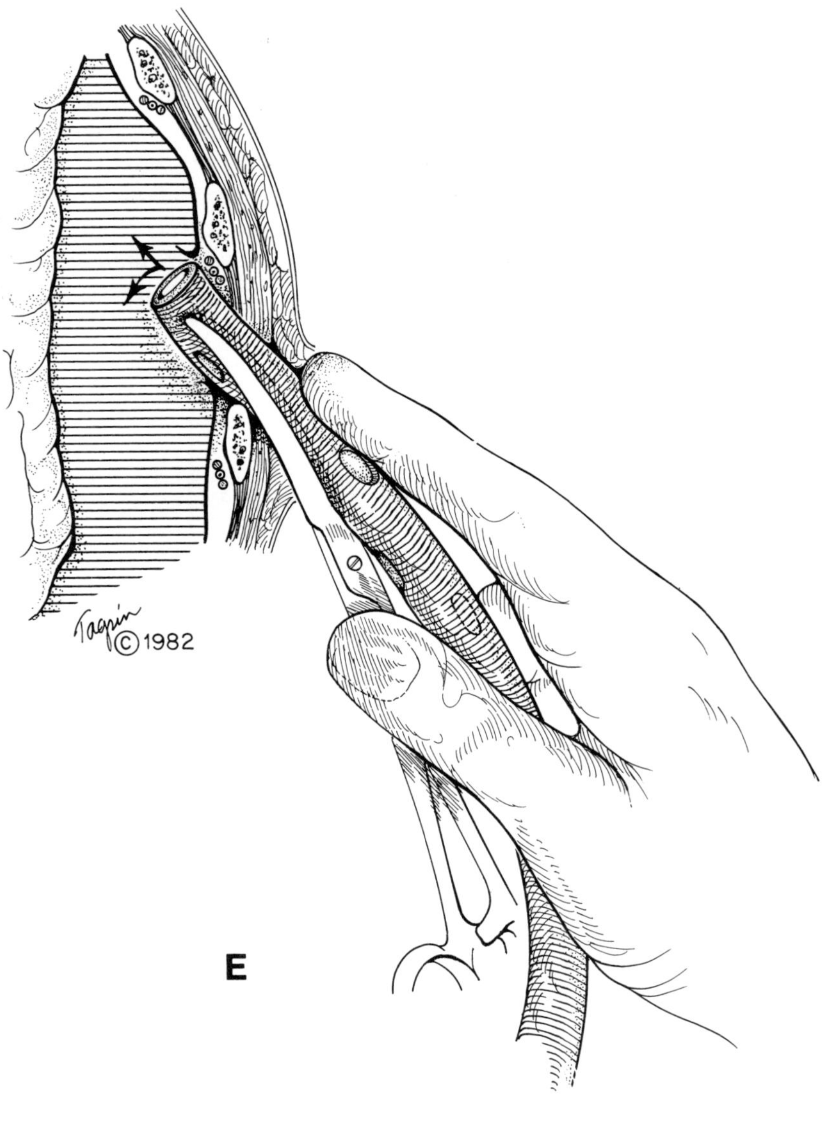

FIGURE D14.1E. After an adequate tract is made using the digit, the chest tube is inserted through the created tract. The chest tube is threaded superiorly or inferiorly within the pleura. The chest tube should be inserted approximately 2–3 cm beyond the last (outer) hole in the catheter. The tube is secured to the chest wall with sutures and connected to the drainage device.

(6) Consider using a drainage system which includes a trap bottle; this prevents any possibility of aspiration of fluid back into the thorax, as when an underwater seal bottle is elevated above the level of the patient.
(7) Always check an X-ray after tube placement.

The section on Special Problems in General Thoracic Surgery is thorough and complete. It does not require comment, except to suggest caution in tube drainage of lung abscess, where early attempts at drainage may convert the abscess to a pyopneumothorax or prolonged tube placement may result in hemorrhage.

Finally, comment must be made about the increasing utilization of radiologic placement of tubes. The great advantage is the imaging guidance (by computer tomography, magnetic resonance, or ultrasound) in the correct placement of the tube. A potential disadvantage is the use of tubes of inadequate calibre. In principle, it is another responsibility in the care of his patient that the surgeon is failing to exercise.

REFERENCE

1 McCabe CJ. Chest tube insertion. In: Wilkins Jr EW (ed.). Emergency Medicine: Scientific Foundations and Current Practice. Baltimore, Williams & Wilkins 1989: pp 1023–1055.

Current Topics in General Thoracic Surgery: An International Series, Vol. 2
Perioperative Care, edited by R.M. Peters and J. Toledo

Chapter 15

Indications for re-exploration thoracotomy

Mario J. Milano

1. GENERAL OVERVIEW

In spite of both technical and biomedical advances in the field of general thoracic surgery, postoperative complications, though limited, still persist. They result from widespread use of surgical procedures of increasing complexity on patients of higher risk, once unsuitable candidates for surgery, plus an inevitable quota of human error, technical and judgmental. Although there is a greater probability of postoperative complications following emergency operation, elective surgery is not free of them.

The majority of complications in general thoracic surgery can be effectively managed by timely nonoperative methods, or by means of minor surgical procedures. However, in certain clinical situations the decision to undertake prompt re-exploration in the early postoperative course may be a real necessity. The implicit hazards of a repeated operation require thoughtful justification of the proposed procedure in terms of (1) a life-saving step resulting from progressive deterioration or severe functional derangement of the patient, (2) preventing or decreasing the likelihood of late surgical sequelae, (3) or avoidance of long hospital stays. Other important circumstances related to complications must also be considered: the high cost of medical care, the possibility of patient death or disability, potential lawsuit, etc. [3] All of these possibilities make it essential that the surgical team adopt an attitude of fully committed and continuing observation of the postoperative patient.

Unexpected complications or adverse results, so distressing in terms of suffering, death and cost, are real challenges to the surgeon [8,10]. It takes a maximum of knowledge, training and experience to deal with them. *Prevention remains the best defense against complications.* It rests on: (1) proper indications for the primary surgery; (2) a basic knowledge of surgical anatomy and pathology; and (3) thorough compliance with essential technical principles.

Specific local or pathologic circumstances, often unavoidable, may contribute to the possibility of complications. Iatrogenic events derive almost exclusively from human error resulting from a lack of basic knowledge, poor training, inexperience and/or fatigue [3,10]. These factors hamper proper therapeutic decisions when complications do occur. Faulty surgical staplers are rarely the cause of complications requiring re-exploration; nevertheless, oversewing of the stapled line may be advisable in certain situations. True surgical mishap or misadventure is a rare cause of postoperative complication.

Awareness of the possibility of a particular complication, close clinical surveillance of the patient, utilization of proper confirmatory diagnostic measures and sound judgment are all essential to support the decision for re-exploration in the overall management of the patient.

It is not the intention of this chapter to provide a review of all theoretical complications requiring early re-exploration in general thoracic surgery. The purpose is to point out the stressful incidents encountered in practice or reported in the literature, emphasizing the indications for repeat thoracotomy. Basic patient management in these situations is also provided.

2. PULMONARY SURGERY

2.1. Postoperative bleeding

This familiar situation is recognized by a clinical picture of hypovolemia with sweatiness, tachycardia, hypotension and reduced urine output. Hematocrit values are not reliable in its early phase. Portable chest X-rays with the patient upright may be helpful in assessing fluid accumulation.

Monitoring the volume and quality of fluid loss through chest tubes, provided they are patent, is the best method for assessing bleeding. This is the reason we prefer to provide a drainage tube in pneumonectomy patients, especially when an extensive mediastinal lymph node dissection has been performed. A tube, placed low, is used for 24 hours. The tube remains clamped and, when indicated, may be unclamped for short periods to assess blood loss or to manage troublesome mediastinal shift.

Blood loss exceeding 100 ml/h following lung resection, when associated with a consistent clinical picture of hypovolemia, 'warm' (open) chest tubes, hematocrit readings of drainage fluid and findings on chest X-ray, should prompt re-operation. Appropriate diagnostic assessment and correction of any altered coagulation factors are mandatory before a decision to re-operate is made.

The sources of bleeding are usually systemic – the azygos vein; bronchial arteries; pericardiophrenic, mediastinal or intercostal vessels; dense parietal adhesions of lung. They almost always provide a margin of time for proper assessment and safe re-operation [22]. If postoperative re-expansion of lung is achieved immediately, pulmonary arteries and veins seldom contribute to blood loss. However, in rare occasions slippage of a ligature, disruption of a suture line or an inadvertent tear may result in massive hemorrhage from a pulmonary vessel. This catastrophic event requires quick re-opening of the incision for manual hemostatic control, even in the intensive unit.

Clotted hemothorax gives rise to a different situation. Blood, retained within the pleural cavity, results from a misinterpretation of the pleural drainage debit, a space-occupying defect, and consumption of coagulation factors and activation of fibrinolytic mechanisms with persistence of bleeding. The space-occupying defect differs with the type of resection. In lobectomy, segmentectomy or local excision, compression of the ipsilateral remaining lung ensues; in pneumonectomy mediastinal shift, often with associated arrhythmias is commonly observed. Emergency re-exploration thoracotomy is imperative to remove the clot and stop the bleeding [22]. Occasionally, unexpected interruption of the hemorrhage is observed after clot removal and pleural lavage with warm saline. Nonetheless, careful exploration is essential before closing to identify a potential source for persisting bleeding.

Postoperative bleeding in cases of pleural decortication without pulmonary resection is fairly common. Thorough intraoperative electrocoagulation hemostasis of all raw surfaces, particularly the parietal, is of utmost importance in preventing blood loss and facilitating immediate lung re-expansion.

Utilization of autotransfusion in thoracic postoperative bleeding has been advocated.

2.2. Air leakage

Postoperative air leak is perhaps the most common and worrisome complication of lung surgery [22]. In general, leaks close spontaneously in a few days and re-expansion is achieved by means of continuous suction and chest physical therapy. The optimum management is prevention: gentle handling of parenchymal surfaces, careful dissection of anatomic planes, reconstruction of lung surfaces and proper positioning of drainage tubes [8]. Stapling of incomplete fissures helps to reduce the incidence of air leaks [18]. Fibrin glue or other sealing adhesives have not proved effective in closing the parenchymal surfaces. Particularly in patients with pulmonary emphysema, the greatest intraoperative technical care is essential to preserve airtight pleuropulmonary surfaces.

The management of non-threatening air leaks has been widely reported in the literature. In such cases, further surgical intervention is discouraged since a meager reduction in air leakage is ordinarily achieved [9]. In the majority of cases conservative management with properly functioning chest tubes is effective. The management of residual air spaces is not within the subject of this chapter.

Massive air leaks, on the other hand, herald a serious problem and deserve careful consideration. An *immediate* excessive leak overloading evacuation drainage capability and producing soft-tissue emphysema indicates either inadequate closure of the bronchial stump or an early disruption of the suture line or row of staples [18,22]. This situation may be worsened by mechanical ventilation with high pressures. Bronchoscopy is helpful in clarifying the possibility of stump breakdown. Early re-exploration thoracotomy is mandatory to attempt resuture of the bronchial stump (resuture reduces the chances of infection in the pleural cavity [22]). Particularly in the pneumonectomy patient, an empyema is otherwise predictable.

The *late* appearance of a major leak is usually indicative of a bronchial fistula [8]. Here the risks of re-operation should be weighed carefully because surgical intervention is seldom useful at this stage. Occasionally, prompt resuture of the bronchus, through viable tissue with stump reinforcement with pericardium, omentum, or intercostal muscle pedicle, produces a satisfactory result [8]. The technical details of prophylaxis and surgical management of bronchial fistula are well described elsewhere [18,22,23].

Disruption of a bronchial anastomosis or bronchoplasty at the level of a main bronchus is managed in a manner as just expressed above relative to the bronchial stump. Dehiscence of a tracheal anastomosis poses a special and difficult problem in management. This severe and often fatal complication is the result of one or more of the following: impaired vascular supply, excessive tension, post-radiation tissue damage, the use of steroids, high pressure ventilatory support, and improper technical detail such as deficient sutures. If endoscopy confirms the diagnosis, an immediate re-operation should follow. Intraoperative findings guide proper surgical management: (1) complete reanastomosis or resuture of a partial dehiscence accompanied by laryngeal and pericardial release, carina and main bronchial mobilization, division of the inferior pulmonary ligament; (2) covering with adjacent muscle, omentum or transposed muscle pedicle; and (3) mediastinal or mural tracheostomy if reanastomosis is not technically feasible. Anastomotic dehiscence close to the carina is not suitable for mediastinal tracheostomy [22]. In general, re-operation in tracheal surgery bears a high rate of morbidity and mortality.

2.3. Acute cardiac herniation

The actual incidence of this critical complication of pulmonary resection is uncertain [5,19]. It has occasionally been reported – with high mortality figures [1]. Since 1956 only two cases of acute cardiac herniation have been recorded in 1600 pulmonary resections representing the entire experience of our group.

Partial excision of pericardium or pericardiotomy associated with lung resection are the causes of this complication. Because clinical and hemodynamic findings may be nonspecific, the differential diagnosis from massive hemorrhage, hypoxic heart failure, airway obstruction or cardiac tamponade is essential [8,19]. Prompt recognition may provide the only opportunity of a salvaging re-exploration thoracotomy before the situation becomes irreversible [4,5,15,17].

Two distinct clinical pictures are observed: (1) central circulatory failure (strangulation of the heart) and (2) acute vena caval syndrome (rotation of the heart) [1,22]. The former is more common in left-sided resections, leading rapidly to compressive and ischemic myocardial damage by the squeezing pericardial edges.

Right-sided herniation with heart volvulus causes twisting or strangulation of the vena cavae with progressive low cardiac output and cyanosis [4,8,20].

Certain factors may precipitate acute cardiac herniation: drainage suction, the lateral decubitus, coughing and positive pressure ventilation [1,20]. Awareness of the possibility of this complication is of the utmost importance in leading to emergency re-exploration thoracotomy which includes prompt reduction of the herniated heart and repair of the pericardial defect by means of direct suture, prosthetic or biologic graft, or myopericardial sutures [4,6,8,15,20]. These techniques are preventive if properly utilized at the initial lung resection whenever a pericardial defect results, regardless of its size. Prevention is crucial.

Placement of the patient on the side opposite the thoracotomy during preparation for re-exploration may temporarily improve hemodynamic conditions [6,19].

2.4. Pulmonary torsion

Postoperative axial rotation of a lobe or a segment results in impairment of venous drainage with a lesser degree of bronchial and arterial obstruction. Consequent congestion produces engorgement of the lung which soon becomes hepatized. Early clinical and radiological recognition is mandatory. Only re-exploration thoracotomy with untwisting of the torsion and fixation of the lobe or segment can reverse the progression toward nonviability.

The clinical picture is characterized by high fever, tachycardia, dyspnea and bloody sputum. A progressively expanding homogeneous density on the side of the pulmonary resection is usually apparent on chest X-ray [22]. Endoscopy may show bronchial obstruction; it also assists in the differential diagnosis from plain atelectasis due to retained secretions.

Intraoperative findings dictate the necessary surgical action, whether conservative or resectional. If the lobe or segment is viable, release of the torsion is preferred with lung fixation by stapling or suture to the adjacent lobe. If necrosis or impending gangrene is evident, lobectomy or completion of the resection is necessary. There have been three cases of postoperative torsion in our series of lung resections and all of them were successfully treated.

Once again, prophylaxis at time of the initial procedure is the action of choice. Every effort should be made to affix any unstable portion of remaining lung before closing the thoracotomy. A middle lobe with complete fissures is particularly prone to torsion after either a right upper or lower lobectomy. Preventive fixation to adjacent lung parenchyma is essential [22].

2.5. Lung gangrene

Lung necrosis is a very uncommon postoperative complication produced by total obstruction of venous drainage or by combined occlusion of the pulmonary artery and bronchial circulation to a portion of remaining lung [8]. Secondary infection may precipitate the ensuing gangrene. The situation may also be produced as the result of a difficult pulmonary dissection which deprives the remaining lung of its circulation [13]. Although the patient's clinical condition may be severely compromised, repeat thoracotomy with excision of affected lung is essential if the patient is to be salvaged [8]. We have documented this troublesome emergency in one instance with a clinical picture as just described.

2.6. Pulmonary artery stump thrombosis

Central progression of a thrombus originating in the stump of a pulmonary artery with repeated embolization to the contralateral lung has been only infrequently reported. Obstruction of the right ventricular flow and right heart failure are the main clinical features of the complication [22]. Particularly in right pneumonectomy, a pulmonary artery stump that is too long has been clinically and experimentally demonstrated [8].

The diagnosis can be established by pulmonary artery angiography. Removal of the thrombus and reamputation of the stump can be carried out through a repeat thoracotomy although, preferably, the approach may be via a median sternotomy with the aid of extracorporeal circulation [22].

3. ESOPHAGEAL SURGERY

3.1. Hiatal hernia repair

Esophageal perforation or leak from a misplaced suture during hiatal hernia repair by the transthoracic approach, although most unusual, requires careful attention to prevent the harmful results of uncontrolled fistula, sepsis and malnutrition [22]. This setback in the management of an otherwise benign disease may occur: (1) during attempts to dilate a stricture at the time of the antireflux procedure; (2) when fundoplicating sutures are placed too deeply in the esophageal muscle; or (3) if there is disruption of a suture line or staple row following a lengthening (Collis) gastroplasty.

If the diagnosis of esophageal leakage is made early, immediate re-operation should be considered. Such active surgical management usually provides a more expedient resolution of the complication and avoids prolonged hospitalization. The site of perforation or leak is first identified and primary suture attempted with reinforcement with viable adjacent tissue. The operation should include appropriate drainage and a feeding jejunostomy.

Small asymptomatic leaks detected on routine follow-up radiologic contrast swallow usually do not require active surgical intervention.

3.2. Esophageal resection and esophageal replacement

Intrathoracic anastomotic or suture leak is a dreaded complication of resectional esophageal surgery which involves both a difficult challenge for the surgeon and a high rate of morbidity or mortality for the patient. There is a wide variation in the reported incidence of this complication with an overall mortality approaching 40% [22].

Anastomotic leaks in the cervical esophagus are usually transient and pursue a benign course without the need for an aggressive therapeutic approach. Spontaneous healing is the rule. Because of this and the oncologic principle of maximal resection, many authors favor subtotal esophagectomy for cancer with replacement by the substituting organ brought to the neck for cervical anastomosis.

Long lesser curvature suture lines, the non-reversed gastric tube [Boerema] and the reversed gastric tube [Gavriliu–Heimlich] are three nonanastomotic sources of leakage in intrathoracic gastric esophageal substitution. One or more fistulae can develop in the extensive suture line. There is little information regarding extent of usage of these techniques.

The occurrence of dehiscence is increased by the following factors, singly or in combination: (1) technical, including impaired blood supply, residual carcinoma at the suture line, excessive tension and faulty surgical technique; and (2) biologic, including malnutrition, post-radiation tissue changes, the use of steroids and autodigestion by gastric secretions.

The clinical and radiologic picture of this complication is characteristic, usually appearing in the early postoperative course with sepsis, shock, and the presence of air and fluid levels on X-ray. The diagnosis is substantiated by a contrast swallow using iodized oil or hydrosoluble media. This may also provide information about the size of the leak. Fiber-optic endoscopy is not a requisite in substantiating the diagnosis. Life-threatening chemical empyema and mediastinitis require urgent re-operation; delay or reluctance in performing re-exploration may result in irreversibility of the patient's condition.

A small, limited intrathoracic leak may sometimes be managed by adequate drainage, gastric decompression and a feeding jejunostomy. If tissue necrosis is not encountered at re-operation, closure may be attempted with resuture reinforced with adjacent tissue [7]. Recurrence of the leak is common in these cases with scant possibility of healing. Persistence of sepsis may force one to sacrifice the entire esophagus in a subsequent operation.

Ischemic necrosis of a transplant, whether gastric, colonic or jejunal, is an established indication for re-exploration thoracotomy. Awareness of the possibility of this complication is essential, so that appropriate action can be taken prior to the development of putrid mediastinitis and rapid deterioration of the patient's condition. Dubious viability of the substituting viscus at the conclusion of the initial operation coupled with a clinical course including toxic appearance of the patient and foul-smelling aspirate suggests necrosis of the transplant. Radiopaque swallow may not be diagnostic. Esophagoscopy is more helpful showing any ischemic mucosal tissue. Cervical re-exploration or even a repeat thoracotomy is advisable to confirm the diagnosis.

When a major, extensive dehiscence is found at re-exploration, a decision should be adopted to perform a salvage procedure. Any attempt to carry out excision and refashioning of the anastomosis in an infected area is doomed to failure. It is necessary to adopt an aggressive approach including: (1) taking down the disrupted anastomosis; (2) exteriorization of the proximal esophagus by cervical esophagostomy; (3) resection of any nonviable portion of the esophageal substitute returning the remnant into the abdomen; and (4) performing a feeding jejunostomy or sometimes a gastrostomy. This extreme procedure may succeed in spite of the adverse clinical situation.

This general scheme may be applied to gastric, colon or jejunal transplants equally well. Particular technical differences should not be overlooked. A plan to restore alimentary tract continuity must be deferred to a later date.

It is clear that preventive action must be taken at the primary procedure to avoid ischemia by excessive handling, clamping, kinking, rotation and impairment of venous return.

3.3. Pediatric esophageal surgery

The failure of an esophageal anastomosis in the transpleural repair of esophageal atresia provides an almost identical situation as seen in adults; similarly, in esophageal substitution for corrosive stricture. The effect of pleuromediastinal soilage resulting from a major disruption in children is disastrous [22]. Thus, the decision for re-intervention is compulsory. The findings at re-operation establish which of the alternative courses of management is appropriate. The options are basically similar to those mentioned for adults.

4. CHYLOTHORAX

Chylothorax is an uncommon complication of thoracic surgery, occurring almost exclusively in cardiovascular and esophageal procedures [2,12,16,22]. It is most frequent in upper thoracic esophageal resection as the result of inadvertent injury to the thoracic duct. When chyle leakage occurs at the hiatal level during diaphragmatic hernia repair, it usually resolves spontaneously with conservative therapy. In esophageal resection, however, spontaneous closure rarely occurs.

Metabolic and nutritional deterioration of the patient despite maximal conservative therapy is an indication for early re-exploration for ligation of the thoracic duct [14,22]. Technical details on the level of surgical approach and identification of the site of leakage are well described in the literature [2,12,14,16].

5. CONCLUSIONS

Perioperative management in thoracic surgery is demanding. It involves both preventive and therapeutic actions. If both are properly exercised, complications when they do occur will be detected early. The majority can be effectively managed by timely nonoperative therapy or by minor surgical procedures.

Complications, however, even those that are apparently minor and insignificant, should never be underestimated. They may pose challenging surgical problems of diagnosis, approach, repair and management. On rare occasions, immediate postoperative complications lead to critical situations in which survival of the patient or further morbidity depend on a well-timed decision to re-intervene surgically.

The therapeutic goals of often hazardous re-exploration are: (1) to save life; (2) to minimize morbidity; (3) to preserve function for a good quality of survival. An understanding of pathophysiology in these infrequent but demanding situations is of the utmost importance in determining the need for prompt re-intervention. It is mandatory to have diagnostic proof and clinical justification before undertaking this course of action. Re-exploration thoracotomy then may allow an expedient solution with recovery of the patient.

The best management is always to anticipate and prevent complications. Basic anatomic, pathophysiologic and surgical understanding is essential in predicting high-risk situations and in utilizing suitable technical approaches at the initial procedure.

REFERENCES

1 Arnot RD, Frank CG, Schmitz AL, Haveson SB. Cardiac Herniation with Volvulus after pneumonectomy. AJR 1978; 130: 155–156.
2 Bessone LN, Ferguson TB, Burford TH. Chylothorax. Ann Thorac Surg 1971; 12: 527–550.
3 Couch NP, Tilney NL, Rayner AA, Moore FD. The high costs of low-frequency events. N Engl J Med 1981; 304: 634–637.
4 Deiraniya AK. Cardiac herniation following intrapericardial pneumonectomy. Thorax 1974; 29: 545–552.
5 Dombey JJ, Delaye A, Metras D, Preciozi MC, Malmejac C, Houel J. Luxation du coeur après pneumonectomie élargie. Ann Chir Thorac Cardiovasc 1971; 10: 155–159.
6 Gates GF, Sette RS, Cope JA. Acute cardiac herniation with incarceration following pneumonectomy. Radiology 1970; 94; 561–562.
7 Inberg MV, Linna MI, Scheinin TM, Vanttinen E. Anastomotic leakage after excision of esophageal and high gastric carcinoma. Am J Surg 1971; 122: 540.
8 Kirsh MM, Rotman H, Behrendt DM, Orringer MB, Sloan H. Complications of pulmonary resection. Ann Thorac Surg 1975; 20: 215–236.
9 Langston HT, Barker WL. Management of prolonged parenchymal air leaks and residual pleural spaces. In: Grillo HC, Eschapasse H (eds.). International Trends in General Thoracic Surgery, Vol 2, Major Challenges. Philadelphia, PA, WB Saunders 1987: ch 36.
10 Mullin MJ, Zumbro Jr GL, Fishbach ME, Nelson TG. Pulmonary lobar gangrene complicating lobectomy. Ann Surg 1972; 175: 62–66.
11 Myers JD. Preventing iatrogenic complications [editorial]. N Engl J Med 1981; 304: 664–665.
12 Robinson CLN. The management of chylothorax. Ann Thorac Surg 1985; 39: 90–95.
13 Salyer JM, Harrison HN. Pulmonary infarction complicating segmental resection. J Thorac Surg 1958; 36: 818–838.

14 Selle JG, Snyder III WH, Schreiber JT. Chylothorax: indications for surgery. Ann Surg 1973; 177: 245–249.
15 Takita H, Mijares WS. Herniation of the heart following intrapericardial pneumonectomy. J Thorac Cardiovasc Surg 1970; 59: 443–446.
16 Teba L, Dedhia HV, Bowen R, Alexander JC. Chylothorax Review. Crit Care Med 1985; 13: 49–52.
17 Tschersich HU, Skopara Jr V, Flemming WH. Acute cardiac herniation following pneumonectomy. Radiology 1976; 120: 546.
18 Vogt-Moykopf I, Meyer G. Management of prolonged parenchymal air leaks and residual air spaces [discussion]. In: Grillo HC, Eschapasse H (eds.). International Trends in General Thoracic Surgery, Vol 2, Major Challenges. Philadelpia, PA, WB Saunders 1987.
19 Wright MP, Nelson C, Johnson AM, McMillan IKR. Herniation of the heart. Thorax 1970; 25: 656–664.
20 Yacoub MH, Williams WG, Ahmad A. Strangulation of the heart following intrapericardial pneumonectomy. Thorax 1968; 23: 261–265.
21 Artz CP, Hardy JD (eds.). Management of Surgical Complications, 3rd Ed. Philadelphia, PA, WB Saunders 1975.
22 Greenfield LJ (ed.). Complications in Surgery and Trauma. Philadelphia, PA, JB Lippincott 1984.
23 Hood RM. Techniques in General Thoracic Surgery. Philadelphia, PA, WB Saunders 1985.

Current Topics in General Thoracic Surgery: An International Series, Vol. 2
Perioperative Care, edited by R.M. Peters and J. Toledo

Discussion of "Indications for re-exploration thoracotomy" by Mario J. Milano

Earle W. Wilkins Jr.

1. INTRODUCTION

One cannot take issue with the statement: "*Prevention remains the best defense against complications*". Indeed, throughout a long career of operating room teaching of general thoracic residents, that has been the cornerstone of my instructions. The most common technical complication in pulmonary surgery is the bronchial stump leak; in esophageal surgery, the anastomotic leak. These are preventable. I have discussed prophylaxis against bronchopleural fistula in Grillo and Eschapasse's *Major Challenges* [1]. Preservation of blood supply, gentle handling of the stump whether by suture or staple, and proper coverage especially under the circumstances of prior radiation, necessity for steroid maintenance, immunosuppression, unusual inflammation or the need for mechanical ventilation – these are the guidelines for prevention. In the case of esophageal anastomotic leakage, the experience at the Massachusetts General Hospital (MGH) is cited [2] where 104 consecutive esophageal resections and primary anastomoses were accomplished without leak, 90% done by residents under supervision. Again, preservation of blood supply, avoidance of tension and meticulous attention to a sutured anastomosis are paramount.

But, this chapter is about indications for re-exploration thoracotomy when complications, despite the best of preventive intent, do occur. The principles of management include: (1) careful surveillance of the patient, particularly early in the intensive care unit or recovery room; (2) expeditious diagnosis of the complication, whether by clinical assessment or radiographic confirmation; and (3) an aggressive approach in the decision regarding the need for re-operation. Delay can often result in a fatal outcome. Another approach to the indications for re-exploration is by the operation performed.

2. PNEUMONECTOMY

Of the commonly performed general thoracic operations, pneumonectomy, particularly right pneumonectomy, carries one of the highest mortality and morbidity rates[3]. Many of the deaths result from failure to address promptly the need for re-exploration thoracotomy.

Major hemorrhage as measured by chest tube drainage and sudden hypotension is one indication. This stems from failure of a suture line or staples on the pulmonary artery or veins. These vessels should never be simply ligated; ligatures slip. This type of bleeding may occur during closure, transfer to the bed, or early in the recovery room. It demands *immediate* re-opening of the thoracic incision and control of the bleeding vessel, often initially with the fingers. Only dramatic action can prevent death.

Lesser hemorrhage characterized by chest tube drainage greater than a continuing 100 ml/h, with or without clinical shock, merits re-operation. This type of bleeding usually originates from a systemic artery (bronchial, intercostal, internal mammary) but may arise from vascular parietal adhesions. In this case, replacement transfusion permits an orderly return to the operating room.

Bronchial stump leak is the second indication for re-exploration after pneumonectomy. Early *dehiscence* demands immediate operation; otherwise, adequate ventilation is not possible. Reclosure must be accompanied by stump coverage with viable tissue (muscle rotation, intercostal, pedicle, omentum). Simple *leak* during hospitalization requires careful endoscopic assessment but in general such leaks after pneumonectomy should lead to re-exploration for completion of closure.

An additional word is necessary regarding the author's thorough discussion of acute cardiac herniation. (This complication is indeed totally preventable with proper pericardial closure.) Review of our MGH experience reveals one fatal case following right pneumonectomy; prolapse of the heart resulted in laceration of both the superior and the inferior vena cava. The unwise use of chest suction with the right decubitus position were unquestionably contributing factors.

Close the pericardium; use water-seal drainage only after pneumonectomy

3. LOBECTOMY

The risk of fatal complication after lobectomy is very much lower than after pneumonectomy. An additional cause of bleeding is the slipped ligature from a branch of the pulmonary artery. Once again, continued bloody drainage in excess of 100 ml/h requires a second look.

Air leaks in general require re-operation only if a bronchial stump leak is visualized by endoscopy. Peripheral parenchymal leaks usually close with time and full expansion of remaining lung. Occasionally in an emphysematous patient it may be necessary to re-operate for closure of leaking blebs or reinforcement of an inadequate parenchymal staple line.

4. ESOPHAGECTOMY

The critical complications following esophagectomy with replacement by stomach, colon or jejunum are anastomotic fistula, anastomotic dehiscence and necrosis of the replacing organ.

A fistula in the neck is likely to heal with simple drainage. One within the thorax, unless an incidental, blind tract found at postoperative radiographic study, requires re-exploration for closure and reinforcing abutment of viable tissue. Actual separation of the anastomosis is uncommon. One dramatic example is recorded at the Massachusetts General Hospital (MGH) when a patient with a full stomach tried to vomit while a bronchoscopy was being performed (an unusual mechanism of a Boerhaave phenomenon – forceful emesis against a closed glottis). Survival in such a dehiscence is possible only with re-exploration and repair.

Necrosis of the replacing viscus is suggested by high fever, septic shock, air within the viscus by X-ray, and the esophagoscopic appearance of devitalized mucosa. Re-exploration should be carried out prior to radiographic evidence of perforation, and it is mandatory for removal of the viscus (more commonly seen when colon or jejunum is the replacing conduit), exteriorization of the esophagus in the neck and a feeding gastrostomy or jejunostomy.

When esophageal leakage is *suspected* in the thorax, a negative re-exploration is preferable to undue delay in managing a leak. The handling of an esophageal leak is an emergency. Time is of the essence!

5. CHYLOTHORAX

Despite the occasional closure of a leaking thoracic duct under conservative therapy, chylothorax most often requires re-operation for ligation of the duct. This re-operation is *not* an emergency. Lymphangiography may be helpful in verifying the diagnosis and localizing the site of leakage. However, a right supradiaphragmatic thoracotomy provides excellent exposure of the lower thoracic duct where it lies between the descending aorta and the azygos vein. Double ligation with non-resorbable ties is adequate. There has been no example at the MGH of chylothorax complicating transthoracic distal hernia repair.

REFERENCES

1 Wilkins Jr EW. Bronchopleural fistual: Prophylaxis. In: Grillo HC, Eschapasse H (eds.). International Trends in General Thoracic Surgery, Vol 2, Major Challenges. Philadelphia, PA, WB Saunders 1987; ch 37: pp 394–397.
2 Mathisen DJ, Grillo HC, Wilkins Jr EW, et al: Transthoracic esophagectomy: A safe approach to carcinoma of the esophagus. Ann Thoracic Surg 1988; 45: 137–143.
3 Wilkins Jr EW, Scannell JG, Craver JG. Four decades of experience with resections for bronchogenic carcinoma at the Massachusetts General Hospital. J Thorac Cardiovasc Surg 1978; 76: 364–368.

Current Topics in General Thoracic Surgery: An International Series, Vol. 2
Perioperative Care, edited by R.M. Peters and J. Toledo

Chapter 16

Prevention and treatment of atelectasis

Robert H. Bartlett

GLOSSARY

CPAP	continuous positive airway pressure	PEEP	positive end-expiratory pressure
IPPB	intermittent positive-pressure breathing	PIP	peak inspiratory pressure

1. INTRODUCTION

Atelectasis is the most common postoperative pulmonary complication. It usually occurs as a primary event, but may be caused by left ventricular failure, aspiration, capillary leak syndromes (ARDS), or extracellular space overload. Atelectasis usually involves specific basilar segments or lower lobes, but may be diffuse or isolated to one entire lung. It may resolve with appropriate re-inflation therapy, or may progress to bacterial pneumonia. The prevention and treatment of atelectasis is based on an understanding of the pathophysiology – hypoventilation, hypoinflation, alveolar collapse, and transpulmonary shunting.

2. PATHOGENESIS OF POSTOPERATIVE ATELECTASIS

After any major operation, changes occur in lung function [1–4]. These changes occur in all patients but are not detected on routine examination. Aside from shallow tidal ventilation and some decreased breath sounds at the lung bases, the patient shows no signs of respiratory abnormality. On direct measurement lung volumes are decreased (particularly residual volume, expiratory reserve volume, functional residual capacity, and vital capacity). Compliance is decreased because of the decrease in FRC. The work of breathing is increased for the same reason (i.e., more pressure is required to inhale a given volume into the decreased lung air

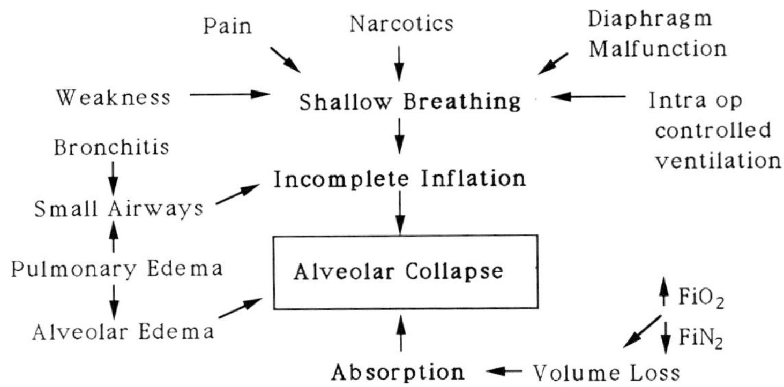

FIGURE 16.1. Pathogenesis of postoperative atelectasis.

space). Further evidence that alveoli are not being ventilated is absolute or relative arterial hypoxemia, which occurs with the patient breathing room air or 100% oxygen, indicating that non-ventilated alveoli are being perfused (transpulmonary shunting).

These changes in lung function are present immediately after operation, progress over 1 to 2 days, and gradually return to normal in most patients. The extent and the duration of these abnormalities are greatest for operations on the thorax and upper abdomen and progressively decrease as the site of operation moves more distally and more superficially on the body structures. These changes may occur after only 1 to 2 hours of general anesthesia if careful attention is not paid to maximal lung inflation during anesthesia [6]. They are superimposed on the patient's pre-existing lung status. If, for example, the patient requires operation for complication of pancreatitis two weeks after the onset of disease, he may already have pleural effusions, increased pulmonary capillary permeability, and existing transpulmonary shunting, and will not tolerate any further deterioration of lung function. Likewise, the patient with pre-existing chronic obstructive lung disease with high airway resistance, maximal work of breathing, and minimal functional lung tissue pre-operatively may proceed to carbon dioxide retention if the work of breathing is only slightly increased after an operation. Advanced age *per se* does not cause lung dysfunction [7]. However the elderly patient is more likely to have chronic lung disease or cardiac disease, which could raise the threshold for pulmonary failure. More important, the elderly patient may be weak, and weakness of respiratory muscles is a major predisposition to alveolar collapse.

Ford et al. [5] have presented evidence that the diaphragm does not function normally in post-laparotomy patients. In their patients, breathing shifted from abdominal to rib cage, and pleural/gastric pressure swings showed decreased diaphragmatic activity during the first postoperative day. Atelectasis occurred in 90% of their cases.

Several factors contribute to these changes in pulmonary function (Fig. 16.1), but shallow breathing with incomplete alveolar inflation is the common denominator. If spontaneous deep breaths to maximal lung inflation are eliminated from the pattern of breathing, alveolar collapse begins within one hour and progresses rather rapidly to produce significant transpulmonary shunting [8,9]. Several studies have shown that patients postoperatively lack the normal pattern of spontaneous deep breaths because of severe pain, anesthetics, or narcotic drugs [1–4]. Further evidence supporting this observation is the fact that the postoperative changes in lung function can be returned toward normal by instituting maximal inflation, deep breathing exercises at regular intervals [4].

If the pattern of decreased lung volume and shunting progresses rather than returns to normal, it becomes clinically evident within 2 to 4 days after operation. Decreased lung volume is detectable as decreased breath sounds on physical examination, and atelectatic areas may be visible on chest X-ray film. Shunt-produced hypoxemia leads to an increased ventilatory rate and the sensation of dyspnea. Severe hypoxemia may cause cyanosis. Atelectasis causes fever and pooling of mucus secretions in non-ventilated areas, leading to an apparent increase in sputum production.

Pulmonary edema migrates to loose aveolar tissue where pulmonary arteries and respiratory bronchioles run side-by-side [10]. The respiratory bronchioles are compressed, leading to decreased ventilation and the chest sounds often called 'cardiac asthma'. As pulmonary edema progresses, airways close completely and alveoli become flooded, creating right to left shunting.

Patients with asthma and bronchospastic pulmonary disease are uniquely protected from atelectasis because of air trapping beyond diseased or spastic airways. These patients have trouble breathing out, not in. They may have serious respiratory failure following operation, but atelectasis *per se* is unusual. The fact that postoperative atelectasis rarely occurs in patients with air trapping and enlarged functional residual capacity suggests an important lesson in pathogenesis: Atelectasis is prevented by alveolar inflation. Conversely, patients with chronic bronchitis, cystic fibrosis, or emphysema with thick mucoid secretions are limited in inspiration (more than expiration) and are at high risk for atelectasis.

In postoperative pulmonary insufficiency due to atelectasis, physical examination shows diminished breath sounds over one or both lung bases. Rales and rhonchi may be heard in the mid and lower lung fields. Although the tidal volume is normal, vital capacity (judged or actually measured) is abnormally small. Chest X-ray demonstrates incomplete lung inflation, usually with overt collapse or consolidation apparent in the lower lobes. If the pathogenesis is predominantly due to lung edema, diffuse increase in lung density is seen, which, when combined with irregular inflation, is often described as diffuse fluffy infiltrates. This radiographic finding can usually be differentiated from cardiogenic pulmonary edema because the latter is more apparent in the lower and middle lung fields when the X-ray is taken when the patient is sitting or standing. Arterial blood gases measured while the patient is breathing air demonstrate hypoxemia, hypocarbia, and respiratory alkalosis.

Supplemental oxygen supplied by nasal catheter or face mask with high flow oxygen (10–20 l/min) supplies approximately 40% inspired oxygen (regardless of the 'settings' on the equipment). Supplemental oxygen results in major improvement in hypoxemia resulting from ventilation – perfusion mismatch, pulmonary embolism, or cardiogenic pulmonary edema, typically resulting in arterial $P_aO_2 > 150$. In contrast supplemental oxygen has a minor effect on hypoxemia due to atelectasis, with P_aO_2 typically rising from the 40's to the 80's.

Fever and mild leukocytosis often accompany atelectasis, and the differential diagnosis between atelectasis and pneumonia is based primarily on continuing signs of infection without another obvious source, combined with pathogenic organisms on sputum culture. Thickened or copious bronchial secretions may be present in any postoperative patient, particularly if the patient has had endotracheal intubation and/or inhalation anesthesia during operation. Bronchial secretions are neither the cause nor the result of atelectasis. However, sputum samples should be acquired from a patient with pulmonary complications for gramstain and culture.

3. DETECTING THE PATIENT AT RISK FOR ATELECTASIS

Identification of the high-risk patient can minimize the incidence of pulmonary complications, so pre-operative assessment of respiratory status is important. The history is the most valuable step. Symptoms that are indications for more detailed study of pulmonary function include exercise intolerance, dyspnea on exertion, wheezing, cigarette smoking, cough, and sputum production. Physical examination should include auscultation and percussion of the lung bases during tidal breathing and maximal inspiration to detect hypoventilation in the weak or debilitated patient and hyperinflation in the patient with chronic airway disease. Wheezing, rales, or rhonchi should trigger further examination. Physical signs of cardiac insufficiency, obesity, clubbing, tobacco stains, and poor oral hygiene are all relative indications for more detailed pulmonary function testing. Chest X-ray should be considered part of the routine physical examination and an integral part of pulmonary function evaluation for any patient with an abnormality detected from the history or physical examination, any patient having a thoracotomy, and any patient over the age of 40.

Part of the physical exam should include instruction to inhale to the maximum, followed by a vigorous forced expiration (a vital capacity maneuver). By observing the chest and the sound of forced expiration the surgeon can make a good guess at the volume of inspiration (should be at least one liter per 50 kg), forced expiration (should be at least two liters per 50 kg), and expiratory flow (most of the exhaled volume should come out in the first second without wheezing). The forced expiratory volume or vital capacity (different names for the same thing) and maximum voluntary ventilation (MVV) can be directly measured with a hand-held turbine spirometer. The ability to climb one or two flights of stairs at a steady pace without dyspnea provides information about the patient that is not available in any other way short of treadmill or exercise testing. A patient who cannot do

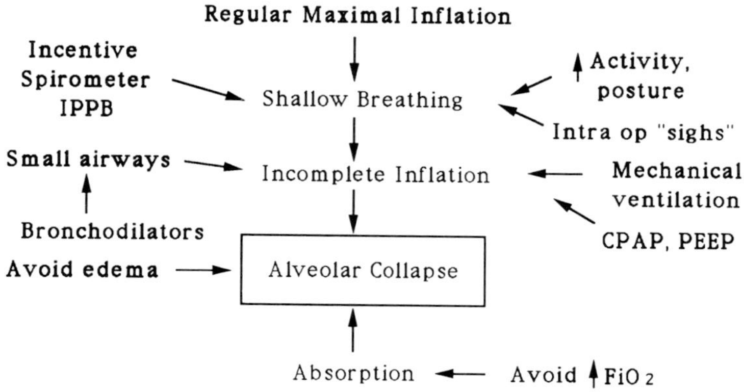

FIGURE 16.2. Prevention of postoperative atelectasis.

this may have respiratory, cardiac, or joint disease, or may be too obese, too weak, too sedentary or too debilitated to manage mild exercise. Whatever the cause, an elective operation should be delayed if the patient cannot do this simple exercise.

Simple spirometry ('pulmonary function tests') and baseline arterial blood gases should be done whenever the history, physical examination, or bedside tests detect the findings of abnormal pulmonary function. Tidal volume, inspiratory capacity, and vital capacity (total and timed intervals) and MVV are measured. The methods and interpretation of spirometric testing are presented in other chapters. The test which correlates best with the incidence of postoperative atelectasis is MVV (formerly maximal breathing capacity) below 50% of predicted. MVV may be abnormally low for many reasons, both pulmonary and non-pulmonary.

In summary, history, physical examination, and chest X-ray is sufficient pulmonary assessment in almost all pre-operative patients. Patients at risk for pulmonary complications as identified by history or examination should have simple spirometry (pulmonary function testing) to identify abnormalities which can be corrected prior to elective operations. Arterial blood gases should be measured pre-operatively in patients with major respiratory dysfunction to serve as a baseline for postoperative management.

3.1. Prevention of atelectasis

Prevention of atelectasis is summarized in Fig. 16.2. The most important factor is to maintain a normal pattern of breathing with regular maximal lung inflation. This can usually be done voluntarily and spontaneously by the patient, taking deep forced inspiratory breaths at least ten times each hour. The incentive spirometer may be used to encourage the patient in this effort and to provide measurement of the volume of inspiration [4]. If the patient cannot take deep breaths spontaneously then mechanical assistance should be utilized. This is usually done intermittently with a mechanical ventilator and mouthpiece (intermittent positive-pressure breathing, IPPB)[11]. In high-risk patients who have had major operations postoperative prophylactic intubation and mechanical ventilation is an appropriate preventative measure[12], continued until the patient can sustain a normal pattern of breathing. Keeping the airway clear by humidification and postural drainage is important in patients with chronic bronchitis. Note that coughing is not a useful measure to prevent postoperative pulmonary complications[13].

Factors that may decrease the efficiency of ventilation should be corrected preoperatively, including cessation of smoking, elective weight loss in grossly obese patients, and treatment of existing bacterial infection (chronic bronchitis) with culture-specific antibiotics, where indicated. Patients with a known tendency to bronchospasm should become accustomed to bronchodilator treatment preoperatively, and the effect of bronchodilators on pulmonary mechanics should be directly measured, particularly in patients with known bronchospastic disorders such as asthma.

The patient with pre-existing lung disease requires special consideration. Preparation related to bronchospasm or chronic bronchitis has been discussed. The patient with acute pulmonary insufficiency, increased lung water, and atelectasis secondary to an acute disorder such as pancreatitis or systemic sepsis will often improve after an operation which solves the primary problem. However, thoracotomy in such a patient should be reserved for life-threatening situations, such as uncontrolled lung diseases.

The patient with severe, chronic obstructive lung disease should be improved as much as possible with bronchodilators, treatment of chronic bronchitis, if present, nutrition, and breathing training. If the pulmonary disorder is very severe (P_aO_2[air] < 50 torr, or carbon dioxide retention), prolonged postoperative intubation and mechanical ventilation should be anticipated and the patient advised accordingly. Such a patient is generally not a candidate for thoracotomy, unless it will improve the physiologic status (such as resection of a totally emphasematous lobe).

Mechanical ventilation should be continued postoperatively until the adequacy of spontaneous ventilation has been clearly established. The action of paralytic drugs should be reversed completely and a vital capacity at least twice the tidal volume documented before extubation.

4. ROUTINE POSTOPERATIVE MEASURES

Postoperatively, both the surgeon and the patient must participate in preventing pulmonary complications. In the recovery room, the endotracheal tube should be maintained in place as long as is necessary, as noted above. Patients with pre-existing pulmonary dysfunction or those at high risk of pulmonary complications may need to be left intubated and maintained on mechanical ventilation for hours or days after operation.

The well-ventilated alveolus is less susceptible to humoral capillary damage than is the atelectatic alveolus. Elderly, debilitated patients, patients following major cardiac esophageal, or pulmonary procedures, and patients with extensive trauma, multiple fractures are often left intubated and maintained on mechanical ventilation 12 hours or more postoperatively. When the patient is fully alert and awake, when his perfusion and cardiac status are stable, and when the blood and extracellular fluid volumes are demonstrated to be normal, then the patient is ready for spontaneous ventilation and extubation.

Special precautions should be taken to prevent atelectasis in the post-thoracotomy patient. Before closing the chest, the lungs should be fully expanded under direct vision by sustained positive pressure. Chest tubes should be placed to evaluate blood and fluid from the posterior gutters and attached to suction. An additional tube should be placed in the anterior apex if air leak is anticipated. Mechanical ventilation should be used until spontaneous breathing with a good inspiratory force (>40 on H_2O) is assured. However, excessive positive pressure increases the risk of air leak, especially when lung tissue has been resected. Peak inspiratory airway pressure (PIP) should be the lowest possible to achieve adequate inflation, generally 20 cmH_2O and never over 40 cmH_2O. Positive end-expiratory pressure (PEEP) is safe and generally indicated, as long as the tidal volume and rate are adjusted to keep the PIP low. The pleural cavity should be maintained free of blood, fluid, and gas by well-placed and well-functioning chest tubes. Tubes should be kept on suction for the first 24 hours postop, at a level of suction sufficient to evaluate the pleural space and keep the lung fully expanded.

Deep breathing exercises, clearing of sputum and mucus, and avoidance of prolonged periods in the supine position should begin in the recovery room. Profound hypoventilation, ventilation–perfusion imbalance, and resultant hypoxemia are the rule in the patient awakening from anesthesia. For this reason, it is common practice to administer moderate amounts (5–10 l/min) of supplemental oxygen to all patients in the recovery room. This is a wise precaution for the first hour or two after anesthesia, but this practice is really prophylactic only against hypoxic arrhythmias and may actually be slightly detrimental to lung function by suppressing whatever deep breathing may result from moderate degrees of hypoxemia. Consequently, supplemental oxygen should not be administered for more than a few hours unless serial blood gas analyses indicate serious hypoxemia.

Airway cleaning, suctioning, expectorant drugs, mist inhalation, and mucolytic agents are all useful in patients with pre-existing chronic bronchitis or thick, tenacious tracheobronchial secretions. The surgeon should have a low threshold for bronchoscopy if these maneuvers do not lead to good basilar inflation, or if there is reason to suspect clots or mucous plugs in the airway. However, these maneuvers and agents may not be necessary in patients who maintain the lung adequately inflated by emphasis on inspiratory maneuvers. A compulsion to force patients to cough dominates much of the thinking on postoperative pulmonary care. Coughing maneuvers are painful in thoracotomy or laparotomy patients and should not be necessary if the lung remains well ventilated.

Breathing maneuvers, and devices designed to encourage those maneuvers, are important adjuncts to postoperative care [14]. Since shallow breathing, the lack of spontaneous deep breaths, and alveolar collapse are the steps that lead to postoperative pulmonary complications, respiratory maneuvers must be those that emphasize maximal lung inflation. Emphasis on breathing out (coughing, tracheal stimulation, 'blow bottles') will do nothing to accomplish alveolar inflation, save the preparatory inspiration the patient may take before that maneuver. The more emphasis that is placed on the inhaled volume and inspiratory pressure, the more effective the maneuver will be.

Several authors have emphasized the ineffectiveness of routine IPPB in preventing pulmonary complications [15,16]. This does not mean that IPPB is not a useful method of treatment. On the contrary, in patients who are too obtunded, in those too weak to carry out spontaneous breathing maneuvers, or in those with already established atelectasis, IPPB is very useful. In those circumstances, however, the device should be used frequently, preferably each hour, and monitored by direct measurement of exhaled volumes, with maximum volume inflation attempted with each breath [11].

Deep inspiratory maneuvers can be done spontaneously but are better done with the use of a device that will record the volume inhaled and 'reward' the patient for his efforts. Such a device is the incentive spirometer. When using this device, the patient can see his inspired volume with each breath, and the total breathing excursions in a period of time are recorded on a counter. Consequently, the physician, respiratory therapist, and patient can all be assured that the proper maneuver is being done, and frequently enough to maintain alveolar inflation. The regular use of deep breathing exercises using an incentive spirometer has been shown to decrease the incidence of pulmonary complications following laparotomy from about 30% to about 10% [4,15,16]. If the incidence of pulmonary complications is already less than 10%, then the addition of spirometry or other devices is not necessary [17]. The incidence of significant atelectic complications following thoracotomy is close to 50%, and deep breathing excercise is well advised but less effective.

Another method of preventing postoperative atelectasis is the application of continuous positive airway pressure (CPAP) with a tight-fitting face mask. Initial reports of this technique show improved alveolar inflation [18]. The potential complications of mask CPAP (gastric distension, vomiting and aspiration, patient discomfort) did not occur in the initial series but remain a cause for concern. This technique, perhaps combined with 'mask' IPPB, may prove useful in patients who are extubated but who cannot or will not breathe deeply.

Whatever method is used to accomplish maximal inflation must be carefully taught to the patient preoperatively. Most patients cannot learn breathing exercises in a painful, narcotized, postoperative state.

Frequent change of position and early ambulation will minimize fluid collection in the dependent portions of the lung. Postoperative nutrition should be maintained. If the patient must go without oral intake for more than 4 or 5 days,

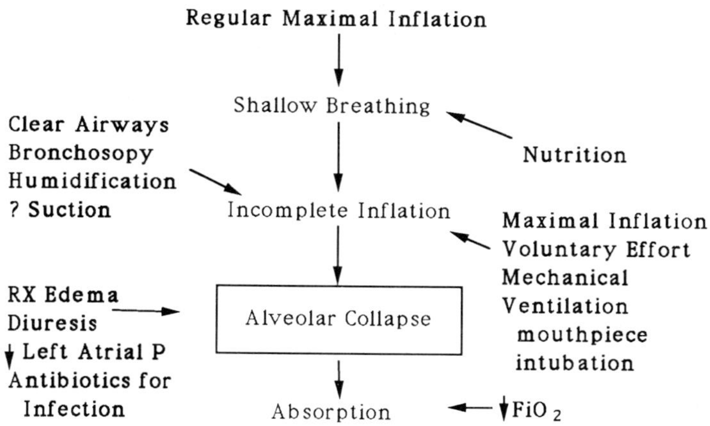

FIGURE 16.3. Treatment of postoperative atelectasis.

total parenteral nutrition is advisable for several reasons, not the least of which is to maintain the strength of the respiratory effort. Fluids must be managed carefully to avoid overloading the extracellular space and diluting the serum proteins. Dehydration must also be avoided because it leads to thickening of secretions.

5. TREATMENT OF ATELECTASIS

While conducting the preliminary clinical and laboratory examinations and making a differential diagnosis the following steps should be taken. Supply supplemental oxygen by nasal catheter or face mask at 10–20 l/min. If the patient has a prior history of limited pulmonary function with hypoxemia and hypercarbia prior to operation, supplemental oxygen may correct the hypoxemia but may diminish the respiratory drive and result in CO_2 narcosis, so special precautions should be taken in the patient with existing chronic lung disease. The patient should be positioned in a way that maximizes diaphragmatic excursion, sitting but not hunched forward with assurance that the stomach and abdomen are not distended.

Treatment aimed at alveolar inflation is outlined in Fig. 16.3. The cornerstone is to establish large volume inflation by instituting deep breathing exercises. The patient should be taught to carry out a sustained maximal inspiration (basically a yawn maneuver). An incentive spirometer will encourage the patient in this manner and quantitate his effort. If adequate volumes cannot be generated by the patient in this manner, then mechanical assistance is necessary, initially with intermittent positive pressure breathing with a mechanical ventilator, without intubation. This must be done with direct exhaled volume measurement, and often requires high pressures with the IPPB device (30 to 40 cm of water). All of the inflation techniques of mechanical ventilation (PEEP, sighs, inspiratory hold, pressure support, CPAP) can be used in the non-intubated patient. Notice that *coughing is not* listed as treatment for pulmonary insufficiency. Forced expiration collapses alveoli, does not clear small airways, and is painful, ineffective activity in the postoperative patient.

When an area of lung is not ventilated, mucus secreted in the bronchi draining from that lung segment may become thickened and impacted, which hinders efforts at re-expansion. This mucus should be cleared by chest physical therapy (percussion) and postural drainage. Hydration and nebulized bronchodilator and mucolytic drugs via the airway may be used. Coughing will help to expel mucus from airways that have been inflated distally. Coughing will not dislodge mucus from airways leading to non-ventilated areas of lung. In this situation mucus must be removed directly with tracheal suction or bronchoscopy. Bronchoscopy is preferred as the initial step in managing any postoperative patient with major atelectasis. This is particularly true in post-thoracotomy patients, who will be limited by pain and edema during both inspiration and expiration. Care must be taken to avoid high airway pressure and direct trauma to an area of resection and bronchial closure.

Routine endotracheal suctioning is practiced on many surgical services. In adults the value of this technique lies primarily in stimulation of deep breathing associated with the vigorous coughing that it induces. If that is the intent, then deep breathing can be easily accomplished by other means without the potential vagal complications associated with tracheal suctioning. In other words, *routine tracheal suctioning has no rational place* in the care of postoperative adult patients.

In infants the size of the airway is such that a very small amount of mucus (which would be insignificant in a larger patient) may cause major tracheal or bronchial occlusion. Infants breathe rapidly with a large ventilation of the dead space, leading to drying of the tracheal secretions, and may have difficulty coughing material from the lower trachea or from the bronchi. Consequently, endotracheal suctioning can be valuable in the postoperative management of infants following operations on the thorax or upper abdomen.

Tracheal suctioning will exacerbate hypoxia if not done properly. The catheter is passed through the nose, verified as passing through the larynx by a change in voice, and connected to oxygen at 5 l/min. Then, 5 cc of saline is injected and the oxygen reconnected for several coughing breaths. Suction is applied for no longer than 10 seconds, then oxygen is resumed. This process is repeated until the suction return is clear (1–5 min). ECG monitoring should be done during and after suctioning. Atropine is given for bradycardia.

In both infants and adults, if adequate ventilation cannot be established with the methods mentioned above, endotracheal intubation and continuous mechanical ventilation are instituted [19]. Mechanical ventilation is indicated when the inspiratory force during a Muller maneuver is less than 20 cm of water, when the vital capacity is less than twice the tidal volume if the respiratory rate is consistently over 30, or if the patient is severely hypoxemic (P_aO_2 less than 50 torr breathing air). If any one of these indications exist and cannot be reversed by the measures mentioned above, intubation and mechanical ventilation are carried out. Intubation with spontaneous breathing and continuous positive airway pressure (5–10 cm of water, CPAP) without mechanical ventilation are standard therapy in the respiratory distress syndrome of the newborn and are commonly used when that condition is complicated by a surgical procedure. However if an adult patient requires intubation, the use of the mechanical ventilator is also indicated (not just CPAP).

The principles outlined above for spontaneous respiration apply equally well to mechanical ventilation. Emphasis is placed on maximum alveolar inflation with every breath. The goal is to return the FRC to normal and to maintain it there. As discussed earlier, PIP must be limited in patients who are susceptible to air leaks. PEEP is acceptable and usually indicated for the ventilated patient with atelectasis, but the tidal volume must be decreased as PEEP is increased to maintain a low PIP and mean airway pressure.

If supplemental oxygen has been instituted as general support of the patient, the amount of oxygen should be kept as low as possible to avoid displacing nitrogen from alveoli and causing absorption atelectasis. Nutrition should be instituted, focusing on positive nitrogen balance to maintain the strength of respiratory muscles and optimize host defenses. The amount of nutrition should be based on measured energy expenditure to avoid overfeeding. Overfeeding with carbohydrate causes conversion of carbohydrate to fat which leads to an excess CO_2 load which may add to the pulmonary insufficiency [20]. Treating lung edema and lung infection are both important steps in improving alveolar inflation, and are discussed below.

Vigorous treatment of alveolar collapse can lead to lung injury and exacerbate lung edema. Specifically inspired oxygen concentration over 60% and airway pressure over 40 cmH_2O should be carefully avoided [21]. With this precaution in mind, efforts at maintaining alveolar expansion are an important component of the treatment of interstitial lung edema. The well-ventilated lung appears to be more resistant to capillary injury than the atelectatic lung.

6. TREATING PNEUMONIA

Bacterial infection often complicates atelectasis and edema, and may occur as a primary event in the postoperative patient. The progression from atelectasis to pneumonia can be difficult to identify, since pulmonary infiltrate and consolidation, fever, leukocytosis, and sputum production occur in both conditions. There is a temptation to institute broad spectrum antibiotics if the diagnosis is uncertain "until sputum culture results are available". There is some rationale in this shotgun approach, because 48 hours delay in treating staphylococcal or pneumococcal pneumonia can be disastrous. On the other hand, two days of unnecessary antibiotics may lead to an equally disastrous infection with candida or resistant gram-negative organisms.

The best approach is to examine the sputum sample under the microscope. The presence of white cells with bacteria indicates active bacterial infection which should be treated with antibiotics based on the gramstain characterization. If bacteria are found without abundant white cells they are most likely contaminants, and antibiotics should not be given. It should be noted however that this differential diagnosis is one of the most difficult in postoperative care and decisions must be based on repeated examination of the patient and the sputum.

7. SUMMARY

Atelectasis is a common complication after surgical operations. Shallow breathing is the common denominator in pathogenesis, and regular maximal inflation is the key to prevention. Treatment of atelectasis includes cleaning the airways, avoiding the supine position, and voluntary or mechanical inflation – all maneuvers aimed at achieving and sustaining alveolar inflation.

REFERENCES

1 Thoren L. Post-operative pulmonary complications: Observations on their prevention by means of physiotherapy. Acta Chir Scand 1954; 107: 193.
2 Zikria BA, Spencer JL, Kinney JM, Broell JR. Alterations in ventilatory function and breathing patterns following surgical trauma. Ann Surg 1974; 179: 1–7.
3 Okinaka AJ. The pattern of breathing after operation. Surg Gynecol Obstet 1967; 125: 785–790.
4 Bartlett RH, Brennan ML, Gazzaniga AB, Hanson EL. Studies on the pathogenesis and prevention of postoperative pulmonary complications. Surg Gynecol Obstet 1973; 137: 925–933.
5 Ford GT, Whitelaw, WA, Rosenal TW, Cruse PJ, Guenter CA. Diaphragm function after upper abdominal surgery in humans. Am Rev Resp Dis 1983; 127: 431–436.
6 Bendixen HH, Bullwinkel B, Hedley-Whyte J, Laver MB. Atelectasis and shunting during spontaneous ventilation in anesthetized patients. Anesthesiology 1964; 25: 297–301.
7 Bartlett RH. Physiology of aging: The respiratory system. In: Meakins, McClaran (eds.). Surgical Care of the Elderly. 1988; 121–128.
8 Caro CG, Butler J, DuBois AB. Some effects of restriction of chest cage expansion on pulmonary function in man: An experimental study. J Clin Invest 1960; 39: 573–583.
9 Pontoppidan H. Mechanical aids to lung expansion in non-intubated surgical patients. Am Rev Respir Dis 1980; 122: 109–119.
10 Staub NC. Pulmonary edema: Physiologic approaches to management. Chest 1978; 74: 559.
11 Welch Jr MA, Shapiro BJ, Mercurio P, et al. Methods of intermittent positive pressure breathing. Chest 1980; 78: 463–467.
12 Shackford SR, Virgilio RW, Peters RM. Early extubation versus prophylactic ventilation in the high risk patient: A comparison of postoperative management in the prevention of respiratory complications. Anesth Analg 1981; 60: 76–80.
13 Bartlett RH, Gazzaniga AB, Geraghty TR. Respiratory maneuvers to prevent postoperative pulmonary complications. A critical review. JAMA 1973; 224: 1017–1021.
14 Bartlett RH. Respiratory therapy to prevent postoperative pulmonary complications. In: Pierson DJ (ed.). Respiratory Intensive Care. Dallas, Daedalus Enterprises 1986: 369–379.
15 Sands JH, Cypert C, Armstrong R, et al. A controlled study using routine intermittent positive pressure breathing in the post-surgical patient. Dis Chest 1961; 40: 128–133.
16 Baxter WD, Levine RS. An evaluation of intermittent positive pressure breathing in the prevention of postoperative pulmonary complications. Arch Surg 1969; 98: 795–798.
17 Schwieger I, Gamulin Z, Forster A, Meyer P, Gemperle M, Suter PM. Absence of benefit of incentive spirometry in low-risk patients undergoing elective cholecystectomy. Chest 1986; 89: 652–656.

18 Ricksten S-E, Bengtsson A, Soderberg C, Thorden M, Kvist H. Effects of periodic positive airway pressure by mask on postoperative pulmonary function. Chest 1986; 89: 774–781.
19 Bartlett RH. Approach to mechanical ventilation. In: Holcroft J (ed.). Pre and Postoperative Manual. New York, Scientific American Medicine 1989.
20 Askanazi J, Rosenbaum SH, Hyman AI. Respiratory changes induced by the large glucose loads of parenteral nutrition. JAMA 1980; 243: 1444–1447.
21 Kolobow T, Moretti MP, Fumagalli R, et al. Severe impairment in lung function induced by high peak airway pressure during mechanical ventilation. Am Rev Respir Dis 1987; 135: 312–315.

Current Topics in General Thoracic Surgery: An International Series, Vol. 2
Perioperative Care, edited by R.M. Peters and J. Toledo

Chapter 17

Analgesia following thoracotomy

Jonathan L. Benumof

1. INTRODUCTION

The treatment of pain following thoracotomy is important not only for patient comfort but also to minimize pulmonary complications by enabling patients to breathe normally (without active exhalation and/or splinting) and deeply (so that they can cough) and to ambulate. Normal and deep breathing require stretching of the skin incision, which is painful. Postoperative patients will normally try to prevent stretching of the skin incision by reflexly contracting their expiratory muscles (splinting), which limits the stretch on the incision during inspiration, and by actively exhaling, which rapidly diminishes whatever stretch there is on the incision. Failing to cough avoids the deep inspiration prior to the forceful exhalation. Splinting, active exhalation, and failing to cough promote retention of secretions, airway closure and atelectasis.

The systemic administration of narcotics can achieve the goals of relieving pain, diminishing splinting, and promoting coughing, but the therapeutic-respiratory depression window is small. Intercostal nerve blocks and thoracic epidural analgesia with local anesthetics are short-term, time-consuming (require repeated injections), higher-risk but efficacious procedures; they can be alternative to, or used in conjunction with, conventional narcotic treatment. Cryoanalgesia is a relatively new, safe, effective and long-lasting (3–4 weeks) pain management technique. Transcutaneous electrical nerve stimulation may have beneficial effects when used as an adjunct to one of the above techniques. However, epidural narcotic administration has become a more frequent pain relief method for post-thoracotomy patients and is, therefore, the technique discussed at greater length in this chapter.

2. CRYOANALGESIA

Extremely long-lasting intercostal nerve block may be obtained by intercostal nerve freezing (cryoanalgesia)[1–8]. Direct application of an ice-ball to the nerve causes degeneration of nerve axons without damage to the support structure of the nerve (the neurolemma), thereby reversibly disrupting nerve activity. Thus, intraneural and perineural connective tissue are preserved, providing a scaffolding for regenerating capillaries, axons and Schwann cells[9]. The area of anesthesia is along the dermatomes treated. During the next two to three weeks after nerve freezing, nerve structure and function begin to recover in parallel. Usually, from one to three months post freezing, there is full restoration of nerve structure and function, without untoward sequelae (neuritis or neuroma formation). The numbness that persists during this time period is not especially bothersome. Young women, however, have admitted to some distress during the period of axonal regeneration due to loss of sensation in the nipple area if the fifth and higher intercostal nerves have been frozen[8].

Currently used cryoprobes are about the size of a pen; the core of the instrument has an exit port that permits rapid expansion of a gas (nitrous oxide). The rapid expansion of nitrous oxide cools a surrounding metal sheath. Since the metal sheath is in contact with a fluid, an ice-ball (temperature= – 60°C) forms at the tip of the cryoprobe. The cryoprobe is applied to the intercostal nerves as far posteriorly as possible from within the chest at the level of the incision, plus two or three interspaces above and below this level, just prior to closure of the thoracotomy wound. The nerves are approached from within the chest since the probe has to pierce the parietal pleura to reach the intercostal nerves in the subcostal groove. This is easily accomplished by the surgeon lifting the nerve out of the groove with a small nerve hook. The cryoprobe is placed directly on the nerve and activated so that the center of the resultant ice-ball encapsulates the nerve. During the freeze, nerve tissue temperature is approximately – 20°C[8]. If 2–3 mm of tissue remains between the tip of the cryoprobe and the nerve to be blocked, the nerve will not become adequately frozen and nerve function might not be totally eliminated. If the pleura is thickened, local peeling of the pleura is advisable[8]. Usually two 30-second freeze cycles, which are separated by a 5-second thaw period, are applied to each of the nerves selected. However, recent experience with one 30-second freeze exposure has resulted in no loss of postoperative pain control with a significantly reduced period of numbness (from 3.0 months to 1.2 months)[8].

The use of cryoanalgesia in this way has effectively reduced postoperative narcotic requirements and improved pulmonary function[1,3–6]. Cryoanalgesia patients have had slight to moderate pain at the end of the first postoperative day, and only slight pain after that (as compared with patients receiving intravenous narcotics who experience moderate to severe pain at 24 hours). Most of the pain experienced by the cryoanalgesia patients has not been incisional discomfort, but rather shoulder or arm pain secondary to chest tube irritation of the pleura. Further advantage of the cryoanalgesia can be gained if the chest tubes can be placed within an intercostal space whose nerve has been subjected to cryoanalgesia [8]. Once the chest tubes are removed, usually on the second or third postoperative day, the pain in the cryoanalgesia patients has become barely noticeable. Consequently, these patients are more able to cooperate with postoperative pulmonary physiotherapy maneuvers. Return of sensation occurs in most patients by the 30th postoperative day. Long-term follow-up for six months has shown no adverse sequelae from the procedure.

Since cryoanalgesia causes temporary nerve damage, and the duration of the nerve damage far exceeds the duration of significant postoperative pain (even with a single 30-second freeze, numbness persisted a mean of 38 days) [8], cryonalgesia cannot be considered a routine post-thoracotomy pain treatment. Cryoanalgesia may be a treatment of choice in thoracic pain situations that are expected to last a long time (e.g., pain from chest trauma) and significantly limit respiratory function.

3. EPIDURAL OPIOIDS

Since the use of epidural morphine for the treatment of pain in man was first reported in 1979 [10], this therapy has rapidly achieved widespread popularity [11]. Treatment of pain after thoracic surgery with epidural narcotics has several very important advantages: (1) there is no sympathetic blockade, and neither motor nor sensory loss; (2) success in relieving pain is usually predictable; and (3) the duration of pain relief is generally much longer than that which results from using parenteral narcotics [10,12–17].

It appears that epidural and intrathecal opiates block the presynaptic and postsynaptic neurons in the substantia gelatinosa of the dorsal horn of the spinal cord. Epidural opiates gain access to the spinal cord by passive diffusion across the dura into the cerebrospinal fluid (CSF) [13,18] and by absorption into arachnoid villi and posterior radicular arteries (which supply the dorsal horn region) [19]. In support of these contentions are the high density of opiate receptors in the substantia gelatinosa of the dorsal horn [20,21]; the high-CSF/low plasma concentration ratio (40–100) of all narcotics after epidural and intrathecal use [13,22]; and the fact that onset of action, potency, and duration of action are related to CSF narcotic concentration rather than plasma narcotic concentration [13,22]. Blockade of the substantia gelatinosa results in a 'selective' spinal block of pain conduction; does not block other sensations, such as external pressure, pin prick, temperature and proprioception; and does not cause a sympathetic or motor block. Consequently, epidural narcotics cannot provide complete anesthesia during surgery [23,24]. In contrast, epidural local anesthetics block nerve impulse conduction in the axons of nerve roots and long tracks in the spinal cord, resulting in blockade of sympathetic, sensory, and motor function, and can be used to provide complete anesthesia.

There is a close relationship between the lipid solubility of epidural narcotics and onset, duration, and extent of analgesia. High lipid solubility means that the narcotic leaves the epidural space and enters the subarachnoid CSF space rapidly;

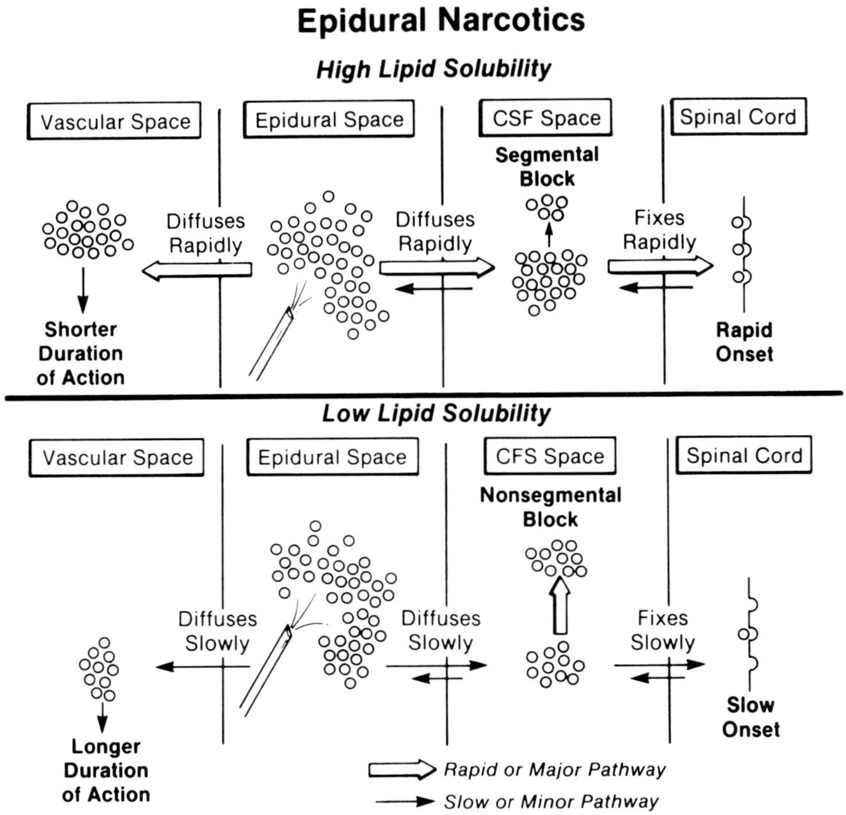

FIGURE 17.1. Epidural narcotics may be either of high or low lipid solubility. Narcotics with high lipid solubility diffuse rapidly into the cerebrospinal fluid (CSF) space and readily fix to spinal cord receptors, resulting in a rapid onset of a segmental block. In addition, high lipid solubility narcotics diffuse rapidly out of the epidural space into the vascular space, resulting in a shorter duration of action. Conversely, low lipid solubility narcotics diffuse into the CSF space and do not readily fix to spinal cord receptors, resulting in a slow onset of a nonsegmental block. In addition, low solubility narcotics diffuse slowly out of the epidural space into the vascular space, resulting in a longer duration of action. The open arrows indicate rapid or major pathways, and the thin solid arrows indicate slow or minor pathways. (Reproduced with permission from Benumof JL. Anesthesia for Thoracic Surgery. Philadelphia, PA, WB Saunders 1987.)

readily fixes to spinal opioid receptors, resulting in a rapid onset of action; does not diffuse widely throughout the epidural and cerebrospinal fluid space; and therefore results in a more segmental block (Fig. 17.1). High lipid solubility also means that the drug is absorbed into the vascular space from the epidural and CSF spaces more rapidly, resulting in a shorter duration of action (Fig. 17.1). The lipophilic narcotics are fentanyl, methadone, and meperidine (in decreasing order of lipid solubility);

when administered in the epidural space at the segmental level of pain in doses of 0.1 mg, 5 mg, and 30–100 mg, respectively, they have a relatively short onset of action of less than 12 minutes, provide nearly complete pain relief in 20–30 minutes, and have a duration of action of 6–7 hours [19,25].

By contrast, morphine has a more complex molecular structure and a low lipid solubility. Low lipid solubility means that the narcotic leaves the epidural space and enters the subarachnoid space slowly; does not readily fix to the spinal opioid receptors, which results in a slow onset of action; diffuses widely throughout cerebrospinal fluid space; and therefore results in a relatively non-segmental block (Fig. 17.1, upper panel). Low lipid solubility also means that the drug is absorbed into the vascular space from the epidural and CSF spaces more slowly, resulting in a longer duration of action (Fig. 17.1, lower panel). With an epidural dose of 5 mg, morphine has a relatively slow onset of action of 15–30 minutes, provides maximal pain relief in 40–60 minutes, and has a duration of action often in excess of 12 hours. Since the lipophobic morphine spreads widely in the epidural and CSF space and causes a non-segmental block, the level of epidural injection is not nearly as important for adequate pain relief (see below) as it is with the lipophilic narcotics. The wider spread of morphine is also responsible for an increased incidence of late respiratory depression compared to the lipophilic narcotics. All the narcotics have a positive epidural dose–response (intensity and duration of pain relief) relationship [17,26,27].

The major advantage of 'selective' blockade of spinal pain with narcotics lies in the avoidance of the major complications of local anesthetic blockade or parenteral narcotic administration described above. Contraindications to the use of both epidural and intrathecal narcotics include elevated intracranial pressure, pre-existing peripheral necrologic disease, allergy to narcotics, infection at the site of injection, and perhaps gross disturbances of coagulation.

The use of intrathecal (subarachnoid) narcotics for pain relief is greatly limited by the inability to give repeated injections owing to the risks involved in leaving an indwelling catheter in the subarachnoid space. In an attempt to partially bypass this problem, single intrathecal injections of morphine have been successfully used preoperatively or intraoperatively to provide 18–24 hours of postoperative pain relief [28–30]. Intrathecal morphine results in extremely high CSF concentrations; subsequent slow (6 hours) passive circulation of CSF allows the lipophobic morphine to reach the cisterns of the brain and the respiratory center [31]. Thus, the use of intrathecal morphine appears to be associated with an increased occurrence of severe late respiratory depression (4–7% compared to $<1\%$ for epidural administration) [31]. Since the epidural route can provide much longer-lasting analgesia with less risk, it has generally replaced the intrathecal route for treating postoperative pain.

The most serious complications of epidural opioids are early and late respiratory depression. The late respiratory depression can be life-threatening and is associated with decreased mentation and confusion; fortunately, the late respiratory depression is a very infrequent occurrence (0.25–0.4% [31] or lower [32] incidence) and is usually gradual in onset, allowing time for diagnosis and treatment [19,31]. The early respiratory depression seems to be directly related to the plasma concentration of narcotic and has occurred in 30 minutes for some of the lipophilic narcotics and in 98 minutes for lipophobic morphine; the late respiratory depression has occurred in 6–10 hours for epidural morphine and is thought to be due to rostral spread of the hydrophilic morphine within the cerebrospinal fluid [33]. Results of quantitative studies of ventilatory responses to carbon dioxide, such as minute ventilation ($\dot{V}_E$) and airway occlusion pressure, performed before and after epidural morphine, are consistent with clinical experience and have shown 20–30% decreases in $\dot{V}_E/CO_2$ and P_{100}/CO_2 slopes [34]. The rapidity of onset, severity, and incidence of respiratory depression may be increased by other factors such as inadvertent dural puncture [17,35], increased dosage and age [31], position of the patient after injection [36], raised intrathoracic and intra-abdominal pressures, and especially the administration of concomitant oral, intramuscular, or intravenous sedatives and/or narcotics [31]. Conversely, chronic administration of systemic opioids protects against the development of respiratory depression; indeed, there are no reports of respiratory depression in chronic pain patients previously made tolerant to opioids [22,37–39]. Naloxone dramatically reverses both early and late respiratory depression.

The other side effects of epidural opioids are urinary retention, pruritus, and nausea and vomiting; these side effects are much more common but also far less serious than late respiratory depression. The incidence of these side effects increases with increasing dosage [40]. Thus, since the relationship between dose and intensity of analgesic response plateaus quickly, the risk/benefit ratio of increasing dosage rises rapidly once effective pain relief levels have been reached [13,29]. The incidence of side effects may be minimized by continuous infusions of low doses of narcotics into the epidural space.

The incidence of postoperative patients requiring bladder catheterization after epidural morphine has generally ranged around 15% [32], although considerable variability in this figure has been reported, and it can be as high as 53% [11,41]. The urinary retention occurs approximately 12 hours after beginning epidural morphine [42], and is probably due to a sympathetically mediated increase in the tone of the bladder detrusor muscle and bladder neck sphincter; the incidence of the complication can be greatly decreased by administration of phenoxybenzamine [41]. The incidence of pruritus has also been variable and has been reported to be as low as 1% [19], although in most series it is considerably higher [14,32,33]. The pruritus is usually generalized [43] but may be confined to just the areas affected by the epidural morphine [44]. The time of onset of pruritus is usually several hours after injection, and therefore histamine release is probably not causative. Nevertheless, the pruritus may occasionally be relieved by promethazine [44]. The mechanism of pruritus is most likely due to a generalized defect in the modulation of cutaneous sensation [45]. The incidence of nausea and vomiting has ranged 17–50% [32,40,46] and is due to morphine reaching the chemoreceptor trigger zone in the fourth ventricle [47]. The incidence decreases with repeated dosing; [37,48]; presumably the brain becomes

TABLE 17.1
Epidural narcotics for postoperative pain management: routes and dosages

Epidural route	Drug	Dosage (diluent saline)	Reference(s)
After thoracotomy			
Thoracic	Fentanyl	1–2 μg/kg (10 ml) → 1–2 μg/kg/h	50, 52
	Methadone	5 mg (10 ml)	52
	Pethidine	30–100 mg (10 ml)	16, 22
	Nalbuphine	10 mg (10 ml)	55
	Morphine	2–4 mg (8 ml); 0.1 mg/h	10, 13, 14, 34, 46–49
Lumbar	Fentanyl	1–2 μg/kg (18 ml) → 1–2 μg/kg/h	50,52
	Morphine	6–8 mg (10–15 ml)	10, 13, 14, 34, 46–49
	Methadone	5 mg (10–15 ml)	53
After abdominal incision			
Lumbar	Fentanyl	1–2 μg/kg (10 ml) → 1–2 μg/kg/h	50,52
	Morphine	2–6 mg (10 ml)	23
	Methadone	4–6 mg (18–20 ml)	53
	Hydromorphone	1.25–1.50 mg (10–15 ml)	54

tolerant to these side effects, as it does to the respiratory depressant effect. Other factors that may contribute to the wide range in reported incidence of epidural morphine side effects are differences in clinical and experimental conditions, such as use of volunteers (increased frequency of complications) rather than patients, patient age, operative site, injection level, and dose of drug administered. Fortunately, the narcotic antagonist naloxone can reverse all of the above side effects. However, repeated injections of naloxone are sometimes necessary to break recurring side effects and suggest that the binding of opiate to receptor is strong. Repeated use of naloxone can reverse the analgesic effects as well, so it must be used cautiously for this procedure.

Epidural opioids have had a moderately extensive trial in relief of post-thoracotomy pain. The epidural catheter may be placed prior to the induction of general anesthesia and checked for correct position by using a small dose of local anesthetic. Alternatively, it may be placed postoperatively prior to emergence from anesthesia, while the patient is still in the lateral decubitus position; the initial injection is made in the recovery room or intensive care unit. Several important clinical points have emerged from the post-thoracotomy epidural opioid analgesia experience.

First, although the thoracic epidural route has been used, the procedure has risks (primarily dural puncture and spinal cord damage), and the lumbar area for catheter insertion has been found to be just as satisfactory for pain relief if a slightly higher dose of morphine and adequate diluent volumes are used[13,16,17,37,49–52]. The reason morphine can be used with a lumbar epidural injection for the relief of thoracic pain is that morphine is lipophobic and will therefore remain in, and have time to spread throughout, the epidural and cerebrospinal fluid spaces. For relief of thoracic pain, instillation of 6 mg of morphine in 10–15 ml of diluent (preservative-free normal saline) in the lumbar epidural region has been used successfully [16,50]. Although studied to a much less degree, fentanyl [53,54], methadone [55], hydromorphone [56], and nalbuphine [57] may also be used by either the thoracic or the lumbar epidural route. Not surprisingly, the lumbar route requires a greater diluent volume to mechanically push the narcotic into a wider distribution, since these lipophilic narcotics will bind too quickly to the spinal cord at, and a few dermatomes above and below, the segmental level of introduction. Since the lumbar route is safer than the thoracic route and since fentanyl has not been associated with respiratory depression [19], the lumbar epidural route with fentanyl is the author's post-thoracotomy pain management technique of choice. However, there remains a wide selection of drugs (and dosages) for use by the lumbar and thoracic epidural route (Table 17.1).

Second, epidural morphine [51] and fentanyl [37] have been reported to be effective following thoracic trauma. In patients with multiple fractured ribs, epidural morphine resulted in well over 6 hours of analgesia with each dose. Alternatively, continuous epidural infusion of fentanyl (1–2 μg/kg/h following 2 μg/kg bolus) would appear to be a good choice in the thoracic trauma situation (as well as for post-thoracotomy pain) because it has a decreased likelihood of causing respiratory depression. Since there is no sympathetic blockade with epidural opioids there is no need to lie the patient supine for top-up doses, and patients with some degree of hypovolemia may be managed more safely than with epidural local anesthetic administration.

Third, in the post-thoracotomy pain relief experience (summarized in Table 17.1) there have been relatively few significant side effects.

Fourth, catheters have been left in-situ and used for as long as five days without the development of tolerance [44].

Fifth, pain relief failures have usually been due to improper catheter location since no pain relief could be demonstrated following injection of local anesthetics [44].

Sixth, the expected increase in the mean post-thoracotomy expiratory flow rate, forced vital capacity, functional residual capacity, and ability to tolerate respiratory care maneuvers following epidural pain relief have been demonstrated to occur [39]. Even larger increases in ventilatory capacity have been demonstrated in the much larger experience with epidural pain-relief after abdominal surgery [43]. These increases are generally greater than, or equal to, those obtained by intravenous narcotics or epidural local anesthetic administration.

Finally, epidural narcotics have been used to treat intractable pain due to thoracic tumors [22]. Less dosage is required and longer duration of analgesia with each intermittent dose is obtained for intractable cancer pain compared to acute postoperative pain [22]. However, although results have been satisfactory after the first few series of injections for intractable pain, tolerance has developed and dosages have had to be increased due to continuously bathing the spinal cord with a CSF concentration of opioid [37]. For treatment of chronic pain, permanent catheters have been implanted in the subarachnoid and epidural spaces and connected to reservoirs or perfusion pumps [37,58]. These implants have been found to be effective, but again tachyphylaxis has been observed [37].

REFERENCES

1 Katz J. The management of pain. In: Benumof JL (ed.). Clinical Frontiers in Anesthesiology. San Diego, Gruen and Stratton 1983.
2 Rooney S, Jain S, McCormack P, et al. A comparison of pulmonary function tests for postthoracotomy pain using cryoanalgesia and transcutaneous nerve stimulation. Ann Thorac Surg 1986; 41: 204–207.
3 Glynn CJ, Lloyd JW, Barnard JDW. Cryoanalgesia in the management of pain after thoracotomy. Thorax 1980; 34: 325–327.
4 Katz J, Nelson W, Forest R, et al. Cryoanalgesia for pain. Lancet 1980; 1: 512–513.
5 Maiwand O, Makey AR. Cryoanalgesia for relief of pain after thoracotomy. Br Med J 1981; 282: 1749–1750.
6 Nelson KM, Vincent RG, Bourke RS, et al. Intraoperative intercostal nerve freezing to prevent post-thoracotomy pain. Ann Thorac Surg 1974; 18: 280–284.
7 Orr IA, Keenan DJM, Dundee JW. Improved pain relief after thoracotomy: Use of cryoprobe and morphine infusion. Br Med J 1981; 283: 945.
8 Maiwand MO, Makey AR, Rees A. Cryoanalgesia after thoracotomy, improvement of technique and review of 600 cases. J Thorac Cardiovasc Surg 1986; 92: 291–295.
9 Myers RR, Powell HC, Heckman HM, et al. Biophysical and pathological effects of cryogenic nerve lesion. Ann Neurol 1981; 10: 478–485.
10 Behar M, Olshwang D, Magora F, et al. Epidural morphine in the treatment of pain. Lancet 1979; 1: 527–529.
11 Torda TA. Management of acute and postoperative pain. Int Anesthesiol Clin 1983; 21(4): 27–47.
12 Torda TA, Pybus DA. Comparison of four narcotic analgesics for extradural analgesia. Br J Anaesth 1982; 54: 291–294.
13 Nordberg G, Hedner T, Mellstrand T, et al. Pharmacokinetic aspect of epidural morphine analgesia. Anesthesiology 1983; 58: 545–551.
14 Pybus DA, Torda TA. Dose-effect relationships of extradural morphine. Br J Anaesth 1982; 54: 1259–1262.
15 Magora F, Olshwang D, Eimerl D, et al. Observations on extradural morphine analgesia in various pain conditions. Br J Anaesth 1980; 52: 247–251.
16 Shulman MS, Brebner J, Sandler A. The effect of epidural morphine on post-operative pain relief and pulmonary function in thoracotomy patients. Anesthesiology 1983; 59: A192.
17 Rawal N, Sjostrand U, Dahlstrom B. Postoperative pain relief by epidural morphine. Anesth Analg 1981; 60: 726–731.
18 Snyder SH. Opiate receptors and internal opiates. Sci Am 1977; 236: 44–56.
19 Cousins MJ, Mather LE. Intrathecal and epidural administration of opioids. Anesthesiology 1984; 61: 276–310.
20 Pert CB, Snyder SH. Opiate receptors: Demonstration in nervous tissue. Science 1973; 179: 1011–1014.
21 Atweh SF, Kuhar MJ. Autoradiographic localization of opiate receptors in rat brains. I. Spinal cord and lower medulla. Brain Res 1977; 124: 53–67.
22 Glynn CJ, Mather LE, Cousins MJ, et al. Peridural meperidine in humans: Analgetic response, pharmacokinetics and transmission into CSF. Anesthesiology 1981; 55: 520–526.
23 Holland AJC, Srikantha S, Tracey JA. Epidural morphine and post-operative pain relief. Can Anaesth Soc J 1981; 28: 453–457.

24 Chayen MS, Rudick V, Borvine A. Pain control with epidural injection of morphine. Anesthesiology 1980; 53: 338–339.
25 Martin J, Lamarche Y, Tetrault JP. Epidural and intrathecal narcotics. Can Anaesth Soc J 1983; 30: 662–673.
26 Crawford RD, Batra MS, Fox F. Epidural morphine dose response for postoperative analgesia. Anesthesiology 1981; 55: A150.
27 Martin R, Salbaing J, Blaise G, et al. Epidural morphine for postoperative pain relief. A dose response curve. Anesthesiology 1982; 56: 423–426.
28 Mathews ET, Abrams LD. Intrathecal morphine in open heart surgery. Lancet 1980; 1: 543.
29 Katz J, Nelson W: Intrathecal morphine for postoperative pain relief. Reg Anesth 1981; 6: 1–3.
30 Fromme GA, Gray JR: A comparison of intrathecal and epidural morphine for treatment of post-thoracotomy pain. Anesth Analg 1985; 64: 185–304.
31 Gustafsson LL, Schildt B, Jacobsen K. Adverse effects of epidural and intrathecal opiates: Report of a nationwide survey in Sweden. Br J Anaesth 1982; 54: 479–486.
32 Reiz S, Westberg M. Side effects of epidural morphine. Lancet 1980; 2: 203–204.
33 Weddel S, Ritter R. Serum levels following epidural administration of morphine and correlation with relief of post-surgical pain. Anesthesiology 1981; 54: 210–214.
34 Knill RL, Clement JL, Thompson WR. Epidural morphine causes delayed and prolonged ventilatory depression, 1981; 28: 537–543.
35 Welch DB. Epidural narcotics and dural puncture. Lancet 1981; 1: 55.
36 Colpaert FC. Can chronic pain be suppressed despite purported tolerance to narcotic analgesia? Life Sci 1979; 24: 1201–1210.
37 Coombs DW, Saunders RL, Gaylor M, et al. Epidural narcotic infusion: Implantation technique and efficacy. Anesthesiology 1981; 55: 469–473.
38 Zenz M, Piepenbrock S, Schappler-Scheele B, et al. Epidural morphine analgesia (PMA). III. Cancer pain. Anaesthetist 1981; 30: 508–513.
39 Zenz M, Schappler-Scheele B, Neuhans R, et al. Long term peridural morphine analgesia in cancer pain. Lancet 1981; 1: 91.
40 Bromage PR, Camporesi EM, Durant PAC, et al. Nonrespiratory side effects of epidural morphine. Anesth Analg 1982; 61: 490–495.
41 Evron S, Magora F, Sadovsky E. Prevention of urinary retention with phenoxybenzamine during epidural morphine. Br Med J 1984; 288: 190.
42 Petersen TK, Husted SE, Rybro L, et al. Urinary retention during I.M. and extradural morphine analgesia. Br J Anaesth 1982; 54: 1175–1177.
43 Bromage PR, Camporesi E, Chestnut D. Epidural narcotics for postoperative analgesia. Anesth Analg 1980; 59: 473.
44 Torda TA, Tybus DA: Clinical experience with epidural morphine. Anaesth Intens Care 1981; 9: 129–134.
45 Bromage PR: The price of intraspinal narcotic analgesia. Anesth Analg 1981; 60: 461–463.
46 Lanz E, Theiss D, Riess W, et al. Epidural morphine for postoperative analgesia: A double-blind study. Anesth Analg 1982; 61: 236–240.
47 Bromage PR, Camporesi EM, Durant PA, et al. Rostral spread of epidural morphine. Anesthesiology 1982; 56: 431–436.
48 Bowen-Wright RM, Goroszeniuk T: Epidural fentanyl for pain of multiple fractures. Lancet 1980; 11: 1033.
49 Welch DB, Hrynaszkiewicz A: Postoperative analgesia using epidural methadone, administration by the lumbar route for thoracic pain relief. Anaesthesia 1981; 36: 1051–1054.
50 Steidl LJ, Fromme GA, Danielson DR. Lumbar versus thoracic epidural morphine for post-thoracotomy pain. Anesth Analg 1984; 63: 277.
51 Johnston JR, McCaughey W. Epidural morphine: A method of management of multiple fractured ribs. Anaesth 1980; 35: 155–157.

52 Fromme GA, Steidl LJ, Danielson DR. Comparison of lumbar and thoracic epidural morphine for relief of postthoracotomy pain. Anesth Analg 1985; 64: 454–455.
53 Lomessy A, Magnin C, Viale J, et al. Clinical advantages of fentanyl given epidurally for postoperative analgesia. Anesthesiology 1984; 61: 466–469.
54 Wolf MJ, Davies GK. Analgesic action of extradural fentanyl. Br J Anaesth 1980; 52: 357–358.
55 Welch DB, Hrynaszkiewicz A. Postoperative analgesia using epidural methadone, Administration by the lumbar route for thoracic pain relief. Anaesthesia 1981; 36: 1051–1054.
56 Wakerlin G, Shulman MS, Yamaguchi LY, et al. Experience with lumbar epidural hydromorphone for pain relief after thoracotomy. Anesth Analg 1986; 65: S163.
57 Mok MS, Louie BW, Hwong BF, et al. Epidural nalbuphine for the relief of pain after thoracic surgery. Anesth Analg 1985; 64: S258.
58 Coombs DW, Saunders RL, Pageau MG. Continuous intraspinal narcotic analgesia, Technical aspects of an implantable infusion system. Reg Anesth 1982; 7: 110–113.
59 Katz J: The management of pain. In: Benumof JL (ed.). Clinical Frontiers in Anesthesiology. San Diego, Gruen and Stratton 1983.
60 Rooney S, Jain S, McCormack P, et al. A comparison of pulmonary function tests for postthoracotomy pain using cryoanalgesia and transcutaneous nerve stimulation. Ann Thorac Surg 1986; 41: 204–207.
61 Glynn CJ, Lloyd JW, Barnard JDW. Cryoanalgesia in the management of pain after thoracotomy. Thorax 1980; 34: 325–327.
62 Katz J, Nelson W, Forest R, et al. Cryoanalgesia for post-thoracotomy pain. Lancet 1980; 1: 512–513.
63 Mainwand O, Makey AR. Cryoanalgesia for relief of pain after thoracotany. Br Med J 1981; 282: 1749–1750.
64 Nelson KM, Vincent RG, Bourke RS, et al. Intraoperative intercostal nerve freezing to prevent post-thoracotomy pain. Ann Thorac Surg 1974; 18: 280–284.

Current Topics in General Thoracic Surgery: An International Series, Vol. 2
Perioperative Care, edited by R.M. Peters and J. Toledo

Chapter 18

Management of post-pneumonectomy empyema of the pleural space

Joseph I. Miller

1. INTRODUCTION

The management of post-pneumonectomy empyema remains a problem to the practicing thoracic surgeon. It is estimated that post-pneumonectomy empyema occurs in approximately 2 to 12% of patients undergoing pneumonectomy[1]. It is associated with a bronchopleural fistula in approximately 40% of patients, and in only 20% of patients does the bronchopleural fistula close spontaneously.

Historical methods used in the treatment of this complication are outlined in Table 18.1. They range from simple rib resection and drainage to complete thoracoplasty. Hippocrates[2], in 229 BC, first proposed an intercostal incision with rib resection for the management of a post-pneumonectomy empyema. Erstlander and Schede proposed various forms of thoracoplasty, and in 1927, Alexander proposed an extrapleural paravertebral thoracoplasty for the management of a post-pneumonectomy empyema[3]. In 1935, Eloesser[4] published a method for creating a cutaneous flap for the drainage of the pleural space, which is still widely used. Perhaps the most important advance in this century in the treatment of this complication was reported by Claggett and Geraci[5] in 1963. They described rib resection with antibiotic irrigation and closure in 6 to 8 weeks. Subsequently, Stafford and Claggett[6] reported a success rate of 75 to 88% utilizing this method, with sterilization of the empyema space and subsequent permanent closure. Our own experience with this method has not achieved that success rate. When the offending organism is *Staphylococcus aureus,* there is a reasonable chance of success. When multiple bacterial organisms are present, the rate of success is only approximately 20%.

Our algorithm for the treatment of post-resectional empyema and, specifically, post-pneumonectomy empyema, is given in Tables 18.2 and 18.3. Once the diagnosis of post-pneumonectomy empyema, with or without bronchopleural fistula, has been established, pleural drainage by closed chest tube thoracostomy

TABLE 18.1
Historical highlights in treatment of post-pneumonectomy empyema[a]

Year	Reference	Treatment
229BC	Hippocrates [2]	Intercostal incision with rib resection
1879	Erstlander[b]	Thoracoplasty
1890	Schede[b]	Thoracoplasty
1927	Alexander[b]	Extrapleural paravertebral thoracoplasty
1935	Eloesser [4]	Eloesser flap
1963	Clagett and Geraci [5]	Open drainage and irrigation
1971	Provan[b]	Closed drainage and irrigation
1975	Miller[b]	Balanced drainage
1983	Pairolero[b]	Flap closure with open drainage
1983	Miller et al. [7]	Complete flap closure without open drainage

[a] Modified from Miller et al. [7].

[b] See Miller et al. [7] for reference.

TABLE 18.2
Post-resectional empyema [8]

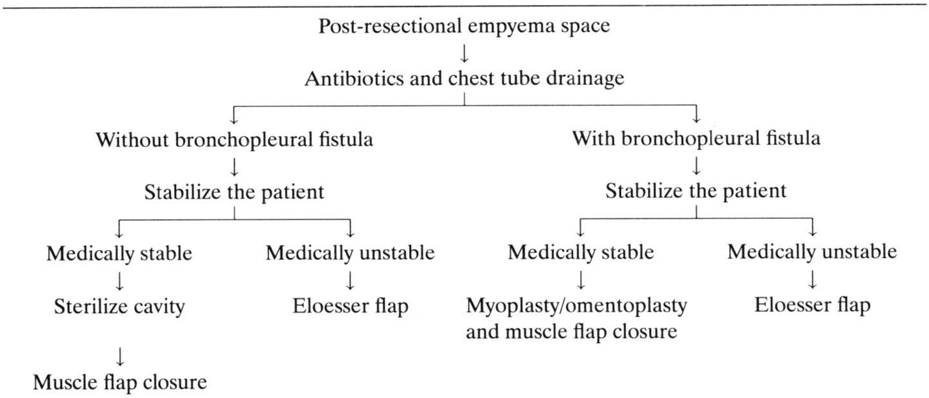

is mandatory. Chest tube thoracostomy is continued until the mediastinum has become stabilized, generally requiring approximately 2 to 3 weeks. Thereafter, open drainage or another modality of therapy for the empyema space can be undertaken safely.

During the acute phase of post-pneumonectomy empyema, the patient is treated with closed chest tube thoracostomy, with or without bronchopleural fistula. Once the patient is medically stable, and has entered into the chronic phase of 3 to 4 weeks, a modified Clagett procedure is performed, if no bronchopleural fistula is present. A second small chest tube is inserted into the second right intercostal space, and a continuous inflow–outflow irrigation system is established through the pleural space. The irrigant is based on antibiotic sensitivities to the pleural drainage. This is generally a cephalosporin with 2 g in 500 cc of D5/0.45 normal saline running at a rate of 50 cc/h through the inflow catheter, with continuous

TABLE 18.3
Post-pneumonectomy space management[8]

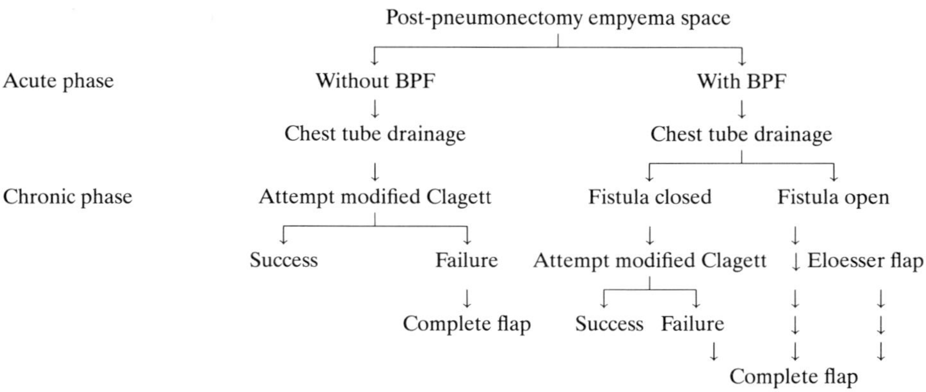

drainage through the outflow catheter. Occasionally, if a gram-negative organism is present, we will utilize 0.25% Neomycin as the irrigant. This method will achieve sterilization of the pleural space in approximately 50% of the patients. If this method is successful, and the return irrigant is negative on three consecutive days after 2 weeks of irrigation, the tubes can be removed, and the space allowed to fill. If the modified Clagett technique fails, a complete muscle flap closure of the pneumonectomy space can be performed.

If the patient is medically unstable, and is not a candidate for a major operation, the post-pneumonectomy space is managed by a simple Eloesser flap procedure.

If a patient with a post-pneumonectomy empyema has a bronchopleural fistula, it is treated during the acute phase with closed chest tube thoracostomy, and converted to open drainage by a chest tube when mediastinal stabilization has occurred. If the fistula should close, one can attempt a modified Clagett sterilization of the cavity, utilizing two chest tubes with inflow–outflow antibiotic irrigation solution, as previously described. If this is successful, and the chest tube drainage is negative on 3 consecutive days after 3 weeks of irrigation, the tubes can be removed. If the pleural fluid is persistently positive, one proceeds with a complete muscle flap closure of the pneumonectomy space. If the patient with the bronchopleural fistula is medically unstable, conversion of the chest tube to an open chest flap by the Eloesser procedure is our procedure of choice.

When the patient is medically unstable, or is not a candidate for single stage muscle flap closure of the post-pneumonectomy empyema space, we feel that the open flap procedure, as originally described by Eloesser[4] in 1935, provides the most satisfactory form of drainage, in that it creates a skin line fistula, and provides drainage without tubes. This is usually done following closed chest tube thoracostomy drainage, or closed rib resection, when long term open drainage is necessary. It can be used to drain a post-pneumonectomy empyema, with or without a bronchopleural fistula, and when open chest tube drainage would be extremely uncomfortable, such as when the tube is located high in the axilla and in the paravertebral area. Symbas et al.[9] modified the Eloesser procedure, and made a significant advance in converting the original U-based shape to an inverted U-based shape flap. In performing the open Eloesser flap procedure, the incision must be planned carefully to be effective. An inverted U-shaped flap of skin is fashioned with a base, approximately 6 to 8 cm in length, and placed parallel to the superior border of the first uninvolved rib above the bottom of the empyema cavity. The curved end of the flap is about 6–7 cm long. The specific technical points in constructing the Eloesser flap are: The base of the flap is usually parallel to the most dependent portion of the empyema cavity. The top of the inverted U-based flap is placed 2 to 3 intercostal spaces, or ribs, above the base of the cavity. The inverted U is placed by incising down through the skin, subcutaneous tissue, and all muscle fascia to the rib cage. Three inches of 2 to 3 ribs are totally resected. The tongue of the flap is completely debrided of all tissue, except underlying subcutaneous tissue. The underlying tongue is tacked down to the bottom of the empyema space, utilizing 0 PDS. The margins of the flap are approximated with interrupted PDS to close over the exposed rib ends.

Open flap drainage by the Eloesser flap is easier to maintain, and generally cleaner than open tube drainage. The cavity is packed daily, depending upon the rate of soilage. Pseudomonas frequently develops, and packing soaked in 1% of acetic acid provides good control of this growth.

Thoracoplasty in the treatment of post-pneumonectomy empyema is discussed briefly for completeness. In general, one should not perform a thoracoplasty unless absolutely necessary, as newer techniques of space obliteration by muscle flap transposition make this mainly of historical significance. Previously, a patient with an empyema of the pleural space had undergone a thoracoplasty, either an extrapleural operation, or one of the Schede–Urstlander type[3]. In the latter group, all underlying ribs, intercostal structures, parietal pleura and peel are removed to allow the space to form granulation tissue. In general, it is fair to say that collapse procedures in the treatment of post-pneumonectomy empyema have been replaced with newer plastic surgical techniques, with transposition of extrathoracic muscle flaps for closure of thoracic spaces.

When post-pneumonectomy empyema develops, the empyema space is inevitably large, and nearly always permanent. In these circumstances, methods of treatment include sterilization by the Clagett technique, permanent drainage, thoracoplasty, and obliteration by muscle flap transposition.

2. CURRENT MANAGEMENT OF POST-PNEUMONECTOMY EMPYEMA

Once the diagnosis of a post-pneumonectomy empyema, with or without a bronchopleural fistula, is made, surgical drainage by closed chest tube thoracostomy and institution of appropriate antibiotic therapy is vitally important. When the patient is medically stabilized, a correct decision in treating the patient can be

TABLE 18.4
Percentage flap coverage of pneumonectomy space [7]

Flap	Percentage
Latissimus dorsi	30–40
Serratus anterior	10–15
Pectoralis major	20–30
Pectoralis minor	0–2
Omentum	5–15
Rectus abdominis	5–15

made. Generally, a period of 10 to 14 days is adequate to stabilize the patient, and the mediastinum.

Once adequate drainage by closed chest tube thoracostomy has been established, and the patient stabilized, the course of management can be determined. If a bronchopleural fistula is present, and the patient is medically stable, the fistula should be closed by a myoplasty or omentoplasty, followed by single stage muscle flap closure of the remaining space. If the patient is medically unstable, the closed chest tube thoracostomy can be converted to an open flap Eloesser procedure.

3. MUSCLE FLAP CLOSURE OF THE POST-PNEUMONECTOMY EMPYEMA SPACE

I believe that the best method of treating the post-pneumonectomy empyema space is by single stage complete muscle flap closure, completely obliterating the pneumonectomy space by the transposition of extrathoracic skeletal muscle.

Intrathoracic muscle transposition was reported by Abrashanoff[10] in 1911 for closure of a bronchopleural fistula. Since then, muscle flaps have been used to obliterate spaces, close bronchopleural fistula, and reinforce tracheal, bronchial, and esophageal anastomosis. In the late 1970s, we used extrathoracic muscle flaps to close bronchopleural fistulas in post-lobectomy empyema cavities, but not until 1980 did we first attempt to fill an entire pneumonectomy space with muscle flaps[7].

Because of their excellent blood supply, and their ability by pedicle flap to reach almost any location in the pleural space, muscle flaps are an ideal tissue to fill the contaminated space. The extrathoracic muscle flaps used in various combinations in our patients, are listed in order of frequency in Table 18.4. These are the latissimus dorsi, the serratus anterior, the pectoralis major and minor, the omentum, and the rectus abdominis. The percentage of flap coverage of the normal pneumonectomy space in the adult by each flap is also shown in the table. These figures are based on clinical estimation of coverage at the time of operation and cadaver studies[7].

Extrathoracic muscle flaps require a route of entry when transposed into the thoracic cavity. Segments from ribs, determined by the blood supply of the muscles, are resected to prevent kinking, constriction, consequent swelling and ischemia in the muscle when the muscle is transposed into the pleural space.

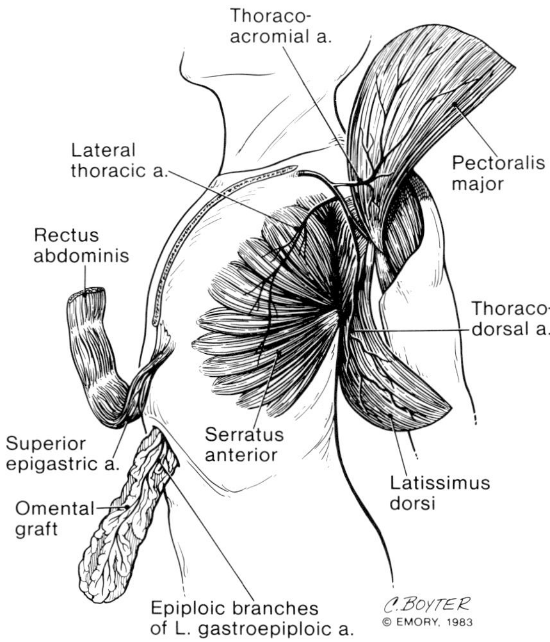

FIGURE 18.1. Extrathoracic muscle flaps that can be utilized in closure of a post-pneumonectomy empyema cavity.

In dealing with a post-resectional space, one must consider the cause of the space, the size of the space, the medical status of the patient, and the options before deciding on the definitive course of management. Options in dealing with the post-resectional spaces are: Chest tube thoracostomy, Clagett procedure, Eloesser procedure, rib resection, decortication, thoracoplasty, and muscle flap closure.

4. SPECIFIC FLAPS (Fig. 18.1)

4.1. Omentum

The omentum can be brought into the pleural space as a flap or free graft. It is the flap of choice to cover an open bronchial stump because of the excellent vascular blood supply. It has been shown that neovascularization is evident in the stump within 48 hours after placement of an omental flap around a closed stump. The omental flap is usually brought up through a separate anterior opening in the diaphragm, and is laid over the bronchial stump; tacking sutures are placed around the flap (Fig. 18.2). Normally, we do not use this flap unless an open bronchial stump is present, or there is not enough muscle to fill the space.

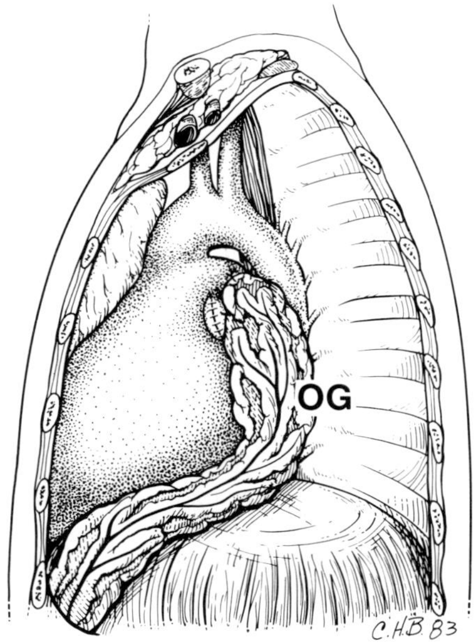

FIGURE 18.2. The omental flap is brought through an anterior opening in the diaphragm and placed over the bronchial stump.

The omentum derives its blood supply from the right and left gastroepiploic vessels. The specific length of the omentum varies from 14 to 30 cm; the lateral width varies from 23 to 46 cm [11]. Division of the left gastroepiploic vessels, and detachment of the gastroepiploic arcade from the greater curve of the stomach, creates a large pedicle based on the intact right gastroepiploic vessels, and allows the mobilized omentum to reach the base of the neck in approximately 88% of patients. The omentum is mobilized by entering the abdominal cavity through an upper midline abdominal incision. The omentum can be brought through an opening on either side of the diaphragm. The opening must be loose enough so that the omentum and its attached blood supply is not compromised.

4.2. Pectoralis major

The pectoralis major flap is one of the two most commonly utilized extrathoracic muscle flaps. It has a dual blood supply from the predominant thoracoacromial artery to the major pedicle; and from the internal mammary artery to the major pedicle and to the secondary pedicle. The pectoralis major muscle has a type-5 blood supply [12] and the flap can be based on its dominant thoracoacromial pedicle, or on the segmental perforators through the internal mammary artery. It may be used as a reverse turnover flap, or may be placed directly into the wound.

4.3. Latissimus dorsi

The latissimus dorsi is our most commonly utilized flap for thoracic defects. The predominant blood supply is from the thoracodorsal artery. It may be used as a turnover flap or placed directly into the wound. It may be brought through the incision or through a separate small rib resection. The flap is generally mobilized through an incision on the posterior axillary line. The skin and subcutaneous tissue are dissected from the latissimus. The muscle is divided distally, and then mobilized from distal to proximal. Based on its dominant thoracodorsal pedicle, it will swing anterolaterally, and may enter the pleural space by a small rib resection. It is an extremely safe and reliable flap.

4.4. Serratus anterior

The serratus anterior is our second choice of flaps for filling a pneumonectomy space, and is particularly good for filling a small space. The entrance into the chest is through the primary chest incision.

4.5. Rectus abdominis

In general, the rectus abdominis is used for closure of defects in the lower third of the sternum. It is reserved for problems involving the pleural space, in case a residual space remains. In general, it is the last flap applied when the post-pneumonectomy space is filled.

The rectus abdominis has a type-3 blood supply [12] and can be based either on its superior pedicle, the superior epigastric artery, or on its inferior pedicle, the deep inferior epigastric artery. Based on the superior epigastric artery, the entire muscle could be turned over upon itself to obliterate the infected median sternotomy, or fill the inferior part of the infected pleural space. The integrity of the internal mammary artery must be established before this flap can be transposed safely, based on the superior pedicle.

5. SURGICAL TECHNIQUE OF SINGLE STAGE COMPLETE MUSCLE FLAP CLOSURE

The empyema, with or without bronchopleural fistula, is managed initially by a closed chest tube in the acute stage. This treatment may be continued, or an Eloesser flap can be performed, depending on the patient's comfort, and the adequacy of drainage. At approximately 3 months for benign disease, and 6 months to 1 year for malignant disease, single stage muscle flap closure is performed.

There are six basic principles for complete flap closure: (1) Appropriate antibiotics are given, based on the sensitivities of the pleural drainage. (2) The original incision is reopened. (3) The cavity is debrided widely so that good

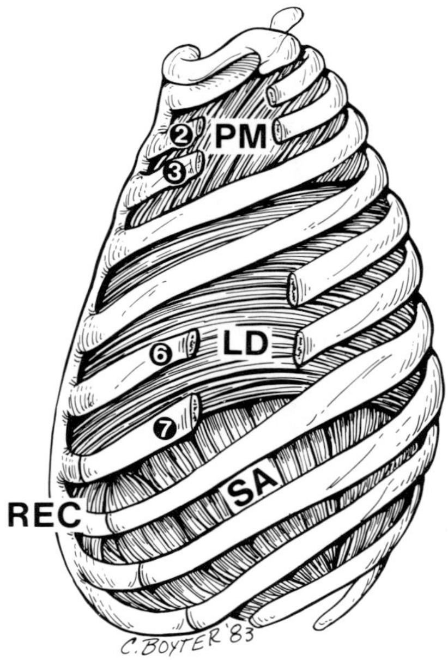

FIGURE 18.3. An entire pleural space filled with muscle flaps and their usual anatomical location. (PM, pectoralis major; LD, latissimus dorsi; REC, rectus abdominis; SA, serratus anterior.)

granulation tissue is present. (4) A bronchopleural fistula is identified, if present, the edges freshened, and the fistula is closed, if technically possible. An omental flap is brought up through the anterior diaphragmatic incision (Fig. 18.2), and is tacked around the fistula with 3–0 prolene suture. (5) Appropriate muscle flaps are then swung to fill the pleural space. (6) We begin with a latissimus dorsi flap, and follow with any necessary flaps to fill the entire space, depending on the anatomical location, and size of the space. The filling of the entire pleural space is shown in Fig. 18.3. The technique of flap mobilization is discussed by Mathis and Nahai [12] in their excellent work on muscle and musculocutaneous flaps.

All extrathoracic muscle flaps require a route of entry into the chest. The location of the opening is usually determined by the blood supply of the muscle, and should be placed so that the blood supply is under no tension after transposition. Generally, 4–5 cm of the appropriate rib is all that must be resected to allow for flap entry. Fig. 18.4 shows the typical site of entry for the pectoralis major and latissimus dorsi flaps. The sine qua non for success with single stage complete muscle flap closure is that the entire space must be filled. If a space is left, it is usually just beneath the 5th or 6th rib in the midaxillary line, and can be closed by a short resection of the ribs over it, without cosmetic deformity. Following transposition of the muscle flaps, the wound is closed primarily, and chest tubes are left to pleurovac suction for 7 to 10 days. Appropriate antibiotics are given.

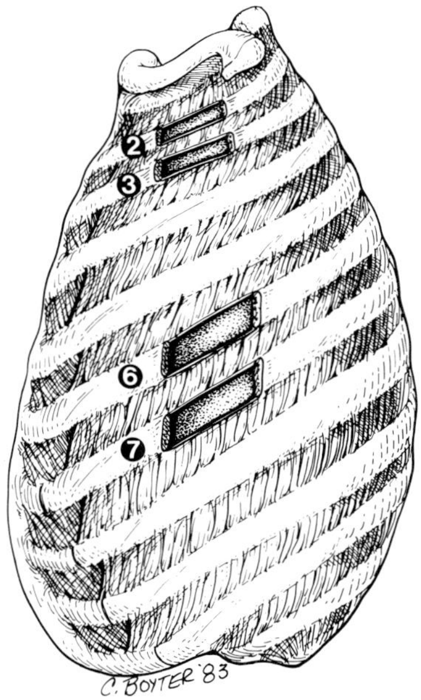

FIGURE 18.4. Usual sites of rib resection for entrance of the pectoralis major (top) and latissimus dorsi (bottom) flaps into the pleural space.

The two predominant points in this surgical technique are as follows: No residual space can be left; and a sufficient number of flaps are available so that any intrathoracic space can be filled. Our schematic approach to the treatment of post-pneumonectomy empyema has been previously given in Table 18.3. We have utilized this technique in over 14 patients, with only 2 failures. In the post-operative period, following closure of the space by muscle flaps, the wound is closed, with chest tube suction drainage in place from 10 to 14 days to allow all flaps to be completely sealed. Following this, assuming there is no abnormal drainage and no evidence of any air leak, the tubes are removed. The patient is surgically dismissed on oral antibiotics, generally a cephalosporin for approximately 1 month. We have experienced no mortality, and essentially no morbidity. The two failures were a matter of the learning curve, and both were performed in patients who had previous mastectomies, and did not have the pectoralis major muscle available for filling the space. In each of these patients, we were left with a small space at the time of the primary flap closure, and a 2 to 3 rib thoracoplasty had been performed in order to fill the space. However, we were left with a persistent small space, and in one patient, a bronchopleural fistula reopened. This was subsequently converted to a permanent Eloesser flap. These two patients have done well in long term follow-up.

6. CONCLUSION

In conclusion, the treatment of post-pneumonectomy empyema continues to plague the practicing thoracic surgeon. The potential consequences are lethal if left untreated, or treated inappropriately. It remains our opinion that in the current era of plastic surgical techniques with transposition of extrathoracic muscle flaps, the single stage complete muscle flap closure remains the primary and definitive method for treating this potentially disabling and life-threatening complication.

REFERENCES

1 LeRoux BT, Mohlala ML, Odell JA, et al. Supporative disease of the lung and pleural space, Part 1: Empyema thoracis and lung abscess. Yearbook 1986; 22: 1.
2 Hippocrates. In: Major Classic Description of Disease. Springfield, IL, CC Thomas 1965.
3 Meade, RH. A History of Thoracic Surgery. Springfield, IL, CC Thomas 1961.
4 Eloesser L. An operation for tuberculosis empyema. Surg Gynecol Obstet 1935; 60: 1096.
5 Clagett OT, Geraci JE. A procedure for the management of post-pneumonectomy empyema. J Thorac Cardiovasc Surg 1963; 45: 141.
6 Stafford EG, Clagett OT. Post-pneumonectomy empyema: neomycin instillation and definitive closure. J Thorac Cardiovasc Surg 1972; 63: 771.
7 Miller, JI, Mansour KA, Nahai F, et al. Single stage complete muscle flap closure of the postpneumonectomy empyema space: A new method and possible solution to a disturbing complication. Ann Thorac Surg 1984; 38: 227.
8 Miller, JI. Infections of the pleura. In: Shields TW (ed.). General Thoracic Surgery, 3rd Ed. Philadelphia, PA, Leg and Febiger 1989.
9 Symbas PN, Nugent JT, Abbott OA, et al. Nontuberculous pleural empyema in adults. Ann Thorac Surg 1971; 12: 69.
10 Abrashanoff. Plastische Methode der Schliessung von Fistelgangen, welche von inneren Organen Kommen. Zentralbl Chir 1911; 38: 186.
11 Jurkiewicz MJ, Rand RP. The omentum in sternal wound reconstruction. In: Van der Salm TJ (ed.). Cardiac Surgery: State of the Art Reviews. Hardy and Belfus 1988; 2: 3.
12 Mathis, SJ, Nahai F. Clinical Applications for Muscle and Musculocutaneous Flaps. St. Louis, Mosby 1982.

Current Topics in General Thoracic Surgery: An International Series, Vol. 2
Perioperative Care, edited by R.M. Peters and J. Toledo

Discussion of "Management of post-pneumonectomy empyema of the pleural space" by Joseph I. Miller

José Mª Borro, Vicente Tarrazona and Francisco París

1. INTRODUCTION

Infection of residual pleural space is one of the most serious post-operative complications following total removal of the lung. Dr. Miller's excellent and schematic work provides a good guide for the management and treatment of post-pneumonectomy empyema.

We agree for the most part with the author, but we would like to emphasize the importance of post-pneumonectomy empyema prophylaxis. There are two principal causes of empyema: (1) the opening of an infected cavity into the pleural space; and (2) the possible devascularization of the terminal bronchial stump in extensive lymph node dissection.

When the pleural cavity is contaminated, prophylaxis of post-operative empyema should be done by irrigating the pleural cavity daily for at least 3 to 4 days with a solution of iodine providone, instilled through a 14 gauge catheter, inserted in the second anterior intercostal space with a basal closed thoracostomy tube for drainage of the irrigation solution. In our unit, in order to prevent local resistances and to avoid their ototoxicity and nephrotoxicity [1], we prefer the local application of antiseptics over the topical use of aminoglycoside antibiotics such as neomycin.

The coverage of the devascularized bronchial stump, with pericardium, parietal pleura, intercostal muscle or omentum becomes essential. Although abdominal omentum is the best tissue to vascularize the terminal bronchus, its disadvantages include the need for a second incision.

Clinical signs of empyema are fever, malaise or increase in the pleural liquid level on X-ray, with or without mediastinal shift. The diagnosis of empyema is made by bacteriological analysis of the pleural fluid, with antibiotic sensitivity tests. If the patient coughs up serosanguinous fluid from the respiratory tract, bronchoscopy will confirm the presence of a concomitant bronchopleural fistula.

In our practice, a similar therapeutic plan to that proposed by Dr. Miller is used: (1) closed tube thoracostomy; (2) open drainage by a chest tube; (3) open skin flap thoracostomy drainage; and (4) muscle flap closure of the post-pneumonectomy empyema space.

We agree with him that it is very difficult to find a patient with post-pneumonectomy empyema being fit enough for an early pleural cavity closure. Surgical approach is contraindicated in patients with unstable clinical condition. On the other hand, we must be sure that the dorsal and serratus muscles remain well revascularized following thoracotomy.

We have seen two cases of spontaneous closure after several months of topical cleaning through an Eloesser thoracostomy. Nevertheless, when the septic period is over and the pleural space macroscopically cleaned, the cavity should be closed. We prefer to have 2–3 sterile wound cultures, but in infection with some nosocomial germs, like *Pseudomonae*, it is difficult to eradicate the microorganisms. In these cases, primary closure with muscle transfer is recommended in spite of positive wound cultures, accompanied by adequate systemic pre- and post-operative antibiotic therapy based on sensitivity tests.

For patients in good condition we always try to close the pleural cavity by surgery, even if we are not sure that the patient is tumor free. This policy gives better quality of life to the patient and the risk of the surgical procedure is low.

2. SURGICAL TECHNIQUE

The operation is started by unroofing the empyema pleural space by resection of the overlying rib fragments, intercostal bundles and subjacent parietal pleural peel. No recess should be left intact. Any osseous or cartilaginous costal fragment showing macroscopic signs of inflammation should be removed (Figs. D18.1 and D18.2). The thoracic cavity is washed several times using iodine providone solution. The first rib should be left intact.

The dorsal, serratus and occasionally pectoral muscles are used, as in Dr. Miller's description, to fill the thoracic cavity with the muscular flaps. Several Redon drainage tubes are placed in the different muscular spaces. Finally, the wound is closed with subcutaneous tissue and skin.

A compression 'bandage' which includes the homolateral arm is maintained for at least 7 days following the operation to exclude the movements of the thoracic muscles and to avoid any residual space remaining (Fig. D18.3).

3. VALENCIA GROUP RESULTS

From March 1981 to November 1989 we have carried out 17 myoplasties in patients with post-pneumonectomy empyema. Eleven had pneumonectomy for neoplastic disease and 6 had infected destroyed lungs (3 tuberculosis). Mean age was 53

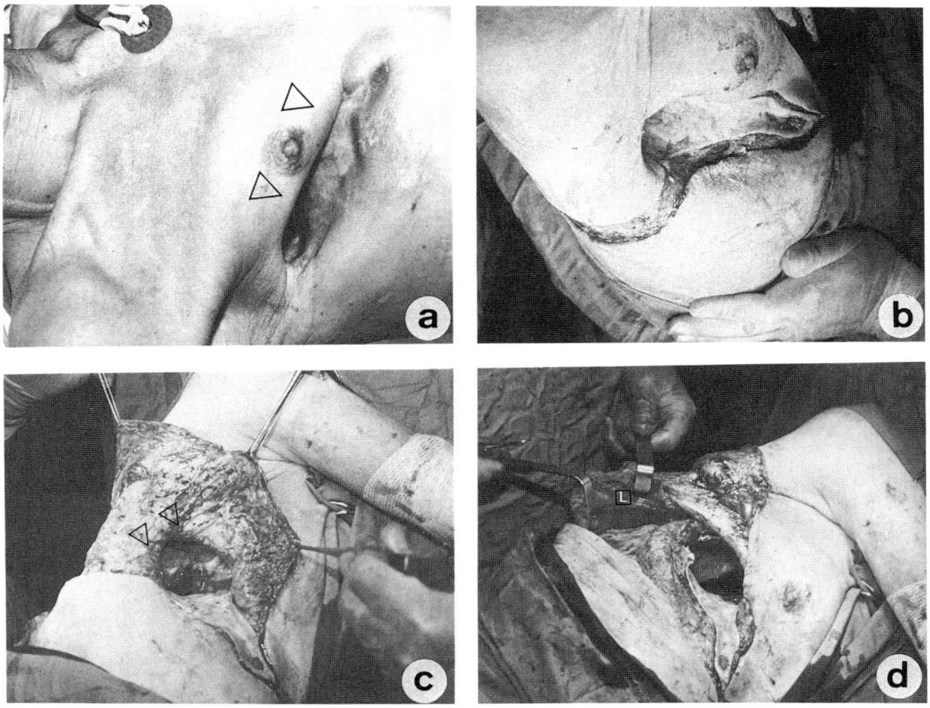

FIGURE D18.1. Operative view: (a) Right post-pneumonectomy empyema showing open drainage thoracostomy wound. (b) Incision resecting a portion of the skin. (c) Open pleural cavity space having had exhaustive 'curettage' of all the infected and necrotic pleural tissues. (d) Open cavity with latissimus dorsi (L) muscle pushed up.

(range 35/70), 9/8 right/left. In only one patient did the pneumonectomy last more than 3 hours. Three cases required intraoperative transfusion but never more than 1000 cc. Two patients had post-operative bleeding and one was submitted to rethoracotomy. No patients had hypoproteinemia or hypoalbuminemia. Seven of the 11 cancer patients had peribronchial dissection for removal of subcarinal and peritracheal nodes, and in 2 of 11, abscessed tumor was open into the pleural space during surgery.

In post-pneumonectomy empyema the most common microorganisms cultured were: *Pseudomona aeruginosa, Enterobacter, Streptococcus, Staphylococcus* and *Serratia*.

The thoracostomy wound was closed within 90 days in five patients (shortest interval: 36 days). In the other seven, the interval between pneumonectomy and closure of the infected thoracic cavity ranged from 3 to 6 months. Five patients waited more than 6 months for the myoplasty; most of these patients refused surgery at first.

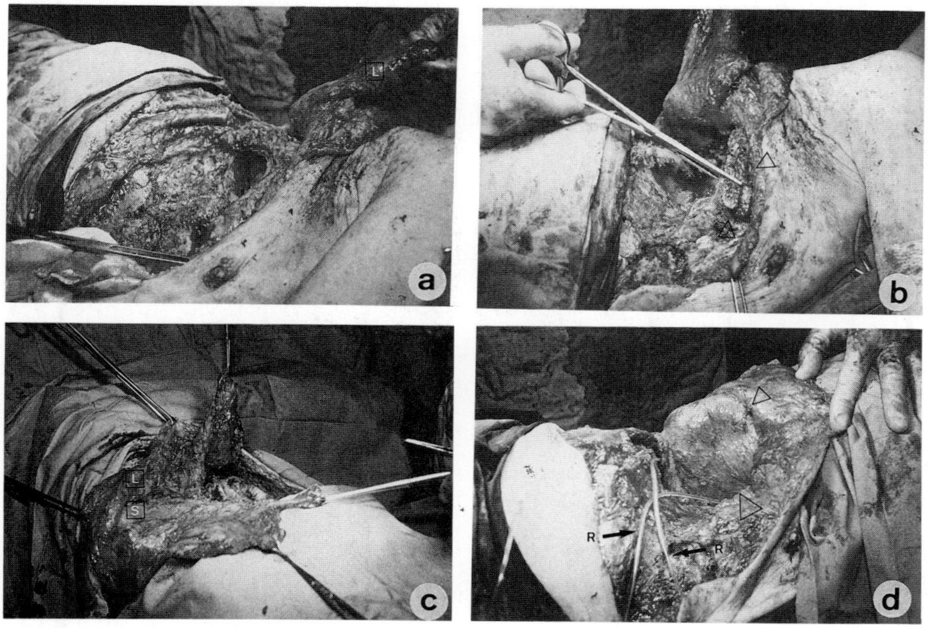

FIGURE D18.2. Operative view: (a) Latissimus dorsi muscle (L) flap dissected, preserving its major vascular supply. (b) Resection of the rib fragments overlying the floor and roof of the thoracic cavity. (c) Serratus anterior (S) and latissimus dorsi (L) muscle flaps. (d) Latissimus dorsi and serratus anterior muscles transferred to fill the remaining post-empyema space. Suction drains (R) placed among the muscles of the obliterated cavity.

In our series, no perioperative mortality occurred and the surgical procedure was well tolerated by all patients. Average hospital stay following myoplasty was 13 days. We have had only one recurrence in a patient with an old post-pneumonectomy empyema. We used the pectoral muscle to fill up the remaining space.

4. DISCUSSION

Whether associated with bronchopleural fistula or not, empyema is very serious and in 1–3% of the patients can be a lethal complication following pneumonectomy. When empyema does occur, the patient shows a greater or lesser degree of general toxicity. When the septic period is over, it is quite important to solve the problem quickly and safely.

The unroofing Schede operation described for obliterating chronic empyema space is a morbid surgical procedure that needs some months for wound healing, and does not give good aesthetic results. Following Pairolero and Arnold[4,5], who emphasized the role of the muscle flaps for treating thoracic reconstructive

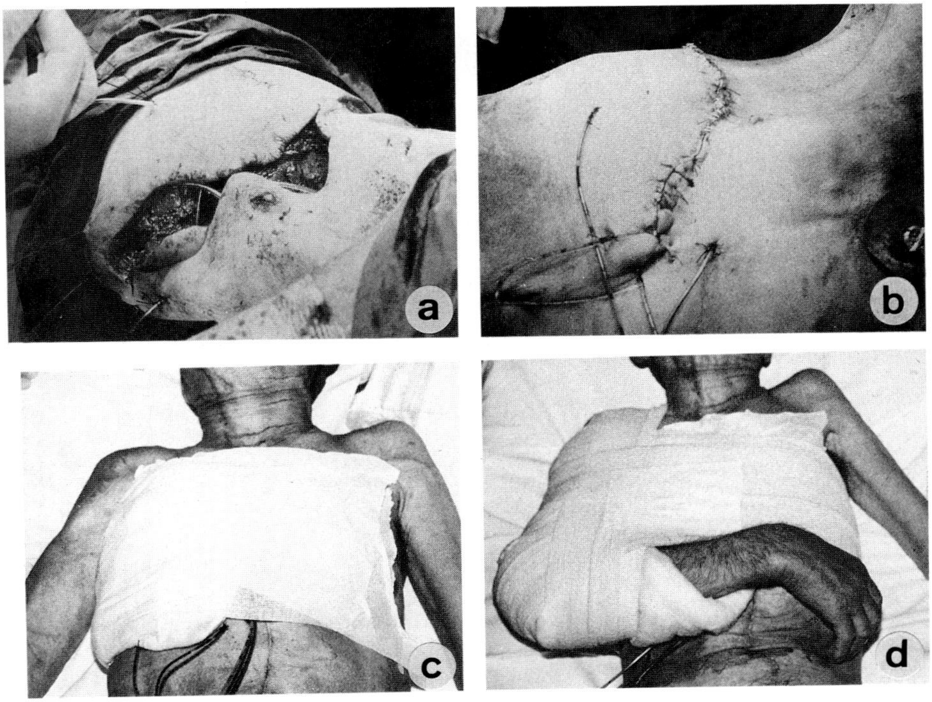

FIGURE D18.3. Operative view: (a, b) Details of the skin closure; suction drains placed for preventing any recess or dead space under the skin. (c) Compressive dressing and suction drainages used in the affected hemithorax. (d) Shoulder compression for restricting thoracic muscle movements.

problems, we have performed muscle transposition to fill up the thoracic space following the removal of ribs and pleural peel in patients with post-pneumonic empyema. In this condition, primary one-stage closure of the pleural cavity using muscle transfer is a good surgical procedure that achieves good results and acceptable cosmetic results[2,3] (Fig. D18.4).

The unroofing-myoplasty technique has some advantages. It is not necessary to wait several months to get the cavity smaller. At the same time, as the thoracic space is reduced surgically, we have never left any residual space, the main cause of recurrence. In our procedure, fewer muscular flaps than in Dr. Miller's operation are needed; rectus abdominis or omentum have never been used. This argument supports our surgical technique because most of these patients are old and have thin muscles. Finally, there is no possibility of vascular kinking of the flap.

In conclusion, we think that it is good to have two types of one-stage primary closure of pleural cavity in post-pneumonectomy empyema, Dr. Miller's and the unroofing-myoplasty procedure. We can choose one of them depending on age, cavity size, condition and muscular mass of the patient. Nevertheless, looking

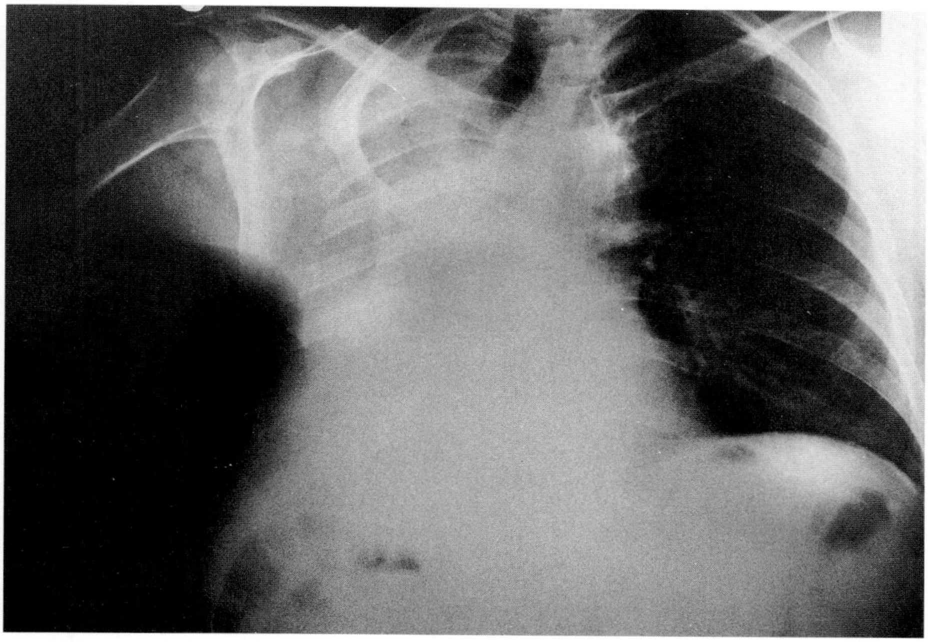

FIGURE D18.4. Chest roentgenogram of a patient with a right post-pneumonectomy empyema who was submitted to our unroofing-myoplasty procedure for closing post-operative pleural space.

at our results we should emphasize our preference for the unroofing-myoplasty operation as it is a safe and nontraumatic procedure which gives good results without recurrences.

REFERENCES

1 Weinstein AJ, McHenry MC, Gavan TL. System absorption of neomycin irrigating solution. JAMA 1977; 238: 152–153.
2 Tarazona V, París F, Chamorro JJ, Baena P, Zarza AG, Mirabet V. Comblement des poches résiduelles après pneumonectomie par transposition complète du grand dorsal, du grand dentelé et du grand pectoral. Ann Chir Thorac Cardiovasc 1981; 35: 681.
3 Baena P, Tarazona V. Bronchopleural fistula: Management with muscle transportion [discussion]. In: Grillo HC, Eschapasse H (eds.). International Trends in General Thoracic Surgery, Vol 2, Major Challenges. Philadelphia, PA, WB Saunders 1987: pp 429–433.
4 Pairolero PC, Arnold PG, Piehler JM. Intrathoracic transposition of extrathoracic skeletal muscle. J Thorac Cardiovasc Surg 1983; 86: 809–817.
5 Arnold PG. Reconstruction of the chest wall. In: Mathes SJ, Nahai F (eds.). Clinical Applications for Muscle and Musculocutaneous Flaps. St. Louis, CV Mosby 1982: pp 236–268.

Current Topics in General Thoracic Surgery: An International Series, Vol. 2
Perioperative Care, edited by R.M. Peters and J. Toledo

Chapter 19

Prophylaxis and treatment of postoperative thromboembolism*

Martín Escribano P.

1. INTRODUCTION

Abundant information in the literature demonstrates the effect of pulmonary thromboembolism (PTE)[a] in human lives, in suffering, in financial expenditures, and also in research. The fundamental aspects of its pathogenesis, diagnosis and treatment are still not completely understood. PTE is, in reality, a complication of another illness, venous thrombosis, which is preventable and treatable[7]. It is estimated that every year in the USA there are 5 million episodes of DVT, 10% of which have PE, and 10% of those die from the same (FPE)[1–8].

In spite of all the work dedicated to the study of PTE, there still exist blank spots in the understanding and treatment of the problem. The clinical diagnosis is not well founded because clear criteria and simple, clinical, diagnostic tests are not available. There is a need for complex technology, used aggressively, and this technology is not always available. Even with the most sophisticated technology, the investigations are not always concordant. All these limitations lead the clinician to insecurity in the evaluation of therapy.

Investigators have designed studies to collect a large quantity of information, epidemiological, clinical, and diagnostic and therapeutic. The investigation has focused on large clinical trials[3,9–12,16], inter-hospital and interdisciplinary,[2,13,14], on the theme of the day[15–17], on official recommendations[18–20], or on critical studies of meta-analysis[21–24].

Less frequently, other forms of pulmonary embolism should be considered: septic, fat, amniotic fluid, hydatid, neoplastic, talc, or air emboli. Air emboli may

*This chapter was translated from the Spanish by Jaime Pacheco-Orosco and the translation edited by Richard M. Peters.

[a] See Table 19.1 for a list of abbreviations used in this chapter.

TABLE 19.1
Abbreviations

Abbreviation	Meaning
LDH	Low-dose heparin
HDHE	Low-dose heparin-dihydroergotamine
IPC	Intermittent pneumatic compression
+FUT	Positive radioactive fibrinogen uptake test
DVT	Deep vein thrombosis
AK DVT	Above-knee deep vein thrombosis
PE	Pulmonary emboli
PTE	Pulmonary thromboemboli
FPE	Fatal pulmonary emboli
IP	Impedance plethysmography

TABLE 19.2
Relative incidence of venous thrombosis and fatal pulmonary emboli[a]

Patient Group	Incidence of venous thrombosis (%)	Incidence of fatal pulmonary emboli (%)
Hip fracture	40–70	1.5
Total hip replacement	40–70	1–2
Total knee replacement	40–70	5
Urologic surgery	15–20	5
General and gynecological surgery	15–20	1
Neurologic surgery	15–20	1
Medical patients	15	1

[a] From Hyers et al. [29].

have a greater relevance to patients subjected to thoracic surgery, for surgical trauma proper or multiple, venous intrusions which may be necessary.

Thoracic surgery always presupposes a certain risk of venous thrombosis and pulmonary thrombosis, fatal or not. Prevention of DVT and the treatment of PE should be systematically foreseen and standardized in this type of surgical unit.

2. EPIDEMIOLOGY OF DEEP VEIN THROMBOSIS AND PULMONARY THROMBOEMBOLISM

Deep vein thrombosis affects primarily the proximal veins of the legs and only exceptionally other venous systems, and results in two types of risks: obstruction and possible limitation or nullification of blood flow, and the dislodgement of thrombotic material and embolization to the lung. Venous thrombosis can occur in asymptomatic form, or it can manifest itself as DVT or PE of an acute form, as pulmonary hypertension, recurring PE, as massive PE, or as simple postphlebitis syndrome.

TABLE 19.3
Incidence of deep vein thrombosis in thoracic surgery

Reference	Year	Number of patients	Percentage DVT
Multi-unit trial [8A]	1974	18	44
Jackaman et al. [106]	1978	183	51
Cade and Clegg [110]	1983	44	18
Rajah et al. [111]	1983	114	26
Gamondès and Defour [112]	1984	128	9.4
Gamondès et al. [115]	1985	82	11

In a recent and extensive study using meta-analysis [23], published incidences from 1976 to August 1986 are given (Table 19.2). Selected patients were adults over 40 years of age, subjected to general surgery, excluding minor surgery, or trauma or orthopaedic surgery. The incidence of diagnosed DVT by radioactive fibrinogen uptake (FUT) was 25.1%, confirmed in 19.1% by phlebography; above-knee thrombosis occurred in 6.9%; pulmonary emboli 1.6%; and fatal pulmonary emboli (FPE) 0.9%. In this analysis there was a difference in the percentage of diagnosed DVTs in the European (29.7%) and North American (16.1%) studies. Even though there does not appear to be a relationship between DVT and climate [24], similar differences appear in other studies [12, 22].

PE almost exclusively (95% [25, 26]) originates from the veins of the lower extremities above the knees, and only rarely from the veins of the upper extremities or other organs, the cardiac cavities, or intravenous perfusion catheters [7]. The localization of thrombi in the legs above the knee corresponds to 15% of the peripheral thrombi, which progress proximally [27], and the rest to injuries in the thigh proper, e.g., hip fracture. There is the possibility of recurring embolism coming from residual venous thrombi or from reservoirs in the right heart [28].

The relative incidences of DVT and total pulmonary emboli in diverse surgical and medical situations are shown in Table 19.3 [29]. The maximum incidence is among those which affect the hip or the knee.

3. DIAGNOSIS OF THE RISK FACTORS

DVT occurs more commonly in patients with hypercoagulability. In some, hereditary risks have been described: Antithrombin III deficiency, Protein C deficiency, Protein S deficiency, defects in the system of fibrinolysis, dysfibrinogenemia, hemocystinuria, and disorders of plasminogen and plasminogen activation. Hypercoagulability risk factors are present in no more than 10% of DVT cases [7].

The risk factors can be listed in order of seriousness [30], isolated or in combinations. For example, hip surgery by itself gives a risk of DVT of 60 to 70% [31], while for the general group submitted to non-orthopaedic major surgery it is of the order of 25% [23], and of the order of 15% for non-surgical patients [29].

Patients at high risk for pulmonary thromboembolism are those with familial antithrombin III deficiency, surgery of the hip, the neck of the femur, and of the knee; hemi- or paraplegia, acute myocardial infarction, and burns covering 20% or more of the body in individuals over 18.

Other conditions have lower risks, but the risk can be greater if more than one risk factor is present. The lesser risks are: age over 40, immobilization for more than three days, congestive cardiac insufficiency; shock, chronic, debilitating illness; acute cerebral vascular accident; post partum; transurethral prostatic resection; surgery of the central nervous system, cardiac surgery, vascular surgery in the lower limbs, and transplants. Minor risks are obesity, varices, neoplasia, pregnancy, arterial hypertension, chronic obstructive airways disease, diabetes, left heart insufficiency, arthritis of the lower limbs, paroxysmal nocturnal hemoglobinuria, polycythemia vera, splenectomy, thrombocytosis, hypoxemia, hyperlipidemia, vasculopathy of whatever kind, hemocystinuria, repeated surgical interventions, anesthesia lasting more than three hours, sepsis, thoracic, abdominal or pelvic surgery, transurethral prostatic resection, and epidural anesthesia.

In surgical patients the risks can be compounded. In addition to the general risks, one can consider as specific risks of surgery the immobility during the intervention and the immediate postoperative period, the surgical position, the diminution of the peripheral venous flow, the action of anesthesia producing peripheral vasodilation, the hypercoagulability, and the blockage of fibrinolytic activity, etc. It has been suggested that half of the DVTs are produced during the operative intervention proper.

The global risk of DVT and PE can be divided into three levels [22, 32]:

Low risk of venous thrombosis: Patients without additional risks, under 40 years of age, who are scheduled for elective abdominal surgery or procedures on the thorax, or patients over 40 who are scheduled for minor thoracic or abdominal surgery, and anesthesia under 30 minutes. For this group, relative incidences have been described of 10% for distal DVT, 1% for proximal DVT, and 0.01% for fatal, pulmonary embolism (FPE).

Moderate risk of venous thrombosis: Patients over 40 years of age, submitted to surgery with anesthesia for longer than 30 minutes and one or more of the following factors: obesity, neoplastic illness, varices, estrogen use, immobility and paralysis. The observed incidences in this group are 10–40% for distal DVT, 2–10% for proximal DVT, and 0.1–0.7% for FPE.

High risk of venous thrombosis: Patients over 40 years of age, submitted to surgery with anesthesia for longer than 30 minutes, for orthopaedic or neoplastic disease, and with a previous history of venous thrombosis or pulmonary embolism. In this group the incidences are 40–80% for distal DVT, 10–20% for proximal DVT, and 1–5% for FPE.

In the pulmonary surgical patient, it is logical that removal of part of the lung decreases the pulmonary vascular bed and increases hemodynamic repercussion of a particular embolism. The small difference between the incidences of massive, fatal PE in lobectomy and pneumonectomy patients minimizes the importance of the vascular bed factor. Since the first published series [33, 34] following surgery for lung cancer, the rate of venous thrombosis and fatal pulmonary embolism is higher than for lung resection for tuberculosis, and other types of thoracotomies. Recently it has been demonstrated that the presence of a particular coagulant factor in advanced bronchogenic carcinoma increases the thrombosis (TIA) which can be contained with heparin [34]. The position during surgery, lateral or prone, which conditions the posture of the legs or the possible thrombosis at the site of vascular sutures, have not been demonstrated to be additional risk factors [35].

According to the above three-level risk classification, the first group contains the minor procedures in thoracic surgery such as endothoracic drainages, tracheotomies or thoracoscopies; the second, moderate-risk group includes the thoracotomies; and the third comprises those interventions with antecedent deep vein thrombosis or previous embolism.

For the PTE the fundamental risk factor is the presence of DVT in the thigh; the silent thrombi of calf veins do not increase risk, but if symptoms are manifested, monitoring for a possible proximal extension of the thrombosis is needed [7].

4. DIAGNOSIS OF VENOUS THROMBOSIS

95% of the pulmonary symptomatic embolisms which are recognized come from the legs, the majority from above the popliteal level [25].

The diagnostic criteria for venous thrombosis, and especially the clinical signs, are highly nonspecific [14]. This necessitates the use of complementary objective techniques, with concomitant expenditure and risk, and requires experience as well as a willingness to use them on the part of the surgeon. The best of these is venous phlebography, but the non-invasive methods are frequently very productive.

In the diagnosis of DVT, contrast phlebography [37] is the reference technique, but it is difficult to perform and to interpret. The criterion of acute DVT is a constantly and repeatedly visualized lack of intraluminal filling. Criteria of probability of the diagnosis are: lack of filling of a segment of the deep venous system with abrupt termination of the contrast column in a point below the segment and reappearance of the contrast above it; or the lack of filling of the deep venous system above the knee [38]. Complications of phlebography are hypersensitivity to the iodide contrasts, local pain, cutaneous ulcers due to the extravasation of the contrast, and phlebitis, including DVT [39,40]. As a result of the complications and complexity of this technique, there have been attempts at non-invasive diagnostic methods.

Radiofibrinogen leg scanning is based on the deposition of tagged fibrinogen in a zone where a venous thrombosis is being produced [41]. This technique is simple and is very sensitive to the detection of thrombi in calf veins and proximal veins up to the mid-thigh. Above this zone false positives are relatively frequent because of the deposition of fibrinogen in the pelvic veins. The mechanism of action makes radiofibrinogenic scanning logically insensitive to the detection of old thrombi or in cases treated with heparin. The specificity is also high, but the deposit of non-thrombotic fibrinogen can be detected, as in the case of local hemorrhage or marked cellulitis [42]. The definitive result is not obtained until 24 hours after the injection, a primary inconvenience, but the depositing can be monitored for the subsequent five days with the same injection. Another diagnostic technique, the incorporation in new thrombi of platelets marked with radioactive indium, has not proved to be useful [43].

Impedance plethysmography (IP) [44] evaluates the degree of obstruction to the venous flow in the leg, measuring the impedance below an obstruction with a pressure cuff and its improvement with the disappearance of this obstruction. During the obstructed phase, as the blood accumulates the impedance diminishes. The test depends on evaluating the velocity with which initial impedance recuperates, or the velocity with which the accumulated blood disappears. IP used in cases with PE can detect 90% of the silent thromboses diagnosed by venography in veins from the popliteals to the iliacs [14]. IP has less value in the isolated detection of calf vein thrombosis (30%). In old thrombi, of more than five days, the possible development of collateral circulation despite the persistence of the central obstruction can result in false negative. In the detection of calf vein thrombosis, the predictive value of IP is increased by associating it with fibrinogen marked by radioactive iodine (^{125}I-fibrinogen leg scanning) or by repeating it serially. The combination or repetition can limit the necessity [14] of phlebography to those cases with false results from plethysmography due to such conditions as congestive cardiac insufficiency or severe peripheral vasculopathy. A negative IP excludes proximal DVT but not calf vein thrombosis, and serial repetition of IP permits detection of the suprapopliteal progression of the thrombus, which converts it from slightly dangerous to potentially emboligenic. Progression of the thrombus can occur in 20–30% of patients, in the first seven days [14]. If IP remains negative during a period of 10 days, the diagnosis of DVT can be excluded.

Other simple techniques have not demonstrated sufficient value in relation to conventional phlebography: With ultrasound the blood flow can be measured, but the technique is very dependent on the ability and experience of the explorer; recently a new avenue within this same line has been opened with the "duplex" technique [45]. The isotopic venography with macro-aggregates or microsphere of albumin tagged with radioactive technetium is easy to perform but has a lamentably poor image resolution.

This type of situation with multiple diagnostic techniques with variable utility and morbidity requires decision making based on the systematic use of algorithms. A good algorithm [14] is the following: Faced with the clinical suspicion of DVT, IP is done. If there are no conditions which might give a false positive with IP, phlebography should be done without IP. If the IP is positive, it confirms the diagnosis of DVT. If the IP is negative, it is repeated the following day, and on days 3, 5, 7 and 10. If the serial tests are positive, the diagnosis is made, but if it remains negative the diagnosis is excluded.

An additional problem in the diagnosis of DVT is recidivism [46], and in this sense it is necessary to consider the sequence of regression of the thrombosis, observed with serial IPs. The percentages of normalization of the IP after an episode of DVT were: in month 3, 67%; month 6, 85%; month 9, 92%; and month 12, 95% [47]. In addition to detecting DVT in the presence of clinical data, like pain in the legs and swelling suggestive of recurrence, IP is also useful in the postphlebitis syndrome, without the necessity of combining it with ^{125}I-fibrinogen leg scanning.

5. DIAGNOSIS OF PULMONARY THROMBOEMBOLISM

PE is a consequence of DVT and establishes the indication for the anticoagulant treatment. In up to 30% of PE cases, DVT is not shown. The negative studies for DVT do not exclude the diagnosis of PE [7].

The clinical criteria suggest the diagnosis of PE if they are accompanied by risk factors of DVT, but in general they are highly unspecific [14] and without logical correlation with the presence or severity of PE. The data causing suspicion are very diverse, and they present with very different frequency [49]: The most frequent symptom is dyspnea and above all its subtle beginning. After this are pleuritic pain, apprehension, cough, calf pain, diaphoresis, hemoptysis, syncope, palpitations, anginal pains, etc. The most common signs are tachypnea and tachycardia, stridor, or local signs of phlebitis. Simple radiology of the thorax, electrocardiogram, and determination of blood gases are always indispensable in the differential diagnosis, although of little use for a specific diagnosis. For example, in contrast to the usual occurrence of hyperventilation, accompanied frequently by hypoxemia, hypoventilation has also occurred in massive pulmonary embolism [49]. Chest radiographs can suggest the diagnosis if there is a loss of volume, laminar atelectasis, loss of vascular lines, vessel narrowing, or pulmonary consolidation. The electrocardiogram can show acute overloading of the right ventricle.

Given the lack of specificity of the clinical data, an objective diagnosis using complementary techniques is necessary, which entails expenditure and some risk, and requires experience and the willingness to use them on the part of the surgeon.

Its accessibility and the lack of morbidity make perfusion lung scanning the primary study for the diagnosis of PE. A normal image excludes the diagnosis of PE and the necessity of anticoagulant treatment, in the absence of indications for DVT [54]. The abnormal images are more difficult to interpret, so it is necessary to complement them with the data of simple radiology or with ventilation scanning. A defect detected with perfusion scanning should be considered not diagnostic of PE if it corresponds with a radiologic infiltration [55]; if the perfusion defects are segmentary, with normal chest radiographs, ventilation scanning should be done [7].

Perfusion scanning is also very useful at discharge from the hospital [7]. It helps to decide the duration of the treatment, and permits early identification of the causes that might lead to chronic pulmonary vascular obstruction.

Ventilation lung scanning completes the perfusion scan [18]. Patients with perfusion defects of a lobe or a segment and without any defect on ventilation scan have a high probability of PE (86 %). If the ventilation defect is similar to the finding on perfusion scan, the probability of PE is low (36%).

Pulmonary angiography [50] is the technique of reference in the diagnosis of PE. It can be necessary in a considerable number of cases. The indications are: intermediate or low probability by ventilation–perfusion scanning with clinical findings suggestive of PE and normal IP; high probability by ventilation scanning; in massive PE, where it is necessary to use thrombolytics, pulmonary embolectomy or interruption of the vena cava. The contraindications of pulmonary angiography are the presence of pulmonary hypertension, a contraindication which is itself relative [51], or severe, uncompensated cardiac or respiratory illness, or hypersensitivity to iodide contrasts [52]. If the technique is carefully done, the pathognomonic signs of PE [53] are: defect of intraluminal filling, or sharp cut-off in vessels larger than 2.5 mm in diameter are constantly and repeatedly visualized. The clinical complications are arrhythmias or cardiac arrest, endo- or myocardial lesions, and cardiac perforation. Probably digital angiography, and perhaps nuclear magnetic resonance, in the future will facilitate the study of PE.

With the available data a strategy diagnostic of PE should be established, depending on the technical capacity and the experience of each unit: One of the possible algorithms could be [14] the following: All the patients with clinical suspicion of PE should be subjected to perfusion lung scanning, excluding the diagnosis if this is normal. If it is abnormal, and the defects are super-segmentary, a ventilation scan should be done, and if there is mismatch between those the diagnosis of PE is very probable and treatment should begin. If the defects are subsegmentary or if there is concordance between both ventilation and perfusion scanning, it is not possible to make a decision and other diagnostic tests should be made. Initially, phlebography or IP would be indicated to demonstrate presence or absence of DVT. If IP is positive, treatment can be initiated. If these tests do not demonstrate DVT, there are various alternatives. In patients with good cardiorespiratory reserves and clinical stability, IP is repeated until DVT is detected, given that the probability of PE is low in the absence of DVT. Another possibility is to do pulmonary angiography, which is the procedure of reference for the diagnosis of PE.

One of our group [30], faced with the suspicion of pulmonary embolism, uses the following algorithms established from the clinical circumstances: Presence of phlegmasia cerulea dolens, as clinical finding of most severe venous obstruction, requires immediate thrombectomy; respiratory or circulatory insufficiency suggestive of massive pulmonary embolism may require a cycle of fibrinolytic treatment or thrombectomy; suspicion of recurring PE or high risk of hemorrhage under anticoagulant treatment requires the best possible diagnosis, by means of pulmonary angiography. If the clinical findings are less clear, isotopic phlebography is always indicated, with perfusion lung scanning, in 4 to 6 positions: If isotopic phlebography and pulmonary perfusion scanning are normal, DVT and PE are ruled out; if the scanning is normal but the phlebography is not, or if high risk factors for venous thrombosis are present before results of scanning are available, or if in the absence of those risk factors the isotopic phlebography is pathologically doubtful, radiological phlebography would be indicated. In the absence of the risk factors and with normal isotopic phlebography, the scan interpretations are scored high, middle, indeterminate or low [4]: *high,* multiple defects on perfusion, at least one of lobar size; *moderate,* unique defects of pulmonary, lobar or segmentary size; or multiple, subsegmentary defects; *indeterminate,* defects of perfusion coincident with abnormal zones in the radiograph of the thorax; and *low,* unique defects of perfusion, subsegmentary or non-segmentary, or multiple defects of perfusion, if not larger than subsegmentary or non-segmentary. Cases with high probability are diagnosed of having PE, while in the remaining cases the diagnosis must be confirmed with pulmonary angiography; the cases with scanning defects of low probability of PE, without evidence of proximal DVT and with good cardiopulmonary reserve should have clinical observation.

6. PREVENTION OF VENOUS THROMBOSIS

Given the clinical characteristics, the utility of the diagnostic tests, and the morbidity of PE, one should have as the preferred objective of the management of DVT and PE, the prophylaxis of VT [18]. There are various modalities of prevention of DVT and its treatment: Drugs can inhibit the coagulation, drugs can inhibit the platelet function, fibrinolytic drugs and techniques can counteract the venous stasis [29]. Within the first hours, and peaking in the first 3 days, after anticoagulants are initiated the thrombus can recanalize; it becomes fixed to the wall, with the resulting diminution of the risk of embolism, and of progression of the thrombosis [56].

The protocols most frequently used are heparin at low dosages (LDH), low molecular weight heparin (LMWH), dihydroergotamine, dextran, warfarin, or aspirin. On the other side, physical prophylaxis uses intermittent pneumatic compression (IPC), or graduated compression elastic stockings. Extensive retrospective analyses reported [12,19,22,23] in a series of published works, have provided a large quantity of information, with diverse degrees of support for the utility of these different protocols for prevention and treatment of DVT and PE.

Sufficient evidence exists to consider that prophylaxis with heparin (LDH) diminishes the incidence of DVT and of PE in patients submitted to major surgery; this protective effect can be estimated for DVT and FPE [12,19,22,23]. Prophylaxis with heparin at low dosages (LDH) [12] was clearly demonstrated to significantly decrease the incidence of DVT (8.7% in the treatment group vs 25.2% in the control), for PE (0.52% vs 1.2%) and for FPE (0.21% vs 0.7%). The dose of subcutaneous heparin was 5000 units 2 hours before surgery, and every 8 or 12 hours during the following 7 days; there was no increase in major complications such as major hemorrhages, but there was an increase in hemorrhage in the surgical incision. There are indications that a different heparin dosage influences the results of prophylaxis of DVT, but not the hemorrhagic complications. For the cases considered higher risk of DVT, an adjusted low-dose subcutaneous heparin has been proposed [57], trying to maintain the APTT at the high-normal level.

Low molecular weight heparin offers interesting potential advantages. It appears to behave like non-fractionated heparin, but is more convenient to use because it requires only one dose daily, and it does not fluctuate between doses, nor does APTT, and as a result there is a lower risk of hemorrhage [7, 22,58–61]. Dihydroergotamine produces a dose-dependent vasoconstriction of venous capacitance vessels with little effect on vascular smooth muscle [62]. The therapeutic guide low-dose heparin-dihydroergotamine (HDHE), adding 0.5 mg of dihydroergotamine to 5000 units of heparin, was compared [23] with LDH: It was considered more useful in the prophylaxis of DVT (9% vs 14.5%) and it produced fewer hematomas (3.2% vs 7.2 %) and major hemorrhages. Nevertheless it is possible that it has contraindications in patients with coronary ischemia, peripheral vasculopathy, hypertension, hypovolemia or sepsis [17]. The addition of dihydroergotamine to heparin should be reserved for patients with high risk, or for those in which hematomas are poorly tolerated.

Dextran was utilized, in both of its molecular weights, 40 and 70, as a venous infusate, 500–1000 ml, during the operation and the following hours, and continuing at dose 500 ml/day from one to seven days. Its administration is more complex than that of LDH and carries additional risks of excessive IV fluids. The results show [23] significant differences for the incidence of DVT (15.6% vs 24.2%), for PE (1.2% vs 2.8%), and for FPE (0.27% vs 1.5%); a significant difference was not shown in the incidence of hemorrhagic complications. The comparison [21] between LDH and dextran showed that LDH offered better protection than dextran against DVT (9.5% vs 21%), but wound hemorrhage was more frequent with heparin (7% vs 3.5%).

Another possibility is the use of warfarin [10,63–65] in a single dose the night before surgery [64] or the two-step warfarin therapy for programmed surgery, initiating the treatment 10 to 14 days before the intervention, and adjusting the dose to the prothrombin time, and reintroducing it the night after surgery [10], or with a very low fixed dose, 1 mg/day, during the preceding 3 weeks [65]. All these studies encounter the problem of the standardization of prothrombin time due to the different activity of the thromboplastins employed. Each requires a local correction, depending on the reagents employed in that moment or place.

Intermittent Pneumatic Compression (IPC) of the calf veins augments the calf venous blood flow [66]. It is applied to the lower legs, with compression of 35–40 mmHg, beginning intraoperatively and then for one to five days postoperative. Using compression for 10 seconds per minute decreased DVT to 9.9% vs 20.3%.

Graduated compression elastic stockings with major pressure in the inferior zone, above the knee [67] were demonstrated useful [23] in the prevention of DVT (9.3% vs 24.5%). This modality can be prescribed for subjects with low risk, or in association with other prophylactic measures [17].

Aspirin as a prophylaxis [23] was not found to give significant prevention of DVT.

Of all these methods, LDH is utilized most, even though dextran has been demonstrated to be as effective. Dextran should be preferred, in spite of the complications of its administration, in cases in which hematomas at the site of the injury are less desirable.

In the joint reports of the American College of Chest Physicians and National Heart, Lung, and Blood Institute, on Antithrombotic Therapy (ACCP–NHLBI) [19, 29, 68, 69], the use of heparin at low dosages, 5000 units subcutaneously during 12 hours, or IPC is recommended, in the cases of moderate risk. Neurosurgery, major knee or urologic surgery patients should have IPC. Patients for elective hip surgery should have adjusted-dose heparin (to prolong the APTT in the upper half of the normal range) or moderate-dose warfarin (to prolong prothrombin time to an INR of 2–3). If the surgery is on fractured hips, moderate-dose warfarin is recommended (to prolong the prothrombin time to an INR of 2–3).

7. PROPHYLAXIS OF PULMONARY THROMBOEMBOLISM

The prophylaxis of PE is the prophylaxis of DVT. In particular circumstances, as in the polytraumatized, where the diagnosis of DVT is not possible, nor the conventional prophylaxis of DVT, if the estimation of risk is high [7], the placement of a Greenfield filter is indicated [70].

8. TREATMENT OF VENOUS THROMBOSIS AND PULMONARY THROMBOSIS

Venous thrombosis and pulmonary thrombosis, once established, have common pathophysiological aspects and treatments. Venous thrombosis is initially a phenomenon of localized vascular obstruction which needs to be unobstructed mechanically or with fibrinolytics. In addition to using anticoagulation or vena caval interruptions to avoid the emigration of emboli, pulmonary embolism requires anticoagulation and/or fibrinolytics, and perhaps in extreme cases pulmonary endarterectomy.

The reference treatment of DVT and of PE is anticoagulant, initiated with intravenous heparin for a few days and followed with oral coumadin or subcutaneous heparin for three months. This protocol is highly effective [23], with recurrence level below 2%, versus 40–50% without treatment. Even though this concept is generally accepted, there still exist many points of dispute [7, 71,72]. Details of drug therapy are not clearly definable – the total antithrombotic level, time at which the intravenous heparin should be replaced by oral coumadin or by subcutaneous heparin, nor the total duration of the anticoagulant treatment [73].

Another possible guide of treatment can be the following [29]: at the moment of suspicion of DVT or PE and simultaneously with the indication of the diagnostic tests, one obtains Thromboplastin and prothrombin time and first administers an intravenous bolus of heparin of 5000 or 10 000 units; once the diagnosis is confirmed, a new bolus of 5000 units is given, and IV infusion is started at approximately 1000 units/h. The activated thromboplastin time is measured at 6 hours, the dosage is adjusted until it reaches 1.5–2 times the control value, and the platelets are measured every 3 or 4 days. Initiate treatment with warfarin on the first or second day with an estimated dose of 4–10 mg for 7–10 days, and after a minimum of 5 days following the addition of warfarin, suspend the heparin and take prothrombin control 4 hours later. Adjust the dose of warfarin so that the prothrombin time becomes 1.3–1.5 times the control [74]. This treatment is maintained for a minimum of three months for the first episode, or while a risk of VT persists; if this risk is maintained indefinitely, so would the anticoagulant treatment. If recurrence of DVT has been demonstrated, the treatment should be maintained for a year.

The recommendation of a total time of duration of the anticoagulant treatment, in a single episode of DVT and PE, has recently passed from six [75] to three months [19, 76]; in fact shorter periods have been proposed even though these suppositions have yet to be confirmed. As an example of this lack of precision, it has been advised [71] to treat proven cases of DVT for 6 weeks to 3 months, and cases of PE for 3 to 6 months.

Intravenous heparin can be administered in separate doses or in continuous perfusion [76]. Another possibility is the use in PE of an initial, higher dose directed to the initial platelet aggregate and to the liberation of vasoactive agents [7]. The control of the therapy with heparin is made with the activated partial thromboplastin test, APTT, taken in the first hours of the morning or before the next dose in the intermittent regimens. The place of low molecular weight heparin [60] must be determined because of the additional difficulty in the measure of its activity which cannot be adequately measured with the APTT [7].

Coumadin is fundamentally [69] antagonistic to vitamin K by inhibiting vitamin K's action in the synthesis of factors II, VII, IX and X. The dose is monitored by sequential measurements of the prothrombin time. Coumadin during the period of induction of the treatment depresses factor VII, while in the period of maintenance it depresses factors II, VII and X. The dose of coumadin should increase PTF by a factor 2–3 × control. In patients with recurrent PE the INR should be 3–4.5 [78].

The alternative to oral anticoagulation, in pregnancy, or faced with the impossibility of making seriated coagulation controls, is the administration of adjusted doses of subcutaneous heparin [79]. This method has been found to be as effective as oral anticoagulants [50, 74]. The dose is adjusted initially by following the intravenous heparin dose adjustment schedule. It is repeated every 12 hours, and after a first adjustment on the third day this dose is maintained indefinitely.

The fundamental inconvenience of all anticoagulant treatments is obviously hemorrhage; its risk is real, even though evidently less than in other diseases, such as ischemic cerebrovascular disease, or ischemic heart disease. Hemorrhages occur with PE in 23% of the treated; of these, 8.1% are major hemorrhages [61, 80]. Hemorrhages depend on specific risk factors. Age is not a specific factor. The risk factors are drug overdose, or increase of its effect by concomitant medication or comorbidity [29]. The list of medications which can interfere with the treatment by coumadin is very large (see the article by Hull and Raskob [14], page 528): Those which enhance the action of warfarin: ethanol, allopurinol, amiorinone, anabolic steroids, cimetidine, disulfiram, erythromycin, metronidazole, non-steroid anti-inflammatorics, phenylbutazone, phenytoin, quinidine and co-trimoxazole. Conversely, those which reduce the action of warfarin: corticosteroids, barbiturates, cholestyramine, diuretics, griseofulvin, oral contraceptives, rifampin. Comorbidity is also important: acute myocardial infarction, diastolic hypertension, or the necessity for intra-aortic balloon pump; hepatic disease, macrocytosis or hyperbilirubinemia; renal insufficiency, or debility, by carcinoma or decline of hematocrit below 30% with previous hemorrhage, traumatic lesions or peptic ulcer.

Another unfavorable effect of heparin is thrombocytopenia [3, 81], which can be important in case of extension or recurrence of thrombosis [82]. Treatment should be suspended if platelet count descends below 50000 [7]. Lastly, osteoporosis may result from long term treatment. Coumadin can produce [29] a vascular purpura with cutaneous necrosis, and should never be used during pregnancy.

The contraindications to anticoagulant treatment can be absolute or relative. Absolute contraindications are: actual active bleeding, intracranial lesions, hemorrhagic diathesis, diastolic arterial hypertension above 120 mmHg, hypertensive or diabetic retinopathy of degree $>$ II, and surgery on the central nervous system within the last 7 days. Relative contraindications are: thrombocytopenia below 10000, systolic arterial pressure above 200 mmHg, bleeding time over 10 seconds, prothrombin activity below 60%, diabetic or hypertensive retinopathy $\leq$ II, surgery within the last 10 days, serum creatinine over 1.4, medication inhibitory to platelet aggregation, potentially bloody lesions including tooth extractions or biopsies, and important trauma [84]. A specific contraindication is the use of coumadin during all periods of pregnancy.

Theoretically the fibrinolytics [35,84,86,87], should be the drug of choice in venous thrombosis at whatever level. Their function is to destroy the existent thrombosis and to facilitate the thrombolysis of those which might occur later, thereby diminishing recurrences and postphlebitic consequences. Nevertheless, its place is not definitively established [7, 88]; its use has high risk of hemorrhages [16], the possibility of recurrence of embolism during the treatment [89], or pulmonary edema by re-perfusion [90]. Fibrinolytics in DVT should be reserved for the following situations: cases of perfectly established diagnosis of recent, severe, proximal venous thrombosis, and of pulmonary embolism with significant hemodynamic effects; evidence of blood flow obstruction to the pulmonary lobar or in multiple segments [17]; or in patients with previous pulmonary or cardiac illness; or in the cases in which there is not improvement within 48–72 hours of anticoagulant treatment with heparin. It is possible that fibrinolytic treatment may improve long-term pulmonary perfusion, avoiding permanent pulmonary hypertension.

The treatment with streptokinase lasts 24 hours for PE and 48–72 hours for DVT, and that with urokinase is 12 hours [29], equally effective for both. This type of treatment demands a strict control of the patient and a risk–benefit evaluation of the therapy. Absolute contraindications are: active hemorrhage, or recent, cerebrovascular accident or other active, intracranial process. Relative contraindications are: major surgery, recent delivery, biopsy of an organ or puncture of an non-compressible vessel in the last few days, recent gastrointestinal hemorrhage, recent significant hemorrhage, severe arterial hypertension, > 200; other minor criteria are recent minor traumas, like those which occur with cardiopulmonary resuscitation, high probability of thrombosis in the left heart, hemostatic defects, pregnancy, age over 75 years or hemorrhagic, diabetic retinopathy. In the future, new less dangerous fibrinolytic agents might be available: recombinant human tissue plasminogen activator (r-TPA), which can be used with heparin [36, 91, 92], an isolated plasminogen–streptokinase activator complex [93], and single-chain urokinase [94]. These new agents are more specific in their action of production of plasmin, and therefore fibrinolysis, without affecting other factors of coagulation, avoiding the tendency for hemorrhaging.

From the point of view of pulmonary embolism the interruption of the vena cava is indicated if there is absolute contraindication to therapeutic anticoagulants, if the recurrence of DVT has occurred in spite of appropriate anticoagulant treatment, or if there is a high risk of a new episode of PE being fatal. Other possible indications are septic or paradoxical embolism. A number of methods of interruption of the cava have been proposed: complete ligature, plication, or the placement of a filter [95,96]; it appears that the most appropriate procedure is the use of the Greenfield filter [97–99]. It has fewer postphlebitic consequences, with a low frequency of patient loss, and does not require concomitant anticoagulant treatment.

Recurrent pulmonary thromboembolism requires special consideration from the diagnostic and therapeutic points of view: If the initial PTE has been treated correctly, and the recurrence appears during treatment with heparin, the efficacy of the treatment should be checked, or interruption of the cava proposed. If the recurrence has developed during oral anticoagulant treatment, a cycle of heparin should be repeated and the treatment should be prolonged up to one year.

The problem of the treatment of calf vein thrombosis is not clear; firstly because of the difficulty of the diagnosis and secondly because of the low incidence of embolisms from that region. Nevertheless there is evidence of progression of the thrombosis to a more proximal vein in, at least, 6% [44], in the two weeks following the acute episode. For this, monitoring is recommended with IPG at 10 to 14 days to identify progression of the lesion, giving treatment if it becomes abnormal [100] or alternatively anticoagulant treatment during three months. Superficial thrombophlebitis is treated efficaciously with non-steroid anti-inflammatory drugs.

9. TREATMENT OF MASSIVE PULMONARY EMBOLISM

Massive pulmonary embolism is defined by production of right ventricular insufficiency with a decrease in the cardiac output, manifested clinically by severe hypoxemia or hypotension. In this grave situation three types of treatment can be contemplated [7]: use of fibrinolytics, placement of a Greenfield filter, or embolectomy.

Thromboembolitic treatment [85, 86, 92] of these patients has not been any more effective than that with heparin [7]. Embolectomy treatment of massive pulmonary embolism has a similar mortality to conservative treatments [101]. The placement of a Greenfield filter [97, 99] is directed to prevention of recurrent embolism.

Thromboendarterectomy is indicated in cases with chronic thromboembolic occlusion of the pulmonary tree, which can occur even after silent pulmonary emboli [102].

10. TREATMENT OF PULMONARY EMBOLISM IN THORACIC SURGERY

Not many studies have been designed specifically to define the epidemiology of PTE and PE in non-cardiovascular thoracic surgery [32,34,103–116].

Le Brigand and Moreaux in 1959 [34] refer to 12048 patients who underwent thoracic surgery with 4.4% of thromboembolic accidents and 0.7% of fatal embolism. There is a great variety of results, from 1.9% of fatal embolism in one of the personal series to 0.25% in others, and equally for thromboembolitic accidents, from 11.2% to 1.99% of 3723 cases. Fatal pulmonary embolism varies in relation with the type of surgery: 4.7% in pneumonectomy, 1.54% in segmentectomies, 1.26% in tuberculosis, 4% in abscesses and 5.9% in bronchogenic cancer. In a poll of thoracic surgeons in the United Kingdom, data were obtained on 11305 resections, with an incidence of fatal postoperative pulmonary embolism of 1.2%. Abbey Smith showed an incidence of PE demonstrated at necroscopy of 3.2% in 1200 pulmonary resections, while there was no mortality in 500 resections for benign pathology.

In a 1981 report [108] pulmonary cancer had not changed the incidence of PE in thoracic surgical patients, even with prophylactic heparinization, but other studies do not agree with this result. Storm [103], reporting his findings following thoracotomies for resection of bronchogenic carcinoma, finds the group treated with prophylaxis of venous thrombosis compared to the controls, had respective rates of PTE of 0–8.7%, and of PE of 1–4.9%, with the overall operative mortality 3.1–16.5%.

Reports of incidence of PTE comparing use of heparin prophylaxis with control therapy show wide variation in the results [106,112,114,115].

The incidence of venous thrombosis, detectable generally with tagged fibrinogen, is very different in the different studies, from 9.4% to 51%. This incidence is higher in patients with neoplasia surgery. The effectiveness of heparin prophylaxis is similar to that for other types of surgery and should be used, as recommended since 1977 by the American Heart Association [117]. Likewise the treatment guides should be similar in the diagnosed cases.

Another very special problem, and one that is difficult to resolve, is surgery in cases with actual demonstrated venous thrombosis or pulmonary embolism, while on anticoagulant treatment. The anticoagulant should be suspended during the surgical procedure, which supposes a very high risk of progression of the thrombosis or the pulmonary embolism [43]. If the surgery can be delayed, it is better to give appropriate anticoagulant treatment for 3 months, and prophylaxis with heparin during the days of the surgery. If the surgery can only wait several days, light anticoagulation is given with an increase of APTT 1.5–2.5 times the basal value, suspending the heparin 8 hours before the surgery and reinstituting it after 24–48 hours. The same regimen is used in the case of urgent surgery without evidence of proximal PTE. If urgent surgery must be done in a patient with proximal PTE, interruption of the cava with a Greenfield filter is indicated, with initiation of anticoagulation 24–48 hours afterwards.

11. CONCLUSIONS

The high incidence of DVT and PE is an important cause of mortality in medical and surgical patients.

There is ample evidence to establish guidelines for prophylactic therapy pertinent to local situation.

Venous thrombosis is avoidable if the risk factors are evaluated and appropriate prophylaxis provided.

Pulmonary embolism is a potentially fatal medical emergency which demands immediate investigation and treatment.

Primary treatment of PE is systemic anticoagulation, and secondly, the use of fibrinolytics, or interruption of the inferior vena cava.

Pulmonary thrombectomy has not demonstrated its utility in an acute pulmonary embolus with hemodynamic compromise.

REFERENCES

1 Freiman DG, Suyemoto J, Wessler S. Frequency of pulmonary thromboembolism in man. N Engl J Med 1965; 290: 1278.
2 Schuman LM. The epidemiolgy of thromboembolic disorders. A review. J Chron Dis 1965; 18: 815.
3 Urokinase pulmonary embolism trial: Phase 1 results. JAMA 1970; 214: 2163.
4 Dalen JE, Alpert JS. Natural history of pulmonary embolism. Prog Cardiovasc Dis 1975; 17: 259.
5 Bergquist D, Lindblad B. A 30-year survey of embolism verified at autopsy: An analysis of 1274 surgical patients. Br J Surg 1985; 72: 105.
6 Rubinstein J, Murray D, Hoffsten V. Fatal pulmonary embolism in hospitalized patients. Arch Intern Med 1988; 148: 1425–1426.

7 Moser KM. Venous thromboembolism. Am Rev Respir Dis 1990; 141: 235–249.

8 Alpert JS, Smith R, Carlson J, et al. Mortality in patients treated for pulmonary embolism. JAMA 1976; 236: 1477–1480.

8A A multi-unit controlled trial: heparin vs. dextran in the prevention of deep venous thrombosis. Lancet 1974: 118.

9 Groote-Schuur Hospital Thromboembolism Study Group. Failure of low-dose heparin to prevent significant thromboembolic complications in high-risk surgical patients. Interim report of a prospective trial. Br Med J 1979; i: 1447.

10 Francis C, Marder V, Evart C, et al. Two-step warfarin therapy: Prevention of postoperative venous thrombosis without excessive bleeding. JAMA 1983; 249: 374–378.

11 Multi Center Trial Committee. DHE/Heparin in prophylaxis of postoperative DTV. JAMA 1984; 2351: 2960–2966.

12 Collins R, Scrimgeour A, Yusuf S, Phil D, Peto R. Reduction in fatal pulmonary embolism and venous thrombosis by perioperative administration of subcutaneus heparine. N Engl J Med 1988; 318: 1162.

13 Hirsh J. Venous Thromboembolism. New York, Grune and Stratton 1981.

14 Hull RD, Raskob GE. Diagnosis and long-term management of venous thromboembolism. In: Will JA, Dawson ChA, Weir EK, Buckner CK (eds.). The Pulmonary Circulation in Health and Disease. Orlando, FL, Academic Press 1987.

15 Moser KM. Pulmonary embolism. Am Rev Respir Dis 1977; 115: 829.

16 Hirsh J, Hull RD. Treatment of venous thromboembolism. Chest 1986; 89: 426S.

17 Mohr DN, Ryu JH, Litin SC, Rosenow III EC. Recent advances in the management of venous thromboembolism. Mayo Clin Proc 1988; 63: 281.

18 Consensus Conference. Prevention of venous thrombosis and pulmonary embolism. JAMA 1986; 256: 744.

19 Sackett DL. Rules of evidence and clinical recommendations on the use of antithrombic agents. Arch Intern Med 1986; 146: 464.

20 Sacket DL. Rules of evidence and clinical recommendations on the use of antithrombic agents. Chest 1989; 95: 2s–4s.

21 Rosenthal R. Meta-analytic procedures for social research. Beverly Hills, Sage Publications 1984.

22 Colditz GA, Tuden RL, Oster G. Rates of venous thrombosis after general surgery; combined results of randomised clinical trials. Lancet 1986; ii: 143.

23 Clagett GP, Reisch JS. Prevention of venous thromboembolism in general surgical patients. Results of meta-analysis. Ann Surg 1988; 208: 227.

24 Reasbeck PG, Guerrini S, Harper J, Sackelariou R, McCaffrey JF. Incidence of deep vein thrombosis after major abdominal surgery in Brisbane. Br J Surg 1988; 75: 440.

25 Havig GO. Source of pulmonary emboli. Acta Chir Scand 1977; 478Supp: 42.

26 Havig GO. Deep vein thrombosis and pulmonary embolism: An autopsy study with multiple regression analysis of possible risk factors. Acta Chir Scand 1977; 479: 1sup.

27 Moser KM, LeMoine JR. Is embolic risk conditioned by location of deep venous thrombosis? Ann Intern Med 1981; 94: 439.

28 Crowell RH, Adams GS, Koipillai CJ, et al. In vivo right heart thrombus. Chest 1988; 94: 1236–1239.

29 Hyers TM, Hull RD, Weg JG. Antithrombic therapy for venous thromboembolic disease. Chest 1989; 95: 37s.

30 Pozo Rodriguez F, Barbosa Ayúcar C. In: Escribano P M, López Encuentra A (eds.). En Diagramas Neumología. Madrid, Idepsa 1989.

31 Salzman EW, Harris WH. Prevention of venous thromboembolism in orthopedic patients. J Bone Joint Surg 1976; 58: 903.

32 Merli GJ, Martínez J. Prophylaxis for deep vein thrombosis and pulmonary embolism in the surgical patient. Med Clin North Am 1987; 71: 377–397.

33 Ravdin IS, Kirby CK. Experiences with ligation and heparin in thromboembolic disease. Surgery 1951; 29: 334.

34 Le Brigand H, Moreaux J. Le risque thrombo-embolique dans la chirurgie du thorax. Poumon 1959; 49: 102.
35 Maruyama M, Yagawa K, Hayashi S, Kinjo M, Nakanishi M, Ogata K, Iwami T, Ichinose Y, Hara N, Ohta M, Shigematsu. Presence of thrombosis-inducing activity in plasma from patients with lung cancer. Am Rev Respir Dis 1989; 140: 778–781.
36 Goldhaber SZ, Heit J, Sharma GVRK, Nagel JS, et al. Randomised controlled trial of recombinant tissue plasminogen activator versus urokinase in the treatment of acute pulmonary embolism. Lancet 1988; ii: 293–298.
37 Rabinov K., Paulin S. Roentgen diagnosis of venous thrombosis in the leg. Arch Surg 1972; 104: 134–139.
38 Salzman EW. Venous thrombosis made easy. N Engl J Med 1986; 314: 847.
39 Bettman MA, Paulin S. Radiology 1977; 122: 101.
40 Albrechtson V, Olsson CO. Thrombotic side effects of lower limb plebography. Lancet 1976; 1: 723–725.
41 Kakkar VV, Corrigan TP. Detection of deep venous thrombosis survey and current status. Prog Cardiovasc Dis 1975; 17: 207–213.
42 Kakkar VV. Deep veins thrombosis; Detection and prevention. Circulation 1975; 51: 8.
43 Moser KM, Fedullo PF. Imaging of venous thromboemboli with labeled platelets. Sem Nucl Med 1984; 14: 188.
44 Huisman MV, Buller HR, ten Cate JW, Vreeken J. Serial impedance plethysmography for suspected deep venous thrombosis in out-patients. N Engl J Med 1986; 314: 823.
45 Lensing AWA, Prandoni P, Brandjes D, et al. Detection of deep-vein thrombosis by real-time B-mode ultrasonography. N Engl J Med 1989; 320: 342–345.
46 Hirsh J. Clinical utility of impedance plethysmography in the diagnosis of recurrent deep-vein thrombosis. Arch Intern Med 1988; 148: 519.
47 Huisman M, Buller HR, ten Cate JW. Utility of impedance plethysmography in the diagnosis of recurrent deep-vein thrombosis. Arch Intern Med 1988; 148: 681.
48 Stein PD, Willis PW, Demetz DL. History and physical examination in acute pulmonary embolism in patients without preexisting cardiac or pulmonary disease. Am J Cardiol 1981; 47: 218.
49 Bouchama A, Curley W, Al-Dossary S, Elguindi A. Refractory hypercapnia complicating massive pulmonary embolism. Am Rev Respir Dis 1988; 138: 466–468.
50 Dalen JE, Brooks HL, Johnson LW, et al. Pulmonary angiography in acute pulmonary embolism: Indications, techniques and results in 367 patients. Am Heart J 1971; 81: 175–185.
51 Nicod P, Peterson KL, Levine MS, et al. Pulmonary angiography in severe chronic pulmonary hypertension. Ann Intern Med 1987; 107: 565–568.
52 Mills SR, Jackson DC, Older RA, Heaston DK, Moore AV. The incidence, etiologies, and avoidance of complications of pulmonary angiography in a large series. Radiology 1980; 136: 295.
53 Bookstein JJ, Silver TM. Radiology 1974; 110: 25.
54 Kipper MS, Moser K, Kortman KE, Ashburn WL. Long-term follow-up of patients with suspected embolism and a normal lung scan. Chest 1982; 82: 411.
55 Mercandetti AJ, Kipper MS, Moser KM. Influence of perfusion and ventilation scans on therapeutic decision making and outcome in cases of possible embolisms. West J Med 1985; 142: 208–213.
56 Moser KM, Guisan M, Bartimmo EE, Longo AM, Harsanxi PG, Chiorazzi N. In vivo and postmortem dissolution rates of pulmonary emboli and venous thrombi in the dog. Circulation 1973; 48: 170.
57 Leyvraz PF, Richard J, Bachmann F, Van Melle G, Treyvaud JM, Livio JJ, et al. Adjusted versus fixed dose subcutaneous heparin in the prevention of deep vein thrombosis after total hip replacement. N Engl J Med 1983; 309: 954–958.
58 Turpie AGG, Levine MN, Hirsh J, Carter Cj, Jagy RM, Powers PJ, Andrew M, Hull R, Gent M. A randomized controlled trial of a low-molecular-weigth heparine (enoxaparin) to prevent deep-vein thrombosis in patients undergoing elective hip surgery. N Engl J Med 1986; 315: 925.

59 Salzman EW. Low-molecular-weigth heparin: Is small beautiful? N Engl J Med 1986; 315: 957.
60 Samama M, Bernard P, Bonnardot JP, Combe-Tamzali S, Lanson Y, Tissot E, et al. Low molecular weigth heparin compared with unfractionated heparin in prevention of postoperative thrombosis. Br J Surg 1988; 75: 128.
61 Levine Mn, Hirsch J. Clinical use of low molecular weigth heparins and heparinoids. Semin Thromb Hemost 1988; 14: 116–125.
62 Shran HF, Bitz DW, DiSerio FJ, et al. The pharmacokinetics and bioavailability of subcutaneously administered dihydroergotamine, heparin and the dihydroergotamine combination. Thrombo Res 1983; 31: 51–65.
63 Poller L, McKernan A, Thomson JM, Elstein M, Hirsch PJ, Jones JB. Fixed mini-dose warfarin: a new approach to the prophylaxis of venous thrombosis after major surgery. Br Med J 1987; 295: 1309–1312.
64 Harris W, Salzman EW, Athanasoulis C. Comparison of warfarin, low molecular weight dextran, aspirin, and subcutaneous heparin in prevention of venous thromboembolism following total hip replacement. J Bone Joint Surg 1974; 56: 1552–1562.
65 Poller L, McKernan A, Thomson JM, Elstein M, Hirsch PJ, Jones JB. Fixed mini-dose warfarin: a new approach to the prophylaxis of venous thrombosis after major surgery. Br Med J 1987; 295: 1309–1312.
66 Salzman EW, Ploetx J, Bettman M, et al. Intraoperative external pneumatic calf compression to afford long-term prophylaxis against deep vein thrombosis in urologic patients. Surgery 1980; 87: 239–242.
67 Seurr JH, Ibrahim SZ, Faber RA, et al. The efficacy of graduated compression stocking in the prevention of deep venous thrombosis. Br J Surg 1977; 64: 373.
68 Levine MN, Raskob G, Hirsch J. Hemorragic complications of long-term anticoagulant therapy. Arch Intern Med 1986; 146: 466.
69 Hyers TM, Hull RD, Weg JG. Antithrombotic Therapy for Venous Thromboembolic Disease. Arch Intern Med 1986; 146: 467.
70 Kanter B, Moser KM. Tne Greenfield vena cava filter. Chest 1988; 93: 170–175.
71 Editorial. Management of venous thromboembolism. Lancet 1988; i: 275.
72 Nielsen HK, Husted SE, Krussell L, et al. Anticoagulant therapy in deep venous thrombosis. A randomized controlled study. Thromb Haemostas 1985; 54: 223.
73 Cebul RD. Suspected pulmonary embolism: Individualized approaches using clinical decision analysis. Semin Respir Med 1989; 10: 242–251.
74 Hirsch J. The optimal intensity of oral anticoagulant therapy. JAMA 1987; 258: 2723–2727.
75 Coon W, Wills PW, Symons MJ. Assessment of anticoagulant treatment of venous thromboembolism. Ann Surg 1969; 170: 559.
76 Hull RD, Raskob GE, Hirsh J, et al. Continuous intravenous heparin compared with intermittent subcutaneous heparin in the initial treatment of proximal-vein thrombosis. N Engl J Med 1986; 315: 1109.
77 Petiti DB, Strom BL, Melmon KL. Duration of warfarin anticoagulant therapy and the probabilities of recurrent thromboembolism and hemorrage. Am J Med 1986; 81: 255.
78 Hirsh J, Poller L, Deykin D, Levine M, Dalen JE. Optimal therapeutic range for oral anticoagulants. Chest 1989; 95: 5s.
79 Hull R, Delmore F, Carter C, et al. Adjusted subcutaneous heparin versus warfarin sodium in the long term treatment of venus thrombosis. N Engl J Med 1982; 306: 189–194.
80 Levine MN, Raskob G, Hirsh J. Hemorragic complications of long-term anticoagulant therapy. Chest 1989; 95: 26s.
81 Bell WR. Heparin-associated thrombocytopenia and thrombosis. J Lab Clin Med 1988; 111: 600–605.
82 Kelton JG, Levine MN. Heparin-induced thrombocytopenia. Semin Thromb Hemost 1986; 12: 59.
83 Makhoul RG, Greenberg CS, McCann RL. Heparin-associated thrombocytopenia and thrombosis: a serious clinical problem and potential solution. J Vasc Surg 1986; 4: 522.

84 Landefeld CS, Cook EF, Flatley M, et al. Identification and preliminary validation of predictors of major bleeding in hospitalized patients starting anticoagulant therapy. Am J Med 1987; 82: 703.
85 National Heart, Lung, and Blood Institute. Urokinase–streptokinase embolism trial: phase-2 results. JAMA 1974; 229: 1606–1613.
86 Bell WR, Simmon TL, Stengle JM, Sherry S. The urokinase–streptokinase pulmonary embolism trial (phase II) results. Circulation 1974; 50: 1070–1071.
87 Marder VJ, Sherry S. Thrombolytic therapy. Current status. N Engl J Med 1988; 318: 1512–1520, 1585–1594.
88 Goldhaber SZ, Buring JE, Lepnick RJ, Hennekens CH. Pooled analysis of randomized trials of streptokinase and heparin in phleblographically documented deep venous thrombosis. Am J Med 1984; 76: 393–397.
89 Shiffman F, Ducas J, Hollet P, et al. Treatment of canine embolic pulmonary hypertension with recombinant tissue plasminogen activator. Circulation 1988; 19: 214–220.
90 Ward BJ, Pearse DB. Reperfusion pulmonary edema after thromboembolic therapy of massive pulmonary embolism. Am Rev Respir Dis 1988; 138: 1308–1311.
91 Goldhaber SZ, Vaughan DE, Markis JE, Selwyn AP, Meyerowitz MF, Loscalzo J, Kim DS, Kessler CM, Danley DL, Sharma GVRK, Sasahara A, Grossbard EB, Braunwald E. Acute pulmonary embolism treated with tissue plasminogen activator. Lancet 1986; ii: 886.
92 Verstraete M, Miller GAH, Bounamedaux H, et al. Intravenous and intrapulmonary recombinant tissue-type plasminogen activator in the treatment of acute massive pulmonary embolism. Circulation 1988; 77: 353–360.
93 Monk JP, Heel RC. Anisoylated plasminogen streptokinase activator complex (APSAC); a review of its mechanism of action, clinical pharmacology, and therapeutic use in myocardial infarction. Drugs 1987; 34: 25–49.
94 Van de Werf F, Vanhaecke J, de Geest H, Verstraete M. Collen D. Coronary thrombolysis with recombinant single-chain urokinase-type plasminogen activator in patients with acute myocardial infarction. Circulation 1986; 74: 1066–1070.
95 Mobin-Uddin D, Callard GM, Bolooki H, et al. Transvenous caval interruption with umbrella filter. N Engl J Med 1973; 55: 286.
96 Greenfield LJ, McCurdy JR, Brown PP, Elkins RC. A new intracaval filter permitting continued flow and resolution of emboli. Surgery 1973; 73: 599.
97 Greenfield LJ, Michna BA. Twelve-year clinical experience with the Greenfield filter. Surgery 1988; 104: 706–712.
98 Tracy Jr T, Posner MP, Drucker DE, Greenfield LJ, Langhan Jr MR, Mendez-Picon G, Krummel TM, Salzberg AM. Use of Greenfield filter in adolescents for deep vein thrombosis and pulmonary embolism. J Pediatr Surg 1988; 23: 529–532.
99 Greenfield LJ, Wakefield TW. Prevention of venous thrombosis and pulmonary embolism. Adv Surg 1989; 22: 301–323.
100 Hull R, Delmore T, Genton E, Hirsh J, Gent M, Sackett D, McLoughlin D, Armstrong P. Warfarin sodium versus low-dose heparine in the long-term treatment of venous thrombosis. N Engl J Med 1979; 301: 855.
101 Cross FS, Mowlem A. A survey of current status of pulmonary embolectomy for massive pulmonary embolism. Circulation 1974; 50: 236–244.
102 Moser KM, Daily PO, Peteson Kl, et al. Thromboendarterectomy for chronic, major vessel thromboembolic pulmonary hypertension in 42 patients. Immediate and long-term results. An Intern Med 1987; 107: 560–565.
103 Storm O. Anticoagulant protection in surgery. Thromb Diath Haemorrh 1958; 2: 484–491.
104 Clarke DB. Pulmonary embolism after surgery. In: Smith RE, Williams WG (eds.). Surgery of the Lung. The Coventry Conference. London, Butterworths 1974.
105 Kiil J, Kiil J, Axelsen F, Andersen D. Prophylaxis against postoperative pulmonary embolism and deep-vein thrombosis by low-dose heparine. Lancet 1978; i: 1115.

106 Jackaman FR, Perry BJ, Siddons H. Deep vein thrombosis after thoracotomy. Thorax 1978; 33: 761–763.
107 Gaillard J, Plante J, Glovaez D, Eschapasse HE. Prévention des accidents thromboemboliques après pneumonectomie. Poumon et Coeur 1979; 35: 71–75.
108 Le Brigand H, Morille P, Garnier B, Bogaty-Yver J, Samana M, Spriet A. Essai de prévention des accidents thrombo-emboliques post-opératoires par les faibles doses d'héparinate de calcium en chirurgie thoracique. Sem Hôp Paris 1981; 57: 972–977.
109 Marchetti V, Beati C, Pogliani EM, Vincre G. Profilassi calcieparinica a basso dosaggio in chirurgia toracica. Sanguinamento, modificazioni della coagulazione e della fibrinolisi. Min Med 1983; 74: 1745–1748.
110 Cade JF, Clegg EA, Westlake GW. Prophylaxis of venous thrombosis after major thoracic surgery. Aust N Z J Surg 1983; 53: 301.
111 Rajah SM, Salter MCP, Donaldson DR, Crow MJ, Rao RS, Watson DA. A clinical trial comprising 2500 IU heparine and 0.5 mg dihydroergotamine (DHE) with 5000 IU heparine in the prophylaxis of deep vein thrombosis following thoraic surgery. Thromb Haemost 1983; 50: 9.
112 Gamondès JP, Defour M. Le dépistage des thromboses veineuses des membres inférieurs par le test au fibrinogène marqué à l'iode 125 dans la chirurgie du thorax. A propos de 140 opérés. Rev Pneumol Clin 1984; 40: 373–376.
113 Ljungström KG. Deep-vein thrombosis after major non-cardiovascular thoracic surgery. Scand J Thorac Cardiovasc Surg 1985; 19: 161–164.
114 Pogliani EM. Eparina a basse dosi nella chirurgia toracica. Min Med 1985; 76: 495–500.
115 Gamondès JP, Defour M, Girard Cl, Normand R, Tartulier M, Devolfe Ch, Clermont A, Amiel M. Le dépistage des thromboses veineuses des membres inférieurs après thoracotomie. Résultats préliminaires á propos de quatre-vingt-deux opérés. Ann Chir. 1985; 39: 150–152.
116 Rizzi A, Radaelli F, Pisano M, Orro S, Nazzari M, Ratti G, Giobbe R, Maggi G. Profilassi con defibrotide delle trombosi venose profonde in chirurgia toracica. Studio multicentrico controllato verso eparina. Min Med 1987; 78: 745–775.
117 American Heart Association. Prevention of venous thromboembolism in surgical patients by low-dose heparin. Circulation 1977; 55: 423.

Current Topics in General Thoracic Surgery: An International Series, Vol. 2
Perioperative Care, edited by R.M. Peters and J. Toledo

Chapter 20

Indications for therapeutic antibiotics following thoracic surgery

James W. Pate

1. HISTORY

Organic compounds such as tar, phenol, creosote, turpentine and acids such as vinegar and old wine were used as *antiseptics* ("against sepsis") from antiquity. By the time of the American Civil War (1861), a wide spectrum of compounds had been identified and were used during and after surgery. These included the halogens – iodine, bromine and chlorine – and metal salts. Lord Lister, in 1867, building upon the discoveries of Pasteur and the old empiric antiseptics introduced a logical theory and practice of antiseptic surgery in which pathogenic organisms were killed by various agents. Antiseptic compounds now also included Dakin's Solution, chlorine bleaches, and organic iodides and numerous organic compounds. Domagk, in 1932, observed the antibacterial effects of the sulfanilamides; further development of these drugs led to the *chemotherapeutic* antimicrobial agents first proven highly effective in the early 1940s. Newer agents include nitrofurantoin, methenamine mandelate, quinolones and metronidazole. Earlier, in 1929, Sir Arthur Fleming had discovered Penicillin, an *antibiotic*, but its clinical application was delayed until the 1940s when the stimulation of wartime injuries and the development of mass microbial cultures led to its clinical use. Penicillin was a serendipitous discovery, but Waksman went about a systematic search for effective antibiotics and developed Streptomycin in 1944. Since that time, hundreds of natural and synthetic antibiotics, antifungal and chemotherapeutic agents have been discovered and developed. In this chapter, we shall use 'antimicrobial' to include natural and synthetic antibiotics and chemotherapeutic agents effective against viruses, bacteria, fungal or protozoa. The occurrence of mutation and resistant strains of bacteria has led to a constant seesaw battle between new antimicrobials and bacterial resistance. The surgeon must be familiar with the various antibacterial, antiviral, antifungal and antiprotozoan drugs, their usage and side-effects. However, detailed consideration of each agent is beyond the scope of this report and reference to current appropriate publications, such as package inserts, U.S. Pharmacopeia or Physician's Desk Reference is recommended.

2. PROPHYLACTIC vs THERAPEUTIC ANTIMICROBIALS

'Medical infections' are characterized by a clinical syndrome produced by a single organism (e.g. typhoid fever, pneumococcal pneumonia, or bacterial meningitis) in which the elimination of this organism usually results in cure of the patient without permanent residuals. 'Surgical infections', in contrast, are characterized more by the *milieu* in which the infection occurs than by the specific organism – a fact early noted by Pasteur. Surgical infections are frequently polymicrobial. Dead tissue, foreign bodies, continual contamination, and collections of pus characterize these infections. As early as the Hippocratic School (600–400 BC) it was noted that drainage of a surgical infection was the treatment of choice. An interesting exception was empyema, where Hippocrates had noted that early drainage (prior to mediastinal fixation) might result in respiratory insufficiency and death.

Prophylactic antimicrobials are given before and during surgery in an attempt to *prevent* the establishment of infection. Prophylactic antimicrobials are used in 80–96% of thoracotomies; almost 90% are cephalosporins. Therapeutic antimicrobials are given to *treat* an established infection. This infection might be present before surgery and continue during the surgical and postoperative periods or it may follow as a complication of surgery. In the former group are such conditions as empyema as an indication for decortication, or lung abscess as an indication for pulmonary resection. These pre-existing diseases indicate the therapeutic use of antibiotics before surgery and their continuance in the postoperative period. In addition to empyema and lung abscess, other disorders, e.g., bronchiectasis, tuberculosis, specific fungal infections, pneumonia requiring lung biopsy, Pneumocystis disease and Legionellosis fall into this category. However, the diagnosis is frequently not clear until the surgical procedure allows for biopsy or microbiological identification of the infection. In such cases, therapeutic drugs must be started at the time of or even after the procedure. Common complications of thoracic surgery requiring antibiotic therapy include gastric aspiration, pneumonia complicating atelectasis, wound infections, bronchopleural fistulae and empyema resulting from pleural space problems. Other conditions, such as esophageal rupture, require continuation of prophylactic antimicrobials into the therapeutic phase of the resulting mediastinitis or empyema. In such cases, differentiation between prophylactic and therapeutic therapy becomes meaningless.

Naturally occurring immunodeficiency such as from congenital disorders, advanced malignancies, AIDS, starvation, and severe metabolic derangements following major burns or multiple organ failure, also require antimicrobials which are both prophylactic and therapeutic. The iatrogenic immunosuppression seen in radiation therapy, chemotherapy for tumors, transplantation, and certain disease processes, likewise leads to a high incidence of postoperative infectious complications and, thus, indicate a prolongation of prophylactic antimicrobials into the therapeutic period. In these immunocompromised states, frequent re-evaluation of both the patient and laboratory data lead to appropriate therapeutic changes.

3. GENERAL CONSIDERATIONS

Indications for the institution of therapeutic antimicrobials in the postoperative period generally relate to either systemic or local evidence of infection.

The utilization of antimicrobials for postoperative therapeutic use depends upon proper understanding of: (a) the indications and circumstances in which antibiotics are needed, (b) the most likely organism to be involved, (c) identification, classification and sensitivity studies on the specific organism, (d) choice of antimicrobials (based upon clinical, empiric and laboratory studies), (e) appropriate dose given by the appropriate route and (f) maintained for a proper duration.

It is generally recognized that the incidence of wound infections in clean surgical operations is 1.5–6%. In clean-contaminated wounds, infection occurs in 8–20%, but averages only about 4–10% for all pulmonary surgery[1]; it may reach 40% for esophageal surgery. In 'dirty' wounds, more than half will probably become infected.

Among the 'causes' of surgical infection are (1) pathogenic organisms (virulence and number), (2) abnormal serum factors, (3) decreased white blood cell phagocytosis and bacterial killing and, (4) surgical factors. In general, simple wound infections result from surface contaminants such as streptococcus, *Staphylococcus epidermidis* and diphtheroids. Traumatic wounds usually show these same organisms but with a higher incidence of *Staphylococcus aureus* and *Streptococcus pyogenes.* It is generally considered that about 10^5 organisms are required for an infection to develop in clean tissues. In the presence of foreign bodies or necrotic tissue, the number of organisms required to establish infection is far less, by orders of magnitude, than the number required in their absence[2].

Abnormal serum factors include opsonins and gamma globulin deficiencies. In addition to host factors, characteristics of the organism influence phagocytosis. Certain organisms, such as *Klebsiella* and pneumococcus, have a capsule which inhibits phagocytosis and others, such as clostridia and streptococcus, produce exotoxins which have dramatic systemic effects. Still others, such as *Histoplasma*, *Neisseria* and HIV live very well within the host cell.

Decreased phagocytosis is present when there is overwhelming infection, shock, foreign bodies, ischemia, low white cell counts from any cause, hematomas, uremia and steroid therapy. Abnormal phagocytosis occurs with uncontrolled diabetes, uremia and certain systemic diseases. Abnormal intracellular killing of organisms is seen in starvation, markedly increased metabolic states, such as severe burns, trauma and sepsis, and in patients who are immunosuppressed.

3.1. Predisposition and inhibition of infections

Clinically, infection is usually heralded by the onset of inappropriate fever, leukocytosis, left shift in the white count and, in the chest, abnormal radiographic and physical findings. Atelectasis, very frequent after thoracotomy, may, by trapping organisms and their toxins in compressed alveoli, be associated with fever. While technically this may be considered early pneumonia, the fever usually subsides within a few hours with good tracheobronchial toilet. Fever may also occur as a complication of transfusion, as a drug fever or with thrombophlebitis. An elevated white blood cell count is usually associated with infection; in the elderly, debilitated, cachectic, or immunocompromised patient or in those with overwhelming sepsis, the white count may be normal or low. Even with a leukopenia there are usually large numbers of immature cells – the so-called left shift. Local signs of infection include the classic redness, tenderness and swelling; these are usually apparent in a wound infection, but are, of course, hidden in deep-seated infections. Predisposing or risk factors for postoperative thoracic wound infection include: obesity, diabetes, length of the operation, length of preoperative hospital stay (more than five days), smoking, COPD, reoperation, bilateral internal mammary artery dissections, ischemic necrotic tissue, anatomical dead space, hematomas and gross contamination. It should again be emphasized that a large percentage of surgical infections are polymicrobial and antimicrobial therapy is only an adjuvant to proper surgical treatment.

Careful repeated physical examination of the chest and review of repeated chest X-rays are the keystones for recognizing early infection. In addition to the usual examination of surgical wounds, the areas around chest tubes, intravenous cannula, electronic wires and other invasive gadgets should be frequently inspected. When such invasive appliances are prolonged (three or four days), they should be cultured.

When a bronchus or the esophagus is opened, organisms from the lumen enter the surgical field leading to a 'clean-contaminated' wound. Consideration of both the microbiologic and physiologic characteristics of these structures is essential to proper use of therapeutic antibiotics for surgical complications. The tracheobronchial tree is usually sterile in its more distal divisions; as one passes more proximally towards the larynx, the numbers and species of organisms increase. In the absence of pulmonary or bronchial disease, the trapping mechanism of the mucus barrier, cilial activity (with its escalator effect), I_gA, alpha-antitrypsin, lysozyme, and complement all tend to keep the numbers of organisms at a low level. Tubes in the trachea increase bacterial adherence to epithelial cells, decrease mucus and ciliary function and exaggerate drying – all of which decrease the natural protective factors in the tracheobronchial tree. Cuffed endotracheal tubes produce an area of stagnant accumulated secretions between the endotracheal cuff and the pharynx; these secretions are not reached by the usual suction catheters. As prolonged accumulation occurs (hours) a very high concentration of organisms results. 'Bolus aspiration' of such material past the cuff, occurring on patient gasps, deep breathing, iatrogenic manipulations and similar events, inoculates the lower bronchial system with these myriad organisms. Smaller bronchi and alveoli are also protected by pulmonary surfactant, cell-surface fibronectin, I_gG and high neutrophil phagocytic concentrations. Protecting the oropharynx are the gag and cough reflexes, I_gA, and cellular fibronectin. The mucosal cells are normally coated with fibronectin which selects for adherence of gram-positive cocci. In the elderly, debilitated, post-operative, or similar patient, fibronectin is decreased with loss of normal gram-positive cocci, leading to an increased colonization of the oropharynx by gram-negative rods. The tracheobronchial tree may take on the microbiological characteristics more typical of the oropharynx with disease (either acute or chronic), anesthetic gases, endotracheal tubes, and in other pathologic conditions. The oropharynx may contain a wide spectrum of organisms, including gram-positive and gram-negative bacteria as well as spirochetes, diphtheroids and anaerobes in the gingival recesses [3]. These organisms pass with the saliva into the esophagus and contaminate the mediastinum and pleural spaces when there is esophageal penetration.

In the severely ill patient, the flora and numbers of organisms in the oropharynx change dramatically so that many more virulent numbers *and* strains of organisms are present. This mechanism plays a part in 'nosocomial pneumonia', which is really more related to abnormal pathophysiology of illness rather than to a specific hospital environment. Nosocomial pneumonia is the most common and most fatal ($>50\%$) of hospital-acquired infections. Inappropriate antibiotic usage facilitates the emergence of more virulent or resistant strains of organisms. Fever alone, without a more specific diagnosis, should not be treated with antibiotics. Only about 40–50% of ICU patients with fever actually have pneumonia. About 5% of normal people have significant gram-negative organisms in the oropharynx, whereas half of the very ill have such bacteria. Good oral hygiene and use of antiseptics or antibiotic pastes in the mouth may reduce risks of pulmonary aspiration of these organisms.

With gastric aspiration, a mixture of esophageal organisms, as well as the acid contents of the stomach, gain access to the tracheobronchial tree. The development of a chemical pneumonia from high acidic fluid may be followed (in 2–3 hours) by a superimposed mixed bacterial infection from these organisms as well as progression to ARDS. About 80% of patients with tracheotomies aspirate, at least intermittently; probably all patients with peroral endotracheal tubes have continuous contamination of the bronchial tree. Gastric contents are usually quite 'clean' of bacterial pathogens due to acid. However, with natural achlorhydria and especially when antacids and/or H_2 blockers are used, this protective mechanism is lost and aspiration of even small amounts of stomach contents may produce a severe, virulent, polymicrobial pneumonia. This is common in ICU patients. Alcoholism, chronic lung disease, airway instrumentation, coma, use of PEEP, sepsis and artificial ventilation for more than three days are each a significant risk factor. ICU's and ventilators are especially dangerous. About half of the cases are related to gram-negative rods (especially *Klebsiella*, pseudomonas, proteus). *S. aureus* (MRSA), enterococcus and anaerobes are also frequent offenders.

Bacterial translocation from the gut lumen to mesenteric nodes and distant organs, such as lung, occurs following shock, general sepsis, immunosuppression, intestinal stasis or bacterial overgrowth, or direct injury to the gut (e.g. trauma)[4]. The lungs may, by this mechanism, also be invaded by organisms usually associated with the gastrointestinal tract.

Ventilator-associated ('respirator-related') pneumonia may be initially empirically treated with Tobramycin (3 mg/kg/day in divided IV doses), which is effective against most pseudomonas, among the more common organisms associated with this disease. However, two-drug therapy is more common, either: aminoglycoside with a semisynthetic penicillin, aminoglycoside with clindamycin, or aminoglycoside with cephalosporin. Simultaneously, adequate bacteriological study of lower airway secretions is followed by appropriate therapy when results of sensitivity testing are known.

Humoral immunodeficiency, such as in asplenic patients, affects the body's ability to control encapsulated organisms, leading to increased risks of infection with *Streptococcus pneumoniae*, *Haemophilus influenzae*, *Neisseria*, and also viruses and *Pneumocystis carinii*. Cell-mediated deficiencies produce a vulnerability to gram-negative organisms such as *Salmonella* and *Escherichia coli*, but also to the 'granulomatous organisms' – *M. tuberculosis* (especially atypical), *Nocardia*, fungi, yeast, and viruses. Pseudomonas infections occur in both humoral and cell-mediated deficiencies. *Candida*, cryptococcus, aspergillus, *Pneumocystis pneumoniae* and herpes are far more virulent in the immunocompromised individual.

4. MICROBIOLOGY

'Empiric' antimicrobials are those given prior to, or even in the absence of, identification of the specific organism involved[5]. The organism may not be identified because of previous antimicrobial therapy, problems in specimen collection and laboratory growth, the polymicrobial nature of the infection, or urgency of the clinical situation. Empiric therapy, while not as 'scientific' as desired, makes up a large part of clinical practice (Table 20.1). Rational choice of empiric therapy rests primarily upon two factors: (a) the probability of certain pathogens being involved in the given case, and (b) the gram-stain of material, when available, from the pathologic lesion. Especially in thoracic surgery, empiric therapy is frequently mandatory; an understanding of these two factors becomes crucial.

Observations of pus and discharge may yield considerable useful clinical information. A thin, watery, slightly sanguineous exudate is typical of streptococcus, especially when associated with cellulitis, bullous formation and dissection along fascial planes and systemic toxicity. Pus which is thick and creamy is typical of *S. aureus*; green thick pus is characteristic of pseudomonas. Pus which is foul smelling results from proteolytic activity, most commonly from anaerobic organisms. Gas occurs with anaerobic and with some streptococcal infections. Sterile pus may result from tissue necrosis, foreign body reaction or chemical

TABLE 20.1
Drugs which are usually effective in post-thoracotomy complications while awaiting cultural identification and sensitivity studies

Complication	Recommended drug	Alternatives and comments
Pus available for stain		
Gram-positive cocci		
clumps (staph.)	nafcillin, cephalotin, erythromycin, vancomycin	Frequently resistant; with anaerobes – clindamycin and gentamicin
chains (strep)	penicillin G; erythromycin	cephalosporins or vancomycin
Gram-negative rods	aminoglycoside and cephalosporin; ampicillin	anaerobic – imipenem
Gram-positive rods	penicillin G; tetracyclines; clindamycin	
Mixed stains	imipenem, vancomycin	(except Pseudomonas)
No stain available		
Pulmonary surgery	nafcillin and aminoglycoside	Allergic, penicillin; MRSA or S. epi. – vancomycin + aminoglycoside
Esophageal contamination	aminoglycoside + clindamycin or cephalosporin	3rd gen. cephalosporin + clindamycin *or* ticarcillin, piperacillin plus aminoglycoside
Immunocompromised	aminoglycoside + cephalosporin	ceftazidine – pseudomonas

irritation without bacteria. Sterile pus may also follow a pre-existing infection which is 'burned out' or in which antibiotic therapy has prevented continued bacterial growth, especially in the laboratory.

Identification and study of the organism responsible for an infection depends upon proper collection of the specimen. With pneumonia or bronchitis, specimens are properly obtained by endoscopy. The protected brush technique and bronchoalveolar lavage yield good specimens from the area of infection; sputum or tracheal aspirants are notoriously non-representative and thus may actually mislead [6,7]. Alveolar macrophages, markers for lower airway specimens, should be seen in properly collected specimens. Brushings with bacteriological study at repeated bronchoscopies may be used to monitor changes in flora. Actually, infection is probably not present unless $> 10^3$ colony-forming units/ml are found on culture.

Collections of pus elsewhere should be sampled by aspiration so that proper representative specimens are collected in a syringe from which air has been excluded, sealed and promptly transported to the laboratory for culturing under anaerobic conditions (as blood gas specimens are handled). Collection by open drainage, swabs and improper aspirations may yield misleading results. In infections in which there is no pus available, actual biopsy of tissues with a scalpel or by needle is indicated. Many infections can only be diagnosed from such tissue samples. It is important that material for culture not be allowed to dry prior to laboratory handling.

All material removed for microbiological study should have an *immediate* gram stain and, when appropriate, acid-fast and fungal stains. Gram stain yields much useful information and is available immediately rather than after several days of delay for culturing. When several organisms are present, the gram stain will demonstrate the predominate organism which may not be the one which grows best in culture. In such circumstances, gram stain may be more useful than culture, which is overly influenced by the organism which grows most easily and rapidly. The gram stain aids in the selection of empiric antibiotics for immediate use prior to cultural identification and sensitivity studies. Such prompt appropriate antibiotic therapy may prevent major surgical complications which could become more serious while awaiting cultures. For example, typical clostridia may be seen on gram-stain of an infected traumatic wound, thus allowing therapy which avoids death which could occur while awaiting cultures. Positive acid-fast smears allow immediate therapy and isolation techniques prior to the several weeks necessary for culture.

A telephone call to the laboratory may lead to more accurate and quicker analysis. Direct communication between the surgeon and the laboratory is much more important than usually practiced. When a patient is seriously ill, the laboratory may be requested to do direct antibiotic disk-sensitivity studies on agar plates *prior* to isolation and identification of the organisms. Such sensitivities may be available in 12 to 24 hours and allow prompt institution of appropriate antibiotic therapy well before the cultures have been identified, replated and had sensitivity studies. Sensitivity tests are usually not necessary with pneumococcus, group-A *Streptococcus*, most anaerobic bacteria, *Neisseria*, *Haemophilus*, and fungi. However, selective sensitivity testing should be done on pneumococcus for penicillin-resistance, on *Haemophilus* for β-lactamase production (ampicillin resistance) and *Bacteroides* for penicillinase production. Sensitivities are critically important with organisms such as gram-negative rods or with coagulase-positive staphylococcus.

The simplest classification of bacteria depends upon their gross morphology and staining characteristics. Cocci, rods, clubs, spores, long slender forms and branching all are significant basic shapes. Diphtheroids, clostridia, yeasts, and some mycelia may be tentatively identified on stain. The ability of the organism to hold gentian violet stain after an alcohol wash – gram-positive stain – defines a group of organisms quite different from the gram-negative ones which lose gentian violet stain on alcohol wash. The ability of an organism to retain its staining after a wash in acid-alcohol characterizes the acid-fast organisms – particularly *M. tuberculosis* and *Nocardia*.

A cultural classification depends upon the organisms' requirement for oxygen. (1) Obligate aerobes require a atmospheric concentration of oxygen for their growth; major organisms of clinical importance include pseudomonas, brucella and mycobacteria. (2) Obligate anaerobes require an oxygen-free environment for their growth; major organisms in this group include *Bacteroides*, *Clostridia* and

Actinomyces. The largest group, (3) the facultative anaerobes, will grow either aerobically or anaerobically. These are the most common pathogens and include the coagulase-positive staphylococci, group-A *Streptococcus*, pneumococcus and various coliform organisms.

Fungi are eukaryotic, i.e. have a nuclei membrane. The cell wall, which is a polysaccharide complex (chitin, similar to shrimp) containing sterols, is affected by the polyene antibiotics such as Amphotericin B. It should be noted that *Nocardia* and *Actinomyces*, while having long mycelia-like structures, are not eukaryotic; they are bacteria.

5. CHOICE OF DRUG

Details of the dozens of antimicrobials and their spectra of activity and actions are beyond the scope of this chapter. Newer drugs are constantly being added. However, the *principles* of choosing antimicrobial are basic. Ideally, the choice of drug depends upon bacteriologic identification and drug sensitivity studies. However, consideration of the specific disease, the host characteristics, common nosocomial organisms at a particular hospital at a certain time, the probability and severity of adverse reactions, cost, and convenience are all important. Very commonly, it is highly desirable to begin empiric therapy prior to bacteriologic identification. In such instances, the clinical diagnosis of the site of infection, the likelihood of certain organisms from the specific source of contamination, and the known nosocomial characteristics of the hospital, all enter into the decision for an empirical drug. The gram stain is extremely important in allowing appropriate selection of antimicrobial prior to culture and sensitivity studies (Table 20.1, above).

The nature of the pathologic process should be considered. In general, blood and pulmonary alveoli contain a high concentration of administered antibiotics, whereas the tracheobronchial secretions, pleural and pericardial spaces will have much lower concentrations. Diffusion into avascular areas (e.g. granulomas) and encapsulated areas (e.g. chronic abscess or empyema) will result in still lower levels. Such factors influence the choice of drug and, especially, the dose and route of administration.

Infection control services of each major hospital usually maintain a running inventory of the common nosocomial organisms found within it, as well as their usual antibiotic sensitivities. This information may be of great practical value.

Antimicrobial dosage is usually started with a 'standard' dose, adjusted by such factors as severity of disease, known or suspected sensitivity of the offending organism, tissue of interest, route of administration, and, especially, toxicity. In cases of low sensitivity of the organisms, with toxic drugs and in the presence of factors which predispose to toxicity (e.g. renal insufficiency, shock, hepatic failure, neurologic problems) it is extremely important to adjust dosage based upon measured peak and trough blood levels of antimicrobial[5]. With poor renal functions, less drug may be necessary or the intervals between doses may be increased to as much as every 12 hours or even once a day, to maintain appropriate peak blood levels. Prolonged high trough levels should also be avoided. Exact dosages and adverse reactions should be determined by reference to current official works. In using cultures and sensitivity studies for selection of antimicrobials, one must critically evaluate the laboratory results in cases in which more than one organism is recovered. The immediate gram stain and clinical picture may indicate which one of the several organisms is probably responsible and should be targeted.

Most pulmonary anaerobes are sensitive to penicillin, erythromycin, and tetracyclines (doxycycline). Therefore, with the onset of postoperative pulmonary or pleural complications, even in patients who received prophylactic cephalosporins, these older antibiotics remain a good choice for empiric selection while awaiting sensitivity studies and specific therapy. Penicillin G remains one of the more valuable antibiotics. In lung abscesses and mediastinitis from esophageal perforations, we prefer **10–14 million** units per day by intermittent intravenous injection. It is highly effective against many of the virulent oral pathogens involved in these infections: *Streptococcus* (pneumoniae, A, B, C and G, and viridans), peptostreptococcus, many staphylococci, clostridia, *Alcaligenes faecalis* and some *Bacteroides* melaninogenicus and oris. There are increasing strains (15–20%) of penicillinase-producing anaerobes. Penicillin-resistant *S. aureus* may be treated with nafcillin, methicillin, oxacillin, or dicloxacillin. These are generally given at 9–15 g/day, intravenously, while awaiting sensitivity studies. Most methicillin-resistent *S. aureus* in hospitals are resistent to cephalosporins; aminoglycosides and vancomycin may be substituted. When patients are severely ill, or fail to respond to penicillin, clindamycin is indicated. Penicillin combined with metronidazole has been used extensively in Europe. For thoracic wound infections empiric antibiotics commonly used include: (a) nafcillin or vancomycin plus an aminoglycoside, (b) cefazolin, (c) newer 'third-generation' cephalosporins.

Human bites, with sputum frequently containing spirochetes, aerobes and anaerobes, develop thick, foul-smelling pus which empirically responds best to high doses of penicillin. *Eikenella corrodeus*, a facultative anaerobe, gram-negative rod is frequently found. It is usually sensitive to penicillin, ampicillin and cephalosporins. Because of the similar bacteriology and previous experience, we use large doses of intravenous penicillin for esophageal perforation or surgical spillage. A third generation cephalosporin *and* clindamycin may be added or even substituted. Infections of vascular catheters are frequently due to enteric organisms, pseudomonas, serratia and, especially, *S. aureus*. Empiric therapy of a third generation cephalosporin *or* a combination of gentamicin and nafcillin is recommended. However, there is increasing frequency ($>50\%$) of *S. epidermidis* and *S. aureus* on plastic catheters, associated with 'slime production' and adherence to plastic. These organisms are frequently methicillin resistant and vancomycin plus gentamicin may be indicated.

Aminoglycosides are especially valuable for most gram-negative facultative anaerobes. They are effective against some pseudomonas and some serratia. In general, streptomycin and neomycin are not indicated in the treatment of systemic gram-negative infections. Tetracyclines are especially useful for *Mycoplasma pneumoniae* and *Haemophilus influenzae*. Erythromycin is a low-toxicity antibiotic useful against streptococcus, staphylococcus, pneumoniae, *Neisseria*, mycoplasma, diphtheria, clostridia and some atypical mycobacteria. It is best used orally. With high, prolonged dosages, secondary bacterial overgrowth in the gut may appear. Legionella is also treated with erythromycin. Both lincomycin and clindamycin have narrower spectrums than erythromycin but are especially active against streptococcus, staphylococcus and *B. fragilis* as well as the anaerobic gram-negative bacteria frequently seen in aspiration pneumonia, lung abscesses and empyemas. Sulfa-trimethoprim drugs act synergistically and are especially useful against gram-negative rods (except pseudomonas); they may be given orally and produce good tissue penetration. These are especially valuable in chronic lung diseases.

The synthetic antibacterial agent, metronidazole, is bactericidal against most obligate anaerobic bacteria, but exhibits little activity against facultative anaerobes or obligate aerobes. It diffuses well into the spinal fluid and is usually given in the intravenous form as an antibacterial drug. However, similar serum and tissue levels are easily reached with oral administration. *Bacteroides* is especially sensitive to this drug, along with anaerobic gram-positive clostridia and anaerobic cocci, peptococcus and *Peptostreptococcus*. Any or all of these organisms may appear in mediastinitis, pulmonary gangrene or, especially, aspiration abscesses, making the drug especially useful in these conditions. Anaerobic hepatic abscess rupturing into pleura or lung is an especial indication for its use, since *Endamoeba* histiolytic, a common etiologic agent, is extremely sensitive.

Rifampin has a very wide spectrum against both gram-positive and gram-negative organisms as well as against mycobacteria. However, it is associated with the development of rapid bacterial resistance and is primarily used for treating tuberculosis. When combined with another antibiotic, it may exhibit considerable synergy and be useful in other bacterial infections.

Adverse reactions from antimicrobials fall into several large groups. The first group is hypersensitivity reaction or *allergy*, varying from a simple skin rash to anaphylactic shock. These sensitivities are best determined by history and are highly individual. The penicillins and, less frequently, the cephalosporins are most important in this regard. *Toxicity*, the second adverse group, is a characteristic of most antimicrobials and usually involves the kidney, liver, neurological structures (especially the eighth cranial nerve) and bone marrow. Aminoglycosides may be associated with auditory, vestibular and more rarely, other neurological toxicity or renal damage. The development of antibiotic *resistance* is an adverse reaction and may occur during therapy, leading to a relapse or exacerbation of the disease in the face of continued antimicrobial therapy. Prolonged and broad spectrum antibiotics may lead to the development of superinfection with secondary growth of organisms which are resistant to the antibiotic and may also be more virulent. These organisms may be yeast or fungi, such as *Candida*. 'Superinfection' pneumonia, for example, may result in a mortality rate that is up to 80% higher than the rate in pneumonia patients who are not receiving antibiotics. Antibiotics may 'mask' an infectious complication and lead to delay in its recognition or even in misdiagnosis.

In myasthenic patients one should avoid aminoglycosides, especially streptomycin and gentamicin, because of associated neuromuscular depression. If the patient is severely ill and these drugs are critical, he may be kept on a ventilator while they are used. Clindamycin (or less commonly any antibiotic) may be associated with *Clostridium difficile* overgrowth and severe colitis from enterotoxins. This organism is sensitive to vancomycin which is used orally or via enteric tube for treatment. Staphylococcal enterocolitis usually occurs following oral broad spectrum antibiotics; it is an emergency and is treated with anti-staphylococcal drugs.

6. ROUTE

During the acute postoperative period, the *intravenous* route is the most reliable method of antibiotic administration. The *intramuscular* route may not be adequate in the face of shock, low tissue perfusion or hypovolemia. The *oral* route is usually reserved for the period during recovery when the patient is on an oral diet. Not all drugs can be given by all routes. For example, only in the spring of 1991 has a quinolone for intravenous use become available.

Topical administration is a frequently overlooked route of therapy[8]. The advantages of topical use include: very high local concentration, usage of drugs which would be too toxic for systemic administration, ability to add other drugs to those used systemically and access of drug to non-vascular spaces (e.g. long standing empyema pockets). Topical antimicrobials have proven highly effective when there is a single large contamination. Long-standing abscesses or spaces with well-developed walls may not allow diffusion of significant antimicrobials into the space when the drug is given systemically. Irrigation and the instillation of topical antibiotics or chemotherapeutic drugs through a tube may be advantageous in such circumstances. When a single large contamination occurs, e.g. spillage of lung abscess or esophageal contents into the pleural space, generous irrigation with saline followed by high concentrations of topical antibiotics may reduce the contamination load to one which the body can adequately handle. For example, studies on rats with contaminated wounds have shown that topical cephalosporins are as good or better than intramuscular cephalosporins in the prevention of wound infections. Studies of appendicitis in the human have shown similar results.

Chronic empyema spaces may be filled with antimicrobial or antiseptic solution, which is left for two or three hours, as often as twice a day. As home treatment, the patient or family can be instructed to instill the solutions into the chest cavity and properly position the patient. A day's dose of antibiotics may be instilled through the tube which is clamped for three hours prior to re-establishment of drainage. A commonly used fluid for irrigation of infected pleural spaces is: 1 gram of kanamycin and 1 gram of cephalosporin or bacitracin per liter of fluid. For small, long-standing spaces, we have used diluted (1:10 to 1:40) povidone–iodine alone, especially when the infection is of fungal or tubercular etiology.

There are three separate regimes of topical applications: (1) high concentration of the same drug which is also used systemically; a drug which could be given systemically is only given locally; (2) drugs which diffuse poorly or whose toxicity limits their concentration when given systemically may be used in high concentration as local irrigation. Examples include neomycin, polymyxin and bacitracin, all of which may be used in very high concentrations for irrigation within the chest either at the time of surgery or intermittently for postoperative spaces; (3) agents which cannot be given systemically may be used by irrigation. We have long used these for fungal diseases. Examples include intracavitary instillation of potassium iodide for aspergilloma and repeated irrigation of empyema spaces, open wounds, chronic osteomyelitis or prostheses with diluted (1:10) povidone–iodine. Povidone–iodine is effective against almost all bacteria, fungi, yeast and protozoa. Dakin's Solution or other chlorine compounds are similarly used.

In our experience, continuous irrigation of infected wounds is less satisfactory than is intermittent irrigation. Studies with pacemaker pockets have shown that within a day or two of continuous irrigation, a 'track of least resistance' exists from the point of entry to the point of exit and the entire pocket is not adequately irrigated. If the exit track is sealed and the space is distended with the antimicrobial solution for an hour or two, all areas of the pocket are irrigated. We have recognized this same principle in other spaces, as have others. Continuous irrigation is probably obsolete.

Echinococcal disease requires a unique topical therapy. Formaldehyde or 10% saline solution is injected into the cyst prior to its manipulation in order to sterilize the organisms in case of spillage during manipulation. Repeated irrigations of any areas of spillage with dilute povidone–iodine is indicated.

7. SPECIFIC INFECTIONS

7.1. Tuberculosis

When a diagnosis of tuberculosis is known prior to surgery, a period of preoperative antibiotic therapy is indicated. The maximum length of this therapy is usually determined by the clinical course of the disease and may be years; the minimum duration of therapy necessary to protect against surgical spread of the disease is not clear. Because of the slow rate of division of the organism and the fact that it frequently resides in relatively avascular areas, most surgeons believe that at least several days of antibiotics are desirable prior to surgery. In the case of long-term antituberculous therapy, the addition of a new effective drug at the time of major surgery is advisable. At the time of operation, the organism is studied again for antimicrobial sensitivities. When specimens, not known to be tubercular, removed at the operating table are positive on culture, or especially upon mandatory *stat.* acid-fast smears, antituberculous drugs should be instituted immediately. We believe that it is good practice to copiously irrigate any areas contaminated at surgery with normal saline and diluted povidone–iodine. At least two drugs should be given systemically and continued until sensitivity studies indicate a change. The primary drugs used are isoniazid, streptomycin, ethambutol, para-aminosalicylic acid, and rifampin. When the organism is resistant to these drugs, the surgical complication rate is more than tripled. Secondary drugs include cycloserine, ethionamide, viomycin, kanamycin, capreomycin and pyrazinamide. Tuberculous empyemas are frequently secondarily infected with bacteria so that other antibiotics are necessary, along with adequate surgical drainage. Following surgery for tuberculosis the incidence of bronchopleural fistula is 20–30%, more than following other pulmonary resections (about 7–10%). When the sputum is positive the incidence of bronchopleural fistula is considerably higher and still higher after pneumonectomy. These observations emphasize the wisdom of good antituberculous therapy prior to surgery, with one or more drugs added at operation. One is actively *treating* disease, not only giving prophylactic drugs.

7.2. Infections with *Actinomyces*

Infections with *Actinomyces bovis* and *A. Israellii* are characterized by dissection along fascial planes, multiple sinus tracts and draining 'sulfa granules', which point to the specific diagnosis. These pathological characteristics are associated with complications after surgical spread. High, prolonged penicillin therapy combined with sulfa drugs is indicated. When surgery is carried out, 20 million units per day of penicillin is given intravenously immediately before and for three months after surgery. Sulfadiazine, 4–8 g/day, or sulfisoxazole, 12 g/day, may be added for shorter perioperative periods. Infections with *Nocardia asteroides* are generally treated the same.

7.3. Chronic mediastinitis

Chronic mediastinitis may be produced by tuberculosis, histoplasmosis, actinomycosis, nocardiosis or blastomycosis. Since these are usually 'burned out' infections, antibiotic therapy is not routinely given. However, when surgery is necessary for obstructive complications or when large numbers of organisms are demonstrated on stain of tissue, consideration should be given to use of antifungal agents for several weeks after surgery. Culture-positive cases should be treated, hopefully to prevent obstruction of superior vena cava, pulmonary vessels and esophagus.

7.4. Fungal infections

Operations for fungal infections in the lung are not common. In many cases, the diagnosis is known and specific therapy has been given prior to operation. In other cases, the organism is recovered from or seen in a small granuloma (coin lesion) or in a very localized pulmonary area. In these cases, if there is good local resection and no spillage into tissues, specific chemotherapy or antibiotics are usually not indicated [1]. However, in the immunocompromised patient, such as transplant recipients or patients receiving chemotherapy, our practice has been to give treatment unless contraindicated by the patient's predisposition to toxicity.

In general, Amphotericin is effective against systemic histoplasmosis, blastomycosis, coccidioidomycosis, cryptococcus, and candida infections [9]. Nystatin is used primarily as a topical agent, while Amphotericin B is given intravenously. However, Amphotericin may produce severe toxic effects on kidneys, liver and bone marrow and frequently produces fever, chills, vomiting, headaches and hypocalemia. Flucytosine is relatively nontoxic but is primarily useful against *Candida* and *Cryptococcus neoformans*. Fluconazole is used for coccidioidomycosis and cryptococcosis. Ketoconazole is effective against blastomycosis and coccidioidomycosis. However, it is not valuable in controlling nervous system involvement due to poor penetration.

When histoplasma organisms are found by smear, do not grow, and there is no evidence of disease outside the granuloma, usually no treatment is given. However, we believe that a full course of Amphotericin B is desirable when there is infiltrative disease or cavity in the lung, organisms within the bone marrow, systemic spread, or organisms in mediastinal pus. Histoplasmosis may be complicated after surgery by new cavitary disease, acute and chronic empyema or bronchopleural fistula. Operative complications occur in about one-fourth of the cases and mortality is considerable. In such cases, Amphotericin B should be given for at least four to six weeks. It is preferable to give four weeks of therapy both before and after surgery in active infections. While this therapy may not have a major effect on the complication rate, it does seem to ameliorate late progression or recurrence. Itraconazole, a new oral drug, may prove equally effective with many fewer side-effects.

Blastomycotic granulomas require no therapy after removal unless there is evidence of lymph node, bone, prostate, skin or other distant involvement. In the fully immunosuppressed transplant recipient, we have given Amphotericin even with small granulomas when the organisms were seen in microscopic sections. Active disease is treated with a 'full' dose (2–4 g) of Amphotericin B (< 1.5 mg/kg/day). There is recent evidence that ketoconazole is the drug of choice for *Blastomycosis*. Two rather unique thoracic infections are aspergillosis and cryptococcosis. *Aspergillus* is a non-virulent organism in most patients but may exist as a saprophyte in a pre-existing space such as a tuberculous cavity or bulla. In such cases, while hemoptysis may be severe, there is no significant invasion of tissues and topical iodine therapy through an indwelling catheter may be effective. Surgical obliteration of the offending space may be required. It is rare for aspergillus to produce invasive pneumonitis or systemic spread requiring specific antibiotic treatment. Aspergillosis has a high incidence of recurrence months or years after surgery particularly in empyema, other residual or pleural space infections or in bullae. Amphotericin B is given systemically in such cases and the space can be irrigated with high concentrations of amphotericin B or iodines. If the pleural space or chest wall is contaminated at surgery, repeated topical irrigations with chlorine or povidone–iodine solutions may be carried out. *Cryptococcus* is frequently fatal when the central nervous system is infected; however, well-localized pulmonary lesions (not a typical coin lesion) may occur without central nervous system involvement. In such cases, our practice has been to widely resect the lesion (which is usually not diagnosed until surgery), monitor the patient carefully after surgery, and withhold antimicrobial therapy unless there are specific indications. Serological monitoring, with latex agglutination tests for capsular antigen [9] for two years should follow immediate perioperative examination of spinal fluid. When spinal fluid India-ink smear and/or repeated serological tests are positive, we believe amphotericin B, with or without flucytosine should be given for several months. Fluconazole may prove to be preferable.

8. DURATION OF ANTIMICROBIOLOGIC THERAPY

In general, therapeutic antimicrobials are given until there is no clinical, laboratory and radiographic evidence of infection. Three or more days without fever and with normal white blood cell and differential counts is desired. At times, the antibiotic itself may produce a low grade 'drug' fever [10]. Other evidence of infection is usually absent in such cases and antimicrobials may be stopped, leading to a normal temperature. Wounds should show no significant areas of cellulitis, undrained pus or fluid collections, and have a good blood supply. When there is rapid and near-complete clinical resolution of signs of infection, adequate drainage and debridement, and the organisms are highly sensitive to the antimicrobials, only 5–7 days of therapy are usually necessary. When there are abscesses, foreign bodies, necrotic tissue and/or infections with coagulase-positive staphylococcus, pseudomonas or proteus, one to three months of antimicrobials may be necessary. For slower-growing organisms such as *Nocardia*, actinomyces and fungi, several months (1–4) of antimicrobials are necessary. Tuberculosis usually requires six to twelve months or more of therapy. Repeated cultures and sensitivity studies are necessary for any bacterial infection which persists after about one week of antibiotic therapy.

When there is 'failure' of antimicrobial therapy, one must search for another organism which is resistant (emerging or superinfection) or a 'surgical' problem. Surgical problems which lead to failure to respond to antimicrobials include: inadequately drained fluid or space with poor antibiotic penetration, necrotic tissue, neoplasm, or foreign body. Obviously, when the response is less than desired, one must always re-evaluate the clinical, laboratory or radiographic status to be certain that there is not a missed diagnosis or onset of new disease. Host factors, such as diabetes, starvation, generalized sepsis, multi-organ failure, massive trauma, or other immunocompromised conditions must be evaluated and addressed.

REFERENCES

1 Sethi GK. In: Cordell, Ellison (eds.). Complications of Intra-thoracic Surgery. Boston, Little, Brown & Co 1979.
2 Alexander JW. In: Textbook of Surgery. Sabiston (ed.). Philadelphia, PA, WB Saunders 1986: pp 259–283.
3 Hunt TK, Jawetz E. Inflammation, infection and antibiotics. In: Current Surgical Diagnosis and Treatment, 8th Ed. Appleton & Lange 1988: pp 99–127.
4 Pingleton SK. The gut and infection. Pulmonary perspectives. Am Coll Chest Phys 1991; 8(1).
5 Klastersky J. Concept of empiric therapy with antibiotic combinations. Am J Med 1986; 80: 2.
6 Maunder R. Recognition and treatment of pneumonia in the intensive care patient. Surg ICU Infect Suppl 1990; November: 18–23.
7 Meduri GU. Ventilator-associated pneumonia in patients with respiratory failure: A diagnostic approach. Chest 1990; 97: 1208–1219.
8 Stringel G, Bawdon R, Savrich M, Guertin L, Horton J. Topical and systemic antibiotics in the prevention of wound infection. J Pediatr Surg 1989; 24: 1003.
9 Medoff G, Kobayashi GS. Systemic fungal infection: An overview. Hosp Prac 1991; Februari 2: 41–52.
10 Marino PL. The ICU Book. Philadelphia, PA, Lea & Febiger 1991.

Current Topics in General Thoracic Surgery: An International Series, Vol. 2
Perioperative Care, edited by R.M. Peters and J. Toledo

Chapter 21

Monitoring of spontaneous ventilation and ventilator support

Richard M. Peters

GLOSSARY

ABG	arterial blood gases
ARDS	acute respiratory distress syndrome
ARF	acute respiratory failure
CI	cardiac index
CO	cardiac output
CPAP	continuous positive airway pressure
D_{O_2}	oxygen delivery to tissues
FEV_1	forced expiratory volume in the first second
F_IO_2	fraction of inspired oxygen
FRC	functional residual capacity
IMV	intermittent mandatory ventilation
MMV	minute mandatory ventilation
O_2ER	oxygen extraction
P_aCO_2	partial pressure of carbon dioxide in arterial blood
P_ECO_2	partial pressure of carbon dioxide in mixed expired air
$P_{et}CO_2$	partial pressure of carbon dioxide in end-tidal air
$P_{(a-et)}CO_2$	partial pressure difference of carbon dioxide between arterial blood and end-tidal air
P_aO_2	partial pressure of oxygen in arterial blood
$P_{(A-a)}O_2$	partial pressure difference of oxygen between alveolar air and arterial blood
$P_{tc}O_2$	transcutaneous partial pressure of oxygen
PEEP	positive end expiratory pressure
P_IMax	maximum inspiratory pressure
P_EMax	maximum expiratory pressure
PS	pressure support ventilation
$\dot{Q}_S/\dot{Q}_{tot}$	intrapulmonary shunt fraction
RR	respiratory rate
S_aO_2	arterial oxygen saturation
$S_{\bar{v}}O_2$	venous oxygen saturation
T_I/T_E	ratio of inspiratory time to expiratory time
$\dot{V}_A/\dot{Q}$	ventilation perfusion ratio
VC	vital capacity
V_{min}	minute ventilation
$\dot{V}_{O_2}$	oxygen consumption
$\dot{V}_{O_2,resp}$	oxygen consumption for respiratory muscle work
V_D	dead space ventilation
V_{Ds}	serial dead space ventilation
V_{Dalv}	alveolar dead space ventilation
V_D/V_T	ratio of dead space to tidal ventilation
V_T	tidal volume
W_{resp}	work of breathing

1. INTRODUCTION

To affect outcome, monitors must capture information that has the potential to affect patient management and present it effectively for decision making. Monitors must be accurate, and the measurements should have high sensitivity, specificity and reproducibility. Presentation should assemble data in a format that enhances clinical decisions. Few monitors of ventilation meet these criteria. The monitoring of lung and ventilator function suffers from a common problem in modern medicine – the need to discriminate between what is possible to measure and what measurements provide useful information.

2. MONITORING OF ADEQUACY OF SPONTANEOUS VENTILATION

Providing ventilator support for patients is necessary only if the muscular effort required for them to breathe exceeds their capacity. The physician's job is, therefore, to monitor whether the patients have the energy stores and strength to continue to support their ventilation or whether fatigue is imminent. Clinical manifestations of impending ventilatory failure are anxious facies and speech limited to a few words between gasps for a breath. These clinical signs represent excessive effort to breathe. The most precise monitors of spontaneous ventilation would assess the work required to breathe and the maximum work capacity of the patient [1,2].

The amount of work for breathing is determined by the force that must be generated during inspiration by ventilatory muscles to stretch the lungs and the chest cage to overcome airways resistance and to meet the gas exchange needs of the patient. The force for expiration, except at vigorous exercise or severe airway obstruction, is provided by elastic recoil of stretched lungs and chest cage. To expand the chest cage requires force for stretching the elastic elements of the chest cage and also for lifting of the muscles and fat that surround the chest cage. The diaphragms must push down on the abdominal contents, lifting the abdominal viscera and any fat on the abdominal wall. The chest cage muscles must displace the muscles and fat attached to the chest cage. A heavily muscled or obese patient must do more work to breathe than an asthenic patient. Measurement of mechanical work done on the chest cage during spontaneous breathing is not feasible, but work done on the lungs can be measured by inserting a catheter with side holes covered by a latex balloon into the esophagus [3–6]. [a] The esophageal catheter permits measurement of pleural pressure. The sum of the products of gas flow times esophageal pressure over the inspiratory cycle is the work of inspiration, the active phase of ventilation that requires muscular work. If the output of electronic monitors connected to (1) the esophageal catheter that records swings

[a] If the patient requires a nasogastric tube, by using a commercial nasogastric triple lumen tube with one lumen leading to an attached esophageal balloon, no additional invasion of the patient is needed.

in pleural pressure and (2) a pneumotachograph to measure air flow at the mouth, are sampled and converted to digits in a computer, work on the lungs per minute or per breath can be calculated. Although facilities to measure work on the lungs are rarely available, an understanding of what causes work to inflate the lungs to increase gives insight into clinical appraisal of work of breathing.

While measurement of work of breathing on the lungs remains a clinical investigative tool, there are clinical measurements which can give useful insight into work requirements and work capacity. These measurements are not continuous and can be misleading. A patient may be capable of performing a test of strength, but this may not predict the ability to maintain the effort. Strength is easier to measure than endurance. Anything which makes the lungs stiffer, fall in lung compliance, will increase the degree of subatmospheric pleural pressure (the force) that must be generated by the muscles of ventilation for a given tidal volume. If the lungs are stiff, the patient will elect to limit the maximum increase in force required to stretch the lungs by taking shallow breaths. With shallow breathing, dead-space ventilation increases so the patient must increase the ventilatory rate to maintain minute ventilation. Tachypnea is one of the most reliable monitors of an excessive force requirement for ventilation. A rate above 25 usually cannot be maintained by an adult for more than a few hours, and above a rate of 30 most individuals will fail in a shorter time.

Lung volumes – tidal volume and vital capacity – can be accurately measured with hand-held instruments at the bedside. In an adult, a tidal volume of less than 300 ml (4–5 ml/kg; normal 6–8 ml/kg) is likely to predict ventilatory failure. Normal vital capacity is between 65–75 ml/kg and vital capacity above 10 ml/kg is needed for the patient to maintain spontaneous ventilation. Unfortunately, the measure of vital capacity is very dependent on patient cooperation and effort, a difficult criterion to meet in an acutely ill postsurgical patient.

3. CHEST X-RAY

An important monitor of pulmonary function which provides specific information about etiology and nature of the problem is the chest X-ray. Change in the lungs on chest X-ray may precede or follow physiologic changes. The chest X-ray is essential for differential diagnosis of the nature of the patient's problem – pneumothorax, hydrothorax, atelectasis, lung congestion, and/or consolidation.

4. MAXIMUM AIRWAY PRESSURES

Maximum airway pressures are measured with a manometer connected to the airway while the patient inspires or expires against an occluded airway. The maximum airway pressure the patient can generate permits estimation of ventilatory muscle strength and is useful, but has only fair correlation with

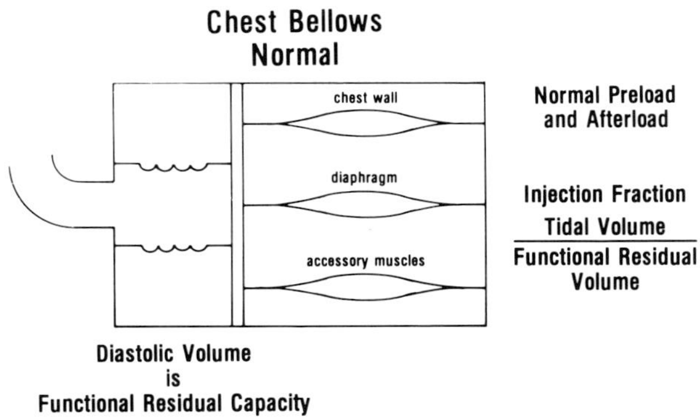

FIGURE 21.1A. The relationships among lung mechanics, functional residual capacity, and work of ventilation. The ventilatory pump is an injection pump; it pulls air into the lungs. Like the heart, it needs an adequate preload stretch of the muscle fibers, and contractility will be opposed by afterload. The functional residual volume is determined by the relative elastic recoil of the lungs and chest wall. The inspiratory muscles pull air into the lung. (From: Peters RM. The lung. In: Peters RM, Peacock Jr EE, Benfield JR (eds.). The Scientific Management of Surgical Patients. Boston, Little & Brown 1983.)

ventilatory muscle endurance. The lung volume at which the pressure measurement is made is important. At low lung volumes the inspiratory muscles are at optimum stretch (maximum preload) and so at maximum potential. Marini et al.[7] have proposed that even when patients cannot cooperate by using a one-way valve system which allows expiration but is occluded on the inspiratory limb for up to 20 seconds, the maximum inspiratory pressure (P_IMax) can be recorded. Normal values for P_IMax for men is $115 \pm 27\,cmH_2O$ and maximum expiratory pressure (P_EMax) $180 \pm 40\,cmH_2O$. Women have values approximately 25% lower. There is about 20% fall-off in P_IMax between 20 and 70 years of age. P_IMax of $30\,cmH_2O$ below atmospheric pressure has gained clinical creditability as the minimum for ventilator weaning. This criterion has both false negative and positive results when used alone as the criterion for weaning.

Vital capacity and maximum pressures give us a measure of the maximum force the patient can generate. They give no information about what effort is required to breathe. The habitus of patients provides some index of the effort needed to expand the chest cage. An obese or heavily muscled patient will have more weight to lift, particularly in the supine position where the weight of the abdomen pushes up on the diaphragm and weights down the chest. A patient with a hyperexpanded chest, as in chronic obstructive airways disease, has requirements for greater work on the chest cage because it is already stretched and so stiffer. In addition, the inspiratory muscles are less efficient because the high end-expiratory volume does not put the inspiratory muscles on stretch (they lack an adequate preload) (Figs. 21.1A–C)[8].

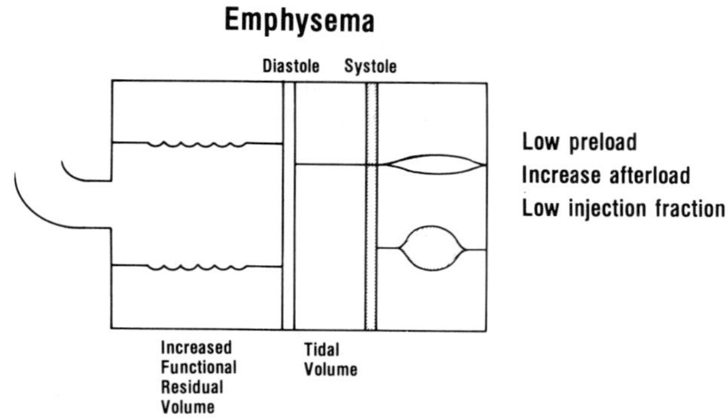

FIGURE 21.1B. With emphysema, muscles are not adequately stretched because of the increased functional residual volume. The preload is inadequate and afterload is up because a hyperexpanded chest is at poor mechanical advantage for further expansion. (From: Peters RM. The lung. In: Peters RM, Peacock Jr EE, Benfield JR (eds.). The Scientific Management of Surgical Patients. Boston, Little & Brown 1983.)

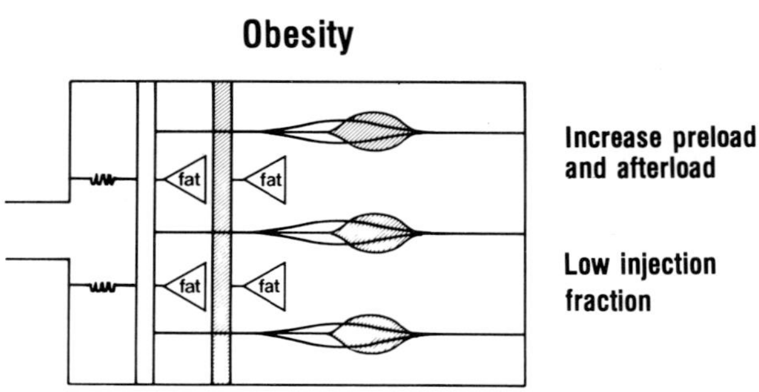

FIGURE 21.1C. Obese patients have a low functional residual capacity and an increased afterload from the weight of the fat. The work is increased for each liter of ventilation. (From: Peters RM. Identification, assessment and management of surgical patients with chronic respiratory disease. In: Greenfield LJ (ed.). Problems in General Surgery. Philadelphia, PA, JB Lippincott 1984; Vol 1, No 3, pp 432–444.)

5. LUNG COMPLIANCE

While chest cage abnormalities alone can lead to ventilatory failure, they are more often an aggravating factor that complicates deteriorations in lung mechanics. Atelectasis, pulmonary edema, and congestion all result in a fall in lung compliance (the lung becomes stiffer). Normal lung compliance is about 200 ml/cmH_2O. The compliance of the chest cage is the same, 200 ml/cmH_2O. Since these compliances are in series, the compliance of lungs and chest cage together is one-half that, 100 ml/cmH_2O.

Compliance of lung and chest cage combined can be measured only when a patient is on controlled ventilation. If the patient makes no effort to assist or oppose the ventilator, the force generated by the ventilator must stretch the lungs and chest cage and overcome airway resistance. During controlled ventilation the compliance is equal to tidal volume divided by the difference between no air flow end-expiratory pressure and plateau inspiratory pressure points. The normal range of lung and chest wall compliance measured in this manner is 60–100 ml/cmH_2O. Below a compliance level of 25 ml/cmH_2O patients can only rarely support spontaneous ventilation[9,10].

Stiff, low compliant lungs are the major cause of ventilatory failure. Lung compliance can be measured if an esophageal balloon is in place to measure pleural pressure. (Airway pressure minus pleural pressure equals transpulmonary pressure, the force stretching the lungs; tidal volume divided by the difference between end-inspiratory and end-expiratory pressure equals lung compliance.)

Lungs with edema, congestion or atelectasis are stiff and also have severe incoordination of ventilation and perfusion. There is perfusion of congested, unventilated portions of the lung. The resulting intrapulmonary shunt leads to fall in P_aO_2 and S_aO_2. The fall in P_aO_2 stimulates the respiratory center and causes the patient to hyperventilate. The combination of tachypnea and stiff lungs markedly elevates work of breathing and ventilatory muscle fatigue results. Some indication of the increase in subatmospheric pressure in the pleura during spontaneous ventilation of low compliance lungs may be seen by the wide respiratory swings superimposed on the vascular pressure if a CVP or Swan–Ganz catheter is in place. A more accurate estimate comes from esophageal balloon pressure measurements.

6. ARTERIAL BLOOD GASES – SPECIFIC DIAGNOSIS OF THE ADEQUACY OF GAS EXCHANGE

Blood gas values are best interpreted by evaluating the pH, first to ascertain whether it is below the normal range (7.38–7.42): acidosis, or above the normal range: alkalosis. The arterial partial pressure of carbon dioxide (P_aCO_2) should then be evaluated to appraise whether it is appropriate to the pH. If the pH is depressed and P_aCO_2 is elevated, the patient is hypoventilating. The clinical examination and chest X-ray are indicated to look for a correctable reason, such as central depression, pneumothorax, pain and splinting, or atelectasis. If pH is low due to low bicarbonate, metabolic acidosis, P_aCO_2 should also be below normal, signifying some attempt to compensate for the metabolic acidosis. If no compensation has occurred, the patient has serious ventilatory compromise as well as metabolic acidosis and a search for the cause for ventilatory insufficiency must be initiated.

Evaluation of P_aO_2 is more complex. If P_aCO_2 is normal or low, a low P_aO_2 is due to ventilation–perfusion incoordination, an intrapulmonary shunt due to lobar or micro-atelectasis or regional underventilation. In a patient with an intrapulmonary shunt, increasing the fraction of inspired oxygen (F_IO_2) has little effect on P_aO_2 because the oxygen does not reach collapsed or flooded alveoli.

A low P_aO_2 also can result, particularly in patients with advanced chronic obstructive lung disease, from hypoventilation of families of alveoli. Low P_aO_2 due to alveolar hypoventilation can be corrected by increasing F_IO_2, but F_IO_2 should be raised to no more than 0.65–0.70. In chronic obstructive lung disease patients, hypoventilation can be aggravated by raising F_IO_2. Increasing F_IO_2 for a patient with chronic obstructive lung disease removes the necessary extra ventilatory drive provided by hypoxaemia to generate the work to ventilate their inefficient lungs. F_IO_2 must be adjusted to minimize hypoxaemia without increasing P_aCO_2.

Blood gases are at best intermittent monitors which are invasive and have built-in time delay. To date, attempts to continuously monitor arterial pH, P_aCO_2, and P_aO_2 are experimental. Available intra-arterial, subcutaneous and surface monitors of P_aCO_2 and P_aO_2 are unreliable and often inaccurate. Transcutaneous continuous monitoring of arterial oxygen saturation (S_aO_2) and pulmonary artery monitoring of mixed venous oxygen saturation (S_vO_2) have reached levels of clinical usefulness.

In the last few years pulse oximeters have provided us with a good noninvasive, continuous monitor of oxygen saturation in patients with intact circulation. These monitors have alarms for low oxygen and disappearance of digital pulse. They are a significant addition to our monitoring capability. If the pulse oximeter measures a drop in oxygen saturation below 90%, supplemental oxygen is usually indicated. Pulse oximeters are also useful during exercise testing of patients and provide indications of the patient's need for supplemental oxygen during the postoperative recovery. If with only moderate levels of exercise oxygen saturation falls below 85–90%, supplemental oxygen is indicated.

The new generation of computerized ventilators has frightened off many physicians and the 'trade union' of respiratory therapists and the ICU physicians have tried to limit privileges to manage ventilators. In fact, these new ventilators are characterized more by their increase in cost than by significant enhancement of the fundamental requirements for ventilator support. The physician responsible for the care of a patient on a ventilator must understand the generic requirements which are applicable to setting up all ventilators. This knowledge should allow them to set up most ventilators regardless of how complex the manufacturers try to make them. There is considerable controversy about which parameters are needed to monitor ventilators and the patients they are ventilating. The process of placing a patient on a ventilator requires setting the controls of ventilator function and the alarm levels for monitors of these functions. A useful way to evaluate parameters needed for monitoring ventilated patients is to review the steps needed to place a patient on a ventilator.

7. VENTILATOR MANAGEMENT

7.1. Tidal volume and rate

The obvious first functions to be set are tidal volume and rate. Tidal volume is set 12–15 cc/kg (a level greater than the usual resting tidal volume of 8–10 cc/kg). The extra volume enhances expansion of dependent area of lung and holds functional residual volume (end-expiratory lung volume) at more normal levels. In a patient on controlled ventilation, to compensate for the increased tidal volume the rate is set at slightly lower than the normal resting spontaneous rate, 10–14.

7.2. Expired tidal volume

There must be a monitor of both rate and expiratory tidal volume. The important question is not how much air the ventilator moved but how much got into the patient. A true excess of inspired over expired tidal volume of any amount over a long time would result in lung hyperexpansion. Water vapor added to inspired air makes expired volume exceed inspired volume by 10% despite a usual respiratory quotient of 0.8 (volume CO_2 produced/volume oxygen consumed); more oxygen is removed from inspired air than carbon dioxide added to expired air. The variations in respiratory quotient and amount of added water vapor in the lungs make monitoring difference between inspired and expired volume useless as a means of controlling total lung volume. The error of measuring methods is too great to use anything but gross differences as clinical monitors. Other methods to avoid hyperexpansion must be used. If expired tidal volume is 10% less than inspired volume, a leak in the system during inspiration is the likely cause. The leak in the system can be around the endotracheal cuff or at any of the tubing connections.

7.3. Peak airway pressure

Lung hyperexpansion is monitored in a simple and effective manner by measuring peak airway pressure, an important information-rich measurement that is seriously underutilized. All safe ventilators have an interrupt system to stop inspiration and alarm when inspired pressure exceeds the preset limit. When the patient is placed on the ventilator, a peak pressure limit of 30 is usually set. If this does not generate an alarm at the chosen tidal volume, this setting is appropriate. If the setting of 30 does generate an alarm at the chosen tidal volume, a check to be certain that there is no obstruction to inspiration or expiration is necessary. The most common reason for patients exceeding the pressure limit is fighting the ventilator or coughing. The patient's muscular effort is opposing the ventilator. Such patients will produce frequent alarms. The response must be to determine the cause of the patient's restlessness.

A complete or partial obstruction of expiration which over the course of a few breaths results in expiration of less air than is pumped into the patient can cause excessive, dangerous peak airway pressure. The obstruction may be at any level of the patient's and the ventilator airways. There is no easy monitor to localize the point of obstruction. Disconnecting the patient from the ventilator determines whether the problem is with the patient or the ventilator. If disconnecting the patient from the ventilator corrects the hyperexpansion, then the problem is ventilator malfunction, most likely a stuck expiratory valve. If after disconnection the patient remains hyperexpanded, the most likely cause is obstruction of the artificial airway by kinking, insertion too far down the airway, or having a mucus plug acting as a ball valve. In these circumstances, the airway cuff must be deflated and, if this maneuver does not work, the tube must be removed and replaced. This type of airway obstruction is one of the most urgent airway emergencies.

An increase in peak airway pressure is also an important indicator of pneumothorax. The chest cage is hyperexpanded by air trapped in the pleural space, the lung is compressed by the pneumothorax. The pressure to force in the preset tidal volume will be excessive (see below).

7.4. Low airway pressure

An alarm is set if during inspiration the airway pressure does not reach a preset limit. This functions as a disconnect alarm. The impedance of lung and chest cage is removed so no pressure is generated. The problem may be partial disconnect of a connector tubing site, airway out of the trachea, or balloon deflated. This is an urgent emergency; the patient is not being ventilated.

7.5. Inspiratory time/expiratory time

A ventilator pumps air into the patient, but the elastic recoil of the stretched lungs and chest cage must push the air out. The amount of force needed to push the air out depends on both the tidal volume and the duration of expiration. The shorter the expiratory time, the greater the force required. The ratio of inspiratory time to expiratory time is an important parameter to set. In a patient with chronic obstructive lung disease (COLD), the expiratory time would be long, with an I:E ratio of 1:2 or 1:3. In a patient with stiff lungs, inspiratory time can be prolonged because the greater recoil force of the lungs is more than adequate for expiration. In the discussion of the interpretation of airway pressure, I shall present how the reader can interpret airway pressure pattern to evaluate the appropriateness of I:E setting.

7.6. Modes of ventilation support

The next setting is mode of ventilation. There are a number of available methods or modes of programming ventilators. The physician makes an often arbitrary decision based on his prejudices and evaluation of the patient about which mode to use.

7.6.1. Controlled ventilation (CMV)

In controlled ventilation, the ventilator rate and volume are set to provide complete ventilator support of ventilation. To put a patient on controlled ventilation requires a ventilator rate, tidal volume, and P_aO_2 set at a level to lower P_aCO_2 to 32–35 mmHg and keep P_aO_2 above 65. Patients will often also need narcotics to suppress the respiratory center. Patients with extremely stiff lungs or CNS dysfunction or a large shunt with low P_aO_2 may need to receive a muscle relaxant. These patients should receive drugs to suppress all knowledge of the paralysis.

7.6.2. Intermittent mandatory ventilation (IMV)

In the intermittent mandatory ventilation (IMV) mode, the ventilator supplies a set number of breaths per minute. The ventilator has a supplemental gas source so the patient can inspire between ventilator breaths while the ventilator bellows is being refilled.

For centrally depressed postoperative patients, intermittent mandatory ventilation can provide complete support by setting the rate or tidal volume high. As the patient recovers from anesthesia, this rate can be lowered as the patient begins to take spontaneous breaths between the ventilator breaths. With each lowering of rate and tidal volume, the increment in spontaneous rate and tidal volume and blood gases should be measured. If spontaneous tidal volume falls and/or rate goes above 20–25, the patient usually will not tolerate lowering of IMV rate. A rise in P_aCO_2 of 5 mmHg also usually requires increase in rate and/or tidal volume.

7.6.3. Assist and assist–control

In *assisted ventilation* the ventilator has a sensor of pressure in the airway. When pressure in the airway drops below a preset level (usually 2.0 cmH_2O) below atmospheric or PEEP level, the inspiratory cycle of the ventilator is triggered and the preset volume pumped into the patient. The interpretation of the significance of the pattern of airway pressure and work in this mode will be discussed below.

The *assist–control* mode is the same as the assist mode with the added function that if the patient does not activate the ventilator within a given period of time, the ventilator will be automatically activated to maintain the preset rate.

Assist control or assisted ventilation and pressure support are popular methods of ventilator support. The rationale is that the patient is setting his own rate. This author sees two problems with this mode of ventilation: (1) If lungs are stiff, the effort required of the patient to turn on the ventilator (create a $-2 cmH_2O$ airway pressure) can be excessive [11]. (We have recorded intrapleural pressures of $-20 cmH_2O$ for patients with stiff lungs to create $-2 cmH_2O$ airway pressure. [12]) (2) The patient gets a fixed volume for all breaths no matter how high the rate. This can lead to excessive airway pressures and hyperexpansion of the lungs due to limitation of expiratory time.

7.6.4. Pressure support

In the pressure support mode, inspiration is activated by the patient as in the assist modes, and inspiratory flow and volume are limited to those achieved by a preset airway pressure and stopped when inspiratory flow falls to a preset level. Pressure support is in essence a reversion to old, discarded pressure-controlled ventilators. With modern computerized ventilators, some gimmicks have been added. The inspiratory cycle is stopped when flow falls to a certain level, not only when peak pressure is reached as in pure pressure-controlled ventilation. In pressure modes of ventilation, the mechanics of lung and chest cage control tidal volume and patient effort, the rate [13]. If lung and chest wall mechanics are near normal and the patient responsive, i.e., the patient is ready to begin the weaning process, pressure support will work and so will most systems.

7.6.5. Inverse ratio ventilation

Inverse ratio ventilation is the newest fad. In most patients, expiratory time needs to be two to three times inspiratory time to assure expulsion of all air pumped in. In patients with pulmonary edema and stiff lungs, elastic recoil is excessive and air is very quickly forced out by the excessive recoil force of the lung. To improve gas distribution and lower airway peak pressure, inspiratory time is set to exceed expiratory time. There is a slow inspiration that is held and the expiratory cycle is brief. This is a logical matching of the ventilator to the impedance of the lungs. It is applying a basic principle of mechanics. Unfortunately, a new term is devised rather than adding this logic to settings of I:E ratio.

8. UNIVERSALLY REQUIRED MONITORS

(1) **Peak inspiratory pressure:** to monitor changes in peak pressure and shut off the ventilator if peak pressure limit is reached during inspiratory cycle. The purpose is to prevent hyperexpansion of lungs due to failure to completely expel previous breaths due to expiratory airway obstruction; to prevent excessive pleural pressure from pneumothorax or hyperexpanded lungs which would decrease venous return and lower cardiac output; to warn of possibility of pneumothorax or inspiratory airway obstruction. *This is a very information-rich monitor.*

(2) **Expired tidal volume:** to assess for leaks or other causes of failure to deliver set tidal volume.

(3) **Low pressure limit:** the minimal airway pressure that must be reached during the inspiratory cycle of the ventilator. This is a disconnect alarm and/or ventilator malfunction alarm. There is no impedance to the ventilator forcing air out of its gas volume.

(4) **F_IO_2 level:** to assure that F_IO_2 remains at preset level.

(5) **End-tidal CO_2:** Some clinicians propose use of an end-tidal CO_2 measurement, using end-tidal CO_2 as an indicator of arterial P_aCO_2 and thus end-tidal CO_2 becomes a measure of adequacy of alveolar ventilation. In sick patients

who need ventilator support, there is usually a significant end-tidal arterial CO_2 difference. The ventilation–perfusion abnormality results in hyperventilation of some alveoli and inadequate to absent ventilation of others. The arterial end-tidal CO_2 difference will vary as the amount of lung dysfunction varies. These monitors are expensive, hard to maintain, and have not proved effective. They cannot differentiate the relative role of alveolar-arterial CO_2 difference and change in P_aCO_2 in altering end-tidal CO_2. A rise in alveolar-arterial CO_2 difference may hide a significant rise in arterial P_aCO_2.

(6) **Pulse oximeter:** this new monitor is a reliable monitor of oxygen saturation in patients with adequate circulation. It is not reliable in patients with hemodynamic compromise. If blood is not being delivered to the finger, the oximeter cannot function. The oximeter, therefore, monitors pulse as well as oxygen saturation. If pulse diminishes, an error signal is displayed. The use of this monitor has improved the safety of patients with compromised gas exchange system. Monitoring oxygenation is useful in making the decision to institute ventilator care, the oxygenation of patients on ventilator, oxygenation with postoperative activity, and in deciding the need for supplemental oxygen during late recovery. Oxygen saturation is less sensitive than PO_2 to clinically marginal shunts or regional alveolar hypoventilation, but the pulse oximeter is an adequate monitor of the level of oxygen in the blood. If cardiac output falls, pulse volume falls and the instruments usually give a no-reading signal. The users often assume the problem is sensor dysfunction. If the signal fails, it is essential to check pulses and blood pressure as well as position of the sensor; if the blood pressure is adequate and peripheral pulses present, sensor dysfunction is the likely problem. If blood pressure is low and/or peripheral pulses weak, perfusion is the problem.

REFERENCES

1 Peters RM. The energy cost (work) of breathing. Ann Thorac Surg 1969; 7: 51.
2 Fiastro JF, Habib MP, Shon BY, Campbell SC. Comparison of standard weaning parameters and the mechanical work of breathing in mechanically ventilated patients. Chest 1988; 94: 232.
3 Hilberman M, Stacy RW, Peters RM. A phase method of calculating respiratory mechanics using a digital computer. J Appl Physiol 1972; 32: 535.
4 Peters RM. Work of breathing and abnormal mechanics. Surg Clin North Am 1974; 54: 955.
5 Peters RM. Routine respiratory care and support. In: JD Hardy (ed.). Textbook of Surgery. Philadelphia, PA, Lippincott 1983: ch 6.
6 Peters RM, Knight MK, Brimm JE, et al. A personal computer system for testing gas exchange, heart, lungs, ventilatory pump. Int J Clin Monitoring Comput 1985; 2: 101.
7 Marini JJ, Smith TC, Lamb VJ. External work output and force generation during synchronized intermittent mechanical ventilation. Effect of machine assistance on breathing effort. Am Rev Respir Dis 1988; 138: 1169.
8 Roussos C, Macklem PT. The respiratory muscles. N Engl J Med 1982; 307: 786.
9 Peters RM, Brimm JE, Utley JR. Predicting the need for prolonged ventilatory support in adult cardiac patients. J Thorac Cardiovasc Surg 1979; 77: 175.
10 Peters RM. Pulmonary physiologic studies of the perioperative period. Chest 1979; 76: 576.

11 Marini JJ, Rodriguez RM, Lamb V. The inspiratory workload of patient-initiated mechanical ventilation. Am Rev Respir Dis 1986; 134: 902.
12 Boom MJ, Lutz P, Hogan JS, Peters RM. An automated method of separating patient from ventilator work on the lungs. Int J Clin Monitoring Comput 1988; 5: 235.
13 Black JW, Grover BS. A hazard of pressure support ventilation. Chest 1988; 93: 333.

Current Topics in General Thoracic Surgery: An International Series, Vol. 2
Perioperative Care, edited by R.M. Peters and J. Toledo

Lung and ventilation monitoring

Discussion of "Monitoring of spontaneous ventilation and ventilator support" by Richard M. Peters

C. Chopin and M. Ribet

1. INTRODUCTION

One event that both surgeons and anesthesiologists fear the most is certainly perioperative acute respiratory failure (ARF). During the last ten years, progress in surgical techniques, anesthesia, and intensive care have permitted an aggressive treatment of critically ill patients who undergo surgery with impaired pulmonary function or of patients whose function is impaired by surgery and who are consequently at risk of an ARF or of a dramatic increase of respiratory dysfunction.

Management of these perioperative conditions depends on the mechanisms thought to be likely responsible for them. These mechanisms can be divided into two groups: ventilatory pump failure and acute gas exchange deterioration.

2. DIAGNOSIS OF ARF MECHANISMS

2.1. Ventilatory pump failure

Ventilatory pump failure, as the unique cause of ARF in previously normal lung patients, is sometimes difficult to assess, and the diagnosis may be overlooked in purely clinical examination. Minute ventilation (V_{min}) is low, depending on the cause of the hypoventilation, and dyspnea is not always evident. Anaesthetic and narcotic drugs are responsible for depression of the respiratory center, and the neuromuscular junction is affected by neuro-muscular blocking agents.

Such a drug-induced hypoventilation is frequently observed during postoperative hours. But cardiac, renal and hepatic failure, obesity and starvation may cause this effect to be prolonged, and may prevent the return of ventilation to an adequate level for more than 12 hours [1].

In the absence of underlying pulmonary disease, respiratory muscle fatigue is usually not involved in acute postoperative ventilatory pump failure. But it must be emphasized that some acute metabolic disorders have deleterious effects on diaphragmatic contractility, such as hypophosphatemia, hypokalemia [2], hypomagnesemia [3], metabolic acidosis [4] and acute hypercapnia [5].

Patients with acute ventilatory pump failure do not present any clinical sign of ARF but show an increased respiratory rate (RR). The diagnosis is clearly confirmed by the arterial blood gas (ABG) pattern. Observed increases in P_aCO_2 and decreases in arterial partial pressure of oxygen (P_aO_2) correspond to the theoretical changes resulting from pure hypoventilation [6]. But it must be kept in mind that ABGs remain at relatively normal levels unless a deep depression of the alveolar ventilation occurs. Analysis of the physiological relationships between P_aO_2, P_aCO_2 and alveolar ventilation shows that P_aCO_2 increases and P_aO_2 decreases dramatically just as $\dot{V}_{min}$ falls below 3.5 l/min [7]. Clearly, these patients require careful monitoring of their spontaneous ventilation: continuous monitoring of hemoglobin saturation is the most useful technique.

2.2. Acute gas exchange deterioration

Acute gas exchange deterioration is most often encountered in patients with pre-existing pulmonary abnormalities, but also in previously normal lung patients. This deterioration primarily concerns alveolar to arterial oxygen difference $P_{(A-a)}O_2$ and the most likely explanation is ventilation–perfusion ($\dot{V}_A/\dot{Q}$) disparities. But a decrease in mixed venous oxygen saturation ($S_{\bar{v}}O_2$) and an increase in oxygen consumption ($\dot{V}_{O_2}$) are possible additional mechanisms. $\dot{V}_A/\dot{Q}$ abnormalities are primarily due to decrease in functional residual capacity (FRC). Tracheal intubation, supine position and respiratory muscle relaxation decrease FRC by about 30% [8] and even more in obese patients [9]. A prolonged supine position induces development of dependent-lung atelectasis [10]. Pneumothorax, pleural effusion and abdominal or peritoneal causes contribute to these phenomena and their diagnosis is not always easy, even with the help of standard chest and abdominal films. CT scans can help. Sedation and muscular relaxation decrease the diaphragmatic and inter-costal muscular tone and reduce the thoracic volume. Infection, pulmonary congestion and edema, pneumonia, pulmonary emboli worsen the $\dot{V}_A/\dot{Q}$ abnormalities. In the presence of $\dot{V}_A/\dot{Q}$, part of the blood flows through scattered underventilated alveoli, causing a venous contamination of arterial blood. A low $S_{\bar{v}}O_2$ increases the consequences of $\dot{V}_A/\dot{Q}$ and decreases the resulting P_aO_2 further.

To compensate for $\dot{V}_A/\dot{Q}$ scattering, the patient should increase the depth and rate of breathing, but he may be no longer able to do that, because of pain and increase of his respiratory work (W_{resp}). W_{resp} is determined by the force the patient must generate to inspire (W_{insp}) and expire (W_{exp}) per liter of gas. W_{resp} increases dramatically when FRC and compliance decrease. Increase of W_{resp} increases $\dot{V}_{O_2}$ by raising the respiratory cost of breathing which in turn is responsible for further decrease of $S_{\bar{v}}O_2$ and arterial oxygen saturation (S_aO_2). When muscular fatigue appears, a ventilatory pump failure occurs and adds its effects, resulting in an acute deterioration of gas exchange.

So, in most of the operated patients, postoperative ARF is the outcome of both ventilatory pump failure and acute gas exchange deterioration. Yet, the problem is how to evaluate the relative importance of each of these mechanisms, since the care and weaning strategy will depend on that differentiation.

3. RESPIRATORY MONITORING

Non-invasive respiratory monitoring techniques are now available and offer the possibility to assess respiratory function during both spontaneous and controlled ventilation.

The methods of monitoring can be divided into three groups: first are the methods specially designed to indirectly assess ABG, then those which evaluate respiratory function, and last those which monitor tissue oxygen delivery.

3.1. Assessment of ABG

3.1.1. Pulse oximeter

Cyanosis is the main sign of hypoxemia, but it is not consistently detected by clinical examination until hemoglobin saturation is lower than 75%. It may be altered by anemia. Pulse oximetry allows accurate assessment of S_aO_2, over a range of 70 to 95% [11,12]. A low blood pressure and a bad peripheral arterial pulse are usual causes of dysfunction. The lowest limit of acceptable pulse oximeter S_aO_2 is clearly 90%, corresponding to P_aO_2 at 60 mmHg. Leftward shift in the hemoglobin–oxygen dissociation curve, due to alkalosis or excessive blood transfusions, results in a lower P_aO_2 for a given S_aO_2. In practice, the pulse oximeter is clearly the most useful device in the operative theater and postoperative ward. Patients with pulse oximeter S_aO_2 below 90% despite adequate oxygen supply and continuous positive airway pressure (CPAP) need mechanical ventilation without delay or are unable to be weaned.

3.1.2. Transcutaneous oximetry

The transcutaneous oxygen sensor measures, with a modified Clark electrode, oxygen diffusion through the heated skin ($P_{tc}O_2$). $P_{tc}O_2$ is well correlated with P_aO_2 in patients without circulatory failure. But when cardiac output falls, $P_{tc}O_2$ no longer correlates with P_aO_2. $P_{tc}O_2$ depends not only on P_aO_2, but also during shock and acute cardiac failure on cardiac output and oxygen delivery to peripheral tissues [13,14]. Interpretation of $P_{tc}O_2$ changes are then difficult and few studies have reported the interest of this monitoring method in adults.

Neither pulse oximeter nor transcutaneous oximetry are able to accurately assess the need for respiratory support. In well oxygenated patients, P_aCO_2 may rise dramatically, owing to subsequent depression of the respiratory center.

Although its value is not admitted by all, capnography appears to us to be a very useful complementary technique.

3.1.3. Capnography

For a long time infra-red capnographers have been available in anesthesia and critical care. They provide useful monitors, sometimes incorporated in electrical ventilators or in bedside monitors. The reason why capnography is largely used in Europe and systematically debated in USA remains unclear. Most investigators [15] surprisingly argue that there is a difference between P_aCO_2 and end-tidal partial pressure of CO_2 ($P_{et}CO_2$), that this difference $P_{(a-et)}CO_2$ varies with the respiratory status and consequently that capnography must be rejected as a reliable monitoring method. The $P_{(a-et)}CO_2$ difference is due to $\dot{V}_A/\dot{Q}$ abnormalities. $P_{(a-et)}CO_2$ can be considered as constant as long as a respiratory and/or cardiac complication does not occur. A constant $P_{et}CO_2$ implies a constant P_aCO_2 but for the unlikely condition where P_aCO_2 and $P_{(a-et)}CO_2$ would change exactly the same amount but in opposite directions. It is true that an observed variation of $P_{et}CO_2$ does not allow prediction of a variation of P_aCO_2 but, on the other hand, a constant $P_{et}CO_2$ indicates that respiratory function, hemodynamics and energetic status are quite stable [16]. In addition, the equation $P_{et}CO_2 < P_aCO_2$ is always true and a $P_{et}CO_2$ higher than 40 mmHg implies a trend towards hypercapnia. Capnography allows detection, determination or calculation of the respiratory rate and breathing pattern, respiratory arrhythmia and pauses [17,18], mechanical conflict between patient and ventilatory support, $\dot{V}_A/\dot{Q}$ scattering by studying the slope of the alveolar plateau [19], the ratio of dead space to tidal ventilation (V_D/V_T), the diagnosis of pulmonary embolism [19], the risk of cardiac arrest and the efficacy of cardiac pulmonary resuscitation [20], the settings of ventilator and PEEP selection in mechanically ventilated patients [21]. Capnography may be included in a computerized bedside monitoring system and, in the near future, in the closed loop of a servo-regulated ventilator as the main controlled variable [22]. In summary, few monitoring techniques provide as many useful guidelines for the management of patients in the perioperative period, but it is clear that the interpretation of $P_{et}CO_2$ variations needs further investigation to be fully understood.

3.2. Assessment of respiratory function

In evaluating the need for mechanical support and the patient's ability to be weaned, the assessment of the functional and mechanical qualities of the lung is essential. Measurements of pulmonary function include mechanics and gas exchange.

3.2.1. Gas exchange

Dead space is defined as the part of the respiratory tract that does not contribute to exchange with blood. Physiologic dead space (V_D) includes serial (V_{Ds}) or anatomic dead space and alveolar dead space (V_{Dalv}). V_{Dalv} corresponds to alveoli that are ventilated and either hypoperfused or non-perfused. A widely accepted criterion for weaning is a V_D/V_T ratio < 0.6 [23]. The V_D/V_T ratio is calculated by the following formula:

$$\frac{V_D}{V_T} = \frac{P_aCO_2 - P_ECO_2}{P_aCO_2},$$

where P_ECO_2 is the mean expired partial pressure of CO_2. P_ECO_2 is measured by an infrared capnograph sampling a Douglas bag or in a mixing box. It is simpler to assess dead space effect from the V_{min} necessary to obtain $P_aCO_2 = 40$ mmHg. The value of V_{min}, corresponding to P_aCO_2 40 mmHg, less than 180 ml/kg/min, has the same significance as a V_D/V_T ratio < 0.6 [23].

Venous admixture ($\dot{Q}_S/\dot{Q}_{tot}$) is responsible for arterial hypoxemia and is defined as the part of the pulmonary blood flow that does not contribute to exchange with alveolar gas; $\dot{Q}_S/\dot{Q}_{tot}$ is generally assessed by calculating the ratio $(C_{c'} - C_a)/(C_{c'} - C_v)$, where $C_{c'}$, C_a, and C_v refer to the O_2 content of end-capillary, arterial, and mixed venous blood. A $\dot{Q}_S/\dot{Q}_{tot} < 20\%$ is a good weaning criterion but it requires a pulmonary arterial Swan–Ganz catheter to sample mixed venous blood and ventilation with pure O_2. Simpler to obtain is the ratio P_aO_2/F_IO_2 (fraction of inspired oxygen) which, when greater than 200 mmHg, has the same significance [23].

Although difficult to measure, $\dot{V}_{O_2}$ will be in the near future a cornerstone of perioperative monitoring. It is now established that $\dot{V}_{O_2}$ must be measured directly by a gas exchange method and that $\dot{V}_{O_2} = \dot{Q}_{tot} \times C_a - C_v$ underestimated the real value of $\dot{V}_{O_2}$ [24] in septic patients. The recent development of a portable system (Deltatrac Datex Finland) facilitates the bedside monitoring of $\dot{V}_{O_2}$.

3.2.2. Mechanics

As gas exchange deteriorates and metabolic demands increase, the patient's ability to sustain an adequate high level of ventilation depends on his ability to generate an adequate muscular force. Among weaning criteria, W_{resp} and muscular fatigue are certainly the most useful. W_{resp} can be directly assessed by calculating the area under the volume/pressure curve. This method requires an esophageal balloon, careful measurements of the tidal volume and a complex electronic system for integration and calculation. It is not very easy to use in a clinical situation. W_{resp} may be determined by the oxygen cost of breathing, corresponding to the difference between $\dot{V}_{O_2}$ during mechanical ventilation compared with $\dot{V}_{O_2}$ during spontaneous ventilation ($\dot{V}_{O_2,resp}$). $\dot{V}_{O_2,resp}$ has been shown to be a reliable indicator of probable weaning success and extubation in a patient recovering from ARF. Normal values for control subjects are less than 4% of whole body $\dot{V}_{O_2}$. $\dot{V}_{O_2,resp}$ can increase at an average of 25% of $\dot{V}_{O_2}$ in patients who are unable to be weaned successfully[25]. $\dot{V}_{O_2}$ measurements might take a place as a monitoring tool during the postoperative period.

$\dot{V}_{O_2}$ is also the main parameter in assessing tissue oxygenation.

3.3. Assessment of tissue oxygenation

3.3.1. Measurement of S_vO_2

Recently introduced as a monitoring technique in critical care, continuous measurement of S_vO_2 has been demonstrated to be of some clinical interest but remains questionable. This invasive method is based on the measurement of reflected light of selected wavelengths, which depends on the color of the blood and therefore on the hemoglobin oxygen saturation. A catheter is inserted in the same way as a flow-directed pulmonary Swan–Ganz catheter and also provides pressure monitoring and thermodilution cardiac output (CO) measurements.

But S_vO_2 depends on several physiological variables such as CO, S_aO_2, oxygen extraction ratio (O_2ER) and $\dot{V}_{O_2}$. As CO decreases, S_vO_2 decreases since O_2ER increases.

However, previous studies failed to demonstrate a consistently good relationship between S_vO_2 and CO[26]. S_vO_2 reflects O_2ER and a value higher than 60% likely indicates good circulatory status and tissue oxygenation, except in sepsis and ARDS patients. Indeed, in sepsis and ARDS it has been demonstrated that oxygen utilization by the peripheral tissues is supply dependent: endotoxins could induce a limitation of oxygen extraction by the cells[27,28]. Therefore the value of S_vO_2 in these patients as an indicator of tissue oxygenation is questionable.

3.3.2. Oxygen supply dependence

Adequate oxygen supply to the tissues is the end point of all care plans in critically ill patients, including postoperative ones. Adequacy of oxygen supply can be assessed by calculating the systemic oxygen transport $\dot{D}_{O_2} = \dot{Q}_{tot}(C_a - C_{\bar{v}})$.

A level of 330 ml min^{-1} m^{-2} is generally admitted as the physiological critical level[29] (anaerobic threshold, $\dot{D}_{O_2,crit}$) in anesthetized man. Nevertheless some authors hypothesized that $\dot{D}_{O_2} > \dot{D}_{O_2,crit}$ might be very insufficient for increased metabolic needs. It has been demonstrated[30] that intra-operatively $\dot{D}_{O_2}$ and $\dot{V}_{O_2}$ fell in all the patients, and that by contrast $\dot{D}_{O_2}$ and $\dot{V}_{O_2}$ increased steadily during the first 12 postoperative hours in survivors and did not significantly change in patients who died. Increases of $\dot{D}_{O_2}$ and $\dot{V}_{O_2}$ are interpreted as a compensatory stress response. Non-survivors fail to achieve the magnitude of the survivors' responses. As a consequence high-risk postoperative patients' therapeutic goals could be defined as: CI 50% greater than normal, $\dot{D}_{O_2}$ over 600 ml min^{-1} m^{-2} and $\dot{V}_{O_2}$ 30% greater than normal[30]. If this hypothesis is substantiated by further cooperative studies, then the need for high-level monitoring systems in postoperative wards will be demonstrated.

4. CARE STRATEGY FOR ARF IN POSTOPERATIVE PATIENTS

The FRC of the operated patient is reduced along with his muscular tone. There is a decrease in the thoracic compliance and a lowering of the ventilatory rest level. The diaphragmatic cephalad displacement is a factor contributing to atelectasis and there is an increase in airway resistance. $C_{(A-a)}O_2$ rises, due to shunts secondary to the reduction of muscular tone supporting the lung. Perfusion modifications are added to ventilation disturbances.

Postoperative hypoxemia should not last longer than 24 hours. After that period, bad oxygenation is due to a preoperative poor respiratory status, to the operation itself or to a complication. Although they concern a minority of cases, acute respiratory failure and gas exchange deterioration are important to diagnose and treat. The preoperative status of the patient and/or the nature of the operation help to predict some of the postoperative difficulties. A significant preoperative decrease of vital capacity VC (<2000 ml), of forced expiratory volume in the first second FEV_1 (<1200 ml) of P_aO_2 (<60 mmHg and associated with hypercapnia) is correlated with an increase of morbidity and mortality, but is insufficient to establish an accurate prognosis. The clinical situation is the most important factor.

If the patient is maintained on a ventilator after surgery, the ventilation parameters are usually: $F_IO_2 = 0.4$, $V_T = 10$ ml/kg, RR = 12–15, $T_I/T_E = 1/2$. Standard monitoring includes EKG and pulse oximetry. A small peripheral arterial catheter facilitates blood gas samples. Weaning from the ventilator goes through a period of oxygen supply (4 l/min) through the tracheal tube, when the patient is awake, not hypothermic, has a good muscular tone and a spontaneous respiratory rate between 12 and 30, is calm, without cutaneous vasoconstriction, without acidosis. The tracheal tube is removed when, at least one hour after weaning, P_aO_2 is ≥ 70 mmHg, P_aCO_2 is ≤ 45 mmHg, the chest film is considered as satisfactory, there is no bleeding from the chest tube(s). The pulse rate and the blood pressure must be steady. If not all of these conditions are met, the tracheal tube is left in place and the patient is put back on the ventilator. Insufficient respiratory function may require prolonged ventilation.

After extubation, oxygen is given through a nasal thin tube, using a humidifier. Sterile aerosol therapy can be used to liquefy bronchial secretions.

As soon as possible the patient is made to sit up in his bed, which helps coughing, increases the FRC, decreases lung edema and avoids inhalation of gastric contents. The day after operation, the patient should stand up for a short period.

The patient's clinical aspect is regularly controlled, looking for restlessness, sweating, and modifications of colour of the skin and nails. Blood pressure, EKG, and pulse oximetry are routinely checked during that period. Central venous pressure and pulmonary artery pressure are monitored in cases of shock, of cardiac failure or if a complication occurs. Blood gases are measured once or twice a day, according to the clinical situation. Hemoglobin, hematocrit, electrolytes, P and Mg and serum proteins are verified. Blood coagulation is tested in cases of abundant losses and replacement or of abnormal bleeding.

The respiratory function is maintained through physical therapy, prevention of pleural effusion, accurate but not excessive maintenance of fluid volume and prevention of pain. Physical therapy is most important, as it evacuates bronchial secretions, opens small bronchioles and alveoli and maintains muscular respiratory strength; it is facilitated by analgesia.

Respiratory complications are most frequent in general thoracic surgery, often due to infection, facilitated by chronic bronchial obstruction, malnutrition and age, also by operative trauma. After surgery, hypervolemia, anemia, pain or excess of analgesia, insufficient movement and physical therapy, abdominal complications, elevation or immobility of the diaphragms, inhalation or intrathoracic complications are all causes of respiratory insufficiency. It can be restrictive (hypoxia–hypercapnia with an eventual acidemia), obstructive (hypoxia–hypocapnia with a frequent alkalemia), or the effect of an intrapulmonary shunt (hypoxia corrected or not by administration of O_2, hypocapnia with alkalemia) or the consequence of ventilatory fatigue (hypoxia–hypercapnia with mixed acidemia). Inspiratory thoracic retraction is a sign of respiratory effort against difficult breathing, tachypnea is a sign of muscular tiredness which is secondary to a respiratory overwork or to extra-respiratory muscular causes. Generally, there is a decrease of the diaphragmatic work and an increase of the chest cage respiratory work.

These disorders influence other organs: the heart, with arrhythmia and low output; the brain, with restlessness and confusion; the kidneys, with oliguria; and the digestive tract, with gastroplegia, hemorrhage and ileus. Repeated clinical examination, along with chest films and monitoring, are necessary.

Simple causes must be looked for and are found in 90% of cases. (1) In the patient: bronchial secretions, pleural effusion, abdominal compression, venous thrombosis (and embolism), cardiac impairment by displacement or compression. (2) In the pleural suction system. (3) In the intra-tracheal tube. (4) In the ventilator mode of function, tubing and connections if the patient is mechanically assisted, fights against the machine or is poorly oxygenated.

A restrictive syndrome is badly tolerated when $P_aO_2 < 60$ mmHg and $P_aCO_2 \geq 50$ mmHg. It may be rapidly aggravated and in this case mechanical ventilation is necessary before the patient becomes exhausted. An intra-pulmonary shunt is tolerated for a longer time if RR is < 40, with no bronchial obstruction and if hypoxemia does not impair other functions. An obstructive syndrome, most frequently observed, can be corrected by physical therapy, endo-bronchial suction, antibiotics, bronchodilators and possibly steroids.

The vicious cycle hypoventilation–bronchial obstruction–infection–aggravated hypoventilation indicates the need for mechanical ventilation. Weaning is possible when, during spontaneous breathing, the following parameters are found: $V_T >$ 5 ml/kg, $V_{min} > 10$ l, inspiratory strength > -25 cmH_2O, $FEV_1 > 15$ ml/kg, $VC >$ 20 ml/kg, $RR < 30$.

If these conditions are not met, a weaning method is necessary. Many ventilator weaning modes are now available: CPAP, Intermittent Mandatory Ventilation (IMV), Minute Mandatory Ventilation (MMV) and, more recently introduced, Pressure Support (PS). Few published data are today available comparing the effectiveness of these different modes of weaning. The following points must be kept in mind: (1) A FRC restored to adequate level by judicious PEEP decreases W_{resp}, decreases intrapulmonary shunt and improves gas exchange. (2) An endotracheal tube dramatically increases W_{resp} [31]. (3) All partially controlled modes of ventilation, like IMV, increase W_{resp} [32] in comparison with controlled ventilation, except PS, which acts as an additive respiratory muscle and decreases W_{resp} proportionally to the PS level [33,34]. Correct values of ABG and $RR < 30$ with a PS level $\leq 8\,cmH_2O$ allow the patient to be extubated without delay [34]. Consequently, in the future PS combined with PEEP should become the most efficient weaning method, replacing IMV.

5. CONCLUSION

Postoperative respiratory insufficiency is not infrequent in general thoracic surgery. Good clinical examination and adequate monitoring should diagnose it at an early stage. It can be prevented in many cases by regular check-ups of the patient and of the surrounding equipment and by good interpretation of the monitored parameters. Among the non-invasive monitoring methods now available, pulse oximetry and capnography seem to be the most useful in a surgical ward but $\dot{V}_{O_2}$ measurement undoubtedly has a promising future, allowing the monitoring to go beyond the respiratory status and reach the level of tissue oxygenation monitoring. Mechanical ventilation is an efficient tool when it becomes necessary but it must obey accurate rules concerning its indications, modes, management and weaning.

REFERENCES

1 Mc Quay HG, Moore RA, Patterson GMC, et al. Plasma concentrations and clinical observations during and after operation. Br J Anesth 1982; 54: 1087–1095.
2 Aubier M, Munciano D, Lecoegnie Y, Viires N, Jacquens Y, Squara P, Pariente R. Effects of hypophosphatemia on diaphragmatic contractility in patients with acute respiratory failure. N Engl J Med 1985; 313: 420–424.
3 Malloy DW, Dhingra S, Solven F, Wilson A, Mc Carthy DS. Hypomagnesemia and respiratory muscle power. Am Rev Respir Dis 1984; 129: 497–498.
4 Fitts RH, Hoelsoszy JO. Lactate and contractile force in frog muscle during development of fatigue and recovery. Am J Physiol 1976; 231: 430–433.
5 Juan G, Calverley P, Tolamo C, Schneider J, Roussos C. Effects of carbon dioxide on diaphragmatic function in human beings. N Engl J Med 1984; 310: 874–879.
6 Nunn JF. Ventilatory failure. In: Applied Respiratory Physics, 3rd Ed. London, Butterworths; ch 20: pp 379–391.
7 Nunn JF. Pulmonary ventilation. In: Applied Respiratory Physics, 3rd Ed. London, Butterworths; ch 5, pp 100–116.
8 Don HF, Wahba WM, Craig DB. Airway closure, gas trapping and the functional residual capacity during anesthesia. Anesthesiology 1972; 36: 533–537.

9 Hedenstierna G, Standberg A, Busmar B, Lundquist H, Svensson L, Tokics L. Functional residual capacity, thoracoabdominal dimensions and central blood volume during general anesthesia with muscle paralysis and mechanical ventilation. Anesthesiology 1985; 62: 247–254.
10 Bierry DR, Marks JD, Schapera A, Autry M, Schlobohm RM, Katz JA. Factors affecting peroperative pulmonary function in acute respiratory failure. Chest 1990; 98: 1455–1462.
11 Yelderman M, New W. Evaluation of Pulse oximetry. Anesthesiology 1983; 59(4): 349–352.
12 Moore FA, Haenel JB. Advances in oxygen monitoring of trauma patients. Med. Instrum (Baltimore) 1988; 22: 135–142.
13 Tremper KK, Waxman K, Bowman R, Schoemaker W. Continuous transcutaneous oxygen monitoring during respiratory failure, cardiac decompensation, cardiac arrest, and CPR. Crit Care Med 1980; 8: 377–381.
14 Lubbers DW. Theoretical basis of transcutaneous blood gas measurement. Crit Care Med 1981; 9: 721–725.
15 Peters RM. Monitoring of spontaneous ventilation and ventilator support. ch 21, this volume.
16 Healey JC, Fedullo AJ, Swinburne AJ, Wahl GW. Comparison of non invasive measurements of carbon dioxide tension during withdrawal from mechanical ventilation. Crit Care Med 1987; 15: 764–768.
17 Carlon GC, Ray C, Miodownik S, Kopec I, Groeger JS. Capnography in mechanically ventilated patients. Crit Care Med 1988; 16: 550–556.
18 Chopin C, Mangolaboyi J, Fournier F, Chambrin MC, Lestavel P. Utilisation de la capnographie en réanimation: intérêt et limites. In: Reanimation et Medecine d'urgence (Paris) Expansion Scientifique Francaise 1985; 102–116.
19 Chopin C, Fesard P, Mangolaboyi J, Lestavel D, Chambrin MC, Fournier F, Rime A. Use of capnography in diagnosis of pulmonary embolism during acute respiratory failure of chronic obstructive pulmonary disease. Crit Care Med 1990; 18: 353–357.
20 Sanders AB, Kern KB, Otto CW, Milander MM, Ewy GA. End-tidal carbon dioxide concentration monitoring during cardio-pulmonary resuscitation: a prognostic indicator for survival. JAMA 1989; 262: 1347–1351.
21 Blanch L, Fernandez R, Benito S, Mancebo J, Net A. Effect of PEEP on the arterial minus end-tidal carbon dioxide gradient. Chest 1987; 92: 451–454.
22 Chopin C, Chambrin MC, Mangoluboyi J, Lestavel P, Fournier F. Carbon dioxide mandatory ventilation (CO_2MV): a new method for weaning from mechanical ventilation. Description and comparative study with IMV and T-tube method in COP D patient. Int J Clin Monitoring Comput 1989; 6: 11–19.
23 Pierson DJ. Indications for mechanical ventilation in ARF. Respir Care 1983; 28: 570–577.
24 Chopin C, Mehdaoui H, Boniface B, Mangolaboyi J, Chambrin MC, Lestavel P, Rime A, Fournier F. Transport consommation et extraction de l'oxygène au cours des états septiques graves. Rean Soins Intens Med Urg 1990; 6: 117–122.
25 Lewis WD, Chwalo W, Benotti PN, Lakshman K, O'Donnel C, Blackburn GL, Bristian BR. Bedside assessment of the work of breathing. Crit Care Med 1988; 16: 117–122.
26 Hassan E, Green JA, Nara AR, Jarvis RC, Kasmer RJ, Pospisil R. Continuous monitoring of mixed venous oxygen saturation as an indicator of pharmacologic intervention. Chest 1989; 95: 406–409.
27 Cain M. Supply dependency of oxygen uptake in ARDS: myth or reality. Am J Med 1984; 288: 119–124.
28 Nelson DP, Beyer C, Samsel RW, Wood LDH, Shumacker PT. Pathological supply dependency of O_2 uptake during bacteremia in dogs. J Appl Physiol 1987; 63: 1487–1492.
29 Shibutami K, Komatsu T, Kubal K, Sanchala U, Kumar K, Riazori D. Critical level of oxygen delivery in anaesthetised man. Crit Care Med 1983; 11: 640–643.
30 Schoemaker W. Haemodynamic and oxygen transport pattern in septic shock; physiological mechanism and therapeutic application. In: Sibbald W, Spring C (eds.). Perspectives on Sepsis and Septic Shock. New Horizons. Calfornia, Society of Critical Care Medicine 1986: pp 203–204.

31 Shapiro M, Wilson RK, Casar G, Bloom K, Teague RB. Work of breathing through different sized endotracheal tubes. Crit Care Med 1986; 14: 1028–1031.
32 Prakash O, Meij SH. Oxygen consumption and blood gas exchange during controlled and intermittent mandatory ventilation after cardiac surgery. Crit Care Med 1985; 13: 556–559.
33 Viale JP, Annat GJ, Bouffard YM, et al. Oxygen cost of breathing in postoperative patients. Chest 1988; 93: 506–509.
34 Brochard L, Harf A, Lorino H, Lemaire F. Pressure support decreases work of breathing and oxygen consumption during weaning from mechanical ventilation. Am Rev Respir Dis 1987; 135: 4 ASI.

Current Topics in General Thoracic Surgery: An International Series, Vol. 2
Perioperative Care, edited by R.M. Peters and J. Toledo

Chapter 22

Cancer surgery on a single lung

Ph. Levasseur, J.F. Regnard, Ph. Dartevelle and Ph. Icard

1. INTRODUCTION

Cancer surgery on a single lung is mainly debated for metachronous cancers, in patients who have already undergone a pneumonectomy. It remains very exceptional considering the total absence of literature published on this specific subject.

At present this surgery poses two problems which are not clearly resolved:

– The specific operative risk of these interventions, closely linked to the extent of the surgery.

– The prognosis of these patients when a curative resection is advisable.

2. PATIENTS

During 30 years at the Marie Lannelongue Hospital, 7 patients underwent cancer surgery on a single lung. One of these patients underwent two consecutive, partial operations with a one year interval. We will study in addition two patients who underwent partial surgery of one lung and later a contralateral pneumonectomy for a second cancer.

These 9 patients represented only 10% of the 84 patients who underwent pulmonary resection for a second cancer either ipsi- or contralateral, synchronous or metachronous, during the same period; these 84 patients in turn represented only 1.5% of the 5000 lung cancer resections carried out during the same period. These numbers emphasize the rarity of these operations.

All 9 patients were male, with a mean age of 59 (51–63 years) at the time of the second operation.

The nature of the operations and the results are presented in Table 22.1. The histology was squamous cell carcinoma in 8 cases and adenocarcinoma in the remaining case. The TNM classification of the first cancer was: 3 stage I, 3 stage II, 2 stage IIIA (N2) and 1 stage IIIB (T4, carina).

TABLE 22.1
Surgical procedures

Patient	First operation	Second operation	Result
1	Left pneumonectomy	Right upper lobectomy	Postoperative death (6 days)
2	Left pneumonectomy	Right wedge-resection	Dead 15 months
3	Right pneumonectomy	Left wedge-resection	Alive 29 months
4	Right pneumonectomy	Bi-segmentectomy	Postoperative death (4 days)
5	Right pneumonectomy	Left wedge-resection	Dead 20 months
6	Right pneumonectomy	Left wedge-resection	Alive 6 months
7	Right pneumonectomy	Left wedge-resection	Alive 12 months (third surgery new left wedge)
8	Right middle lobe	Left pneumonectomy	Dead 24 months
9	Right inferior lobe	Left pneumonectomy	Dead 6 weeks

TABLE 22.2
Pulmonary function in patients with previous pneumonectomy

Patient	CV[a]	FEV_1[a]	Second resection	Postoperative cause
1	77	71	Right lobectomy	Postoperative death
2	50	40	Wedge-resection	Benign
3	53	49	Wedge-resection	Benign
4	59	55	Bi-segmentectomy	Postoperative death
5	72	60	Wedge-resection	Benign
6	60	60	Wedge-resection	Benign
7	50	42	Wedge-resection	Benign

[a]Percentage of predicted.

The second cancer was always diagnosed by a systematic chest X-ray. It was synchronous in one case and metachronous in 8, with a mean interval between the two cancers of 4 years and 8 months (2–17 years).

Of the 7 patients with previous pneumonectomies, 5 had a second cancer which was small and peripheral without evidence of disease at bronchoscopic study; 2 patients had a larger peripheral tumor which was located by endoscopic study at a segmental bronchial level. On the other hand, the two patients who had partial resection first and a secondary pneumonectomy, had proximal tumors, confirmed by endoscopic examinations.

The respiratory function for the 7 initially pneumonectomized patients is presented in Table 22.2.

The respiratory tests of the two patients with secondary pneumonectomies showed for one patient (case 8, Table 22.1), a vital capacity of 100% and a FEV_1 of 79% of the predicted values; the ventilation–perfusion on scintigraphy examination of the lung which should be removed was 46%. The other patient (case 9, Table 22.1), had a vital capacity of 79% and a FEV_1 of 35%. However the ventilation–perfusion test showed the total loss of function of the affected lung which should be removed.

With regard to the nature of the second resection it can be noted from Table 22.1 that 5 patients had wedge resection associated with a pneumonectomy, 2 patients had a contralateral lobectomy associated with a pneumonectomy, one patient a bi-segmentectomy and a pneumonectomy, and the last patient a pneumonectomy and a medium right lobectomy.

The histological type of the second cancer was in all cases identical to that of the first.

Finally the TNM classification of the second cancer was: 6 stage I, 2 stage II, and 1 stage IIIA (extension to parietal pleura).

3. RESULTS

3.1. Perioperative mortality

Two patients died in the immediate postoperative course. One who had a left pneumonectomy 17 years previously, died of refractory hypoxia 6 days after a right superior lobectomy. Nevertheless this patient had satisfactory preoperative respiratory function with a FEV_1 at 71% of predicted. The refractory hypoxia occurred without evidence of infection and/or pulmonary emboli.

The second patient, with a previous right pneumonectomy, died 4 days after a left bi-segmentectomy, due to acute respiratory failure without evidence of infection. The preoperative FEV_1 value was 55% of predicted.

3.2. Secondary deaths

One other death occurred 6 weeks after surgery in a patient who had undergone a left pneumonectomy after having a previous right inferior lobectomy. This patient was therefore breathing with his superior right lobe and his medium lobe. The immediate postoperative period was difficult, marked by a pulmonary embolus, and a vena cava filter was inserted. The patient then left the hospital and was readmitted two weeks later with a serious cardiorespiratory failure which caused a rapid death. It is important to know that this patient had a FEV_1 of 35% of predicted before the left pneumonectomy, but his left lung was not functional with a pulmonary ventilation–perfusion scintigraphy of 0%.

3.3. Morbidity

The 6 other patients had simple postoperative courses with, in one case, repeated bronchial obstructions which were treated by endoscopic aspirations.

3.4. Long term results

Three patients died, probably of cancer recurrence, 15, 20 and 24 months later. Three patients are alive at the time of writing, 6, 12 and 29 months after surgery.

TABLE 22.3
Cancer surgery in a single lung: literature available)

Reference	Year	Resection on single lung	Multiple resections for bronchogenic carcinoma in general
Abbey Smith [1]	1976	0	15
Salerno [9]	1979	3	12
Jensik [3]	1981	7	64
French national survey [4]	1987	7	88
Mousset [6]	1989	1	36
Levasseur (this chapter)	1992	9	84

One of these patients was recently reoperated for a third cancer on his remaining lung.

4. COMMENTS

Cancer resection on a single lung is exceptional both in our experience and in the literature (Table 22.3).

It usually concerns surgery of a second metachronous cancer. Multiple lung cancer resections, synchronous or metachronous, are rare: 1.5% of lung cancer interventions in our experience, and 1–4% in the literature [1–3,5,6,8].

Recurring lung cancers are generally erroneously considered as metastases and consequently not operated.

According to Martinia and Melamed [5], a second lung tumor in a patient previously operated for lung cancer, should be considered as a second cancer and not as a metastasis when the interval between the two lesions exceeds two years, in the absence of other distant tumor localizations.

As well, single synchronous contralateral localizations are considered as a second cancer, in the absence of other neoplastic localization, especially when there is endobronchial evidence of tumor. On the other hand, histology cannot usually help to differentiate between a second cancer or a metastasis, because both tumors are generally of the same type: squamous cell carcinoma.

The second limiting factor for performing a second operation is the limited respiratory function resulting from the first intervention in conjunction with the predicted extent of surgery necessary to remove the second cancer. Thus only 25–50% of diagnosed metachronous cancers can be removed [6,8].

A previous pneumonectomy or the need to perform a pneumonectomy in a patient who has already undergone a partial contralateral surgery are considerable limiting factors which explain the rarity of these interventions.

In case of a previous pneumonectomy, only peripheral and small tumors without endoscopic detection can usually be removed in a satisfactory manner.

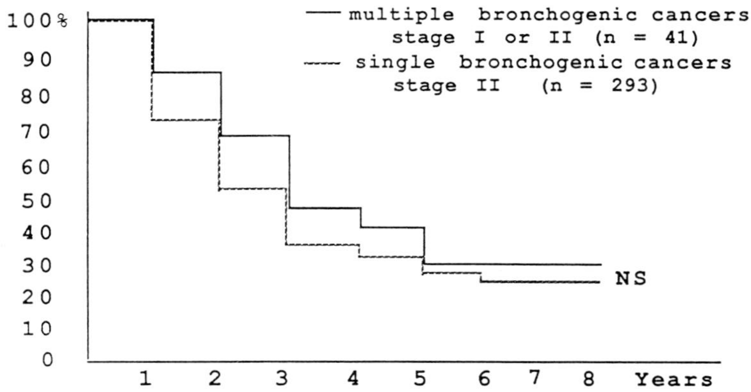

FIGURE 22.1. Actuarial survival of multiple and single resected bronchogenic cancers at the same stage.

This emphasizes the importance of extended and rigorous follow-up of all resected lung cancer patients, knowing that metachronous cancers occur with an average interval of 4 years after the first cancer [6] and according to Razzuk et al. [7] and Shields and Robinette [10] many occur 10 or more years later.

Two problems remain incompletely resolved:

The operative risk of cancer surgery on a single lung seems higher and directly related to the extent of the surgery. In fact surgery for recurring lung cancer is already a higher-risk operation than for a first lung cancer resection [3,4,6], even if the first resection was not a pneumonectomy.

The operative mortality rate for cancer surgery on a single lung is difficult to evaluate due to the small number of cases.

In Jensik's experience [3], 7 wedge resections for cancer on single lung resulted in no mortality. In our experience, we had 2 early postoperative deaths due to refractory hypoxia and a precocious death at 6 weeks due to cardiorespiratory failure.

It should be noted that all these deaths occurred in patients who had associated pneumonectomy and lobectomy or a contralateral bi-segmentectomy.

On the other hand, no deaths were observed in patients with pneumonectomy associated with contralateral wedge resection.

Consequently this perioperative mortality seems more related to the extent of surgery than to preoperative respiratory function, as the three deceased patients had satisfactory preoperative respiratory function. These lethal hypoxias could be related to a pulmonary arterial hypertension, but this could not be proven.

Finally, the extent of cancer surgery on a single lung should be limited to wedge resection of peripheral tumors without endoscopic evidence, or to segmentectomy. Lobectomy is probably inadvisable for these patients even if pulmonary function is very good. This emphasizes, once again, the importance of early diagnosis of these recurring cancers through a rigorous follow up.

The long term results of cancer surgery on a single lung remain also unclear. In general, in our experience, the prognosis of multiple lung cancer resection seems equivalent to those of first lung cancer resection, and remain mainly a function of the TNM stage of the cancer, which leads us to recommend this repeated surgery (Fig. 22.1).

These results are in accordance with those published elsewhere [2–4,6,8–10].

In case of cancer surgery on a single lung, experience is very limited, but in Jensik's experience [3] and in our experience some patients had a good outcome, so these resections can be performed in patients in good condition, but further results should be reported.

REFERENCES

1 Abbey Smith R, Nigam BK, Thomson JM. Second primary lung cancer. Thorax 1976; 31: 507–516.
2 Gabler A, Liebig S. Reoperation for bronchial carcinoma. Thorax 1980; 35: 668–670.
3 Jensik RJ, Faber LP, Kittle CF, Meng RL. Survival following resection for second primary bronchogenic carcinoma. J Thorac Cardiovasc Surg 1981; 82: 658–668.
4 Levasseur Ph, Delambre JF. Les cancers bronchiques métachrones opérés (à l'exclusion des récidives). Résultats de l'Enquête Nationale 1987. Ann Chir Thorac Cardio-Vasc 1984; 43(2): 130–132.
5 Martini N, Melamed MR. Multiple primary lung cancers. J Thorac Cardiovasc Surg 1975; 70: 606.
6 Mousset X, Deslauriers J, Beaulieu M, Despres JP, Piraux M, Fournier B, Lavallee J, Saint-Pierre C. Le cancer bronchopulmonaire successif. Importance du diagnostic précoce et survie après nouvelle exérèse chirurgicale. Ann Chir Thorac Cardio-Vasc 1989; 43(8): 658–662.
7 Razzuk MA, Puckey M, Urschel HC, Paulson DL. Dual primary bronchogenic carcinoma. Ann Thorac Surg 17: 425.
8 Roeslin N, Wintringer P, Vergeret J, Taytard A, Witz JP. Analyse de 64 cancers métachrones des bronches. Ann Chir Thorac Cardio-Vasc 1989; 43(2): 125–129.
9 Salerno TA, Munro DD, Blundell PE, Chiu RCJ. Second primary bronchogenic carcinoma: Life table analysis of surgical treatment. Ann Thorac Surg 1979; 27(1): 3–6.
10 Shields TW, Robinette CD. Long term survivors after resection of bronchial carcinoma. Surg Gynecol Obstet 1973; 136: 759.

Current Topics in General Thoracic Surgery: An International Series, Vol. 2
Perioperative Care, edited by R.M. Peters and J. Toledo

The second primary lung cancer

Discussion of "Cancer surgery on a single lung" by Ph. Levasseur, J.F. Regnard, Ph. Dartevelle and Ph. Icard

Gordon F. Murray

Multiple synchronous and metachronous primary bronchogenic cancers have been reported with increasing frequency in recent years. Logically, the incidence of a second primary lung tumor is higher in patients with more favorable initial lesions. The second primary tumor has a greater chance of appearing in patients who have survived a certain period of time following the resection of the first tumor. When the entire population with carcinoma is observed, 0.5% of patients will have a second primary lung cancer diagnosed before death [1]. When the population is limited to those patients who have undergone successful resection, the risk increases to about 2% [2]. For those patients surviving more than 30 months after resection, the incidence increases to 6.4% [3]. Pairolero and colleagues [4] recently reported a remarkable 26% incidence of second primary lung cancers in their patients with Stage-I disease followed a median of 7 years. Indeed, the incidence may be even higher in patients whose resected tumor was initially occult – cytologically positive but roentgenographically negative.

Although bilateral and multiple unilateral synchronous lesions have been reported, most second primary lung tumors present nonsynchronously. The new metachronous tumor usually arises in the opposite lung, but may occur in the remaining ipsilateral lung following lobectomy. In the former instance, a distinction must be made between a possible metastatic lesion or a new primary lung cancer. In the latter instance, the new lesion must be differentiated from a local recurrence of the initial cancer. Distinction between these three types of recurrent cancer may be difficult, but certain developed criteria have proven helpful [5]. A cancer is considered a local recurrence when the new lesion is histologically similar to the original tumor and occurs in an area anatomically contiguous to the resected area and its regional lymphatics. A neoplasm is considered a second lung primary when a cancer of a different cell type develops, or when a similar cell type occurs outside the area defined as local recurrence, and there is no evidence of extrathoracic cancer, and the new lesion is solitary. A reasonable clinical assumption can usually be made by consideration of these factors. Notably, a recent analysis has demonstrated that in two-thirds of patients with prior aerodigestive tumors, the new lesion within the lung is in fact a second primary lung cancer [6]. Further, permanent pathologic diagnosis is needed to confirm that the new lesion is not a second primary carcinoma of the lung. Unless definitely proved otherwise, it is my approach to consider the new tumor a second primary lung cancer, and manage the patient accordingly.

From a practical viewpoint, definition of the type of recurrence is of secondary importance. If non-regional metastatic disease can be excluded and the patient will tolerate it, resection remains the cornerstone of therapy for lung cancer. Unfortunately, in an estimated two-thirds of these individuals the pulmonary status or the extent of the new disease precludes resection. As noted in this volume by Levasseur and co-authors, respiratory insufficiency is a major factor in postoperative morbidity and mortality following *cancer surgery on a single lung.* On the other hand, the prognosis is bleak for patients with a pulmonary malignancy whose tumor cannot be resected, and any decision to withhold operation on the basis of pulmonary function tests must be made with full knowledge of the predictive ability of those tests. Three widely used tests of pulmonary function – FVC, FEV_1, and FEV_1/FVC ratio – have been shown by us [7] to have no correlation with postoperative morbidity and mortality in 90 patients undergoing pneumonectomy for carcinoma of the lung. Another method of evaluating pulmonary function is the combination of spirometric tests with ventilation/perfusion scans [8]. The latter gives some indication of effective gas exchange in various areas of the lung parenchyma, and the information appears superior to that of spirometry testing alone. Reichel [9] found that preoperative evaluation of cardiac performance was more useful in estimating surgical risks in patients undergoing lung resection than were pulmonary function studies. Eugene and colleagues [10] compared maximum oxygen consumption, which measures both cardiac and pulmonary function, with routinely used spirometry tests. The former was significantly superior as a predictor of postoperative mortality. Thus, tests that measure both the cardiac and pulmonary reserve seem to offer better preoperative evaluation than measurements of lung function alone.

As early as 1936, Gibbon and Churchill [11] showed that occlusion of 60% of the pulmonary vascular bed was required before a reduction of cardiac output or a fall in arterial pressure was observed. More recently, Ebert et al. [12] confirmed in the canine that aortic and pulmonary blood flows show little change until 60% of the pulmonary vasculature is occluded. Pulmonary vascular resistance decreases in a manner such that 75% of the normal pulmonary flow can be perfused through 18% of the lung. Mean right ventricular pressure increases stepwise and reflects the degree of pulmonary vascular bed occlusion. Right ventricular failure was demonstrated by a rise in end-diastolic pressure, but the mean ventricular pressure fell for only a brief period prior to complete circulatory collapse. Del Guerico [13] had previously emphasized that a mean right ventricular pressure of 22 mmHg or above in patients having pulmonary embolus indicated a fatal outcome. Clinical experience with the performance of sequential resections for second primary lung cancer reflect the experimental data. Levasseur et al., in the current series, note that all deaths occurred in patients who had associated pneumonectomy and lobectomy or a contralateral bi-segmentectomy. It is probable that the most extensive resection of pulmonary tissue that can be performed safely would be a pneumonectomy with a contralateral limited resection wedge or segment. With careful patient selection and prudent surgical judgment, operations can be performed safely for patients undergoing a second or even third resection. Mathisen and colleagues [14] reported an 8% perioperative mortality following the second operation in seven of ninety patients, and there were no deaths in those patients undergoing a third resection.

Appreciation of the true magnitude of the problem of the second primary tumor has emphasized the importance of preservation of lung tissue in the initial treatment. Several authors have concluded that wedge resection may be performed on high-risk patients with non-small cell Stage-I bronchogenic carcinoma with acceptable operative mortality and morbidity [15,16]. Further, the incidence of local recurrence and survival rate do not appear to be significantly different from those of patients who are better operative risks who underwent lobectomy for similar lesions. Subsequently, a policy of limited resection has prevailed at Rush-Presbyterian-St. Luke's Medical Center, where pulmonary resection less than a lobectomy has been performed and has been considered a 'mini' resection [17]. A low perioperative mortality emphasizes the safety of the lesser resection and probably reflects the greatest benefit to the patient. Importantly, a conservative resection not only permits a more favorable functional result, but also, in those patients who develop a second primary, it increases the likelihood of an appropriate and effective second resection. Accumulating experience with second primary lung cancers continues to show a trend toward better survival among those patients undergoing initial segmentectomy [14]. In light of these recent reports and ongoing studies (the Toronto group), we may find that early disease (T1N0) may be treated most adequately by a more limited resection than lobectomy, allowing preservation of pulmonary tissue.

When resection is successful, it is followed by satisfactory survival. Even long-term survival may be anticipated as pointed out by Salerno et al. [18] in an accumulated series of 38 patients who underwent surgical resection for both the first and second primary bronchogenic carcinoma. One year after resection of a second lung primary tumor, the cumulative survival rate was 70%; two years later, it was 55% and three to five years later, 27%. At 2 years following detection of recurrent lung cancer, Pairolero et al. [4] reported that 52% of patients with second primary lung cancer had survived lung cancer compared with 23% for those with local recurrence and only 9% for those with metastases. While the 52%, 2-year survival following detection of a subsequent primary lung cancer was far less than the 85%, 2-year survival for all 346 patients with postsurgical Stage-I bronchogenic carcinoma reported in their series, Pairolero and colleagues point out that patients with subsequent primary lung cancers were seen with all three clinical stages at detection. It may well be that more careful surveillance will provide patients with subsequent primary lung cancer a more favorable prognosis. Close follow-up is clearly mandatory in the first 3 years, since a second primary develops in 50% of patients during this time [18]. Whereas local and metastatic recurrence diminish with time, there is little change in the rate of subsequent primary cancer during the first 5 years of observation [4]. Temeck and associates [19] have shown a 16% incidence of second lung primaries in those patients who have survived 10 years. Importantly, in approximately 80% of the patients with a second primary lung cancer, the lesion was found by chest roentgenogram at a time when the patient was asymptomatic [14].

Clinical and roentgenographic examination at least four times a year throughout the remaining lifespan of the patient is most appropriate, as the patient will remain at risk for the development of subsequent primary lung cancer.

REFERENCES

1 Lehman Jr JA, Cross FS. Bilateral multiple carcinoma of the lung. Cancer 1966; 19: 1931.
2 Shields TW, Drake CT, Sherrich JC. Bilateral primary bronchogenic carcinoma. J Thorac Cardiovasc Surg 1964; 48: 401.
3 Le Gal Y, Bauer WC. Second primary bronchogenic carcinoma: a complication of successful lung cancer surgery. J Thorac Cardiovasc Surg 1961; 41: 114.
4 Pairolero PC, Williams DE, Bergstralk EJ, et al. Postsurgical Stage I bronchogenic carcinoma: Morbid implications of recurrent disease. Ann Thorac Surg 1984; 38: 331.
5 Cortese DA, Pairolero PC, Bergstralk EJ, et al. Roentgenographically occult lung cancer: a ten-year experience. J Thorac Cardiovasc Surg 1983; 86: 373.
6 Lefor AT, Bredenberg CE, Kellman RM, et al. Multiple malignancies of the lung and head and neck. Arch Surg 1986; 121: 265.
7 Keagy BA, Schorlemmer GR, Murray GF, et al. Correlation of preoperative pulmonary function testing with clinical course in patients after pneumonectomy. Ann Thorac Surg 1983; 36: 253.
8 Ali MK, Mountain CF, Ever MS, et al. Predicting loss of pulmonary function after pulmonary resection or bronchogenic carcinoma. Chest 1980; 77: 337.
9 Reichel J. Assessment of operative risk of pneumonectomy. Chest 1972; 62: 570.
10 Eugene J, Brown SE, Light RW. Maximum oxygen consumption: a physiologic guide to pulmonary resection. Presented at the Surgical Forum, 68th Annual Clinical Congress of the American College of Surgeons, Chicago, October 24–29, 1982.
11 Gibbon Jr JH, Churchill ED. The physiology of massive pulmonary embolism. An experimental study of the changes produced by obstruction to the flow of blood through the pulmonary artery and its lobar branches. Ann Surg 1936; 104: 811.
12 Ebert PA, Allgood RJ, Jones HW, et al. Hemodynamics during pulmonary artery occlusion. Surgery 1967; 62: 18.
13 Del Guerico L. Shock and pulmonary embolism. Clin Anesth 1965; 2: 167.
14 Mathisen DJ, Jensik RJ, Faber LP, et al. Survival following resection for second and third primary lung cancers. J Thorac Cardiovasc Surg 1984; 88: 502.
15 Errett LE, Wilson J, Chiu RC, et al. Wedge resection as an alternative procedure for peripheral bronchogenic carcinoma in poor-risk patients. J Thorac Cardiovasc Surg 1985; 90: 656.
16 Jensik RJ, Faber LP, Milloy FJ, et al. Segmental resection for lung cancer. J Thorac Cardiovasc Surg 1973; 66: 563.

17 Jensik RJ. Minisections of small peripheral carcinomas of the lung. In: Martini N (ed.). The Surgical Clinics of North America. Philadelphia, PA, WB Saunders 1987, pp 951–958.
18 Salerno TA, Munro DD, Blundell PE, et al. Second primary bronchogenic carcinoma: Life-table analysis of surgical treatment. Ann Thorac Surg 1979; 27: 3.
19 Temeck BK, Flehinger BJ, Martini N. A retrospective analysis of 10 year survivors from carcinoma of the lung. Cancer 1984; 53: 1405.

Subject Index